# Lecture Notes in Electrical Engineering

## Volume 898

The book series *Lecture Notes in Electrical Engineering* (LNEE) publishes the latest developments in Electrical Engineering - quickly, informally and in high quality. While original research reported in proceedings and monographs has traditionally formed the core of LNEE, we also encourage authors to submit books devoted to supporting student education and professional training in the various fields and applications areas of electrical engineering. The series cover classical and emerging topics concerning:

- Communication Engineering, Information Theory and Networks
- Electronics Engineering and Microelectronics
- Signal, Image and Speech Processing
- Wireless and Mobile Communication
- Circuits and Systems
- Energy Systems, Power Electronics and Electrical Machines
- Electro-optical Engineering
- Instrumentation Engineering
- Avionics Engineering
- Control Systems
- Internet-of-Things and Cybersecurity
- Biomedical Devices, MEMS and NEMS

For general information about this book series, comments or suggestions, please contact leontina.dicecco@springer.com.

To submit a proposal or request further information, please contact the Publishing Editor in your country:

**China**

Jasmine Dou, Editor (jasmine.dou@springer.com)

**India, Japan, Rest of Asia**

Swati Meherishi, Editorial Director (Swati.Meherishi@springer.com)

**Southeast Asia, Australia, New Zealand**

Ramesh Nath Premnath, Editor (ramesh.premnath@springernature.com)

**USA, Canada:**

Michael Luby, Senior Editor (michael.luby@springer.com)

**All other Countries:**

Leontina Di Cecco, Senior Editor (leontina.dicecco@springer.com)

**** This series is indexed by EI Compendex and Scopus databases. ****

More information about this series at https://link.springer.com/bookseries/7818

Triwiyanto Triwiyanto · Achmad Rizal ·
Wahyu Caesarendra
Editors

# Proceedings of the 2nd International Conference on Electronics, Biomedical Engineering, and Health Informatics

ICEBEHI 2021, 3–4 November, Surabaya, Indonesia

Springer

*Editors*
Triwiyanto Triwiyanto
Department of Electromedical Engineering
Poltekkes Kemenkes Surabaya
Surabaya, Indonesia

Achmad Rizal
School of Electrical Engineering
Telkom University
Bandung
Jawa Barat, Indonesia

Wahyu Caesarendra
Faculty of Integrated Technologies
Universiti Brunei Darussalam
Gadong, Brunei Darussalam

ISSN 1876-1100 ISSN 1876-1119 (electronic)
Lecture Notes in Electrical Engineering
ISBN 978-981-19-1803-2 ISBN 978-981-19-1804-9 (eBook)
https://doi.org/10.1007/978-981-19-1804-9



This Springer imprint is published by the registered company Springer Nature Singapore Pte Ltd.
The registered company address is: 152 Beach Road, #21-01/04 Gateway East, Singapore 189721, Singapore

# Organization

## Organizing Committee

Dr. Triwiyanto Triwiyanto, Poltekkes Kemenkes Surabaya (Chairman)
Dyah Titisari, Poltekkes Kemenkes Surabaya (Vice Chairman)
Sari Luthfiyah, Poltekkes Kemenke Surabaya (Secretary I)
Anita Miftahul Maghfiroh, Poltekkes Kemenkes Surabaya (Secretary II)
Dr. Endro Yulianto, Poltekkes Kemenkes Surabaya (Technical Program Committee Chair)
Triana Rahmwati, Poltekkes Kemenkes Surabaya
Farid Amrinsani, Poltekkes Kemenkes Surabaya
Syaifudin, Poltekkes Kemenkes Surabaya
Ridha Mak'ruf, Poltekkes Kemenkes Surabaya
Levana Forra Wakidi, Poltekkes Kemenkes Surabaya
Singgih Yudha Setiawan, Poltekkes Kemenkes Surabaya
Lusiana, Poltekkes Kemenkes Surabaya
Syevana Dita Musvika, Poltekkes Kemenkes Surabaya
Deenda Putri Duta Natalia, Poltekkes Kemenkes Surabaya

## Proceeding Editorial Board

Dr. Triwiyanto Triwiyanto, Poltekkes Kemenkes Surabaya, Indonesia
Dr. Achmad Rizal, Telkom University, Bandung, Indonesia
Wahyu Caesarendra, Ph.D., Universiti Brunei Darussalam, Brunei Darussalam
Dr. Endro Yulianto, Poltekkes Kemenkes Surabaya

## Scientific Program Committee

Achmad Rizal, Telkom University, Indonesia
Agung triayudi, Universitas Nasional, Indonesia
Anggara Trisna Nugraha, Politeknik Perkapalan Negeri Surabaya, Indonesia
Ahmad Habib, University of 17 Agustus 1945 Surabaya, Indonesia
Alfin Hikmaturokhman, IT Telkom Purwokerto, Indonesia
Alfian Pramudita Putra, Biomedical Engineering, Faculty Science and Technology, Universitas Airlangga, Indonesia
Alfian Ma'arif, Universitas Ahmad Dahlan, Indonesia
Bambang Guruh Irianto, Poltekkes Kemenkes Surabaya, Indonesia
Candra Zonyfar, Universitas Buana Perjuangan Karawang, Indonesia
Dwi Oktavianto Wahyu Nugroho, Institut Teknologi Sepuluh Nopember, Indonesia
Devi Handaya, Politeknik Negeri Jakarta, Indonesia
Dwi Ely Kurniawan, Politeknik Negeri Batam, Indonesia
Dodi Zulherman, Institu Teknologi Telkom Purwokerto, Indonesia
Eka Legya Frannita, Universitas Gadjah Mada, Indonesia
Haresh Pandya, Saurashtra University, India
Harikrishna Parikh, Saurashtra University, India
Henderi, Universitas Raharja, Indonesia
Indah Nursyamsi Handayani, Poltekkes Kemenkes Jakarta II, Indonesia
Jasten Keneth D. Treceñe, Eastern Visayas State University—Tanauan Campus, Philippines
Jans Hendry, Universitas Gadjah Mada, Indonesia
Johan Reimon Batmetan, Universitas Negeri Manado, Indonesia
Kharudin Ali, UC TATI, Malaysia
Mas Aly Afandi, Institut Teknologi Telkom Purwokerto, Indonesia
Manas Kumar Yogi, Pragati Engineering College (Autonomous), India
Mera Kartika Delimayanti, Politeknik Negeri Jakarta, Indonesia
Mohammad Rizki Fadhil Pratama, Universitas Muhammadiyah Palangkaraya, Indonesia
Michael G. Albino, President Ramon Magsaysay State University, Philippines
Novia Susianti, Research and development agency, Jambi Province, Indonesia
Nada Fitrieyatul Hikmah, Institut Teknologi Sepuluh Nopember, Indonesia
Pradeep N., Bapuji Institute of Engineering and Technology, Davangere, India
Raja Siti Nur Adiimah Raja Aris, UC TATI, Malaysia
Ramen A. Purba, Politeknik Unggul LP3M, Medan
Rendra Gustriansyah, Universitas Indo Global Mandiri, Indonesia
Riky Tri Yunardi, Universitas Airlangga, Indonesia
Rismayani, STMIK Dipanegara Makassar, Indonesia
Salahudin Robo, Universitas Yapis Papua, Indonesia
Sidharth Pancholi, Indian Institute of Technology Delhi, India
Shajedul Islam, Health Sciences University of Hokkaido, Japan
Syahri Muharom, Institut Teknologi Adhi Tama Surabaya, Indonesia

Vishwajeet, NIT Jalandhar, India
Vijay Anant Athavale, PIET, India
Wahyu Pamungkas, Institut Teknologi Telkom Purwokerto, Indonesisa
Wan Faizura Wan Tarmizi, UC TATI, Malaysia
Yohanssen Pratama, Institut Teknologi Del, Indonesia
Yuant Tiandho, Universitas Bangka Belitung, Indonesia

# Preface

2nd ICEBEHI-2021, the 2nd International Conference on Electronics, Biomedical Engineering, and Health Informatics, took place during 3–4 November 2021 on virtual platforms (Zoom app). The conference was organized by the Department of Medical Electronics Technology, Health Polytechnic Ministry of Health Surabaya (Poltekkes Kemenkes Surabaya), Surabaya, Indonesia, and co-organized by Panipat Institute of Engineering and Technology (PIET), India, Institut Teknologi TELKOM Purwokerto, Indonesia, Institut Teknologi TELKOM Surabaya, Indonesia, Saurashtra University, India, with aim of bringing together as family all leading scientists, academicians, educationist, young scientist, research scholars and students to present, discuss and exchange their experiences, innovation ideas and recent development in the field of electronics, biomedical engineering and health informatics.

Taking into account the COVID-19 pandemic, ICEBEHI-2021 was held virtually as agencies around the world are now issuing restrictions on travel, gatherings and meetings in an effort to limit and slow the spread of this pandemic. The health and safety of our participants and members of our research community are of top priority to the organizing committee. Therefore, ICEBEHI-2021 was held online through Zoom software. More than 100 participants (presenter and non-presenter) attended the conference, and they were from India, Malaysia, Turkey, Pakistan, Brunei Darussalam, Peru, Iran, Taiwan Belgium and USA. The scientific program of this conference included many topics related to electronics and biomedical engineering as well as those in related fields. In this conference, two distinguished keynote speakers and one invited speaker had delivered their research works in area of biomedical engineering. Each keynote speech lasted 50 minutes.

ICEBEHI-2021 collects the latest research results and applications on electronics, biomedical engineering and health informatics. It includes a selection of 42 papers from 119 papers submitted to the conference from universities all over the world. All of the accepted papers were subjected to strict peer reviewing by 2–3 expert referees. All articles have gone through a plagiarism check. The papers have been selected for this volume because of quality and relevance to the conference.

We are very grateful to the committee which contributed to the success of this conference. Also, we are thankful to the authors who submitted the papers; it was quality of their presentations and communication with the other participants that really made this web conference fruitful. Last but not least, we are thankful to the Lecture Note in Electrical Engineering (Springer) Publishing for their support; it was not only the support but also an inspiration for organizers. We hope this conference can be held every year to make it an ideal platform for people to share views and experiences in electronics, biomedical engineering, health informatics and related areas. We are expecting you and more experts and scholars around the globe to join this international event next year.

Surabaya, Indonesia

Dr. Triwiyanto Triwiyanto
triwi@poltekkesdepkes-sby.ac.id

# Contents

# Analysis of Educational Data Mining Using WEKA for the Performance Students Achievements

**Agung Triayudi, Wahyu Oktri Widyarto, and Vidila Rosalina**

**Abstract** Various scenarios to improve the education system have been carried out. One of them is the application of educational data mining to gain the student's academic achievement, also decreasing the risk of drop out. The data was collected from three private universities in Jakarta, where it consists of academic, social, and economic information, as the demographics of 350 students with 23 attributes. Educational Data Mining applied a WEKA's tool that takes a rule in this study, while the classification phases applied PART, BayesNet, Random Tree, and J48 as their methods of classification. Attributes that have a significant influence on the classification process are selected as a medium of classification. The end of this study explained that Random Tree plays a significant part in classifying all possibilities related to predicting students' academic performance. The accuracy level is relatively high, and the misclassification rate is also low. Besides, the Apriori algorithm also plays a significant role in finding association rules of educational data mining of all the best attributes and rules available.

**Keywords** WEKA · Educational data mining · Student's performance · Classification methods · Algorithm

## 1 Introduction

In the fields of science, there are known competitive educational settings. Educational Data Mining also implements data mining methods in such a data visualization, exploration and analysis of student's performance, and prediction of their

A. Triayudi (✉)
Department of ICT, Universitas Nasional, Jakarta, Indonesia
e-mail: agungtriayudi@civitas.unas.ac.id

W. O. Widyarto
Department of Industrial Engineering, Universitas Serang Raya, Serang, Indonesia

V. Rosalina
Informatics Department, Universitas Serang Raya, Serang, Indonesia

 
T. Triwiyanto et al. (eds.), *Proceedings of the 2nd International Conference on Electronics, Biomedical Engineering, and Health Informatics*, Lecture Notes in Electrical Engineering 898, https://doi.org/10.1007/978-981-19-1804-9_1

work achievement. It is implemented to prevent the possible dropouts and gain the academic performance optimally, also the feedback for the best faculty infrastructure and development. Currently, educational institutions desperately need the application of this data mining to strategize and plan their future [1, 2]. Considering the performance of the students is very closely related to various factors they have, such as personal, economic, social and environmental, and much more. The authority of advanced educational institutions can utilize experimental results obtained in understanding a student's trends and performance to obtain a pedagogical strategy plan for the bright future [3, 4].

Sometimes, Data Mining can also be referred to as Knowledge Data Discovery (KDD). However, while similar, there are still some things that distinguish the two. Data Mining is used to find a subset in d that meets the formula by reducing the matrix. If data mining does not produce any conclusions, KDD will be obtained. It also applies to the opposite possibility. The main features of this study aim to obtain general characteristics that the elements are all set. Knowledge Data Discovery and data mining included ways to extract large amounts of information from data in a database. The result of the application of the resulting algorithm can be called rule discovery. There are two sorts of rules, namely production and association rules [5, 6]. Per Quinlan, production rules are a typical style of expressing knowledge by expert systems. Where the choice Tree Rules can even be considered production rules. Association rules were first discussed to seek out a link between selling different goods by analyzing massive amounts of information. There are many fields applied during this case, one of which is Educational data processing (EDM) [7, 8].

There are a variety of classification algorithms, such as Neural Network, Decision tree, k-Nearest Neighbour, AdaBoost, Support Vector Machine, Random Forest. During the study, several of them are going to be used associated with academic student performance mining efforts: BayesNet, Random Forest, PART, and J48 classification algorithms. On the opposite hand, the Apriori, as a part of unsupervised learning, became one of all the popular algorithms within the data processing association rules employed in terms of unveiling the hidden rules of a dataset. All things are done by comparing each algorithm's supported accuracy in selecting the most straightforward performing algorithm for employment [9, 10].

## 2 Materials and Methods

A study is known to focus on designing a framework that predicted the academic achievement of computer science undergraduate students. The dataset encompasses six years of data ranging from July 2014/2015 to July 2019/2020. Various aspects of student records are collected during this data, like students' academic history, family background, and demographics. Classification methods like Naïve Bayes, Rules-Based classifiers, and Decision Trees are applied to predict students' performance. The results of the experiment show that the classifier of this classification method showed significant results, with 71.3% data accuracy. In other studies, predictions of the success rate of first-year students were made by developing a data model based on the dataset of senior students. A comparison of data mining classification algorithms was conducted to find the J48 algorithm that is best suited for research according to the data they have [11–14].

Other researchers conducted studies in finding the fact that attributes have a strong influence on the prediction. In this case, the selection of features can be used before the classification of the work begins, and the methods used are Decision Tree and Bayesian Network. Subsequent studies have shown that classification models built using decision trees and artificial neural network techniques can help in accessing students' strengths and weaknesses to boost their learning performance [15–17]. Besides, some studies focus on the use of WEKA to evaluate the performance of students. The Bayesian Network, Naïve Bayes, ID3, J48, Neural Network methods were used in this study. It is known that the Bayesian Network excels in terms of the accuracy of the predictions generated. Other experiments also suggest that if a variety of factors have been theoretically explored, a qualitative model that can be used to analyze a student's performance is based on the personal and social factors of the student. Many studies also predict the achievement of students who are divided over graduating or failing by implementing classification models on student achievement outcomes and regression models to predict student scores. In this case, the classification model can extract patterns, but the regression model is unable to change the lines on a simple chart [18–20].

## 3 Result and Discussion

### 3.1 *Stage of Data Preprocess*

The study focused on a dataset of 350 instances with 23 attributes. The following of the proposed framework is represented in Table. 1. This study consist of a dataset from three private universities in Jakarta. Datasets of the 23 most likely attributes were collected to conduct this research. By implementing features in WEKA, the use of features on attribute discovery with significant influence on various evaluations can certainly be done. Through this method of selection of features, it is known that 12 features are very influential in the effort to classify the students' academic performance in this study. Here is a representation of the data in the ARFF format, shown in Table 1.

### 3.2 *Specify the Selected Algorithm*

Once a classification algorithm is established regarding feature selection, i.e., by using the following classification methods: Decision Tree, Naïve Bayes, Random

**Table 1** Description of the datasets

| Attr | Description | Values |
|---|---|---|
| GE | Gender | (Man, Woman) |
| CST | Caste | (Public, ST, SCs, OBCs, MOBCs) |
| TN | Percentage of class Y | (Top, very well, well, sufficient, fail) |
| TWP | Percentage of class XII | If % > = 80 then top<br>If % > = 60 but less than 80 then very well<br>If % > = 45 but less than 60 then well<br>If % > = 30 but less than 45 then sufficient<br>If % < 30 then fail |
| IA | Percentage of internal assessment | (Top, very well, well, sufficient, fail) |
| ESP | Percentage of end semester | (Top, very well, well, sufficient, fail) |
| AR | Whether student had publish a paper | (Yes, No) |
| MS | Marital status | (Married, unmarried) |
| LSA | Lived in town or village | (Town, village) |
| AST | Admission category | (Free, paid) |
| Attr | Description | Values |
| FM | Family month income (in IDR) | (Top, big, tall, average, small)<br>If FM > = 10.000.000 then top<br>If FM > = 8.000.000 but less than 10.000.000 then big<br>If FM > = 5.000.000 but less than 8.000.000 then tall<br>If FM > = 3.500.000 but less than 5.000.000 then Av<br>If FM < 3.500.000 then small |
| FSS | Family size | If FSS > 12 then big |
| | | If FSS > = 6 but less than 12 then medium |
| | | If FSS < 6 then little |
| FQ | Father qualification | (IL, UM, 10, 12, degree, PG)<br>IL = Illiterate, UM = under class X |
| MQ | Mother qualification | (IL, UM, 10, 12, degree, PG)<br>IL = Illiterate, UM = under class X |
| FOA | Father occupation | (Service, business, retired, farmer, others) |
| MO | Mother occupation | (Service, business, retired, farmer, others) |
| NF | Number of friends | (Large, average, small) |
| TS | Time of study | > = 6 h Well, > = 4 h medium, < 2 small |

(continued)

**Table 1** (continued)

| Attr | Description | Values |
|---|---|---|
| SS | Class X level school's student attended | (Govt, private) |
| MEA | Medium | (Bahasa, english) |
| TT | Travel time from home to college | (Well, medium, weak)<br>> = 3 h Well, > = 2 h Medium, < 1 Weak |
| ATDA | Percentage of student class attendance | If % > = 80 then top<br>If % > = 60 but less than 80 then medium<br>If % < 60 then weak |

Forest, k-Nearest Neighbor, Neural Network, Adaboost [21–23]. Several unique algorithms are also implemented related to student academic performance data-mining efforts that we can find in weka programs: BayesNet, PART, J48, and Random Forest. Where BayesNet is an algorithm that generates random instances based on the Bayes network, PART is an algorithm with a divider-and-conquering mechanism in building c4.5 decision trees, J48 is a C4.5 decision tree-producing algorithm that is intact/uns pruned. Random Forest is a type of group classification that is widely used in the method of randomly classifying features. Method's accuracy performance that compared to the best algorithms can be applied in this study [24, 25].

## 3.3 *Classification Result*

WEKA has various algorithms that can be applied when we do the classification stage. Among the studies are BayesNet, PART, J48, and Random Forest. Table 2 below shows a comparison between the four types of methods.

Besides, we also compare classification using Random Tree, either with or without feature selection. The following is presented in Table 3.

Random Forest has a large number of correct instances compared to other classification methods, where the percentage accuracy is 97%. The following is a representation that the random forest classifier shows a slight error, shown in Figs. 1, 2, 3, and 4.

**Table 2** Accuracy comparison of various classifiers

| Classifiers | Accuracy (%) | Correctly instances | Incorrectly instances |
|---|---|---|---|
| J48 | 70 | 245 | 105 |
| PART | 71.33 | 250 | 100 |
| BayesNet | 57.33 | 201 | 149 |
| Random forest | 97 | 340 | 10 |

**Table 3** Comparison of Random forest (RF) classification

| Classifiers | Accuracy (%) | Correctly instances | Incorrectly instances |
|---|---|---|---|
| RF 12 selected attributes | 97 | 340 | 10 |
| RF all attributes | 82.33 | 288 | 62 |

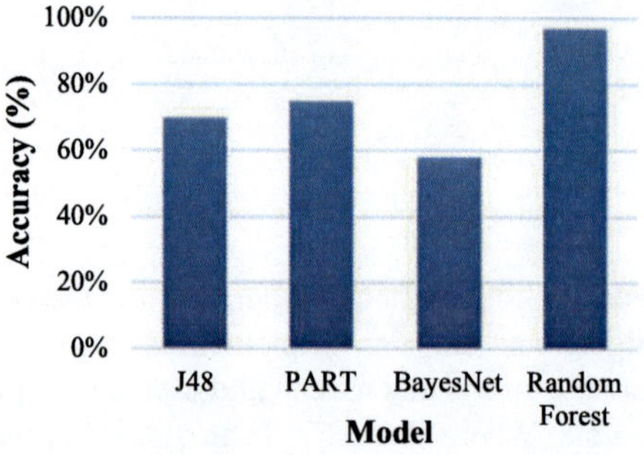


**Fig. 1** Comparison of various classification models

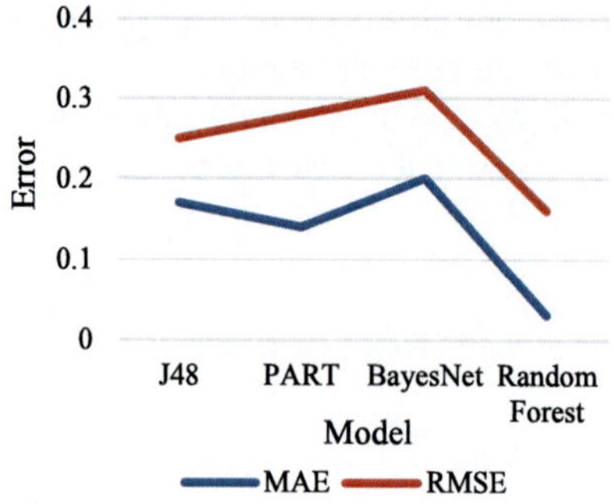


**Fig. 2** Classification Errors MAE and RMSE

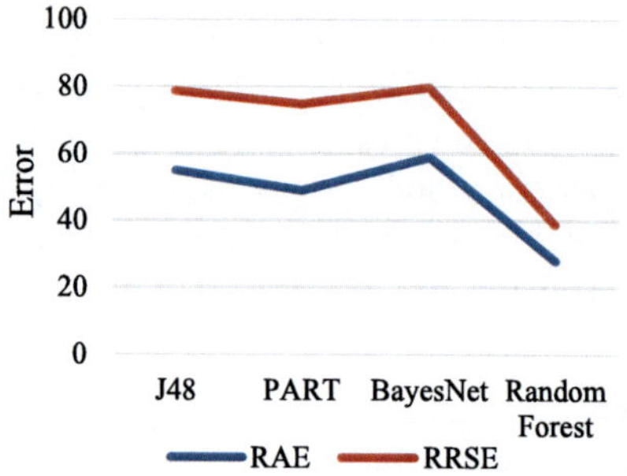


**Fig. 3** Classification error

**Fig. 4** Visualization tree of J48

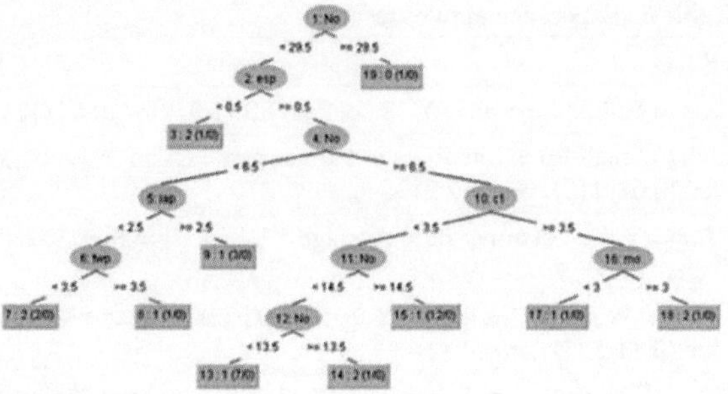

## 3.4 *Association Rules Results*

It is identified that the association rules contain two things, namely antecedent and its consequences. In this case, the Apriori algorithm is often used in an attempt to find correlations in data mining. Therefore, we intend to apply the Apriori algorithm to the available data sets we have using WEKA. Our minimum support is 0.8 (280 instances), with the minimum metric being 0.87 and the number of cycles performed by 11. The best rules we have obtained are as follows (Table 4).

Then, the Re-research continues with the next experiment according to the selected attribute. At this time, the minimum support available is 0.1 (40 instances), with the minimum metric being 0.87 and the number of cycles performed by 23. The best rules we have obtained are as follows (Table 5):

**Table 4** Experimental rules results

| Rules |
|---|
| lsa = V 263 = = > msa = Unmarried 263 < conf:(1) > lift:(1) lev:(0) [0] conv:(0.75) |
| lsa = V moa = Housewife 255 = = > msa = Unmarried 255 < conf:(1) lift:(1) lev:(0) [0] conv:(0.73) |
| fss = Little 178 = = > msa = Unmarried 178 < conf:(1) > lift:(1) lev:(0) [0] conv:(0.51) |
| ast = Free 170 = = > msa = Unmarried 170 < conf:(1) > lift:(1) lev:(0) [0] conv:(0.49) |
| fss = Little mo = Housewife 158 = = > msa = Unmarried 158 < conf:(1) > lift:(1) lev:(0) [0] conv:(0.45) |
| lsa = V ss = Govt 237 = = > msa = Unmarried 237 < conf:(1) > lift:(1) lev:(0) [0] conv:(0.68) |
| moa = Housewife 289 = = > msa = Unmarried 288 < conf:(1) > lift:(1) lev:(-0) [0] conv:(0.41) |
| ss = Govt 235 = = > msa = Unmarried 234 < conf:(1) > lift:(1) lev:(-0) [0] conv:(0.39) |
| moa = Housewife ss = Govt 250 = = > msa = Unmarried 249 < conf:(0.99) > lift:(1) lev:(-0) [0] conv:(0.42) |
| mea = Asm 211 = = > msa = Unmarried 210 < conf:(0.99) > lift:(1) lev:(-0) [0] conv:(0.3) |

**Table 5** Experimental rules results

| Rules |
|---|
| esp = Fail 38 ==> ar = Y 38 conf:(1) lift:(1.97) lev:(0.05) [21] conv:(16.81) |
| Fm = Small fm = Small foa = Farmer mea = Asm 38 ==> ast = Free 38 conf:(1) lift:(1.47) lev:(0.04) [15] conv:(12.21) |
| Arr = Y foa = Farmer nf = Average 37 ==> ast = Free 37 conf:(1) lift:(1.67) lev:(0.04) [15] conv:(13.48) |
| Twp = Well ia = Well ar = Y foa = Business 38 ==> mea = Asm 37 conf:(0.97) lift:(1.63) lev:(0.03) [33] conv:(4.81) |
| Tn = Well fm = Small mea = Asm 37 ==> ast = Free 36 conf:(0.97) lift:(1.43) lev:(0.03) [33] conv:(6.83) |
| Arr = Y nf = Average mea = Asm 70 ==> ast = Free 68 conf:(0.96) lift:(1.38) lev:(0.05) [13] conv:(5.86) |
| Twp = Well ia = Well ast = Free foa = Retired 55 ==> mea = Asm 52 < conf:(0.95) lift:(1.32) lev:(0.05) [14] conv:(6.22) |
| Fm = Small foa = Service 53 ==> ast = Free 51 < conf:(0.95) lift:(1.37) lev:(0.05) [14] conv:(6.08) |
| Ia = Well ar = Y foa = Farmer 53 ==> ast = Free 51 < conf:(0.95) lift:(1.37) lev:(0.05) [14] conv:(6.06) |
| Ia = Well ar = Y foa = Retired mea = Asm 50 ==> ast = Free 48 < conf:(0.95) lift:(1.42) lev:(0.04) [18] conv:(4.68) |

# 4 Conclusion

This study was conducted by evaluating the prediction from student achievement based on data sets collected from 3 private universities in Jakarta. The data set consists of 350 participants and 23 attributes. After going through various stages of selection, 12 attributes were found to have the most significant influence on the classification process conducted in this study. Thus, the implementation uses four algorithm methods in doing, among them J48, PART, BayesNet, and Random Forest. This study uses WEKA as a data mining tool in the process of classifying. The conclusion that can be drawn from the experiments that have been carried out is that the Random Tree method is very suitable to be applied to the available data sets. It can be seen from the results of the study that the accuracy of Random Forest is higher than other methods, namely 97%, this far outperforms the PART method 71%, J48 70%, or BayesNet 57%. Also, in-depth trials of data sets can be conducted to predict students' performance for a better future. Because, at the end of the prediction, it is possible to get various reports related to the characteristics of the students, so efforts in improving their achievement so that learning activities will run even better.

## References

1. Fang Y, et al (2017) Online learning persistence and academic achievement. Int Educ Data Min Soc
2. Ahuja R, Jha A, Maurya R, Srivastava R (2019) Analysis of educational data mining. In: Harmony search and nature inspired optimization algorithms. Springer, Singapore pp 897–907
3. Baker RS (2019) Challenges for the future of educational data mining: the baker learning analytics prizes. JEDM, J Educ Data Min 11(1):1–17
4. Mitrofanova YS, Anna AS, Olga AF (2019) Modeling smart learning processes based on educational data mining tools. In: Smart education and e-learning 2019. Springer, Singapore pp 561–571
5. Asif R, Merceron A, Ali SA, Haider NG (2017) Analyzing undergraduate students' performance using educational data mining. Comput Educ 113:177–194
6. Triayudi A, Sumiati S, Dwiyatno S, Karyaningsih D, Susilawati S (2021) Measure the effectiveness of information systems with the naïve bayes classifier method. IAES Int J Artif Intell 10(2)
7. Silva C, Fonseca J (2017) Educational data mining: a literature review. In: Europe and MENA cooperation advances in information and communication technologies. Springer, Cham pp 87–94
8. Hung HC, Liu IF, Liang CT, Su YS (2020) Applying educational data mining to explore students' learning patterns in the flipped learning approach for coding education. Symmetry 12(2):213
9. Kumar AD, Selvam RP, Kumar KS (2018) Review on prediction algorithms in educational data mining. Int J Pure Appl Math 118(8):531–537
10. Salloum SA, Alshurideh M, Elnagar A, Shaalan K (2020) Mining in educational data: review and future directions. In: AICV pp 92–102
11. Heath MK (2021) Buried treasure or Ill-gotten spoils: the ethics of data mining and learning analytics in online instruction. Educ Tech Res Dev 69(1):331–334
12. Sánchez-Sordo JM (2019) Data mining techniques for the study of online learning from an extended approach. Multi J Educ, Soc Technol Sci 6(1): 1–24
13. Agung T, Widyarto OW, Vidila R (2020) CLG clustering for mapping pattern analysis of student academic achievement. ICIC Express Letters 14(12):1225–1234
14. Devasia T, Vinushree TP, Hegde V (2016) Prediction of students performance using educational data mining. In: 2016 international conference on data mining and advanced computing (SAPIENCE). IEEE pp 91–95
15. Njeru AM, et al (2017) Using IoT technology to improve online education through data mining. 2017 international conference on applied system innovation (ICASI). IEEE
16. Gan G, Ng MKP (2017) K-means clustering with outlier removal. Pattern Recogn Lett 90:8–14
17. Kimmons R, Veletsianos G (2018) Public internet data mining methods in instructional design, educational technology, and online learning research. TechTrends 62(5):492–500
18. Jie W, et al (2017) Application of educational data mining on analysis of students' online learning behavior. 2017 2nd international conference on image, vision and computing (ICIVC). IEEE
19. Wang R (2021) Exploration of data mining algorithms of an online learning behaviour log based on cloud computing. Int J Continuing Eng Educ Life Long Learn 31(3):371–380
20. Islam O, Siddiqui M, Aljohani NR (2019) Identifying online profiles of distance learning students using data mining techniques. In: Proceedings of the 2019 the 3rd international conference on digital technology in education, pp 115–120
21. Gonçalves AFD, Maciel AMA, Rodrigues RL (2017) Development of a data mining education framework for data visualization in distance learning environments. In: International conference on software engineering and knowledge engineering
22. Xu Y, Zhang M, Gao Z (2019) The construction of distance education personalized learning platform based on educational data mining. In: International conference on applications and techniques in cyber security and intelligence. Springer, Cham pp 1076–1085

23. Ferraz RRN, da Silva MVC, da Silva RA, Quoniam L (2019) Implementation of a distance learning program focused on continuing medical education with the support of patent-based data mining. Revista de Gestão
24. Rong L (2021) Remote case teaching mode based on computer FPGA platform and data mining. Microprocess Microsyst 83:103986
25. Qi Z (2018) Personalized distance education system based on data mining. Int J Emerg Technol Learn 13(7)

# IoT-Based Distributed Body Temperature Detection and Monitoring System for the Implementation of Onsite Learning at Schools

**Indrarini Dyah Irawati, Akhmad Alfaruq, Sugondo Hadiyoso, and Dadan Nur Ramadan**

**Abstract** During the Covid-19 pandemic, teaching and learning activities were carried out virtually. It has been running for more than one year. When the trend of Covid-19 cases decreased, onsite learning began to be trialed by implementing strict health protocols. One of the important parameters for the first screening is body temperature because 99% of Covid-19 patients have fever. Therefore, a student temperature measurement mechanism is needed before entering the school area. A number of temperature detectors should be located to prevent queues. A distributed real-time monitoring system as well as data records are required for daily evaluations. Therefore, in this study, a distributed system for measuring body temperature was designed and implemented with data recording. This system runs online real-time on an internet network client server application. This system consists of four temperature detectors connected to a mini-computer as data control and an access point to a dedicated network. All sensor nodes can send data simultaneously. A web server application is provided for data storage and access to the client. From testing the proposed system, it is known that the system can send real-time data with a delay of <150 ms on several measurements and other measurements >150 ms because it really depends on the quality of internet service. The application can run an alarm function if it finds a temperature exceeding the threshold. This system has been implemented in one of a private school in the city of Bandung. With this system, it is hoped that it can support onsite learning activities in schools.

**Keywords** Onsite learning · Temperature detectors · Real-time · Monitoring

I. D. Irawati (✉) · A. Alfaruq · S. Hadiyoso · D. N. Ramadan
School of Applied Science, Telkom University, Bandung, Indonesia
e-mail: indrarini@telkomuniversity.ac.id

A. Alfaruq
Multi Solusindo Agung, Bandung, Indonesia



T. Triwiyanto et al. (eds.), *Proceedings of the 2nd International Conference on Electronics, Biomedical Engineering, and Health Informatics*, Lecture Notes in Electrical Engineering 898, https://doi.org/10.1007/978-981-19-1804-9_2

## 1 Introduction

The Indonesian government requires educational institutions to provide Covid-19 health protocol facilities before reopening their schools as an effort to prevent the spread of the Covid-19 virus. In preparing for the reopening of the school, the head of the education unit is responsible, among others, the availability of sanitation and hygiene, implementation of thermo gun, the application of mandatory area mask. Several tool used to handle body temperature that describes a person's health status, a temperature check is an initial detection to screen people who have a fever during an outbreak of the corona virus [1, 2]. According to [3], the average body temperature of a feverish person at <60 years of age is higher (36.69 ± 0.34) and if the temperature is measured on the tympanic then fever is expressed at a higher (36.64 ± 0.44) temperature. Another study stated that contactless forehead measurements resulted heat temperature greater than (34.71 ± 0.392) [4].

All schools that will open learning activities onsite are required to provide thermos gun. It becomes the most popular thermometer used during the Covid-19 pandemic because it is convenient, fast, and easy to use [5]. Thermo gun shaped like a gun to measure the temperature in the forehead skin surface without touching. However, thermos gun measurement requires officers to operate it manually with a close distance to the object being measured [6]. The use of thermos gun becomes ineffective for the school environment. Especially if it is applied to several measurement nodes, it will require many operators.

During the Covid-19 pandemic, many studies began to develop contactless body temperature measurement systems. Rahimoon et al. designed real-time temperature monitoring data made using a temperature sensor in the form of Arduino controllers, LM-35 (S1), MLX-90614 (S2), CT-UNO controller as data collection and ESP-wifi shield. Measurement data can be shown and monitored directly by authentic observers by utilizing the internet of things (IoT) application [7]. In [8], the authors developed automated social distancing gate and contactless body temperature monitoring using Arduino uno R3, infrared distance sensor GP2YOA21YK for screening the arrival of people who enter at the social distance gate, ultrasonic sensor for monitoring 1-m social distance between visitors inside the gate, IR thermometer sensor MLX90614ESF-BAA-000-TU-ND for measuring the body temperature, LCD module for displaying, buzzer for alerting and speaker for sending alarm. Research by [6] made a body temperature measurement system using the MLX 90614 temperature sensor to detect early symptoms of COVID-19 with an average error of 0.6% and a standard deviation of 0.078. Another study developed by Abirami, et al. conducted experiments for detecting temperature and mask and security guard on smartphone application [9]. The systems are built using IR thermal camera to measure the body temperature of people, computer vision based on Raspberry Pi camera module to detect mask of people, the Wi-fi module ESP8266 to transmit information to edge server and security guard mobile application to send warning messages for people with high temperatures using the MQTT protocol. Another study [10] made a prototype for monitoring body temperature for the elderly using the DS18B20 temperature sensor, Arduino Nano ATmega328, and the ZigBee module to send measurement results. The measurement results are comparable to measurements using a medical thermometer. Study [11] implemented a simple application to monitor patient health using body temperature sensors, ECG for heart rate, proximity for movement and Raspberry Pi. Sensor readings are sent via Raspberry Pi and can be monitored by anyone. An anomaly detection system monitoring the patient's body temperature that can be controlled in real time via the internet was developed by [12]. This system uses a temperature sensor, microcontroller and Xbee module. The sensor measurement results are compared with the readings on a conventional thermometer. Some urgently research right now is the implementation of IoT-based body temperature monitoring for Covid-19 detection [13–16]. However, most studies have not applied a distributed monitoring system where there are several sensor nodes that work simultaneously in a centralized monitoring application. Another issue is processing time as reported in study [16], a body temperature measurement required time up to 3.000 ms.

Therefore, in this study, we propose the IoT-based distributed non-contact body temperature system to reduce direct contact between officers and the measured object. The system consists of four sensor nodes with a central monitoring application. This system has been implemented and tested in a private school in Bandung. The temperature gauge will display the measured temperature information as well as provide a warning if the measured temperature is abnormal. The measured temperature is sent to a cloud server so that it can be accessed online and in real-time via a web application. With the proposed system, it is hoped that it can support the implementation of health protocols, especially in the school environment if later learning activities are carried out onsite.

## 2 System Design and Implementation

### *2.1 Proposed System*

The proposed temperature detection system in this study consists of a number of sensor nodes that are integrated with the cloud server via a computer hub. Figure 1 shows a distributed network for a temperature monitoring system. The system consists of four K3Pro sensors (wall thermometer standard), data concentrators, server, and web application. The K3Pro sensor will detect the temperature, then the measured temperature data is sent to the data concentrator. The data concentrator is a mini-PC which then sends data to the server (MQTT Broker) using the MQTT protocol in JSON format [17–19]. Communication between K3Pro and data concentrator using UART serial communication via USB. On the server, the data received at the broker is then parsed and stored in the database. Web monitoring is used to view temperature data and the number of visitors at each node.

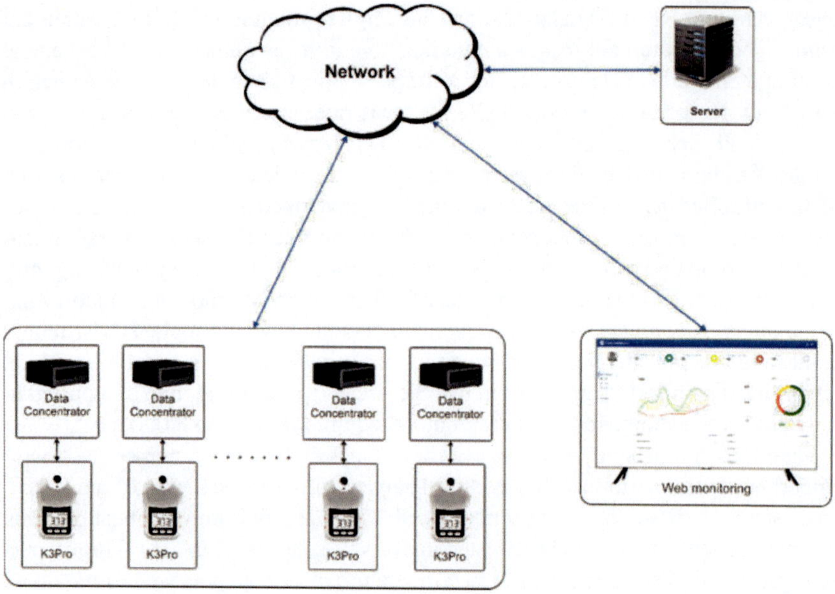


**Fig. 1** Proposed distributed temperature monitoring system

## 2.2 *Data Concentrator*

The data concentrator in this system is designed using a mini-PC Latte Panda. In the data concentrator, a software application is installed which has functions as a data collector as well as a configurator. In this proposed system, the data concentrator is built using CPP + Qt Language. Figure 2 illustrates the communication process between the data concentrator with the sensor and the MQTT broker.

If any object is detected by K3Pro sensor, K3Pro will send data via UART to the data concentrator. Then from the data concentrator the temperature data will be formatted in JSON form and then sent to the server using the MQTT protocol. Snippet code 1, Snippet code 2, and Snippet code 3 are the snippet code of the MQTT configuration and JSON format. Based on Table 1, in the MQTT client configuration, "s6.akh.al" is the host/brokers name used with the port number "1883". Table

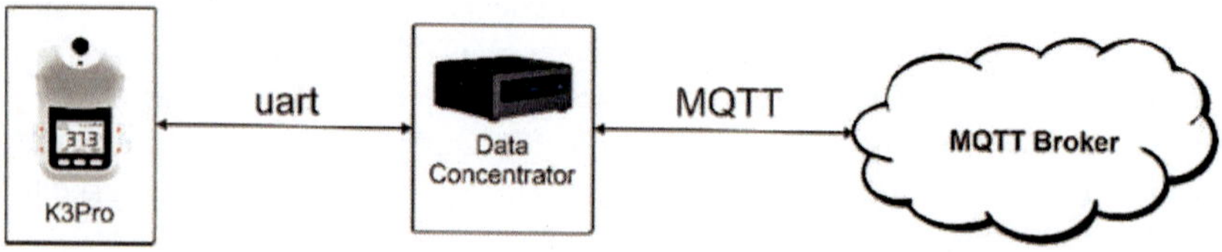


**Fig. 2** Data retrieval flow

**Table 1** Data format for K3Pro configuration

| Header (FIX) | Temp format | Work mode | Limit alarm | | Volume control | Output signal type |
|---|---|---|---|---|---|---|
| | | | °C | F | | |
| 4 hex data | 1 hex data | 1 hex data | 1 hex data | | 1 hex data (%) | 1 hex data |
| 55 AA 0D 02 | 00: °C<br>01: F | 00: Surface mode<br>01: Body mode<br>02: Count mode | 68: 36.0<br>69:36.1<br>6A: 36.2<br>…<br>86: 39.0 | C8: 96.8:<br>CA:97.0<br>CC: 97.2<br>…<br>FC: 102.0 | 00: 0<br>01: 25<br>02: 50<br>03: 75<br>04: 100 | 00: Switch mode<br>01: Pulse mode |

2 describes the JSON functions in parsed including: identification of the sending sensor device/node for example "0001" and retrieval of temperature data "temp". Meanwhile, Snippet code 3 describes the MQTT protocol code for delivery with the header format and data ""K3Pro/"+id+"/data";".

Snippet code 1: '*Config. Mqtt*'

```
qMqttClient = new QMqttClient(this);
qMqttClient - > setHostname("s6.akh.al");
qMqttClient - > setPort(1883);
```

Snippet code 2: '*JSON format*'

```
QJsonObject obj;
obj.insert("temp", temp);
obj.insert("ambience", tempAmb);
QJsonDocument Doc(obj);
mqttPublish("00001", Doc.toJson());
```

Snippet code 3: '*MQTT delivery*'

```
qint32 MainWindow::mqttPublish(QString id, QString message;
{
QString topic = "K3Pro/" + id + "/data";
int ret = qMqttClient- > publish(topic, message.toUtf8();
Return ret;
}
```

### 2.3 Configuration Flow

On the K3Pro, several parameters can be configured, such as backlight, volume level, temperature format, output signal type, work mode, and alarm threshold. To configure these parameters, by sending HEX data to K3Pro via UART with a certain data format as presented in Table 1 [20, 21]. The header consists of 4 Hex data, temperature format, work mode, limit alarm, volume control, backlight, output signal type, fix, and CRC each of 1 Hex data. For example, format: 55 AA 0D 02 00 01 6A 01 00 01 00 01 88. The configuration data can be interpreted as follows: temperature in Celsius, Body mode (sensor is used to scan body temperature), alarm threshold 36.2 °C, volume control: 0, backlight: on, output signal: switch mode.

### 2.4 Cloud Server

The server is an important part of this system to provide real-time monitoring services from sensors to web applications. Server applications are built on a virtual cloud computer. The cloud server specifications used in this proposed system include: MQTT broker using a virtual private server (VPS) with Ubuntu 20.04.2 LTS operating system, meanwhile the application on the personal computer side uses CPU: Intel i7-1065G7, RAM: 16 Gb, Storage: 512 GB SSD, and OS: Windows 10 Pro.

## 3 Results

Testing the functionality and performance of the proposed system was carried out in one of the private schools in the city of Bandung. Four body temperature detectors are placed at the main entrance of the school to avoid queues and maintain health protocols. Figure 3 shows the implementation of the proposed system. In the experiment, we measured the body temperature of students consisting of 2 male students and 2 female students, aged between 13 and 15 years, and all of them were in good health.

The accuracy test of the temperature detector is not performed because it uses standardized and certified devices. In this study, testing on proposed system is more focused on data distribution, delay, and monitoring application functionality. As a reminder, this system consists of four sensors which are connected to a mini-PC via USB (COM port) for data transmission. Data will be sent automatically using a serial protocol after the sensor reads the temperature. Figure 4 shows the data which is sent by one of the sensor nodes in the serial monitor application. From Fig. 4, there is a number of information from each data transmission by the sensor node. However, only body temperature data (the red box) will be sent to the cloud server.

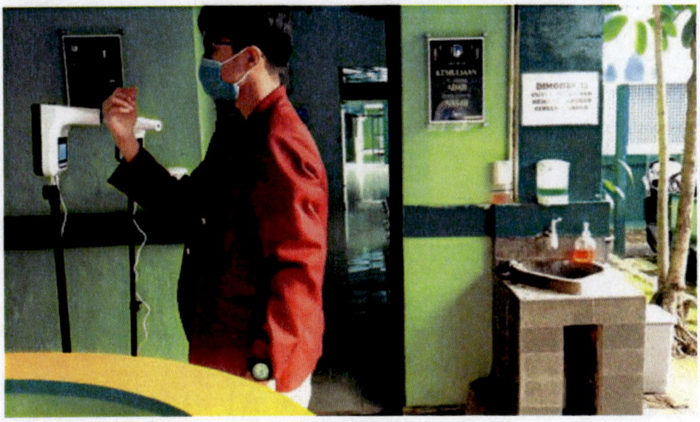

**Fig. 3** System implementation

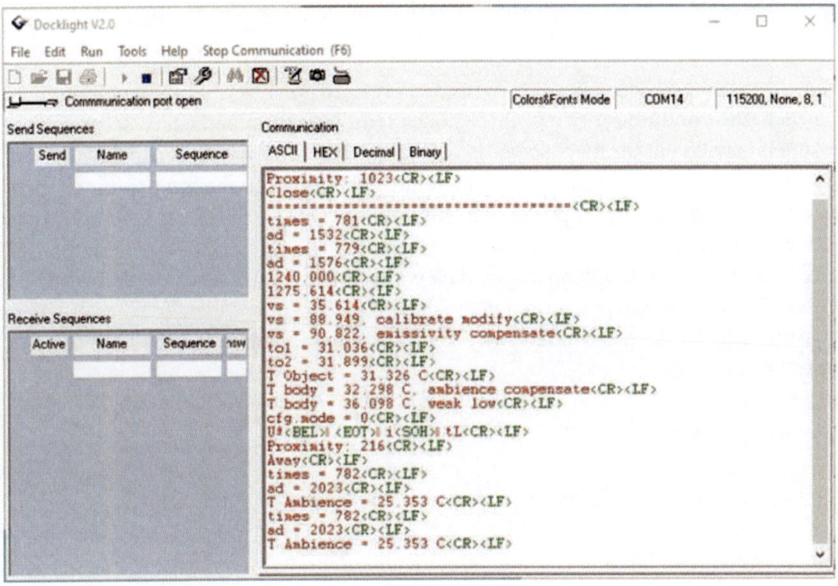


**Fig. 4** Capture temperature data from one of the sensor nodes

Since the system is distributed with four sensors, a test scenario is also carried out where four sensors read the temperature simultaneously. This evaluation is carried out using a serial monitor application. This test aims to observe whether the data can still be received by the mini-PC and in accordance with the sensor data. The serial monitor shows the data transmission line includes, the 1st sensor is on the COM3 serial port, the 2nd sensor is on the COM7 serial port, the 3rd sensor is on the COM5 serial port, meanwhile the 4th sensor is on the COM9 serial port. It is known that data

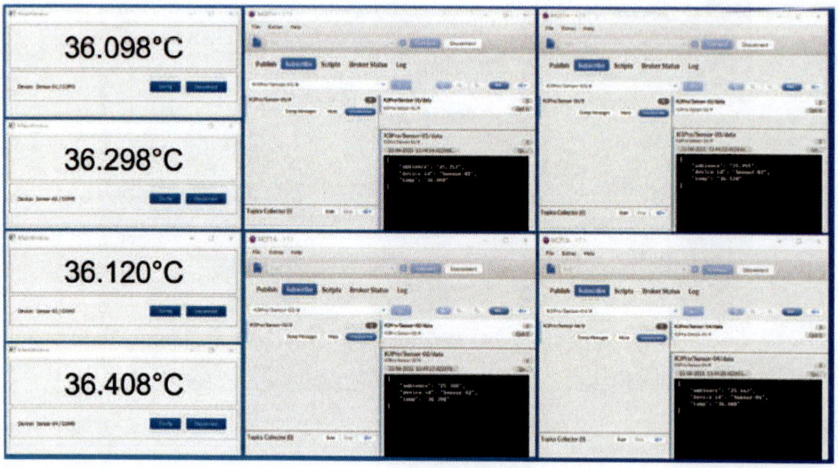


**Fig. 5** Capture PC and server applications while four sensors are sending the data

from all sensor nodes can be received and interpreted correctly. This test is thought to represent the condition if two or three nodes send data simultaneously, so no further testing is carried out for these scenarios. Furthermore, the application on the mini-PC (data concentrator) will parse the temperature data and send the temperature data to the server using the MQTT protocol in JSON form. MQTT data in JSON format can be seen in Fig. 5.

The next process, the temperature data which is sent to the server with the MQTT protocol will be parsed and stored in the database. The database table consists of the measurement number, device identity, measured temperature, and the time the data was sent.

Snippet Code 4: Reading the sensor

```
function updateData() {
  $.get(baseUrl+"api.php", function(message, status){
    if(status=="success") {
      var arr = message.data;
      for(var i=0; i<arr.length;i++) {
        var sensor = arr[i];
        var temp = 'temp_'+sensor["device_id"];
        var count = 'count_'+sensor["device_id"];
        var ts = 'ts_'+sensor["device_id"];
        if(document.getElementById(temp)!=null) {
          document.getElementById(temp).textContent = sensor.temp;
          document.getElementById(count).textContent = sensor.count;
          document.getElementById(ts).textContent = sensor.timestamp;
        }
      }
    }
  });
}
```

On the website page, the data in the database will be retrieved using an AJAX script and displayed on the dashboard. Snippet code 4 is a snippet of the AJAX script implemented in this study. AJAX on the client runs a function to read data sent by the server. These main functions include identification of the sending node, parsing of temperature data, and number of measurements. The web application developed in this study as shown in Fig. 6 display the temperature which has been read by all

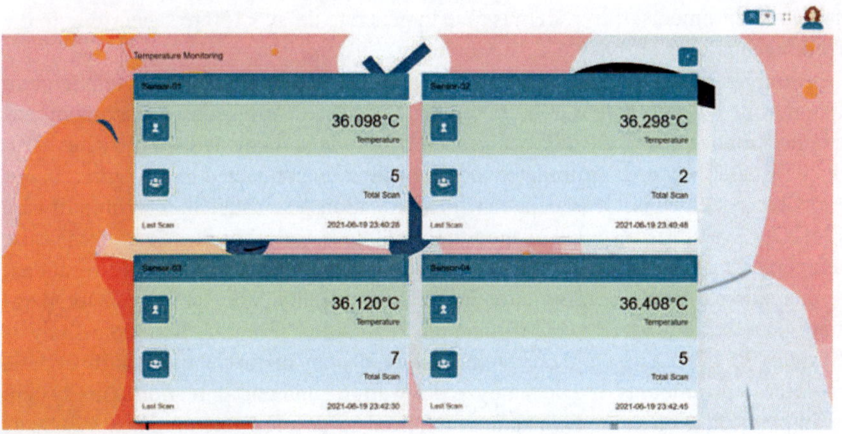


**Fig. 6** Dashboard page display

sensors. The application will also calculate and display the number of temperatures scanned. The results of this test indicate that there is no error in data interpretation, both the temperature value and the number of scans is like the query data on the server.

## 4 Discussion

The following is a system performance test scenario in the form of delay testing. Delay is one of the success parameters in network-based services, especially real-time monitoring applications. In this study, the delay is calculated based on the time of sending data from the mini-PC to the server by retrieving the data of the time of delivery (time taken from the mini-PC) and data of the time when the message is received on the server. Delay testing is performed when all sensor nodes are active and sending the data. Assuming if all sensor nodes are active, it will get the highest delay which represents the best performance when all nodes are active. The server_timestamp column represents the time data from the server. While device_timestamp is the time data obtained from the mini-PC server_timestamp when sending data to the server [22, 23]. This test can be seen in Fig. 7. So, the calculation of the delay in this study is the delta between server_timestamp and device_timestamp. The delay test was carried out 30 times. From the test results, the average delay in sending from the sensor to the application is 1.292 s with a minimum delay of 19 ms, a maximum delay of 9124 s, and a standard deviation of 2438 s. From this test, it is also known that the standard deviation is quite high because in some measurements the generating delay is high. Traffic conditions on the internet network greatly affect the delay. From this test, it shows that the average delay is quite high because in some measurements it generates a delay of >1 s. This can be because the quality of the internet network when the test was carried out was unstable. But at least, in some measurements, this system is able to generate delay <150 ms according to the recommendations of the real-time monitoring system.

Although this study has succeeded in designing and implementing a temperature monitoring system, there is a limitation that this system still uses a minicomputer as a concentrator to send the data to the server. To reduce delay and simplify the hardware installation, the thermometer should be directly connected to the server. In our proposed system, it is not associated with notifications via instant messaging software [24]. Our system is installed at the school entrance and only functions to measure temperature, whereas in [24], the system is installed in each class to measure student temperatures while recording attendance automatically. The Intelligent Temperature Measurement System (ITMS) and the Pandemic Prevention Situation Analysis System (PPAS) can measure body temperature, display historical traceability of data, monitor large amounts of data, analyze pre-warning and post-infection. This system is implemented on campus. The cost required to develop this complex system is almost 300USD [25]. Our simple system is installed in a small area at school to monitor 4 thermometers with a total cost of less than USD 250.

| | no | device_id | timestamp | server_timestamp | device_timestamp |
|---|---|---|---|---|---|
| 63 | 101 | Sensor-01 | 2021-06-23 14:15:53 | 2021-06-23 14:15:53.701 | 23/06/2021-06-23 14:15:53.676 |
| 64 | 102 | Sensor-01 | 2021-06-23 14:15:58 | 2021-06-23 14:15:58.723 | 23/06/2021-06-23 14:15:58.686 |
| 65 | 103 | Sensor-01 | 2021-06-23 14:16:04 | 2021-06-23 14:16:04.379 | 23/06/2021-06-23 14:16:03.689 |
| 66 | 104 | Sensor-01 | 2021-06-23 14:16:08 | 2021-06-23 14:16:08.722 | 23/06/2021-06-23 14:16:08.695 |
| 67 | 105 | Sensor-01 | 2021-06-23 14:16:14 | 2021-06-23 14:16:14.106 | 23/06/2021-06-23 14:16:13.698 |
| 68 | 106 | Sensor-01 | 2021-06-23 14:16:18 | 2021-06-23 14:16:19.034 | 23/06/2021-06-23 14:16:18.703 |
| 69 | 107 | Sensor-01 | 2021-06-23 14:16:23 | 2021-06-23 14:16:23.734 | 23/06/2021-06-23 14:16:23.702 |
| 70 | 108 | Sensor-01 | 2021-06-23 14:16:28 | 2021-06-23 14:16:28.752 | 23/06/2021-06-23 14:16:28.729 |
| 71 | 109 | Sensor-01 | 2021-06-23 14:16:34 | 2021-06-23 14:16:34.177 | 23/06/2021-06-23 14:16:33.737 |
| 72 | 110 | Sensor-01 | 2021-06-23 14:16:38 | 2021-06-23 14:16:38.774 | 23/06/2021-06-23 14:16:38.745 |
| 73 | 111 | Sensor-01 | 2021-06-23 14:16:44 | 2021-06-23 14:16:44.109 | 23/06/2021-06-23 14:16:43.756 |
| 74 | 112 | Sensor-01 | 2021-06-23 14:16:49 | 2021-06-23 14:16:49.127 | 23/06/2021-06-23 14:16:48.760 |
| 75 | 113 | Sensor-01 | 2021-06-23 14:16:54 | 2021-06-23 14:16:54.163 | 23/06/2021-06-23 14:16:53.760 |
| 76 | 114 | Sensor-01 | 2021-06-23 14:17:07 | 2021-06-23 14:17:07.458 | 23/06/2021-06-23 14:16:58.758 |
| 77 | 115 | Sensor-01 | 2021-06-23 14:17:07 | 2021-06-23 14:17:07.960 | 23/06/2021-06-23 14:17:03.772 |
| 78 | 116 | Sensor-01 | 2021-06-23 14:17:17 | 2021-06-23 14:17:17.901 | 23/06/2021-06-23 14:17:08.777 |
| 79 | 117 | Sensor-01 | 2021-06-23 14:17:17 | 2021-06-23 14:17:17.972 | 23/06/2021-06-23 14:17:13.788 |
| 80 | 118 | Sensor-01 | 2021-06-23 14:17:18 | 2021-06-23 14:17:18.828 | 23/06/2021-06-23 14:17:18.799 |
| 81 | 119 | Sensor-01 | 2021-06-23 14:17:25 | 2021-06-23 14:17:25.083 | 23/06/2021-06-23 14:17:23.820 |
| 82 | 120 | Sensor-01 | 2021-06-23 14:17:29 | 2021-06-23 14:17:29.268 | 23/06/2021-06-23 14:17:28.816 |
| 83 | 121 | Sensor-01 | 2021-06-23 14:17:34 | 2021-06-23 14:17:34.992 | 23/06/2021-06-23 14:17:33.819 |
| 84 | 122 | Sensor-01 | 2021-06-23 14:17:38 | 2021-06-23 14:17:38.858 | 23/06/2021-06-23 14:17:38.829 |
| 85 | 123 | Sensor-01 | 2021-06-23 14:17:43 | 2021-06-23 14:17:43.874 | 23/06/2021-06-23 14:17:43.848 |
| 86 | 124 | Sensor-01 | 2021-06-23 14:17:48 | 2021-06-23 14:17:48.884 | 23/06/2021-06-23 14:17:48.859 |
| 87 | 125 | Sensor-01 | 2021-06-23 14:17:53 | 2021-06-23 14:17:53.888 | 23/06/2021-06-23 14:17:53.858 |
| 88 | 126 | Sensor-01 | 2021-06-23 14:18:00 | 2021-06-23 14:18:00.090 | 23/06/2021-06-23 14:17:58.864 |
| 89 | 127 | Sensor-01 | 2021-06-23 14:18:03 | 2021-06-23 14:18:03.901 | 23/06/2021-06-23 14:18:03.876 |
| 90 | 128 | Sensor-01 | 2021-06-23 14:18:08 | 2021-06-23 14:18:08.916 | 23/06/2021-06-23 14:18:08.891 |
| 91 | 129 | Sensor-01 | 2021-06-23 14:18:18 | 2021-06-23 14:18:18.620 | 23/06/2021-06-23 14:18:13.891 |
| 92 | 130 | Sensor-01 | 2021-06-23 14:18:19 | 2021-06-23 14:18:19.281 | 23/06/2021-06-23 14:18:18.898 |

**Fig. 7** Transmission delay test

# 5 Conclusion

The distributed temperature monitoring system has been successfully implemented in a private school in the city of Bandung. The system is built with four K3Pro sensors, data concentrators and an MQTT server. It has been tested on limited face-to-face learning to students who attend. The test results on 30 measurements show that the monitoring system developed can work simultaneously and in real time. Web monitoring succeeded in displaying information from the four sensors simultaneously regarding body temperature, the number of students whose temperature was measured, and the last scan. The resulting average delay is 1292 ms. The proposed system is very useful in reducing physical contact between temperature measuring officers and students during the Covid-19 pandemic. In addition, it helps schools to monitor the condition of students, detect students whose temperatures are above normal, and reduce queues to enter school. On IoT-based systems and without IoT, the thermometer will produce the same measurement results. However, an IoT-based system has advantages, including efficiency in collecting measurement results for several devices, efficiency of monitoring processes because it can be done remotely via the Internet cloud. Further research is needed to reduce the resulting transmission delay. It is also necessary to develop applications that support notifications on student communication devices.

## References


1. Yi-Chi W, Cing-Sung, Yu-Jiun C (2020) The outbreak of COVID-19. J Chin Med Assoc 83(3):217–220
2. Vulpe A, Lupu C, Mihai C (2020) Research on infrared body temperature measurement—virus spreading prevention. Int Conf Electron, Comput Artif Intell (ECAI) 12:1–4
3. Geneva II, Cuzzo B, Fazili T, Javaid W (2019) Normal body temperature: a systematic review. Open forum infectious diseases. Oxford University Press on behalf of Infectious Diseases Society of America pp 1–7
4. Chen HY, Chen A, Chen C (2020) Investigation of the impact of infrared sensors on core body temperature monitoring by comparing measurement sites. Sensors
5. Adams DS, Valentine A, Bucknall T, Kouzani AZ. Technologies for fever screening in the time of COVID-19: a review. IEEE Sens J
6. Rusimamto PW, Harimurti ER, Anistyasari Y, Anifah L (2020) Design and implementation of thermal body system employing thermal sensor MLX 90614 for Covid-19 symptoms early detector. Int Joint Conf Sci Eng (IJCSE) 317–321
7. Rahimoon AA, Abdullah NM, Taib I (2020) Design of a contactless body temperature measurement system using Arduino. Indonesian J Electr Eng Comput Sci 19(3):1251–1258
8. Alvarez GAA, Garcia MB, Alvarez DU (2020) Automated social distancing gate with non-contact body temperature monitoring using Arduino Uno. Int Res J Eng Technol 19(7):4351–4356
9. Abirami M, Saundariya K, Senthil RK, Yamuna I (2021) Contactless temperature detection of multiple people and detection of possible corona virus affected persons using AI enabled IR sensor camera. Sixth international conference on wireless communications, signal processing and networking. pp 166–170
10. Saha R, Biswas S, Sarmah S (2021) A working prototype using DS18B20 temperature sensor and Arduino for health monitoring 2(1):33
11. Kumar R, Rajasekaran PM (2016) An IoT based patient monitoring system using raspberry Pi. International conference on computing technologies and intelligent data engineering. pp 1–4
12. Mansor H, Shukor HMA, Meskam SS, Rusli NQAM, Zamery NS (2013) Body temperature measurement for remote health monitoring system. 2013 IEEE international conference on smart instrumentation, measurement and applications. pp 1–5
13. Costanzo S, Flores MA (2021) IoT noncontact body temperature measurement system implementing access control for COVID-19. Trends and applications in information systems and technologies. WorldCIST 2021. Advances in intelligent systems and computing (1368). Springer
14. Hoang ML, Carratù M, Paciello V, Pietrosanto A (2021) Body temperature indoor condition monitor and activity recognition by MEMS accelerometer based on IoT alert system for people in quarantine due to COVID-19. Sensors, MDPI 21 (2313)
15. Thermal cameras are being outfitted to detect fever and conduct contact tracing for COVID-19. IEEE Spectrum. https://spectrum.ieee.org/news-from-around-ieee/the-institute/ieee-member-news/thermal-cameras-are-being-outfitted-to-detect-fever-and-conduct-contact-tracing-for-covid19. Accessed 25 Dec 2020
16. Ruffin T, Steele J, Acquaah Y, Sharma N, Sarku E, Tesiero R, Gokaraju B (2021) Non-invasive low cost fever detection systems. SoutheastCon 2021:1–7
17. Kodali RK, Gorantla VSK (2017) Weather tracking system using MQTT and SQLite. 3rd International conference on applied and theoretical computing and communication technology (iCATccT). pp 205–208

18. Rana M, Mittal V (2019) Design and development of wearable sensor system using MQTT protocol for real time kinematics analysis. 2019 global conference for advancement in technology (GCAT). pp 1–6
19. Hijazi G, Habaebi MH, Al-Haddad A, Zyoud AM (2021) Stress testing MQTT server for private IOT network. Int J Electr Telecommun 67(2)
20. Harutyunyan S, Kaplanyan T, Kirakosyan A, Momjyan A (2020) Design and verification of autoconfigurable UART controller. IEEE 40th international conference on electronics and nanotechnology (ELNANO). pp 347–350
21. Gupta AK, Raman A, Kumar N, Ranjan R (2020) Design and implementation of high-speed universal asynchronous receiver and transmitter (UART). 7th international conference on signal processing and integrated networks (SPIN). pp 295–300
22. Wu H, Liu H, Wang B, Xin G (2017) Accurate traffic replay based on interactive sequence and timestamp. IEEE 9th international conference on communication software and networks (ICCSN). pp 1107–1110
23. Siddique B, Akhtar N (2017) Temporal hierarchical event detection of timestamped data. International conference on computing, communication and automation (ICCCA). pp 783–788
24. Yen PY, Fanjiang YY, Hung CH, Zhang MT (2021) Design and implement a roll call system with body temperature measurement and the instant messaging software. IEEE international conference on consumer electronics (ICCE). pp 1–2
25. Lin LW, Hsieh HC, Chen ST, Chen J, Lee LJ, Chen CW (2021) Apply IOT technology to practice a pandemic prevention body temperature measurement system: a case study of response measures for COVID-19. Int J Distrib Sens Netw 17(5):1–13

# Improving the Quality and Education Systems Through Integration's Approach of Data Mining Clustering in E-Learning

**Agung Triayudi, Iskandar Fitri, Wahyu Oktri Widyarto, and Sumiati**

**Abstract** Educational Data Mining (EDM) is a discipline developed by focusing on improving independent and adaptive learning methods to find hidden education patterns. In this area, heterogeneous data is known to continue to develop in a big-data paradigm. Several specific data mining techniques are required to extract information with an adaptive value from the available educational data. Therefore, this study aims to present a grouping approach related to partitioning students into a different group or cluster based on the students' behavior during lessons. Then, the architecture related to the e-learning system will be personalized to detect and provide suitable teaching methods and content according to each student's learning ability so that students can improve their quality and learning ability. The grouping methods that can be done in this educational data mining include K-Means, K-Medoids, Agglomerative Hierarchical Cluster Trees, Noise-Based Application Density-Based Spatial Clustering, and Fast Search and Density Peak Findings through Heat Diffusion (CFSFDP-HD) Shows the average compute time with different student count benchmarks: 600, 1200, 1800, 2400, 3000, 3600. Then, it has been found that the CFSFDP-HD method has strong results compared to other methods.

**Keywords** Educational data mining · Big data · Clustering · Profile learning · e-Learning

A. Triayudi (✉) · I. Fitri
Department of ICT, Universitas Nasional, Jakarta, Indonesia
e-mail: agungtriayudi@civitas.unas.ac.id

W. O. Widyarto
Industrial Engineering Department, Universitas Serang Raya, Serang, Indonesia

Sumiati
Informatics Department, Universitas Serang Raya, Serang, Indonesia



T. Triwiyanto et al. (eds.), *Proceedings of the 2nd International Conference on Electronics, Biomedical Engineering, and Health Informatics*, Lecture Notes in Electrical Engineering 898, https://doi.org/10.1007/978-981-19-1804-9_3

## 1 Introduction

The Educational Data Mining method is concerned with modern and up-to-date adaptive studies and developments, where available instruments are used to analyze and visualize hidden patterns of educational datasets. [1]. The educational data also depends on the geographical conditions, most of which are structured, semi-structured, and unstructured [2]. EDM appears as an intrinsic data analysis research field also has a function in extracting information related to hidden pattern predictions to obtain information related to the educational data set. EDM is considered as an effort to implement educational data mining methods that can generate new patterns also analyze the big data artificially with efficient results [3, 4].

Nowadays, technology such as Artificial Intelligence (AI), Internet of Things, Sensor, and various social networks are integrated into education systems to improve teaching and learning activities [5]. At an educational level, the amount of data or information available can provide new insights in prediction or decision-making efforts that can improve learning skills by both teachers and learners. It is why educational data mining plays a significant role to improve the quality and education systems, through: (1) the discovery of new perspectives related to experimental data, (2) the discovery of of knowledge along with associations from various fields, and (3) the improvement of the quality of individual-based education. Along with the development of increasingly advanced and fast-paced communication technology, much use of sensors and intelligent devices are implemented into the education systems to observe the patterns and behaviors from all elements involved in the education system, where it has a variety of information related to thoughts and events that are present in the form of semi-structured or unstructured. Thus, in a virtual-based education system, there is a need for improvement efforts by implementing all techniques available in data mining to meet the needs of an educational institution effectively [6, 7]. There are many models and data mining met hods that can be implemented into an education field, where these methods can be categorized as classification, clustering, relationship mining, and neural networks. *Grouping* is the primary unattended method that is useful for partitioning data sets into a separate cluster based on estimates of intrinsic characteristics or similarities. This method can also be categorized by partition-based, model-based, density-based and hierarchical. The grouping methods that can be done in this educational data mining include K-Means, K-Medoids, Agglomerative Hierarchical Cluster Trees, Noise-Based Application Density-Based Spatial Clustering, and Fast Search and Density Peak Findings through Heat Diffusion (CFSFDP-HD) [8, 9].

## 2 Literature Review

### 2.1 *Techniques of Education Data Mining Clustering*

EDM serves as a research area involving a series of collaborations between psychological and computational methods [10]. Research related to educational data mining has also been done to find techniques in analyzing learning related to big data to know the adaptive learning systems (ALS) model [11]. This ALS model seeks to empower teachers to always quickly understand the needs and adjustments that need to be made to keep up with the changes that continue to occur related to this educational unit. Other research also states that the exploration that has been done on various studies and data sets related to the field of EDM can be used in recognizing students who have a risk of failure in learning, distinguishing adaptation methods of groups or individual students, increasing the number of graduations, and improving the quality and quality of educational institutions [12, 13].

Related to the various benefits that can be obtained from the implementation results, K-means, as one of the partition-based grouping algorithms commonly applied to EDM, can understand student behavior based on available data, as well as consider the impact of self-characteristics on the performance of students, so that it will present clear types of classifications [14, 15].

### 2.2 *Personalized E-Learning System and Data Mining Clustering Approach*

The architecture of e-learning systems focuses on individual needs and makes predictions of references or interests from users. Considering e-learning not only focus on teachers or students to meet virtually but also creates other electronic resources. In Fig. 1, the following is the architecture of a personalized e-learning system, where the steps in PESA are described as follows [16, 17]:

- Student's Profile
- Data Mining Clustering Approach
- Recommendations
- Database
- Virtual Systems
- Considering the big data set of academic databases implemented by educational data mining methods in this study, a virtual display containing all the needs of an institution is presented to students in the form of electronic documents [18].

**Key Steps Involved in The Recommended Educational Data Mining Approach.** The data mining approach recommended in this study (CFSFDP-HD) was implemented using the tools available in data mining to analyze students' patterns and behaviors and simulate them into educational data. The simulated educational

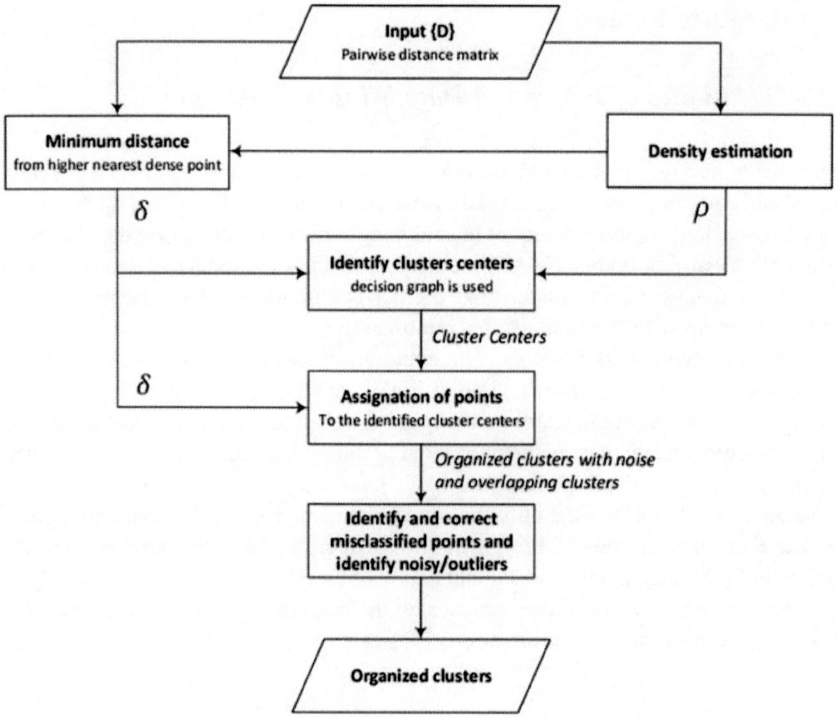


**Fig. 1** Key steps involved in the recommended educational data mining approach [17]

data contains: (1) the grades obtained by each student and (2) attendance in the classroom. The indicators on the grades obtained by each student consist of: (1) two quizzes, (2) four assignments, (3) midterm exam, and (4) final semester exam.

## 3 Result and Discussion

In this study, there was a dataset containing 600 characteristics of students from different classes and sessions, which were then simulated using the approach of CFSFDP-HD to partition them into groups according to the similarity of characteristics and other indicators based on the scores obtained (quizzes, assignments, midterm exams, final semester exams) and attendence in the classroom (Table 1).

This effort is necessary to design suitable teaching methods according to each student's characteristic needs so that an effective learning process will be realized and improve the quality and performance of each individual's learning. In the image below, the decision graph is defined as follows:

**Table 1** Dataset

| Subject | Students | Datasets | Posts | Times |
|---|---|---|---|---|
| Computer security | 280 | Submission (assignment) | 189 | 90 |
| | | Course modul (forum) | 443 | 120 |
| Knowledge management | 320 | Discussion (forum) | 108 | 25 |
| | | Course view | 692 | 234 |
| | | Observe | 85 | 27 |

The decision graph shown is based on (1) estimation through heat diffusion and (2) calculating the minimum distance of $\delta i$ points closest to higher density. At this stage, the cluster center identification process is obtained by implementing the decision graph as shown in Fig. 3a, where the outlier acts as a potential cluster center and is shown by a different color. The clusters that have been found are displayed with various color schemes according to Fig. 3b, where 2D non-classical multidimensional scaling applies to visualizing datasets. In this process, the recommended CFSFDP-HD approach is adaptive, so the available parameters do not need to be explicitly set.

Based on the categories of students obtained through classification based on Figs. 3a and b, the approach of teaching methods can begin to be adapted to each student's learning needs. So there will be improvements related to student performance because the methods they face to improve performance quality are following their characteristics. The student achievement index can also be further analyzed to improve the quality of an educational institution's system.

The grouping method implemented in this study consists of K-means, K-medoid, AHCT, and DBSCAN, which are then simulated through a dataset of 600 students and outlined in Table 2 below.

Based on the comparison of approaches recommended by CFSFDP-HD through K-Means, K-Medoids, AHCT, and DBSCAN, the resulting decision graph is proven to help provide information in-depth insights to select clusters that have the potential to meet all needs related to educational aspects. The implementation of K-means

**Table 2** Clustering method based on the indicator value

| Method | Indicator |
|---|---|
| K-means | The number of clusters (k = 7)<br>The number of iterations (n = 40) |
| K-medoids | The number of clusters (k = 5)<br>Predefined the number of iterations (n = 40) |
| DBSCAN | Epsilon (eps = 0.5)<br>Minimun points (minPts = 10) |
| AHCT | The number of clusters (k = 6) |
| CFSFDP-HD | Does not require the number of clusters and iterations |

and K-medoids has been done repeatedly with various input settings (such as cluster count and iteration) to get the most optimal cluster and provide the right solution of multiple iterations that have been done. Meanwhile, the AHCT approach explicitly defines the number of clusters, making it easier to check, visualize, and compare, as shown in Fig. 2b. This is in contrast to the data visualizations presented in Fig. 3a–d.

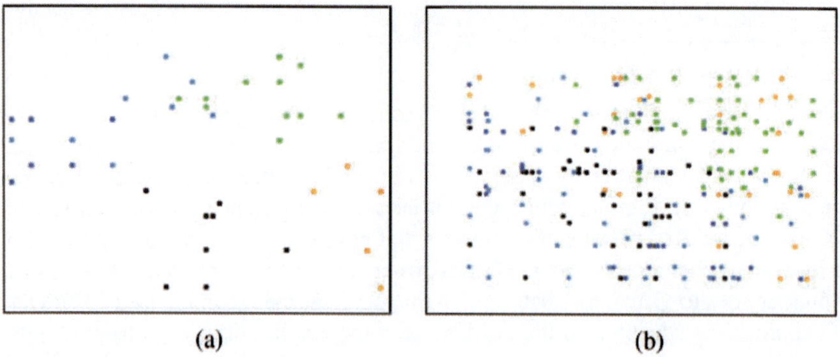


**Fig. 2** **a** Decision graph with adjusted parameters, **b** Identify clusters with different color schemes

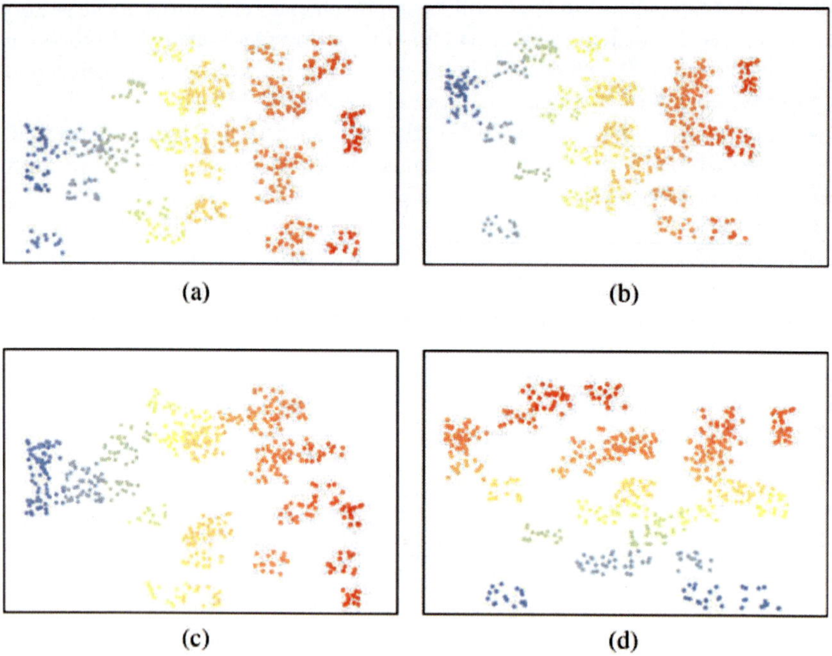


**Fig. 3** Visualization of **a** K-means clustering, **b** K-medoids clustering, **c** AHCT clustering, **d** DBSCAN clustering

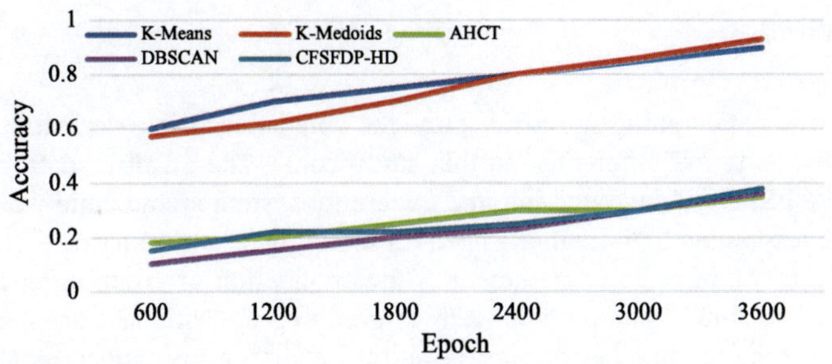


**Fig. 4** Time execution comparison based on the different number of students

The representated data point in Fig. 2b with Fig. 3 is also different given the differences in the location of the data displayed. Based on ρ and δ grades, students with exemplary achievements are on the upper side in Fig. 2b. While in Fig. 3, students who have exemplary achievements are on the right side. To get the cluster form with the implemented approach in this study, it's important to know the number of existing clusters and the possibility of difficulties in detecting low or below average student performance. Of course, this possibility can lead to limitations in finding hidden patterns that are present in the process of classifying data. On that basis, the CFSFDP-HD method is recommended to find hidden patterns without even knowing the technicalities related to the data referenced by the study.

In this study, it was also found that the CFSFDP-HD method is known to be more adaptive and has significant results when compared to some previous approaches. The study also calculated the estimated time in executing the CFSFDP-HD approach and determining whether optimization efforts are required to predict the number of big data sets clusters accurately. Figure 4 below shows the average compute time of K-means, K-medoids, AHCT, DBSCAN, and CFSFDP-HD approaches with different student count benchmarks: 600, 1200, 1800, 2400, 3000, 3600. Each available approach has been run several times to take the required average time. In Fig. 5 below, the number of students is displayed on the x-axis, while the y-axis displays the execution time (in seconds).

Based on the results represented in Fig. 4, it is known that the recommended approach, namely CFSFDP-HD, runs quite effectively and efficiently compared to K-means and K-medoids. The recommended approach also takes less time than AHCT on smaller datasets. Although the DBSCAN approach takes less time on smaller data sets, AHCT and DBSCAN methods are not recommended because they are less efficient when applied to larger data sets. Through this consideration, the CFSFDP-HD approach is recommended to accurately measure the patterns and behaviors of students and present execution results related to significant and real datasets.

## 4 Conclusion

The available data mining approach provides convenience in e-learning systems to run effectively and efficiently. In this study comes the adaptive data grouping approach "CFSFDP" integrated into the e-learning system architecture where most queries are responded to without the need for intelligence and heuristics. This study has also been conducted an assessment of the application of grouping in big data. Experiments to find a suitable approach to grouping educational data need to be done by knowing the number of clusters and the shortcomings concerning the size of the identified data cluster. In this case, the approach recommended in this study, "CFSFDP" is considered capable of analyzing big data to strengthen the education system. This study also shows that the approach has formed a real cluster with less execution time compared to other approach methods. Besides, this approach also serves in solving various obstacles and needs related to elements in the field of education.

**Acknowledgements** This research is the result of the basic research scheme of the Indonesian Dikti grant B/112/E3/RA.00/2021.

## References

1. Hamoud A, Hashim AS, Awadh WA (2018) Predicting student performance in higher education institutions using decision tree analysis. Int J Interact Multimedia Artif Intell 5:26–31
2. Triayudi A, Sumiati S, Dwiyatno S, Karyaningsih D, Susilawati (2021) Measure the effectiveness of information systems with the naïve bayes classifier method. IAES Int J Artif Intell 10(2)
3. Lu OH, Huang AY, Huang JC, Lin AJ, Ogata H, Yang SJ (2018) Applying learning analytics for the early prediction of students' academic performance in blended learning. Educ Technol Soc 220–232
4. Zaffar M, et al (2017) Performance analysis of feature selection algorithm for educational data mining. 2017 IEEE conference on big data and analytics
5. Zhang W, Li J (2015) Extended fast search clustering algorithm: widely density clusters, no density peaks. arXiv preprint arXiv:1505.05610
6. Yang F, Cao J, Zhou K, Zhang P, Wang Y (2018) An adaptive clustering algorithm based on CFSFDP. In: 2018 33rd youth academic annual conference of Chinese association of automation (YAC). pp 404–408
7. Xu H, Yao S, Li Q, Ye Z (2020) An improved k-means clustering algorithm. In: 2020 IEEE 5th international symposium on smart and wireless systems within the conferences on intelligent data acquisition and advanced computing systems. pp 1–5
8. Wang Y, Chen Q, Kang C, Xia Q (2016) Clustering of electricity consumption behavior dynamics toward big data applications. IEEE Trans Smart Grid 7(5):2437–2447
9. Sheng K, Liu Z, Zhou D (2017) An adaptive resampling algorithm based on CFSFDP. In: 2017 2nd IEEE international conference on computational intelligence and applications (ICCIA). pp 41–45
10. Silva C, José F (2017) Educational data mining: a literature review. In: Europe and MENA cooperation advances in information and communication technologies. Springer, Cham, pp 87–94

11. Nakayama M, Mutsuura K, Yamamoto H (2018) Using note taking instructions to reform student's note taking activities and improve learning performance in a blended learning course. Int Conf Inf Visualisation 326–331
12. Hernández-Blanco A, Herrera-Flores B, Tomás D, Navarro-Colorado B (2019) A systematic review of deep learning approaches to educational data mining. Complexity 2019
13. Salloum S, Muhammad A, Ashraf E, Khaled S (2020) Mining in educational data: review and future directions. In: Joint European-US workshop on applications of invariance in computer vision. Springer, Cham pp 92–102
14. Agung T, Widyarto OW, Vidila R (2020) CLG clustering for mapping pattern analysis of student academic achievement. ICIC Express Lett 14(12):1225–1234
15. Ahuja R, et al (2019) Analysis of educational data mining. In: Harmony search and nature inspired optimization algorithms. Springer pp 897–907
16. Baker RS (2019) Challenges for the future of educational data mining: the baker learning analytics prizes. JEDM, J Educ Data Min 11(1):1–17
17. Kausar S, Huahu X, Hussain I, Wenhao Z, Zahid M (2018) Integration of data mining clustering approach in the personalized e-learning system. IEEE Access 6:72724–72734
18. Fynn A et al (2018) A comparison of the utility of data mining algorithms in an open distance learning context. S Afr J High Educ 32(4):81–95
19. Rosalina V, et al (2020) Measuring citizen readiness to adopt electronic citizen relationship management (E-CIRM) using technology readiness index (TRI). J Theor Appl Inf Technol 98(21): 3416–3425
20. Ferraz R, Marcus V, Renan A, Luc Q (2019) Implementation of a distance learning program focused on continuing medical education with the support of patent-based data mining. Revista de Gestão
21. Wang R (2021) Exploration of data mining algorithms of an online learning behaviour log based on cloud computing. Int J Continuing Eng Educ Life Long Learn 31(3):371–380
22. Islam O, Siddiqui M, Aljohani NR (2019) Identifying online profiles of distance learning students using data mining techniques. In: Proceedings of the 2019 The 3rd international conference on digital technology in education. pp 115–120
23. Qi Z (2018) Personalized distance education system based on data mining. Int J Emerg Technol Learn 13(7)
24. Gonçalves AFD, Maciel AMA, Rodrigues RL (2017) Development of a data mining education framework for data visualization in distance learning environments. In: International conference on software engineering and knowledge engineering
25. Xu Y, Miao Z, Zhigang G (2019) The construction of distance education personalized learning platform based on educational data mining. In: International conference on applications and techniques in cyber security and intelligence. Springer, Cham pp 1076–1085

# A Survey of Deep Learning on COVID-19 Identification Through X-Ray Images

Ledya Novamizanti and Tati Latifah Erawati Rajab

**Abstract** New Coronavirus 2019 (COVID-19) is a virus that causes severe pneumonia and affects many organs of the body. This infection was initially discovered in one of the cities in the Republic of China, Wuhan, in December 2019 and since then has been spread throughout the globe as a global pandemic. To prevent the virus from spreading, positive cases must be identified early and infected persons must be treated as soon as possible. As new instances emerge regularly, many developing countries are experiencing COVID-19 testing kit scarcity because the demand for testing kits has soared. As an alternative, radiological imaging techniques such as X-ray images have been proven to help in COVID-19 diagnosis because images from X-ray provide valuable information about the COVID-19 virus disease. This paper presents a survey of Deep learning-based methods in identifying COVID-19 with X-ray input images, and classifies these images into several categories, namely: no findings, normal, COVID, and pneumonia. Several studies have been included with details about their datasets, methodologies, and findings. A total of thirteen popular datasets and fifteen articles are reviewed in this paper. Research challenges and recommendations for future research directions are also provided as an evaluation of previous research. Search for research articles in well-known digital libraries, namely Scopus, IEEE Xplore, Springer, and ScienceDirect, was carried out to obtain a list of studies relevant to the scope of research. Related articles that have a high impact are considered in the list of studies. Also, in selecting studies related to the research scope, we apply some inclusion and exclusion criteria. The list of studies used in subsequent research is imported to the library. Then, studies that did not match the criteria for inclusion were eliminated. The clinical application of artificial intelligence, i.e., DL in diagnosing COVID-19, is promising, and further research is

L. Novamizanti (✉) · T. L. E. Rajab
School of Electrical Engineering and Informatics, Institut Teknologi Bandung, Bandung, Indonesia
e-mail: ledyaldn@telkomuniversity.ac.id

L. Novamizanti
School of Electrical Engineering, Telkom University, Bandung, Indonesia

Human Centric (HUMIC) Engineering, Telkom University, Bandung, Indonesia



T. Triwiyanto et al. (eds.), *Proceedings of the 2nd International Conference on Electronics, Biomedical Engineering, and Health Informatics*, Lecture Notes in Electrical Engineering 898, https://doi.org/10.1007/978-981-19-1804-9_4

needed. Convolutional Neural Network (CNN) approaches could be used in collaboration through X-ray pictures to identify diseases quickly and accurately, reducing the shortage of testing equipment and their restrictions. It is expected that this work can help researchers understand the general picture and existing research gaps to decide on the appropriate architecture and approach in developing deep learning-based covid identification research.

**Keywords** COVID-19 · Deep learning · Identification · X-Ray

## 1 Introduction

On December 31, 2019, coronavirus disease (COVID-19) epidemic began in Wuhan, Hubei Province, China [1, 2]. The World Health Organization (WHO) originally named the epidemic SARS-CoV-2 and then renaming it COVID-19. It only takes 30 days for the new virus to spread from Wuhan to other regions of China [3]. The COVID-19 epidemic was officially designated as a global public health emergency on January 30, 2020. Following that, the WHO selected it as a pandemic on March 11, 2020. COVID-19 had been confirmed in over 160 million people worldwide as of May 13, 2021, and it resulted in over 3 million deaths [4]. The COVID-19 pandemic with exponential infection rates has burdened healthcare systems in all countries around the world [5].

The virus of COVID-19 is discovered frequently in bats and cats and spreads from wild animals to human beings because of its animal-infectious nature and ultimately spread human-to-human. In the past, two kinds of coronaviruses were guilty of serious respiratory diseases and human mortality, namely the Severe Acute Respiratory Syndrome (SARS) and the Middle East Respiratory Syndrome virus (MERS) [6]. The COVID-19 genome has transformed a lot in its short lifespan. According to a study conducted by experts at University College London (UCL), the number of genetic mutations in the COVID-19 virus has reached 198 [7]. A COVID-19 virus mutation analysis research at the University of Glasgow found that these alterations are not identical to other strains of the virus, but that just one strain of the virus is presently circulating [8]. Fever, sore throat, coughing, shortness of breath, headache, and weakness, are some of the most frequent symptoms of COVID-19 [9].

The COVID-19 virus can cause pneumonia in patients. The infection then spreads and makes the patient die due to the COVID-19 virus, which causes lung pneumonia, causing the patient to be unable to breathe and reduces the patient's chances of life. The reverse transcription-polymerase chain reaction (RT-PCR), which operates in a real-time, is the most extensively used approach for identifying COVID-19. According to the WHO, RT-PCR should verify the coronavirus diagnosis as the standard indicator for hospitalization prediction [10]. However, the devices involved are time-consuming and less sensitive to virus detection [11]. Furthermore, earlier studies showed that the vast majority of doctors and nurses caught COVID-19 during saliva sampling using RT-PCR devices [12]. This equipment is also globally limited and requires shipping costs. According to studies, using this RT-PCR equipment to diagnose COVID-19 risks doctors, and nurses to the virus and also is not cost-effective. As a result, to treat and control COVID-19, a quick diagnosis is required [13].

Another approach is using a chest scan for detecting COVID-19 infection [14]. Some chest imaging techniques are computed tomography scans (CT scans) and X-ray images. Fractures, lung infections, pneumonia, and malignancies can all be diagnosed via X-ray images. Organs, bones, and tissues may be seen in greater detail with CT scans. On the other hand, CT scans are not widely available and more expensive than X-ray images. For that reason, currently, X-ray images are generally used in doctors' early stages of diagnosis. X-ray images are a faster, simpler, less expensive, and safer alternative to CT scans [14]. X-ray images are more widely available to the general public than CT scans, particularly in rural and distant regions. After getting a chest X-ray (CXR), the doctor will need to visually diagnose an infection, such as a bacterial, viral, or COVID-19 infection. Visual inspection-based diagnostics are cumbersome, time-consuming, and frequently wrong due to fatigue and the necessity for specialized staff, resulting in poor diagnostic accuracy. There are certain limits to the consistency of CXR images, such as blurring boundaries, overlapping organs, and low contrast. These limitations have a significant influence on the diagnosis of CXR pneumonia [15]. Therefore, in recent studies, automatic detection of viral strains based on chest imaging, such as the COVID-19 virus, has received much attention. The identification of the COVID-19 virus automatically by the computer system is not only speeds up the diagnosis. It also reduces the doctor's workload, allowing for timely treatment and lowers patient mortality.

Several deep-learning-based computational approaches for automatic COVID-19 detection and analysis using X-ray images are currently under development. Deep learning (DL) is a compound of the machine learning methods used to extract and classify pictures automatically. The principal benefit of DL is that it can transform the data from non-linear separable to linear separable through a series of transformations (hidden layers). DL can also find non-linear decision boundaries and simulate non-linear interactions between features. Detection, segmentation, and classification of medical image are some of the most frequent DL applications. Researchers have been able to do basic and in-depth analyses of X-ray images using various deep learning techniques over the past few years [16]. However, from multiple searches, no paper has reviewed deep learning to detect COVID via X-rays. This white paper provides comprehensive information on data sets, methodologies, evaluation indicators, and cutting-edge research in DL in identifying COVID-19 through X-ray images. Lessons learned from the research challenges and the latest research are expected to lead to the improvement of DL models for detecting COVID-19 with better performance, figuring out which models are best suited for use on X-ray datasets. During this pandemic, it can aid in the battle against COVID-19.

The next chapter of this white paper is: Sect. 2 provides basic information about DL. The application of DL for COVID-19 detection via X-ray pictures is discussed in Sect. 3. Next, Sect. 4 presents research challenges and provides recommendations for further research directions. This article ends with a conclusion and future work in Sect. 5.

## 2 Materials and Method

This study offers a comprehensive assessment of the literature on utilizing DL to analyze COVID-19 in CXR images. The goal of this research is to figure out how DL algorithms can be used to detect COVID-19 during this pandemic. To get a list of research that has a high impact and is relevant to the scope of research, research articles are searched in well-known digital libraries, namely Scopus, IEEE Xplorer, Springer, and ScienceDirect. Several selected papers were taken from ArXiv, related to the CXR image dataset. Related articles with high impact are considered in the list of studies. In selecting studies related to the research scope, we applied several inclusion and exclusion criteria. The list of studies used in subsequent research is imported to the library. Then, studies that did not match the criteria for inclusion were eliminated. The most used keywords for the search criteria in this survey paper were ("COVID-19"), ("Deep Learning"), ("Convolution Neural Network"), ("CNN"), (("COVID-19" AND "chest X-ray" AND "Deep Learning"), ("COVID-19" AND "chest X-ray" AND "Deep Learning" AND ("detection" OR "classification")).

From the results of a review of popular research articles published in 2020 and 2021, fifteen articles were reviewed in this paper. From the selected research articles, this paper is further divided into three parts, namely: (1) presenting the working stages of a classification system with DL, (2) making a list of datasets, methodologies, and findings from several selected research articles, (3) presenting research challenges and recommendations for future research directions.

## 3 Result and Discussion

This literature review includes data set collection, application of DL algorithms, and development from findings from previous studies. Discussions and challenges for further study are also underway. This step is helpful for artificial intelligence researchers, particularly those working in DL, who want to research the COVID-19 identification on CXR images. Figure 1 shows the workflow of DL techniques in detecting COVID-19 via X-ray images. Details about each step of the process are described below.

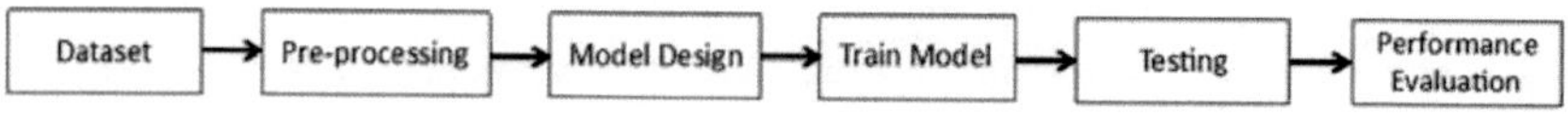


**Fig. 1** General stages of detecting COVID-19 using deep learning

## 3.1 Dataset Collection

In general, the collection of the COVID-19 infection datasets was created by combining and modifying publicly available dataset repositories. Table 1 shows the source of the X-Ray image dataset repositories that researchers widely use for investigating COVID-19 detection. Figure 2 shows four sample images of the COVID-R public dataset [17, 18].

**Table 1** Dataset of X-ray image

| No | Reference | Dataset | Source link |
|---|---|---|---|
| A | [17] | Covid-chestxray | https://github.com/ieee8023/covid-chestxray-dataset |
| B | [18] | COVID-19-radiography-database | https://www.kaggle.com/tawsifurrahman/covid19-radiography-database |
| C | [19] | Chest-X-ray-pneumonia | https://www.kaggle.com/paultimothymooney/chest-xray-pneumonia |
| D | [20] | COVID-19 local hospitals | https://data.mendeley.com/datasets/2fxz4px6d8/4 |
| E | [21] | COVID-19 X-rays | https://www.kaggle.com/andrewmvd/convid19-X-rays |
| F | [22] | COVIDx | https://github.com/lindawangg/COVID-Net |
| G | [23] | Actualmed-COVID-chestxray | https://github.com/agchung/Actualmed-COVID-chestxray-dataset |
| H | [24] | COVID-19-X-ray-10000 | https://www.kaggle.com/nabeelsajid917/covid-19-x-ray-10000-images |
| I | [25] | Kermany | https://data.mendeley.com/datasets/rscbjbr9sj/2 |
| J | [26] | COVID-19-X-ray-dataset-train-test-sets | https://www.kaggle.com/khoongweihao/covid19-xray-dataset-train-test-sets |
| K | [27] | ChestX-ray8 | https://www.cc.nih.gov/drd/summers.html |
| L | [28] | RSNA | https://www.kaggle.com/c/rsnapneumonia-detection-challenge/data |
| M | [29] | COVID-19 | https://www.sirm.org/category/senza-categoria/covid-19/ |

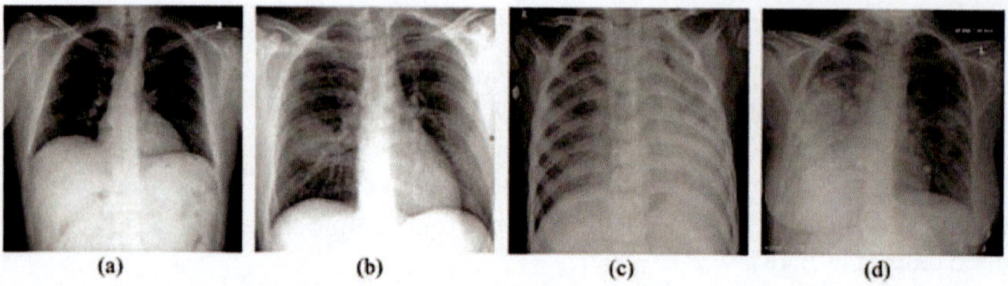

**Fig. 2** Representative of CXR images **a** Normal, **b** COVID-19, **c** Pneumonia-viral, **d** Bacterial pneumonia [17, 18]

A normal chest radiograph or a P-A chest radiograph with normal chest wall size and form, as well as normal trachea, heart, and mediastinum position and appearance is shown in Fig. 2a. No focal opacities, air-fluid levels, hyperlucency, or elevated broncho-vascular symptoms were found. Angles costophrenic and cardio-phrenic are also unrestricted. Figure 2b is a P-A picture of a COVID-19 patient's chest radiograph with hyperlucent lung fields. It suggested that the lungs are hyperinflated due to minor airway blockage. This airway blockage is due to bronchiolitis or bronchitis. Both lung fields had some unequal opacities, indicating bacterial coinfection-induced consolidation. A blunt costophrenic angle indicates a para-pneumonic pleural effusion. Figure 2c displays a non-COVID viral pneumonia X-ray image with diffuse alveolar damage, bilateral diffuse Ground Glass Opacities (GGO), and septal thickening. Figure 2d displays an X-ray of bacterial pneumonia with a focal opacity in the upper lobe of the right lung. This Fig. 2d indicates a consolidation without cavitation, but also the costophrenic and cardio-phrenic angles are free with air-fluid levels are normal.

In the classification and performance evaluation stages, public databases and acquired X-ray images provide diversity and enrichment.

- Dataset A is an open-source collection [17] containing 237 CXR images of COVID-19 patients from Australia, Canada, Germany, Iran, Belgium, Israel, Italy, Taiwan, Korea, Spain, Vietnam, China, Egypt, and the USA on 12 May 2020. A database of patient's chest scans with COVID-19, SARS 1, SARS 2, MERS, and acute respiratory distress syndrome (ARDS) can be found in this open repository.
- Dataset B is an open-source collection [18] comprising 2905 CXR pictures, 219 of which are COVID-19 photos, 1345 of which are viral pneumonia images, and 1341 of which are normal chest images. COVID-19 data is freely available on the Kaggle website and comes from varying sources, including CXR images containing COVID-19 from the Italian Society of Medical and Interventional Radiology COVID1-19 Database (SIRM) and the Novel Corona Virus Dataset 2019 created by Cohen et al. on Github [17], and also several recently published papers. The Kaggle Chest X-Ray Pneumonia dataset [19] included pictures of both viral pneumonia and normal chest.
- Dataset C is an open-source collection [19] with 5848 images of people with pneumonia and normal (healthy) people's CXR scans. CXR number of healthy

images, bacterial pneumonia, viral pneumonia in this data set are 1583, 2772, and 1493, respectively.

- Dataset D is an open-source collection [20] from three different hospitals that the authors compiled from two country in India.
  - 188 pictures were obtained from King George's Medical University (KGMU) in Lucknow, Uttar Pradesh, India. The images consist of 28 COVID-19, 83 abnormal, and 77 normal.
  - 68 pictures of COVID-19 patients were obtained from the Uttar Pradesh University of Medical Sciences, India.
  - 543 X-ray pictures from the Government Medical College in Kota, Rajasthan, India. The images consist of 326 COVID-19, and 217 abnormal.

## 3.2 Preprocessing

One of the most important prerequisites for designing a detection system that produces better results is preprocessing on the input image. The initial processing generally carried out by researchers is in the form of uniformity of the spatial size to the desired size. The image is then transformed from three layer (i.e., red, green, blue) to grayscale for uniformity and normalizing across different data sets. The image is subsequently subjected to min–max normalization to speed up the convergence condition [30]. In several studies, improving image quality is also carried out, one of which is by using the histogram equalization technique.

The imbalanced ratio of the data set's class distribution has a substantial influence on the model's performance when applying DL and classical machine learning approaches to tackle classification difficulties. Data imbalance can affect CNN classification performance [31]. The CNN model performs well when a big amount of training data image is utilized, allowing the computer to learn how to recognize the image more precisely. Augmentation is done to increase the data set, provide resilience to the trained model and minimize the likelihood of overfitting issues. Some of the augmentation methods used in building the model to boost the capability of test images in varied orientations include rotation, shifting of images in affine form, scaling, inverting, increasing brightness, and decreasing brightness.

## 3.3 Model Design

Deep learning (DL) is an application of the core principles of machine learning. This network is referred to as a deep neural network because of the number of hidden layers used by the input and output layers. DL has shown good performance in recent years. It is aided by more powerful computational variables, massive data sets, and techniques for training deeper networks, and all contribute to this [32].

Convolutional Neural Network (CNN) is DL approach that is used to discover and recognize an object in a digital image. CNN has proved to be effective in medical image analysis, for example: X-ray, CT scan, MRI, Ultrasonography, and others. CNN is claimed to be the best model for solving object detection and recognition issues. This approach is widely used because of its uncomplicated structure, flexibility, fewer feature parameters, and low network model complexity, this technique is highly popular. However, like other DL models, CNN has disadvantages, such as the considerable time to train the algorithm. But, this deficiency can be solved with rapid hardware improvement by using Graphical Processing Unit (GPU) technology and high-spec PC. Figure 3 provides an illustration of a CNN architecture in COVID-19 classification.

The convolution stage, which uses a kernel of a specific size, is the first step in the CNN architecture. The number of kernels used is determined by how many features are generated. The following process is the activation function, which in most cases employs the Rectifier Linear Unit's activation function (ReLU). The next stage is the pooling process. This procedure is continued until a sufficiently detailed feature map is created to proceed to a fully connected neural network. The output of a fully connected network is the output class.

In the convolution layer, feature extraction is applied to the image by performing a convolution process between the input image and the filter matrix. Sharpening, smoothing, noise removal, and edge detection are some of the imaging techniques used by the convolution matrix. Images are utilized as input and as a way to extract specific information [33].

The pooling layer aims to decrease the feature matrix's size and preserve important features, thereby reducing computational costs. The pooling layer is also intended to avoid overfitting conditions, namely conditions where the model predicts training data accurately but does not recognize other than training data. Max and average pooling are the most widely used types of pooling approaches. Max pooling means taking the maximum value in a given area while average pooling means taking the average value.

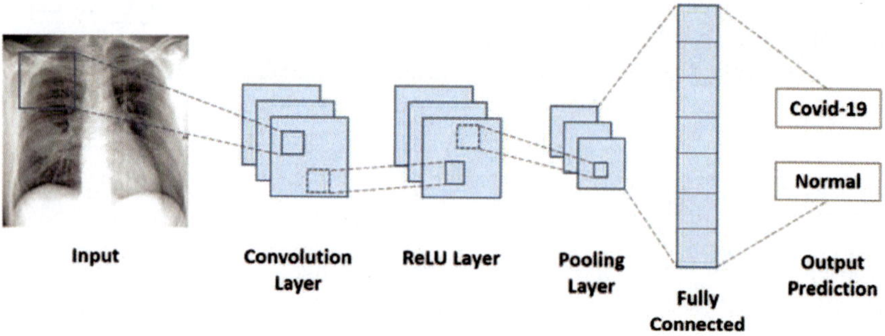


**Fig. 3** Convolutional neural network architecture

A fully connected layer method is used to transfer the output of the smoothing layer to one or more neural layers so that classification predictions are obtained [34].

## 3.4 Model Training and Testing

The training process aims to train the CNN algorithm in recognizing the dataset so that a model is formed based on training. The testing process aims to evaluate the model built on training resistance. At this stage, the model is tested with various images from the training process to test whether the model has performed well in classifying an image.

## 3.5 Performance Evaluation

The metrics used to evaluate the model are accuracy, precision, sensitivity, specificity, and F1 score. To calculate this statistic, a confusion matrix is needed, which is shown in Fig. 4. True positive (TP) is defined as positive predicted to be positive. True negative (TN) is defined as negative that is predicted to be negative. While false negative (FN) is the opposite of false positive (FP), where FN is positive predicted to be negative, and FP is negative predicted to be positive [33].

The variables TP, TN, FN, and FP can be used to compute statistics such as accuracy, precision, recall or sensitivity, specificity, and F1 score. Accuracy is defined as the ratio between the number of rightly predicted data and the total amount of data. Accuracy is used as a parameter of how accurately a model performs classification. Precision describes the ratio of TP to the total data predicted to be positive. In other words, precision describes how accurately a model predicts positive events in a series of predictive activities. While the F1 score is the average of harmonics between precision and memory. The calculations in Eqs. (1–5) are for accuracy, precision, recall or sensitivity, specificity, and F1 score [35].

$$\text{Accuracy} = \frac{\text{TP} + \text{TN}}{\text{TP} + \text{TN} + \text{FP} + \text{FN}} \tag{1}$$

| | | Prediction | |
|---|---|---|---|
| | | Positive (P) | Negative (N) |
| Actual | Positive (P) | TP | FP |
| | Negative (N) | FN | TN |

**Fig. 4** Confusion matrix

$$\text{Precision} = \frac{\text{TP}}{\text{TP} + \text{FP}} \quad (2)$$

$$\text{Recall} = \frac{\text{TP}}{\text{TP} + \text{FN}} \quad (3)$$

$$\text{Specitifity} = \frac{\text{TN}}{\text{TN} + \text{FP}} \quad (4)$$

$$\text{F1-score} = \frac{2 \times \text{precision} \times \text{recall}}{\text{precision} + \text{recall}} \quad (5)$$

In computer science, artificial intelligence refers to the intelligence displayed by machines. The traditional machine learning methods require hand-designed functions extracted from input, while DL methods learn these functions directly from the data. CNN is the most dependable DL model among the several available. Pneumonia is one of the fatal lung diseases. CXR images are read by a radiologist and used to diagnose pneumonia. Human-assisted diagnosis has constraints, such as availability of experts, cost, etc. [35].

Table 2 summarizes the findings of a review of numerous studies that used a DL approach to detect COVID-19. Apostolopoulos et al. [36] assessed five CNN transfer learning architectures (i.e., VGG19, Xception, Inception, Inception ResNet v2, MobileNet v2) for coronavirus disease identification. The study included X-ray images of people with common bacterial pneumonia, COVID-19 disease, and healthy people without infection. The MobileNet v2 model is most effective in differentiating cases of COVID-19 from viral and bacterial pneumonia cases. The detection of numerous abnormalities in a small collection of medical imaging data is an attainable goal for transfer learning. Some drawbacks of this work are that fewer images are used for COVID-19 patients. Subsequently, several cases considered to be pneumonia symptoms were taken from old medical records, so there was no match between the descriptions and images gathered from COVID-19 patients.

Ucar et al. [37] presented a deep Bayes-SqueezeNet decision system based on radiographs for the diagnosis of COVID-19. SqueezeNet includes a lightweight network design that is optimized for COVID-19 diagnosis, as well as Bayesian optimization enhancements.

Fine-tuned hyper-parameters and large data sets enable the proposed network to outperform existing network invents and achieve greater COVID-19 diagnosis accuracy. This research includes a DL method that is easy to implement and has an accuracy of 98.3% (on the classification of three classes, namely: normal, pneumonia, and Covid cases), as well as 100% accuracy for the single recognition of COVID-19 (in addition to others). In further work, this model could be designed to act cellularly, which is of interest to healthcare professionals for the diagnosis of COVID-19.

In the study proposed by Ozturk et al. [38], you only look once (YOLO) with the DarkNet classification model was used for the automatic detection of COVID-19 using raw chest radiographs. There are 17 convolutional layers in total, with distinct filtering on each layer. The proposed model provides a precise diagnosis for binary

**Table 2** DL application survey for COVID-19 identification via CXR images

| Reference | Author and year | Technique | Dataset | Number of class | Number of images | Performance |
|---|---|---|---|---|---|---|
| [36] | Apostolopoulos et al., (2020) | MobileNet v2 | A, E, I | 2 | COVID-19 (224), Normal (504) | Accuracy = 96.78 |
| | | | | 3 | Total = 1442. COVID-19 (224), Normal (504), Pneumonia (400 bacteria & 314 viral) | Accuracy = 94.72, Sensitivity = 98.66, Specificity = 96.46 |
| [37] | Ucar et al., (2020) | COVIDiagnosis-Net (Deep Bayes-SqueezeNet) | F | 3 | Total = 5310. COVID-19 (66), Normal (1349), Pneumonia (3895) | Accuracy = 98.3, Specificity = 99.1, F1-score = 98.3 |
| [38] | Ozturk et al., (2020) | DarkcovidNet | A | 2 | 125 COVID-19 (+), No Findings (500) | Accuracy = 98.08 |
| | | | | 3 | 125 COVID-19 (+), Pneumonia (500), No Findings (500) | Accuracy = 87.02 |
| [39] | Khan et al., (2020) | CoroNet | A, C | 2 | COVID-19 (284), Normal (310) | Accuracy = 99, Sensitivity = 99.3, Specificity = 98.6, Precision = 98.3, F1-score = 99 |

(continued)

**Table 2** (continued)

| Reference | Author and year | Technique | Dataset | Number of class | Number of images | Performance |
|---|---|---|---|---|---|---|
| | | | | 3 | COVID-19 (284), Normal (310), Pneumonia | Accuracy = 95, Sensitivity = 96.9, Specificity = 97.5, Precision = 95, F1-score = 95 |
| | | | | 4 | COVID-19 (284), Normal (310), Pneumonia viral (327), Pneumonia bacterial (330) | Accuracy = 89.6, Sensitivity = 89.92, Specificity = 96.4, Precision = 90, F1-score = 89.8 |
| [40] | Toraman et al., (2020) | Convolutional CapsNat | A, K | 2 | COVID-19 (1050), No-Findings (1050) | Accuracy = 97.24 |
| | | | | 3 | COVID-19 (1050), No-Findings (1050), Pneumonia (1050) | Accuracy = 84.22 |
| [41] | Shibly et al., (2020) | Faster R-CNN | A, F, L | 2 | Total = 13,800. COVID-19 (183), non-COVID (13,617) | Accuracy = 97.36, Sensitivity = 97.65, Precision = 99.28 |
| [42] | Afshar et al., (2020) | COVID-CAPS | K | 2 | (+) COVID-19, (-) COVID-19 | Accuracy = 98.3, Sensitivity = 80, Specificity = 98.6 |
| [43] | Ouchicha et al., (2020) | CVDNet | B | 2 | COVID (219), non COVID | Accuracy = 97.2 |

(continued)

**Table 2** (continued)

| Reference | Author and year | Technique | Dataset | Number of class | Number of images | Performance |
|---|---|---|---|---|---|---|
| | | | | 3 | COVID-19 (219), Normal (1341), Viral Pneumonia (1345) | Accuracy = 96.69, Sensitivity = 96.84, Precision = 96.72, F1-score = 96.68 |
| [44] | Abbas et al., (2020) | DeTraC | A | 3 | Normal (80), COVID-19 (105), SARS (11) | Accuracy = 93.1, Sensitivity = 100, Specificity = 85.18 |
| [45] | Goel et al., (2020) | OptCoNet | B | 3 | COVID-19 (219), Normal (1341), Pneumonia (1345) | Accuracy = 97.78, Sensitivity = 97.75, Specificity = 96.25, Precision = 92.88, F1-score = 95.25 |
| [46] | Gupta et al., (2020) | InstaCovNet-19 | A, B | 3 | COVID-19 (361), Normal (365), Pneumonia (362) | Accuracy = 99.08, Sensitivity = 99.3, Precision = 99 F1-score = 99 |
| | | | | 2 | COVID, non COVID | Accuracy = 99.52 |
| [47] | Hussain et al., (2020) | CoroDet | A, B, G, H, J | 2 | COVID-19 (500), Normal (800) | Accuracy = 99.1 |

(continued)

**Table 2** (continued)

| Reference | Author and year | Technique | Dataset | Number of class | Number of images | Performance |
|---|---|---|---|---|---|---|
| | | | | 3 | COVID-19 (500), Normal (800), Pneumonia bacterial (800) | Accuracy = 94.2 |
| | | | | 4 | COVID-19 (500), Normal (800), Pneumonia viral (400), Pneumonia bacterial (400) | Accuracy = 91.2 |
| [34] | Sheykhivand et al., (2021) | Inception V4, LSTM, GAN | A, B, C, E | 4 | COVID-19 (371), Normal (2923), Pneumonia viral (2840), Pneumonia bacterial (2778) | Accuracy = 99.5, Sensitivity = 100, Specificity = 99.02 |
| [48] | Rajpal et al., (2021) | Resnet + NN | A, B, G | 3 | COVID-19, Normal, Pneumonia (viral&bacterial) | Accuracy = 97.4 ± 2, Sensitivity = 98.7 ± 05 |
| [49] | Nigam et al., (2021) | EfficientNet | Private | 3 | COVID-19 (795), Normal (795), Others (711) | Accuracy = 93.48 |

category (COVID versus No Finding) and multiclass categorization (COVID versus No Finding versus pneumonia). The accuracy of binary and multiclass categorization is 98.08% and 87.02%, respectively. The radiologists review the model's performance and are ready to be evaluated with a more extensive database. Other breast-related disorders, such as TB and pneumonia, can be diagnosed using the model. The study's utilization of COVID-19 X-ray pictures is limited, which is a restriction. In further work, the model can be made more accurate and robust by utilizing additional similar images from nearby hospitals.

Khan et al. [39] proposed CoroNet, a Deep CNN model that uses CXR images to diagnose COVID-19 infection. The suggested model is built on the Xception architecture, which has been end-to-end trained using ImageNet datasets. The suggested model achieves an overall accuracy of 89.6%, with precision and recall rates for COVID-19 instances of 93% and 98.2% in case 4 classes, respectively (COVID versus bacterial pneumonia vs viral pneumonia vs normal). A CoroNet is less computationally intensive and shows promise on small data sets. However, CoroNet still requires study and clinical testing. Then the performance of specificity and precision is still low for bacterial pneumonia.

To detect COVID-19 disease using CXR images, Toraman et al. [40] proposed Convolutional CapsNet. Using two classifications (COVID-19 and No-Findings) and multiclass classification (COVID-19 and No-Findings and pneumonia), the proposed method intends to give a speedy and reliable diagnosis of COVID-19 disease. For binary and multiclass categories, the suggested technique achieves 97.24% and 84.22% accuracy, respectively. The results show that the capsule network can beneficially classify even within a limited data set. However, while processing large images, the suggested capsule network necessitates a lot of hardware resources, resulting in a longer processing time. The size of the input image must be the same in this model for the capsule network to classify it. As a result of differences in image size in different datasets, preprocessing is required before images are entered into the model. Models can be trained with larger data sets for more advanced work, resulting in success rates that can aid doctors in diagnosing coronavirus disease. The training process with large data sets is critical for assessing the system's validity and reliability.

Shiby et al. [41] proposed a Faster Region with CNN (Faster R-CNN) framework based on the VGG-16 network to detect COVID-19 infection on a radiographic basis. Obtaining 97.36% accuracy, 97.65% sensitivity, and 99.28% precision, this autonomous system can perform binary classification. However, the picture of cases infected with COVID-19 is too small, and the class is unbalanced. Then the model only tests the performance of two categories, namely COVID and non-COVID.

Afshar et al. [42] proposed COVID-CAPS, an alternative system that remains on Capsule Networks that can process tiny data sets. COVID-CAPS offers a substantially smaller number of parameters that can be trained and achieves 95.7% accuracy, 90% sensitivity, 95.8% specificity, and 0.97 area under the curve (AUC). COVID-CAPS has a good performance despite having a small number of trainable parameters. Normal cases accounted for 54% of false positives, while bacterial and non-COVID cases only contributed for 27% and 19% of false positives, respectively. The sensitivity of the resulting model is lower than the prior art. The model becomes inefficient, because the pass is too small, so a lot of redundant data.

Ouchicha et al. [43] proposed CVDNet, a Deep CNN model for classifying three classes, i.e., normal, COVID-19, and pneumonia infections using CXR images. The suggested architecture uses a residual neural network and comprises two parallel layers with different kernel sizes to capture global and local and input features. Experimental results show that this CVDNet has promising classification performance on small data sets. CVDNet classification efficiency was determined using k-fold cross-validation. CVDNet detected COVID-19 with an average accuracy of 97.20% and classified three classes (COVID-19, normal and viral pneumonia) with an average accuracy of 96.69%. Research development by developing this CVDNet to detect cases of COVID-19 from other lung diseases. Furthermore, the suggested model must be validated by utilizing additional images from various hospitals. The CVDNet model's performance should be evaluated while processing CT scan images to identify COVID-19 and when compared to results obtained with CVDNet trained on X-ray images.

For the classification of COVID-19 CXR images, Abbas et al. [44] introduced a deep CNN called Decompose, Transfer, and Compose (DeTraC). DeTraC can process irregularities in image data sets by inspecting class boundaries with the class decomposition mechanism. The experimental results demonstrate DeTraC's ability to detect COVID-19 cases using a comprehensive picture data set collected from hospitals all over the world. DeTraC detected COVID-19 X-ray images of normal and SARS with high accuracy of 93.1% (with a sensitivity of 100%). Continuing work with validation methods with larger datasets and adding components that can improve model performance. To increase efficiency, model trimming, quantization and deployment can be performed on wearable devices.

To classify three classes, i.e., normal, COVID-19, and pneumonia patients based on CXR images, Goel et al. [45] proposed the OptCoNet architecture. An optimized CNN model, this OptCoNet consists of feature extraction and an optimized classification component. All test images will be resized to $224 \times 224$ pixels during the data magnification phase. The CNN hyperparameter is adjusted using Gray Wolf Optimizer (GWO) algorithm to avoid overfitting and collapse mode issues and provide the best performance outcomes on X-ray images. According to the model performance evaluation, the accuracy, sensitivity, specificity, precision, and F1 were 97.78%, 97.75%, 96.25%, 92.88%, and 95.25%, respectively. The suggested CNN model might help in the automated screening of COVID-19 patients and minimize the strain on the healthcare framework. However, the position orientation of the input image is not encoded by the OptCoNet model. Because this is one of the model's weaknesses, numerous preprocessing procedures are required. Moreover, spatially OptCoNet not invariant to the input image. Eventually, GWO has several controller parameters that must be carefully selected when applied to problems with a very large number of functions and parameters.

An integrated nested deep convolution network, InstaCovNet-19, was suggested by Gupta et al. [46]. To compensate for the limited amount of training data, the recommended model uses various trained models, including Xception, InceptionV3, ResNet101, NASNet, and MobileNet. The suggested model identifies COVID-19 and pneumonia by detecting anomalies induced by the disease on infected people's CXR images. The suggested model achieves 99.08% accuracy in the three-class categorization (COVID-19, pneumonia, normal) and 99.53% accuracy in the two-class categorization (COVID, NON-COVID). In future COVID-19 detection research, DL techniques could be used to detect other symptoms of COVID-19, which causes anomalies in human organs. According to a COVID-19 specialist or expert, various features such as age, gender, patient history, geolocation data, and genetics can increase the effectiveness of computer-aided diagnosis.

Hussein et al. [47] proposed the CNN 'CoroDet' model using chest radiographs and CT scan images for the automatic detection of COVID-19. CoroDet has been developed as an accurate diagnosis for two class classifications (COVID and Normal), three class classifications (Normal, COVID, and non-COVID pneumonia), and four class classifications (Normal, COVID, non-COVID viral pneumonia, and non-COVID bacteria pneumonia). The classification accuracy for two class is 99.1%, for three class is 94.2%, and for four class is 91.2%. This study also prepares the largest data set for the evaluation of the classification algorithm. Further research overcomes hardware limitations that allow using a larger set of images to train the suggested CoroDet model. When the output is not centered on zero, a vanishing gradient problem occurs. Therefore, gradient updates diverge too much in the other direction, making optimization more difficult.

Sheykhivand et al. [34] introduced a deep neural network for the automatic identification of pneumonia (including COVID-19). The proposed architecture uses Generative Adversarial Networks (GANs) in collaboration with a combination of deep transfer learning and LSTM networks to classify pneumonia without the requirement for feature extraction or selection. Healthy, viral, bacterial, and COVID-19 classes are used to differentiate between 2 and 4 classes in 7 diverse and functional scenarios using CXR pictures. The experimental study reveals that the model achieves better than 90% accuracy in all but one scenario and 99% accuracy in distinguishing COVID-19 from the healthy group. In comparison to existing deep transfer learning systems, the suggested network performance shows promise in terms of accuracy, precision, sensitivity, and specificity. Nevertheless, this network has not proven very efficient in distinguishing other cases of pneumonia, including bacteria from viral samples. Then the computational complexity is moderate, not yet the lowest compared to other networks. Due to the limitations of the COVID-19 sample, clinical validation studies using larger datasets with larger COVID-19 samples are required to assess the recommended network performance.

Rajpal et al. [48] proposed a new classification framework containing a carefully selected feature set obtained from deep CNNs. The framework is divided into three modules, the first of which creates 2048 functions using ResNet-50-based transfer learning. The second module identifies 252 carefully selected functions using frequency and texture domain functions, which are then reduced to a set of 16 functions using PCA and feed-forward neural networks. In classification, the combined feature set is transferred to the dense layer, followed by the softmax layer of the third module. The use of self-selected functions through transfer learning with ResNet50 has increased the learning capabilities of the model. For the effectiveness of the suggested model, tenfold cross-validation was used. For the COVID-19, normal, and pneumonia classes, the model had on the whole classification accuracy of 0.974 $\pm$ 0.02, sensitivity of 0.987 $\pm$ 0.05, 0.963 $\pm$ 0.05, and 0.973 $\pm$ 0.04 with 95% confidence intervals, respectively. Further research could be done to determine the effect of segmentation on the localization of the COVID 19-affected lung area. Furthermore, clinical data such as symptoms, age, and patient medical history can be combined to improve COVID-19 disease detection.

Nigam et al. [49] evaluated the architectures of VGG16, DenseNet121, Xception, NASNet, and EfficientNet to classify three types of patients: COVID-19 positive patients, normal patients, and others. The EfficientNet model has the best recognition accuracy, 93.48%. However, system performance can be improved by experimenting with other DL models and expanding the data set. From the literature review described above, CNN models in DL have been developed to detect COVID-19 on X-ray images.

Yan and Chen [50] introduced various convolutional neural networks to generate composite feature maps. The experimental results display that the accuracy rate is 89% for the model with one feature map. As for the feature map stitched from four convolutional neural networks, the accuracy rate is 91%.

Arya et al. [51] analyzed the performance of VGG19 from X-ray images of the lungs to diagnose COVID-19. There are two test scenarios; (1) experiments for three-class datasets (normal, COVID-19, and viral pneumonia), (2) experiments for four-class datasets (normal, COVID-19, viral pneumonia, and bacterial pneumonia). The accuracy of VGG19 for 3 classes and 4 classes is 98.2% and 94.4%, respectively.

Aulia et al. [52] developed the DL Convolutional Neural Network (CNN) for the classification of lung diseases from CXR images. The datasets were collected for three class categories, namely normal, tuberculosis, COVID-19. The experimental results obtained an accuracy of 88.37% from 208 CXR datasets.

## 4 Challenges

At the start of the pandemic, many countries, including China, had a large number of false-negative cases due to a lack of test kits and a shortage of skilled lab technicians. Consequently, clinicians are encouraged to base their choices primarily on the results of CXR and CT scans [53]. In countries without testing equipment, CT and X-ray images are commonly used to identify COVID-19. The combination of clinical imaging findings and laboratory results, according to researchers, may aid in the initial diagnosis of COVID-19 [54]. AI technologies, especially DL, appear to offer viable solutions to many of today's issues. So far, DL approaches have yielded fairly satisfactory results. However, there are still many improvements and new areas where DL can be done in COVID-19 research. This section reviews the problems these systems face and any suggestions or ways to manage them.

- New approaches to dealing with small data sets must be investigated.
- To diagnose COVID-19, artificial intelligence algorithms that combine chest imaging with clinical symptoms, history of exposure, and laboratory tests are required.
- One problem with implementing DL algorithms is that large amounts of data are required to provide accurate results. DL algorithms can easily overfit. Which the single platform used for researchers should be provided by the community to share data at an early stage. It is also critical to establish the criteria for data collection, such as data format, collection data type, labeling, and code. This is particularly the problem with hospitals not easily distributing data.
- The type and structure of data gathered might vary greatly from hospitals and institutions to different data collection protocols. Building a data set requires adopting a data fusion approach. As for drawing a line for future research, it is necessary to explore different data fusion methods.
- Commonly, COVID-19 tests based on the RT-PCR method are less accurate. Blood and urine tests and other data can show disease-like symptoms including fever, muscle aches, loss of smell, as well as CT and X-ray images. For more accurate testing, it is recommended to develop an ensemble method in which each type of identification data is entered in different tests. This idea has not been used in the literature.
- Datasets continue to grow rapidly in almost all regions. In some cases, new data and findings appear daily that contradict previous data. In this case, incremental learning can be used.
- To improve scan quality and reduce radiation dose to the patient, an artificial intelligence technique can be used in the image acquisition process. This is important since the number of patients who require X-ray imaging in hospitals is increasing, enhancing the danger of exposure. For example, one approach is to match the number of X-ray images applied to the patient with the patient's body parameters, such as fat or muscle and body circumference.
- Many of the data set collected are affected by noise, where the type of noise varies from application to application. For example, X-ray images are usually subject to noise in the form of imaging device noise or noise from recording labeling when processing images. Sound signals collected from the patient, such as coughing, can cause noise, thus significantly impacting the data obtained for the number of cases. Since many patients tend to be asymptomatic, not all of them are recognized, so reported issues underestimate the actual statistics. As a result of the inaccuracy of COVID-19 testing methodologies, many cases are misclassified. To construct successful artificial intelligence algorithms, more research is required in the field of noise reduction.
- Optimization problems are common problems in machine learning. Existing approaches using gradient methods tend to get stuck in the local optima. Because global search algorithms are less likely to become stuck in local optimization, they can be helpful [55]. As future work, we recommend that you train this engine using a global search algorithm when addressing issues related to COVID-19.

- DL algorithms are used in all of the approaches discussed in this article, and they cannot account for the majority of the recommended technical efforts. An important part that needs explanation is whether the planned system can provide information and insight on how decisions are reached by the algorithm [56], especially in diagnosing artificial intelligence systems to help practitioners. Since the system functions as a consultant, understanding why the artificial intelligence algorithm accepts a particular decision or diagnosis is important in providing the final decision-maker.
- Bridging the gap between research and impact is a significant challenge. There is a lot of research and new ideas on the development of new artificial intelligence systems, but seeing them implemented in the real world is another matter. Close collaboration between researchers and practitioners is required.

While there is a lot of exciting work in applying artificial intelligence to dealing with the challenges posed by the pandemic, there is still a lot to explore. This pandemic has presented an opportunity for artificial intelligence to demonstrate its usefulness in unprecedented real-world situations. If artificial intelligence in solving fundamental problems is determined successful, it will get more social acceptability.

## 5 Conclusion

This publication already gives review of Deep learning (DL) use to identify COVID-19 in X-ray images, future research fields, research challenges and recommendations. The therapeutic of artificial intelligence application, especially DL, in the diagnosis of COVID-19 appears promising, but more research is required. Significant advances in deep CNN for medical image classification have been made thanks to the availability of large-scale annotated picture datasets. CNNs enable the direct learning features of local image from data with a highly representative and hierarchical order. However, the most difficult obstacle in addressing COVID-19 actual cases from X-ray images is because of the irregularities in the continued annotated data. DL is used to interpret radiological images, allowing for faster and more accurate diagnosis while also optimizing the radiologist's workflow. Despite its low sensitivity in comparison to CT, efforts to improve X-ray diagnostic outcomes are of particular interest because they are the most popular and commonly utilized imaging method. Its use makes it possible to monitor disease progression, provide objective assessments based on quantitative information, reduce subjectivity and variability and enable resource optimization due to its potential ability to predict the length of hospital stay. When used as a supplement to clinical practice and in conjunction with other diagnostic procedures, it can assist improve COVID-19 infection management efficiency. Further work needs to be done to develop research on COVID-19 detection from patients in various countries and various variants of COVID-19, such as alpha, beta, gamma, delta, lambda, and kappa. Then, it is necessary to develop research in the form of a COVID-19 detection application via mobile devices.

## References

1. Huang C, Wang Y, Li X, Ren L, Zhao J, Hu Y, Cao B (2020) Clinical features of patients infected with 2019 novel coronavirus in Wuhan, China. The Lancet 395(10223):497–506
2. World Health Organization (2020) Pneumonia of unknown cause–China. Emergencies preparedness. Response, Disease Outbreak News, World Health Organization (WHO)
3. Wu Z, McGoogan JM (2020) Characteristics of and important lessons from the coronavirus disease 2019 (COVID-19) outbreak in China: summary of a report of 72 314 cases from the Chinese center for disease control and prevention. JAMA 323(13):1239–1242
4. World Health Organization: coronavirus (COVID-19) data. https://www.who.int/data#reports. (Accessed May. 14, 2021)
5. World Health Organization, "WHO updates on COVID-19," Available: https://www.who.int/emergencies/diseases/novel-coronavirus-2019/events-as-they-happen. (Accessed September. 26, 2021)
6. Kong W, Agarwal PP (2020) Chest imaging appearance of COVID-19 infection. Radiology 2(1)
7. van Dorp L, Acman M, Richard D, Shaw LP, Ford CE, Ormond L, Pang CJJ, Tan CC, Boshier FA, Ortiz AT (2020) Emergence of genomic diversity and recurrent mutations in SARS-CoV-2. Infect, Genet Evol 83:104351
8. MacLean OA, Orton RJ, Singer JB, Robertson DL (2020) No evidence for distinct types in the evolution of SARS-CoV-2. Virus Evol 6(1):veaa034
9. Singhal T (2020) A review of coronavirus disease-2019 (COVID-19). Indian J Pediatr 87(4):281–286
10. Corman V, Bleicker T, Brünink S, Drosten C, Zambon M. Diagnostic detection of 2019-nCoV by real-time RT-PCR. World Health Organization
11. Yan G, Lee CK, Lam LT, Yan B, Chua YX, Lim AY, Phang KF, Kew GS, Teng H, Ngai CH, Lin L (2020) Covert COVID-19 and false-positive dengue serology in Singapore. Lancet Infect Dis 20(5):536
12. Bai HX, Hsieh B, Xiong Z, Halsey K, Choi JW, Tran TML, Pan I, Shi LB, Wang DC, Mei J, Jiang XL (2020) Performance of radiologists in differentiating COVID-19 from non-COVID-19 viral pneumonia at chest CT. Radiology 296(2):E46–E54
13. Esposito A, Palmisano A, Scotti GM, Morelli MJ, Vignale D, De Cobelli F, Tonon G, Tacchetti C (2020) Why is chest CT important for early diagnosis of COVID-19? Prevalence Matters. medRxiv
14. Ai T, Yang Z, Hou H, Zhan C, Chen C, Lv W, Tao Q, Sun Z, Xia L (2020) Correlation of chest CT and RT-PCR testing for coronavirus disease 2019 (COVID-19) in China: a report of 1014 cases. Radiology 296(2):E32–E40
15. Wu H, Xie P, Zhang H, Li D, Cheng M (2020) Predict pneumonia with chest X-ray images based on convolutional deep neural learning networks. J Intell Fuzzy Syst, (Preprint) 1–15. https://doi.org/10.3233/jifs-191438
16. Zhang Z, Cui P, Zhu W (2020) Deep learning on graphs: a survey. IEEE Trans Knowl Data Eng
17. Cohen JP, Morrison P, Dao L, Roth K, Duong TQ, Ghassemi M (2020) COVID-19 image data collection: prospective predictions are the future. arXiv preprint arXiv:2006.11988
18. Chest X-Ray Images (Pneumonia). https://www.kaggle.com/paultimothymooney/chest-xraypneumonia
19. COVID-19 local hospitals datasets. https://doi.org/10.17632/4n66brtp4j.1 (Mendeley database)
20. Rahman T, Chowdhury MEH, Khandakar A, Mazhar R, Kadir MA, Mahbub ZB, Islam KR, Khan MS, Iqbal A, Al-Emadi N, Ibne Reaz MB (2020) COVID-19 chest radiography database. [Online] Available: https://www.kaggle.com/tawsifurrahman/covid19-radiography-database
21. Kaggle. https://www.kaggle.com/andrewmvd/convid19-X-rays
22. Wang L, Wong A (2020) COVID-net: a tailored deep convolutional neural network design for detection of COVID-19 cases from chest radiography images. ArXiv 2200309871

23. Chung AG (2020) GitHub—agchung/actualmed-COVID-chestxray-dataset: actualmed COVID-19 chest X-ray dataset initiative. https://github.com/agchung/Actualmed-COVID-chestxray-dataset
24. Sajid N (2020) COVID-19 patients lungs x ray images 10000, [Online]. Available: https://www.kaggle.com/nabeelsajid917/covid-19-x-ray-10000-images
25. Kermany D, Zhang K, Goldbaum M (2018) Labeled optical coherence tomography (OCT) and chest X-ray images for classification. Mendeley Data V2. https://doi.org/10.17632/rscbjbr9sj.2
26. Khoong WH (2020) COVID-19 x-ray dataset (train & test sets) with COVID-19CNN pneumonia detector. [Online]. Available: https://www.kaggle.com/khoongweihao/covid19-xray-dataset-train-test-sets
27. Wang X, Peng Y, Lu L, Lu Z, Bagheri M, Summers RM (2017) ChestX-ray8: hospital scale chest X-ray database and benchmarks on weakly-supervised classification and localization of common thorax diseases. In: Proceedings of conference on computer vision and pattern recognition. pp 2097–2106. https://doi.org/10.1109/CVPR.2017.369
28. Radiological Society of North America: RSNA pneumonia detection challenge (2019). https://www.kaggle.com/c/rsnapneumonia-detection-challenge/data
29. Societa Italiana di Radiologia Medical Interventistica: COVID-19 database, (2020). [Online]. Available: https://www.sirm.org/category/senza-categoria/covid-19/
30. Jain A, Nandakumar K, Ross A (2005) Score normalization in multimodal biometric systems. Pattern Recogn 38(12):2270–2285
31. Buda M, Maki A, Mazurowski MA (2018) A systematic study of the class imbalance problem in convolutional neural networks. Neural Netw 106:249–259. https://doi.org/10.1016/j.neunet.2018.07.011
32. Goodfellow I, Bengio Y, Courville A, Bengio Y (2016) Deep learning 1(2). MIT press, Cambridge
33. Alzubaidi L, Zhang J, Humaidi AJ, Al-Dujaili A, Duan Y, Al-Shamma O, Santamaría J, Fadhel MA, Al-Amidie M, Farhan L (2021) Review of deep learning: concepts, CNN architectures, challenges, applications, future directions. J big Data 8(1):1–74
34. Sheykhivand S, Mousavi Z, Mojtahedi S, Rezaii TY, Farzamnia A, Meshgini S, Saad I (2021) Developing an efficient deep neural network for automatic detection of COVID-19 using chest X-ray images. Alex Eng J 60(3):2885–2903
35. Labhane G, Pansare R, Maheshwari S, Tiwari R, Shukla A (2020) Detection of pediatric pneumonia from chest X-ray images using CNN and transfer learning. In: 2020 3rd international conference on emerging technologies in computer engineering: machine learning and internet of things (ICETCE). pp 85–92. IEEE
36. Apostolopoulos ID, Mpesiana TA (2020) COVID-19: automatic detection from x-ray images utilizing transfer learning with convolutional neural networks. Phys Eng Sci Med 43(2):635–640
37. Ucar F, Korkmaz D (2020) COVIDiagnosis-net: deep bayes-SqueezeNet based diagnosis of the coronavirus disease 2019 (COVID-19) from X-ray images. Med Hypotheses 140:109761
38. Ozturk T, Talo M, Yildirim EA, Baloglu UB, Yildirim O, Acharya UR (2020) Automated detection of COVID-19 cases using deep neural networks with X-ray images. Comput Biol Med 121:103792
39. Khan AI, Shah JL, Bhat MM (2020) CoroNet: a deep neural network for detection and diagnosis of COVID-19 from chest x-ray images. Comput Methods Programs Biomed 196:105581
40. Toraman S, Alakus TB, Turkoglu I (2020) Convolutional capsnet: a novel artificial neural network approach to detect COVID-19 disease from X-ray images using capsule networks. Chaos, Solitons Fractals 140:110122
41. Shibly KH, Dey SK, Islam MTU, Rahman MM (2020) COVID faster R–CNN: a novel framework to diagnose novel coronavirus disease (COVID-19) in X-ray images. Inf Med Unlocked 20:100405
42. Afshar P, Heidarian S, Naderkhani F, Oikonomou A, Plataniotis KN, Mohammadi A (2020) Covid-caps: a capsule network-based framework for identification of COVID-19 cases from x-ray images. Pattern Recogn Lett 138:638–643

43. Ouchicha C, Ammor O, Meknassi M (2020) CVDNet: a novel deep learning architecture for detection of coronavirus (COVID-19) from chest x-ray images. Chaos, Solitons Fractals 140:110245
44. Abbas A, Abdelsamea MM, Gaber MM (2020) Classification of COVID-19 in chest X-ray images using DeTraC deep convolutional neural network. Appl Intell 1–11
45. Goel T, Murugan R, Mirjalili S, Chakrabartty DK (2020) OptCoNet: an optimized convolutional neural network for an automatic diagnosis of COVID-19. Appl Intell 1–16
46. Gupta A, Gupta S, Katarya R (2021) Instacovnet-19: a deep learning classification model for the detection of COVID-19 patients using chest x-ray. Appl Soft Comput 99:106859
47. Hussain E, Hasan M, Rahman MA, Lee I, Tamanna T, Parvez MZ (2021) CoroDet: a deep learning based classification for COVID-19 detection using chest X-ray images. Chaos, Solitons Fractals 142:110495
48. Rajpal S, Lakhyani N, Singh AK, Kohli R, Kumar N (2021) Using handpicked features in conjunction with ResNet-50 for improved detection of COVID-19 from chest X-ray images. Chaos, Solitons Fractals 145:110749
49. Nigam B, Nigam A, Jain R, Dodia S, Arora N, Annappa B (2021) COVID-19: automatic detection from X-ray images by utilizing deep learning methods. Expert Syst Appl 114883
50. Yan S, Chen B (2021) Coronavirus disease (COVID-19) X-ray film classification based on convolutional neural network. In: Artificial intelligence in China. Lecture notes in electrical engineering vol 653. Springer, Singapore pp 508–515. https://doi.org/10.1007/978-981-15-8599-9_58
51. Arya M, Sehgal A, Agrawal R (2021) Performance analysis of deep transfer learning for manifestation of COVID-19 using chest X-ray. In: Advances in smart communication and imaging systems. Lecture notes in electrical engineering vol 721. Springer, Singapore pp 117–130. https://doi.org/10.1007/978-981-15-9938-5_13
52. Aulia S, Hadiyoso S, Mengko TL, Suksmono AB (2021) COVID-19 and tuberculosis classification based on chest X-ray using convolutional neural network. In: Proceedings of the 1st international conference on electronics, biomedical engineering, and health informatics. Lecture notes in electrical engineering vol 746. Springer, Singapore pp 407–420. https://doi.org/10.1007/978-981-33-6926-9_35
53. Long C, Xu H, Shen Q, Zhang X, Fan B, Wang C, Zeng B, Li Z, Li X, Li H (2020) Diagnosis of the coronavirus disease (COVID-19): rRT-PCR or CT?. Eur J Radiol 126:108961
54. Shi H, Han X, Jiang N, Cao Y, Alwalid O, Gu J, Fan Y, Zheng C (2020) Radiological findings from 81 patients with COVID-19 pneumonia in Wuhan, China: a descriptive study. Lancet Infect Dis 24(4):425–434
55. Tayarani MH (2020) Applications of artificial intelligence in battling against COVID-19: a literature review. Chaos, Solitons Fractals 110338
56. Arrieta AB, Díaz-Rodríguez N, Del Ser J, Bennetot A, Tabik S, Barbado A, García S, Gil-López S, Molina D, Benjamins R, Chatila R (2020) Explainable artificial intelligence (XAI): concepts, taxonomies, opportunities and challenges toward responsible AI. Inf Fusion 58:82–115

# Half Bridge Operational Testing and Optimization for Chemiresistive *Escherichia Coli* Bacteria Sensor Application

**Nurliyana Md. Rosni, Kusnanto Mukti Wibowo, Royan Royan, Fani Susanto, Atqiya Mushlihati, Rudi Irmawanto, and Mohd. Zainizan Sahdan**

**Abstract** Balanced bridge circuits widely used in many electronics applications such as to measure changes in electrical magnitude, light intensity, pressure or strain. The wheatstone bridge is used in many applications for sensing a range of mechanical and electrical properties, but one that is very useful and critical in research area by using Wheatstone bridge is in the biosensor application. Many biosensors to detect harmful bacteria have been developed in the last few years, but the structure and application of the circuit operation still lacking in research publication. In this research, the simple circuit system was developed using half bridge operational with a stand-alone user interface. An Arduino microcontroller was used to operate the new device. The circuit was functionalized to detect resistance change with the help of Wheatstone bridge with half bridge operational principle for device calibration. The result shows that resistivity change that can be detected by the device was as low as 0.0426 Ω. Finally, by dropping the 1000 CFU/ml of *E. coli* bacteria sample

N. Md. Rosni · Mohd. Z. Sahdan
Department of Electronic, Faculty of Electrical and Electronic Engineering, UTHM, Parit Raja, 86400 Batu Pahat, Johor, Malaysia

N. Md. Rosni
Microelectronics and Nanotechnology Shamsuddin Research Center (MiNT-SRC), UTHM, Parit Raja, 86400 Batu Pahat, Johor, Malaysia

K. M. Wibowo (✉) · R. Royan
Department of Electromedical Engineering, Universitas Muhammadiyah Purwokerto, Banyumas, Purwokerto 53182, Indonesia
e-mail: kusnantomuktiwibowo@ump.ac.id

F. Susanto
Department of Radiologic Imaging Technology, Universitas Muhammadiyah Purwokerto, Banyumas, Purwokerto 53182, Indonesia

A. Mushlihati
Faculty of Applied Science and Technology, UTHM, Panchor, 84600 Johor, Malaysia

R. Irmawanto
Department of Electrical Engineering, Universitas Muhammadiyah Surabaya, Mulyorejo, 60113 Surabaya, Indonesia

 
T. Triwiyanto et al. (eds.), *Proceedings of the 2nd International Conference on Electronics, Biomedical Engineering, and Health Informatics*, Lecture Notes in Electrical Engineering 898, https://doi.org/10.1007/978-981-19-1804-9_5

in the sensing platform, the magnitude of change of 0.23 V was detected from the circuit reading with high stability obtained.

**Keywords** Biosensor · Whetstone bridge · Half bridge · *Escherichia coli* · Arduino · Conductometric

## 1 Introduction

The interface between the electronic signal and the biological system is a critical factor to facilitate further development of biosensors. The measurement of resistance changes for electrical signals was continuously developed and implemented for the detection of targeted viruses or biomolecules [1–3]. The conductometric-based approach is a possible technique for the identification and quantification of *E. coli* bacteria [4]. The method is based on the connection between the conductance parameter and bio-recognition elements. The chemiresistive methods are now getting a lot of attention due to the ease and direct conversation between the targeted biological signal and the readable electrical signal on the surface [5, 6]. Muhammad-Tahir and Alocilja developed a conductometric biosensor that successfully detects bacteria such as *E. coli* and *Salmonella* [7]. The research work shows high specificity, low sample volume used, high limit of detection and near real-time assay mechanism.

In order to operate the chemiresistive or conductometric principle, the user need a proper operation system such as voltage reader known as an analogue-digital-converter (ADC) [8]. The resistance must be converted into a voltage by connecting another resistor known as fixed resistor in series [9]. Previous research by Wibowo et al. stated that employing graphene as a sensing layer can impact the resistivity change toward different concentrations of *E. coli* bacteria by using voltage divider principle [10]. Unfortunately, voltage divider was not sufficient for device accuracy since the operation principle not come with the calibration function. Another parallel resistor needs to connect to the series resistor known as Wheatstone bridge connection for calibration instrument.

A Wheatstone bridge is an electrical circuit used to determine an unknown electrical resistance by balancing two legs of a bridge circuit. In contrast with a simple electrical circuit like voltage divider, the advantage provided by Wheatstone bridge is it has an ability to provide extremely precise measurements. Because of its exclusive structure, which allows reduced temperature sensitivity, the Wheatstone bridge technique is widely used in numerous measurement applications such as strain gauges, resistance measurements, and sensors applications such as pressure sensor [11, 12]. The design of the Wheatstone bridge gives benefits for improving the operational versatility, due to the ability to monitor the output signal very sensitively. Figure 1 illustrates the Wheatstone bridge circuit with the following expression describing the relationship between the changes of the four resistances and the diagonal output voltage, as in Eq. (1).

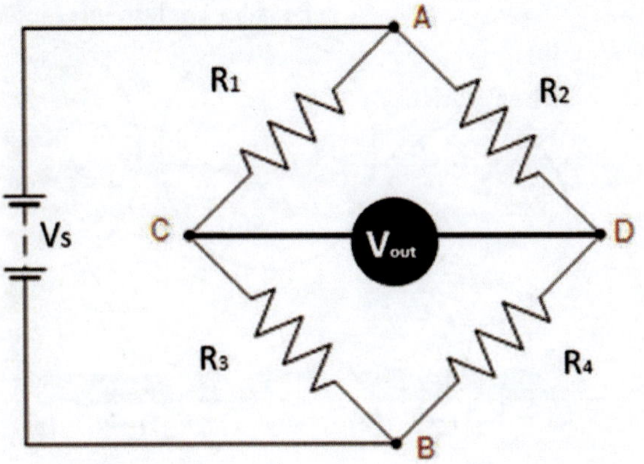


**Fig. 1** Schematic of standard wheatstone bridge

$$V_{out} = \frac{R_1 R_3 - R_2 R_4}{(R_1 + R_2)(R_3 + R_4)} V_s \tag{1}$$

The Wheatstone bridge is used for achieving high voltage changes with respect to relatively small changes in one or more resistors, while requiring only a very simple conduction path. There has the difference between half and full bridge in Wheatstone bridge application. In a full bridge, four resistors are varied, while in a half bridge, only two are subject to such variations. Since the sensor need to operates by detecting a small change in voltage, the Wheatstone bridge circuit is adopted as the basis for a new sensor architecture. The Wheatstone bridge circuit converts a small change in resistance into a voltage measurement, which can be read easily with a voltmeter [13].

The Wheatstone bridge is used in order to achieve high changes in the output voltage with respect to relatively small changes in one or more resistor, while requiring very simple conducting path. The Wheatstone bridge is used in order to achieve high changes in the output voltage with respect to relatively small changes in one or more resistor, while requiring very simple conducting path. Therefore, this research is to integrate half bridge circuit and principle in order to read the electrical changing behaviour of *E. coli* biosensor.

## 2 Literature Review

Generation of chemiresistive sensors. However, the fact that carriers (electrons or holes) are intrinsically charged and can give large interfering signals from a variety of polar and ionic species is a general issue that this field continues to face. Evolving designs provide a plenty of possibilities to incorporate new frameworks to achieve high sensitivity. The mechanism for chemiresistive biosensors is shown in Fig. 2. Electrical detection method using a semiconductor material has the ability to vary

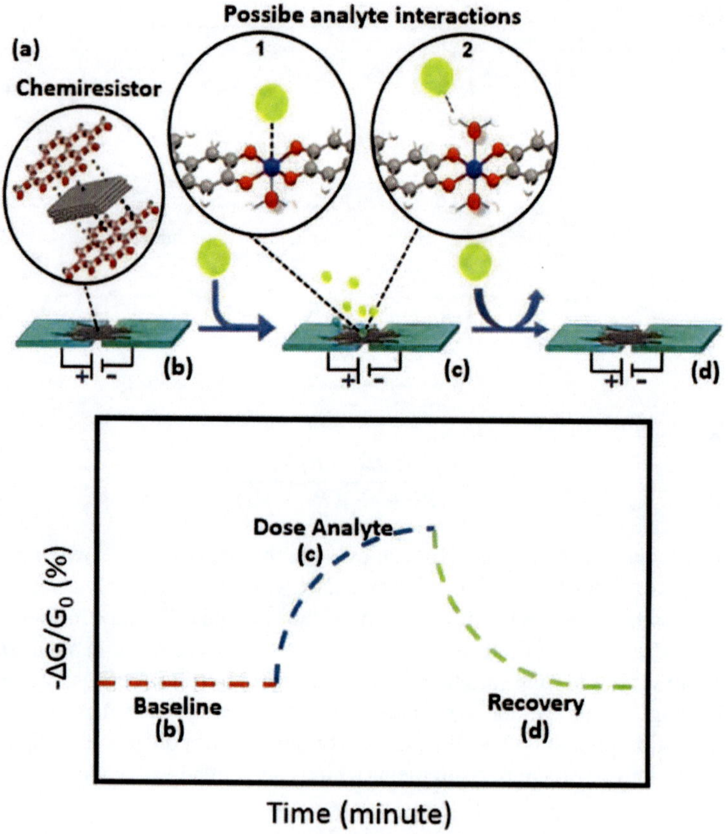


**Fig. 2** Chemiresistive biosensor mechanism **a** integrated sensor array **b**, **c**, and **d** readout interface

its conductivity of the P- or N-type $SiO_2$ material when a charge is applied on the surface. Hence, compared to the other techniques, the chemiresistive or conductometric principle method provides an effective and desirable medium for pathogen detection due to its robustness, less time-consuming, efficiency and simplicity [14].

Morgenshtein et al. is successfully present a novel readout configuration for ion-sensitive field-effect transistor (ISFET) sensors that allows on-chip integration by using Wheatstone bridge connection. In the application, the conversion of pH changes within the respective channel resistance is carry out using the ISFET sensor's operation. The Wheatstone bridge structure is a good candidate for sensor application at which temperature-compensated detection of resistance is required. The equivalent sensitivity of ISFET is regulate by controlling the DC levels of the gate voltage. Wheatstone Bridge Readout Interface proves to be a reliable alternative to ISFET integration in complementary metal-oxide semiconductor (CMOS) process [15].

Behkam and Sitti et al. used a force sensor circuit that contains Wheatstone bridge circuit and a differential amplifier for detecting the flagellar motion of *E. coli* bacteria.

In order to stabilize the output voltage, two voltage followers were used before the differential amplifier. The system consists of strain gauges that has a resistance of ~360 Ω, one resistors of the bridge has a resistance of ~320 Ω, and the other resistor in the Wheatstone bridge is made variable so that the zero value of the bridge when no load is applied could be adjusted [16, 17].

A full Wheatstone bridge for giant magnetoresistive (GMR)-based magnetic sensors was successfully designed and fabricated by Yan et al. which is suitable for various application such as compasses, electrical current measurement, detection of biologic antibodies labelled by magnetic beads, or nondestructive testing. The advantages of this research design are it is quite precise with high and independent frequencies to a parallel resistance and capacitance. As a compromise, the present bridge has a grounded point but is designed for rapid substitution measurements where high accuracy is required. The construction is relatively simple and the operation quite rapid. The bridge, which has been described in previous research has proven to be a very practical substitute for the ideal instrument in the measurement of electrical signals of biological materials [18].

## 3 Methodology

The Wheatstone bridge principle was used in this application to perform the calibration and to detect small change of resistance. Wheatstone bridge is circuit that consist two series resistor know as voltage divider that connected in parallel as shown in Fig. 3 [19]. It has two balance fixed resistor at point 1 and point 2 labels as $R_1$ and $R_2$ respectively. The calibration resistor ($R_C$) has the adjusting function to varying the value of resistance to be same with resistor of the sensor ($R_S$). Hence, can make the device reading which is $V_{out}$ to null value on the initial reading. In this sensor, a change in the charge magnitude was expected to turn the resistance value. It can reach several orders of magnitude within the working range of the sensor. The sensor chips

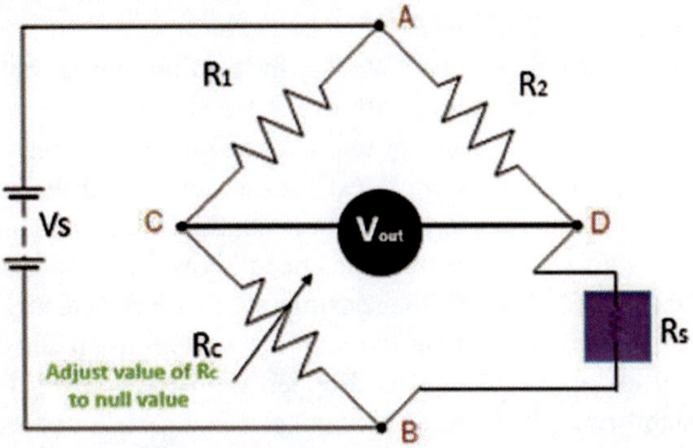


**Fig. 3** Two voltage divider that connected in parallel to form wheatstone bridge

($R_S$), which was functionalized with the anti-*E. coli* antibody on graphene/$SiO_2$, has been utilized as selective sensing material toward anti-*E. coli* measurement [19].

### 3.1 Circuit Design

The electrical part for this research consists of four main parts: microcontroller, user interface (LCD and push button), sensor and power supply. The circuitry was designed using Proteus 7.8 Professional software. The microcontroller is required to control the operation process for whole device and system [20]. Using the Arduino Nano 3.x ATmega328P controller the coding was created in order to generate the system on the circuit. The microcontroller was chosen due to its small size and also being breadboard-compatible, so it was easy to fit on the PCB. The *E. coli* bacteria sensing layer was detected using chemiresistive sensor principle. In this sensor, a change in the concentration of *E. coli* bacteria concentration was expected to turn the resistance value. It can reach several orders of magnitude within the working range of the sensor. All the electronic components in the designed circuit associated the proper operation system. The constructed device consists of two-layer PCB manufactured. The full schematic circuit, as shown in Fig. 4a, was designed before converting it into PCB form, as shown in Fig. 4b.

### 3.2 Electrical Device Testing

The measurement was performed by a comparative test using the device measurement along with the plate-culturing method for identifying the *E. coli* bacteria concentration. The negative charge of the bacteria can produce changes in the electrical properties of the graphene sensing layer, which can be monitored using the developed device. Before the measurement of the device was conducted, the evaluation methods on the device were performed based on its sensitivity, stability, respond time and user interface performance.

Sensitivity was evaluated by the minimum resistivity change that can be detected by the device reading with every 1.0 Ω of resistance change in the simulation and the device measurement using a known variable resistor value that was applied on the device. The stability test for the device and the sensing layer was evaluated in four phases. The first phase, was conducted to evaluate the stability of the device by using a fixed resistor that has been known to have a very stable resistor value [21]. In the second phase, the sensing layer with the electrode assembly was inserted into the device to evaluate the stability of the initial sensing layer. In the third phase, 1.0 ml of DI water was dropped onto the sensing layer. The last phase was the stability evaluation of the device after bacteria exposure on the sensing layer. The device reading with the response time using a serial monitor on the Arduino IDE software was utilized throughout this stability test. The response corresponding to

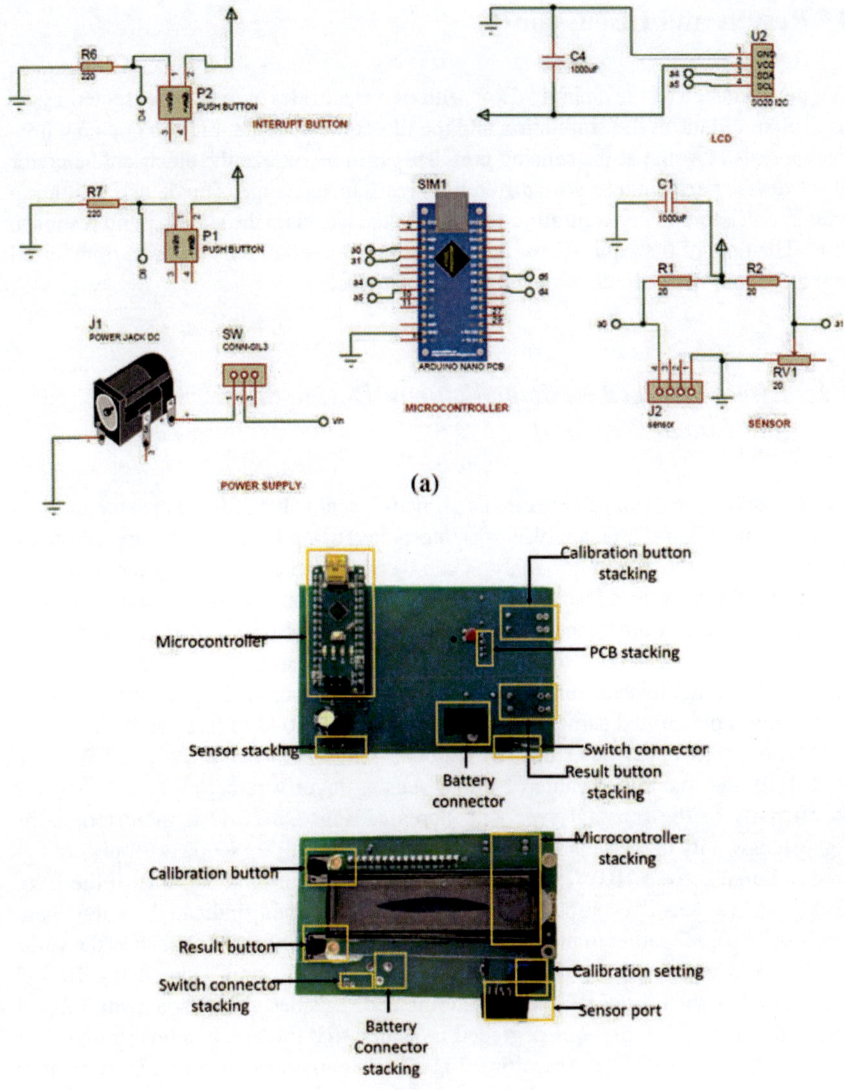


**Fig. 4** Electrical circuit design **a** circuit schematic **b** PCB assembling

the bacteria in the device reading with response time was evaluated. Lastly, the reader/user interface of the device was evaluated based on the proposed software programming. The coding in the programming needs to be adjusted until the desired display on the LCD was attained with the responses to the final input correlation between the device reading and the *E. coli* bacteria concentration.

# 4 Results and Discussion

The performance of the chemiresistor with two electrodes, can be represented by an equivalent circuit in the simulation and the direct measurement in the device with a known resistor value at the sensing port. This is to recognize the electrical behavior of the device performance with differences resistance change. The device validation with *E. coli* bacteria concentration was conducted based on the stability and response time. The data of the equivalence circuit were generated one by one and transferred into the graph for validation and analyzing purpose.

## *4.1 Effect of Fixed Resistor Valueon Device Sensitivity and Linear Respond*

To analyze the sensitivity of the circuit using different value of fixed resistor analysis methods, the computation analysis was interpreted using Proteus software. Based on Adelman et al., the sensitivity analysis can be evaluated by observing the impact of change from the proposed variable solution [22]. The results of simulation sensitivity can be estimated by analysing the gradient of the graph from the different outcomes since the sensitivity is refer to the smallest fractional change in a device that can be measured. In order to determine the sensitivity of the outcome, the gradient sensitivity analysis was performed using 10.0 Ω, 20.0 Ω, and 100.0 Ω of fixed resistor.

According to a previous study by Wu et al. [23], Akbari *et al.* [24] and Wibowo et al. [10], the maximum value of initial sensing layer was below 10.0 Ω and the conductivity of the sensing layer will increase. Hence, 10.0 Ω is indicated as the highest resistivity of the sensing layer. Therefore, the analysis scope was only configured in range zero to 10.0 Ω. Figure 5 shows that with a smaller value of the fixed resistor, more sensitive output voltage change is obtained, indicated by the sharp gradient of 10.0 Ω rather than 100.0 Ω. However, 10.0 Ω was not chosen as the value for the fixed resistor in the Wheatstone bridge circuit design, since using 10.0 Ω make the resistor on the device become heated. Besides, the gradient in Table 1 shows that the sensitivity was degraded indicated that the graph is not straight-line graph from zero to 10.0 Ω. Therefore, 20.0 Ω was chosen as the optimum resistance that can cope with the heat dissipation of the power circuit and give a straight-line graph for the changing resistivity value between zero to 10.0 Ω within tolerance up to three decimal places. Simulation results show that by using the 20.0 Ω resistor, a resistance change of 1.0 Ω on the sensing port can deviate the output voltage by 0.125 V. Results from the small graph in Fig. 5 show a decreasing gradient. Hence, the sensitivity decreases when a high change of resistance is measured. Therefore, by referring to the graph, the circuit is not suitable to detect a high range of resistivity change because the result will not accurate due to the degradation effect when the resistance value of the changeable sensing layer is higher than the value of the fixed

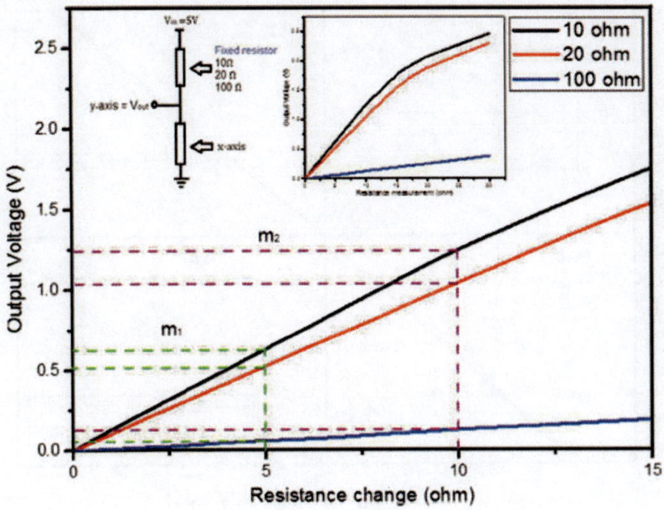


**Fig. 5** Optimisation results from simulation with difference value of fixed resistor

**Table 1** Gradient results of simulation with difference value of fixed resistor

| Fixed resistor (Ω) | $m_1$ | $m_2$ |
|---|---|---|
| 10 | 0.12516 | 0.12444 |
| 20 | 0.10324 | 0.10344 |
| 100 | 0.01302 | 0.01302 |

resistor. This concluded that the designed circuit is only suitable for detecting low resistance change.

## 4.2 *Comparison Between Simulation and Device Measured Reading*

In addition, the comparison between simulation and device measurement reading was evaluated on the device performance. In order to qualify the performances of the device, the feasibility and accuracy using standard variable resistor in simulation and experimental was verified. Figure 6 shows the relationship between changes of resistance and output voltage reading on the device experimentally. It indicates when the $R_S$ has change by 0.1 Ω, the voltage reading was changed from 0.00 V to 0.0115 V on device simulation while the measurement device change from 0.00 V to 0.0112 V. Despite the reading of the device was different from the simulation data, which indicated a more sensitive reading, the sensitivity was still acceptable since it still can detect the resistance change as low as 0.04259 Ω. The changes of resistance

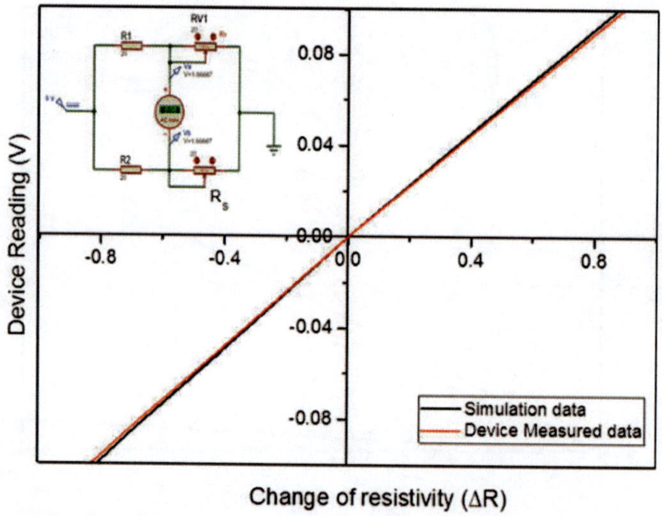


**Fig. 6** Evaluation between Proteus software simulation and device measurement

of the sensing layer when incubated with *E. coli* bacteria needed to be a minimum as low as 0.04259 Ω in order to be detected by the device due to the minimum voltage change on the device is 0.00477 V. Experimental results show a decreasing gradient slope. Hence, the sensitivity decreases compared with the simulation. The deviation percentage between the measurement of the device and the simulation of the device is 2.68%. It was due to the drop-in power supply voltage that did not supply exactly 5.0 V.

## 4.3 Circuit Testing

The stability of the device was tested by inserting a fixed resistor into the sensing port. Then, the sensing electrode's stability was tested by inserting it into the sensing port. Both components showed constancy in their readings. This showed that the device and the sensing layer were in a stable state and the sensor was ready to be used. When the sensing area was in contact with DI water, no deviation was detected by the device since there was no charge distribution on the DI water molecules [25]. In addition, when DI water was dropped onto the sensing layer, the device reading also showed a steady state, which shows that there was no effect of disturbance in the device reading when the water was dropped onto the sensing layer.

The initial device reading without any *E. coli* bacteria showed a very stable reading compared with previous research conducted by Wibowo et al. [10]. In his research, stated that the device needs some amount of stability time before device operation. In this research, since the bypass capacitor was applied in the circuit, any AC noise

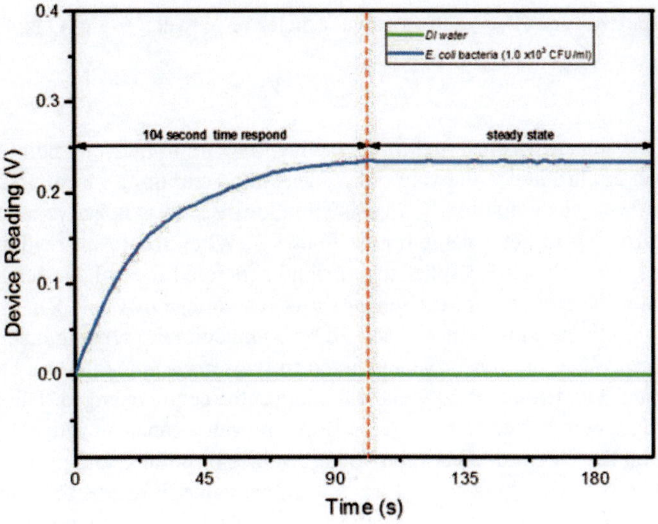


**Fig. 7** Calibration and *E. coli* bacteria testing

that was present on the DC signal was eliminated [26]. Meanwhile for the *E. coli* bacteria sample, the reading showed the significant change for both concentrations. The *E. coli* bacteria with 1000 CFU/ml concentration showed the constant device reading with device reading of 0.23 V with 104 s time respond (Fig. 7).

## 4.4 Analysis of User Interface Performance with Half Bridge Operation

A system display was successfully integrated from the software development for the simple user interface using LCD. In this application, the varying resistance on *Rs* by the graphene sensing layer would vary the output voltage according to the relationship in Eq. (2), (3) and (4). The range of $R_C$ was varied to fit with the value of resistance of *Rs* so it can be adjusted to balance the Wheatstone bridge.

The value of voltage at point D is depend on value of $R_S$

$$V_D = \frac{R_S}{(R_2 + R_S)} V_S \tag{2}$$

While the value of voltage at point C is depend on value of $R_C$ that was adjusted manually using conventional variable resistor.

$$V_C = \frac{R_C}{(R_1 + R_C)} V_S \tag{3}$$

The output voltage ($V_{out}$) across galvanometer or between C and D is,

$$V_{out} = V_C - V_D \tag{4}$$

Before the sensor was inserted in the device, the circuit between point D and B was an open circuit, hence the value of $R_S$ was huge and up to infinity. Therefore, the value of $V_D$ was equal to $V_S$. In this situation, $V_{out}$ was negative since it was impossible for $V_C$ to get a value higher than $V_D$. When the result-reading button was pressed, the unbalanced Whetstone bridge generated the voltage reading with negative value. The reading of the sensor showed a voltage of $V_C - V_D$.

The prototype measurement was started by connecting the sensing layer adaptor to the device. When the sensor was inserted to the sensor port that was connected between point B and point D, the voltage reading at the centre changed. This is due to the $V_D$ reading being affected by the $R_S$ value. The value can be negative or positive depending on the magnitude between voltage values of point C and point D. Based on the equation, if the value of $V_{out}$ has a negative value, it means that the resistor for the sensor, $R_{S,}$ is greater than the calibrating resistor, $R_C$ and vice versa.

The calibration of this device took place before measuring the effect of change in the device. For calibration purposes, $V_{out}$, which is the voltage between the two midpoints (C and D) was adjusted until it reached the null value by varying the $R_C$ value. The voltage difference of the sensor was adjusted to the null value by turning the potentiometer while long-pressing the calibration button. After ensuring the value was stable, which was when only zero value was shown, the calibration button was released. This showed that the bridge at the centre was balanced and no current was flowing at that point. The ratio of the two resistance which are $R_1$ and $R_C$ is equal to the ratio of the two resistors ($R_2$ and $R_S$).

Then, when 1.0 ml of water sample was dropped onto the sensing layer. The result-reading button was pressed. With the absence of *E. coli* bacteria in the water sample, there was no change in the value of $R_S$. Therefore, the value of the output voltage remained the same. Figure 8 shows the readings displayed from the prototype when *E. coli* bacteria were absent and present in the water sample. If *E. coli* bacteria from the water sample were captured by anti-*E. coli* antibodies on the sensing material,

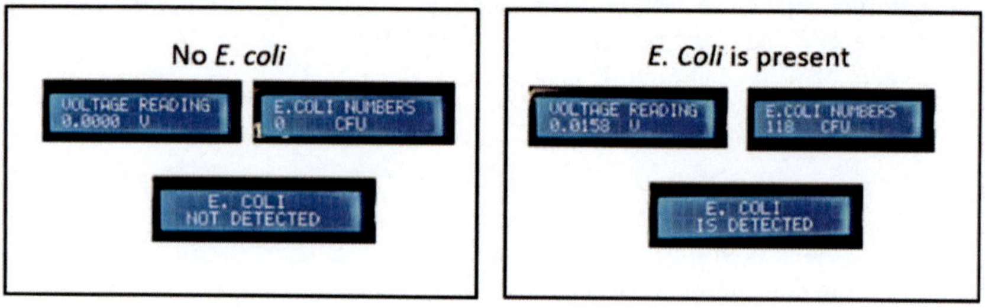


(a) (b)

**Fig. 8** Device display **a** present of *E. coli* bacteria and **b** absent of *E. coli* bacteria the resistance of the graphene change its value. The reading of the voltage difference varies based on the resistance value. The result shows the $V_{out}$ of the Wheatstone bridge reading and number of *E. coli* bacteria with CFU/ml appearing on the screen. Results from the device's display show the success of the circuit's operation.

## 5 Conclusion

Simple system and algorithm are crucial for understanding and built more sophisticated system in future. In this study, the relationship between Wheatstone bridge system and application can be understanding in detail. From the simulation evaluation, it can be concluded that the value of fixed resistor in the half bridge also can contribute to the device sensitivity. The optimum resistance value for detected low resistivity in this research is 20 Ω, which can detect resistivity change as low as 0.0426 Ω. From the evaluation, the system can detect the low amount of resistance change from the sensor chips (RS) which was functionalized with the anti-E. coli antibody on graphene/$SiO_2$ with high stability. In this research, the full system was developed with a standalone user interface and does not require any alternating current (AC) outlet or personal computer (PC) connection. Due to the device simplicity, it can give beneficial for end users to provide information in water quality.

## References

1. Saucedo N, Gao Y, Pham T, Mulchandani A (2018) Lectin-and saccharide-functionalized nano-chemiresistor arrays for detection and identification of pathogenic bacteria infection. Biosensors 8(3):63
2. Wibowo KM, Sahdan MZ, Ramli N, Muslihati A, Rosni N, Tsen VH et al (2018) Detection of Escherichia coli bacteria in wastewater by using graphene as a sensing material detection of Escherichia coli bacteria in wastewater by using graphene as a sensing material. J Phys Conf Ser 995:1–6
3. Mukti K, Muslihati A, Zainizan M, Mad N, Basri H, Fudholi A (2020) A novel, portable Escherichia coli bacteria sensor using graphene as sensing material. Mater Chem Phys 254(3):123459
4. Nurliyana MR, Sahdan MZ, Wibowo KM, Muslihati A, Saim H, Ahmad SA, et al (2018) The detection method of Escherichia coli in water resources: a review. J Phys: Conf Ser
5. Zhao W, Xing Y, Lin Y, Gao Y, Wu M, Xu J (2020) Monolayer graphene chemiresistive biosensor for rapid bacteria detection in a microchannel. Sens Actuators Rep 2(1):100004
6. Huang C, Huang T, Chiang C, Huang W, Lin Y (2020) Biosensors and bioelectronics A chemiresistive biosensor based on a layered graphene oxide/graphene composite for the sensitive and selective detection of circulating miRNA-21. Biosens Bioelectron 164(5):112320
7. Muhammad-Tahir Z, Alocilja EC (2003) Fabrication of a disposable biosensor for Escherichia coli O157: H7 detection. IEEE Sens J 3(4):345–351
8. Blum J (2013) Exploring Arduino: tools and techniques for engineering wizardry. Wiley

9. Fransiska RW, Septia EMP, Vessabhu WK, Frans W, Abednego W (2013) Electrical power measurement using arduino uno microcontroller and labview. In: 2013 3rd international conference on instrumentation, communications, information technology and biomedical engineering (ICICI-BME). IEEE pp 226–229
10. Wibowo KM (2018) Fabrication of graphene-based resistive sensor For Eschericia coli bacteria sensing
11. Castro HF, Correia V, Pereira N, Costab P, Oliveiraa J, Lanceros-méndez S (2018) Printed Wheatstone bridge with embedded polymer based piezoresistive sensors for strain sensing applications. Addit Manuf 20(2):119–125
12. Meena KV, Mathew R, Leelavathi J, Sankar AR (2017) Performance comparison of a single element piezoresistor with a half-active Wheatstone bridge for miniaturized pressure sensors. Measurement 111(April 2016):340–350
13. Figliola RS, Beasley DE (2006) Theory and design for mechanical measurements. Wiley
14. Whitaker CJ (2005) The electronic handbook
15. Morgenshtein A, Sudakov-Boreysha L, Dinnar U, Jakobson CG, Nemirovsky Y (2004) Wheatstone-bridge readout interface for ISFET/REFET applications. Sens Actuators B Chem 98(1):18–27
16. Behkam B, Sitti M (2004) E. coli inspired propulsion for swimming microrobots. In: ASME 2004 international mechanical engineering congress and exposition. American Society of Mechanical Engineers pp 1037–1041
17. Ko M, Aykanat A, Smith M, Mirica K (2017) Drawing sensors with ball-milled blends of metal-organic frameworks and graphite. Sensors 17(10):2192
18. Cole KS, Curtis HJ (1937) Wheatstone bridge and electrolytic resistor for impedance measurements over a wide frequency range. Rev Sci Instrum 8(9):333–339
19. Hoffmann K. Applying the Wheatstone bridge circuit
20. Birns NE, Mizrahi-Shalom OK (1999) Microcontroller system for performing operations of multiple microcontrollers
21. Church HF (1962) The long-term stability of fixed resistors. Proc IEE-Part B Electron Commun Eng 109(21S):19–27
22. Adelman HM, Haftka RT (1986) Sensitivity analysis of discrete structural systems. AIAA J 24(5):823–832
23. Wu G, Meyyappan M, Lai KWC (2016) Graphene field-effect transistors-based biosensors for Escherichia coli detection. In 2016 IEEE 16th international conference on nanotechnology (IEEE-NANO). IEEE pp 22–25
24. Akbari E, Nikoukar A, Buntat Z, Afroozeh A, Zeinalinezhad A (2015) Escherichia coli bacteria detection by using graphene-based biosensor. IET Nanobiotechnol 9(5):273–279
25. Jacobs HO, Whitesides GM (2001) Submicrometer patterning of charge in thin-film electrets. Science 291(5509):1763–1766
26. Toyoda N (1988) Semiconductor integrated circuit device having an integrally formed bypass capacitor

# Vital Sign Monitor Based on Telemedicine Using Android Application on Mobile Phone

**Bambang Guruh Irianto, Anita Miftahul Maghfiroh, Anggit Ananda Solichin, and Fabian Yosna Bintoro**

**Abstract** The price of vital sign machines on the market is very high. Currently, the technology used is still very complicated and ineffective, and the vital sign machine cannot be connected to other devices. Health monitoring with Android is currently increasingly developing for monitoring vital signs of the body to simplify the process of examining patients. Therefore, this research aims to develop a low-cost vital sign machine with a customized design to integrate the machine with other devices via Android. In this study, the main controller of the Vital Sign machine is the Arduino Nano microcontroller which is used to measure body temperature, respiration, blood pressure, and heart rate. To do this, take the heart rate using the index finger of the hand with the fingertip sensor, for respiration using the FC-04 as a breath detector, and body temperature using the DS18b20 sensor mounted on the armpit. The performance of sending vital sign data via android on the BPM measurement obtained an error value of 0.62%, for the measurement of the respiratory rate an error value of 4.87% was obtained and the temperature measurement obtained an error value of 0.43 0C. The results obtained from this study can be implemented for diagnostic purposes and this tool is suitable for use.

**Keywords** Heart rate · Temperature · Respiration · Android

## 1 Introduction

Vital signs of human health can be identified from body temperature, respiration, oxygen saturation, blood pressure, pulse, and heart rate [1]. The unit for checking heart rate is called Beat Per Minute (BPM) [2]. This condition is very important to use for monitoring patients in hospitalization [3] with the risk of harm. In the era of the global pandemic due to the covid-19 virus, telemedicine technology is very important to use to monitor the condition of patients in isolation rooms/ICU to reduce the risk of transmission to medical personnel in hospitals [4]. Telemedicine

B. G. Irianto · A. M. Maghfiroh (✉) · A. A. Solichin · F. Y. Bintoro
Poltekkes Kemenkes Surabaya, Jl. Pucang Jajar Tengah No. 56, Surabaya 60283, Indonesia
e-mail: anitamiftah@poltekkesdepkes-sby.ac.id

 
T. Triwiyanto et al. (eds.), *Proceedings of the 2nd International Conference on Electronics, Biomedical Engineering, and Health Informatics*, Lecture Notes in Electrical Engineering 898, https://doi.org/10.1007/978-981-19-1804-9_6

is the use of information technology and communication technology provided to participants when there is a distance that separates them to support health care [5]. Health monitoring with telemedicine has been developed by several researchers [6–10]. IoT systems are also used in telemedicine technology [11–13]. The IoT system is equipped with a camera and controlled by a raspberry pi 3 then the data is sent to the cloud to be sent to the web and can be accessed via cellphone made for patient monitoring by Alvee Rahman et al., the parameters monitored are ECG signals and body temperature [12]. This method is very effectively used for monitoring patients in the ICU, but the monitored vital sign parameters are still incomplete. Prof. M.T. Hasan et al. developed pulse monitoring taken from heart signals using a wireless system [14]. Wireless systems can be implemented well, but continuous development requires more parameters to increase monitoring of biomedical system efficiency [15, 16]. Pu Zhang et al. mobile phone system implemented as part of telemedicine [17]. The remote monitoring system uses a Java-enabled 3G Mobile Phone with Java jiggles installed on the mobile phone, this system is very helpful for doctors in monitoring the patient's condition but the time it takes to start the application is quite long and the ECG signal image sent sometimes disappears because other than that mode can't be used globally. Several researchers have implemented a telemedicine system using wireless [18–20]. This system is widely used by researchers for central monitoring of vital signs and is still being developed. Roy Abi Zeid Daou et al., have made vital sign monitoring with an android application with a Bluetooth connection to send/receive data between platforms and android [21]. This system is quite good with an accuracy value of 95%. However, a high power system results in lower battery life and no data storage so that when offline data cannot be sent.

Based on the research methods that have been discussed in previous researchers, as far as the author's knowledge, the parameters on vital sign equipment made based on telemedicine are not complete. The parameters made on the tool do not cover all vital signs. Therefore, in this study, the authors added several parameters for telemedicine-based vital sign monitoring. The vital signs monitored were heart rate, body temperature, and breathing.

The purpose of making monitoring of heart rate, body temperature, and respiration based on telemedicine via android is to make it easier for health workers to monitor the condition of patients in the inpatient room/ICU/isolation room at a low price and affordable by the public with accurate measurement results.

## 2 Material and Method

### *2.1 Participant*

In this study, the subjects used were 10 males with an age range of 30–48 years. The participants were given consent so that they understood and studied the experimental protocol. The experimental protocol passed the Ethics Committee of the

Surabaya Health Polytechnic, the Health Ethics Committee of the Indonesian Ministry of Health (No: 035/S/KEPK/V/2017). The test results with the subject are then compared with standard tools.

## 2.2 *Data Acquisition*

In this study, the number of heart beats (BPM) was obtained from the Finger Tip Sensor that was installed on the finger consisting of infrared with a wavelength of 850–1000 nm and a photodiode to capture the infrared light that passed through the finger. The output of the photodiode is then forwarded to the instrument amplifier circuit with a gain of 101 times. Meanwhile, to obtain the respiratory rate in this study, the FC-04 sensor was used which consisted of a condenser mic and an analog signal conditioning module. The FC-04 sensor converts breath sound vibrations captured by the condenser mic into digital data via an analog signal conditioning module. The output produced when the breath is detected has an amplitude ranging from 3.3 to 5 V. To get the body temperature, this study used the DS18b20 sensor which is a digital sensor with 16-bit data processing (4 bits to determine the positive or negative temperature value and 12 bits as the temperature data value). The DS18b20 sensor can be configured with bits ranging from 9 to 12 bits to read temperature data values. Digital data from the DS18b20 sensor can be read in the form of decimal data using the program listing. 1 degree of temperature is equal to 15,996 decimal places. Figure 1 describes the overall system of Vital Sign Monitor Based on Telemedicine via Android. There are three inputs from the 3 sensors, namely heart rate, a respiratory rate signal, and body temperature. In several studies, for data retrieval, BPM is taken from the lead ECG signal [22]. While in this study BPM was taken from the photoplethysmogram signal [23–25]. The output of each sensor is a series of instruments and analog signal conditioning which will be controlled by a microcontroller to produce information in the form of heart rate, several respiratory rates, and body

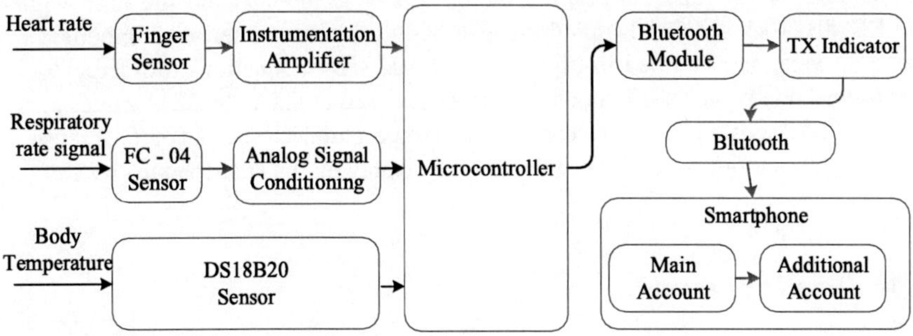


**Fig. 1** The diagram block of the proposed methods

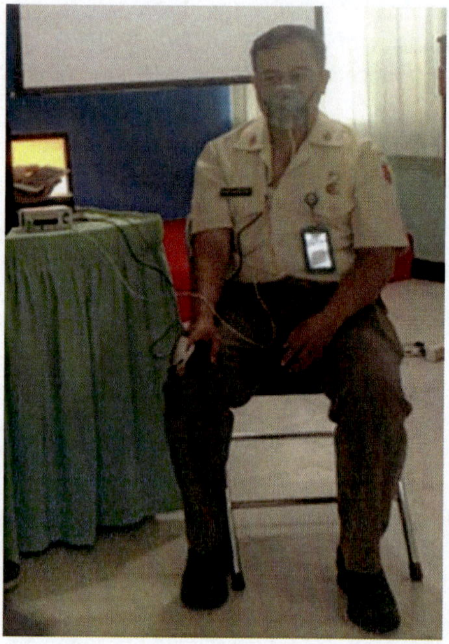

**Fig. 2** Data collection on the subject

temperature which will be sent by Bluetooth system then the data is received via smartphone.

## 2.3 Data Collection

The data collection process was taken from 10 respondents for measurement of heart rate, respiratory rate, and body temperature based via android. The finger sensor is clamped on the index finger, the FC-04 sensor is mounted on the nose while the DS18B20 sensor which functions as a body temperature sensor is mounted in the axial area, as described in Fig. 2. The FC-04 sensor functions to intercept the respiratory rate signal, while the finger sensor is used to generate BPM values , and the DS18B20 sensor is used to measure body temperature. The output of the 3 sensors is sent by Bluetooth which is received by the display on the smartphone.

## 2.4 Data Processing

After the data collection process, to get the error value and accuracy of each measurement including the number of heart beats (BPM), respiratory rate and body temperature, it is necessary to calculate based on Eq. 1, Eq. 2 and Eq. 3 [26]:

$$\text{Mean} = \frac{\sum_{i=1}^{n} X_i}{n} = \frac{X_1 + X_2 + X_3 \ldots\ldots X_n}{n} \quad (1)$$

where x is the retrieval of data to and n is the number of data retrieval

$$Stdv = \sqrt{\frac{1}{n-1}\sum_{i=1}^{n}(V_i - Mean)^2} \quad (2)$$

where V is the retrieval of collected data and mean is the average value

$$\text{Ua} = \frac{\text{Stdev}}{\sqrt{\text{n} - 1}} \quad (3)$$

where Ua uncertainty of readability and n is the number of data.

## 2.5 *Statistical Analysis*

In this study, the performance of the system is calculated based on the ability to send telemedicine-based data via Android. Performance measurements are carried out on each parameter, namely heart rate, respiratory rate, and body temperature. Sensitivity is calculated from the number of indications BPM, Temperature, and Respiration parameter values detected from delivery results on android by reading data on the tool that is made as a reference. Testing system performance used 10 respondents, each respondent data took 6 times. Then the T-Test was carried out to determine if there was a significant difference between the reading of data transmission based on telemedicine via android. An alpha value of 0.05 was used in this study. So, if the P-value is more than 0.05, then this indicates that there is no significant difference between the two groups, On the other hand, if the P-value is less than 0.05, this indicates that there is a significant difference between the two groups.

# 3 Results

Following the purpose of this study, namely telemedicine-based monitoring of vital signs via android, data collection on respiratory rate, BPM, and body temperature was carried out 6 times for each respondent, and the data were analyzed using T-Test.

## 3.1 *Test Results of Data Transmission Based on Telemedicine via Android*

To test the performance of sending data based on telemedicine via Android, performance measurements were carried out on each parameter, namely heart rate, respiratory rate, and body temperature. Performance measurement is carried out by taking data from 10 respondents with each subject taking data 6 times. Figure 3 shows the display of BPM, respiratory rate, and body temperature based on telemedicine via android. We conducted the same test of 10 respondents.

Figure 3 explains that Figure (a) is a screen display of a smartphone from a device that is not connected to the Android system, while Figure (b) is a screen display of a Smart Phone from a device that is connected to the Android system.

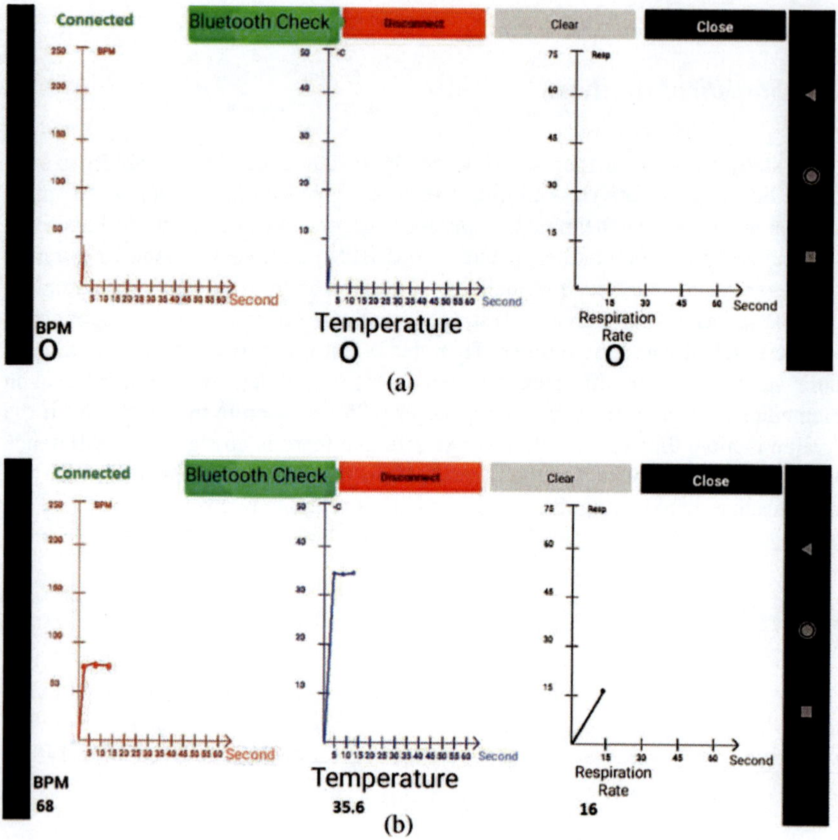


**Fig. 3** Display on a smartphone screen **a** not connected with android **b** connect with android

It is explained in Table 1 that the results of telemedicine performance with heart rate (BPM) parameters indicate the average value of the measurement, the standard deviation value, the uncertainty value, and the error value of the BPM parameter.

In Table 1 it is shown that the measurements were carried out on 10 subjects with each measurement 6 times. The subject's average breathing was 87 BPM. The highest standard deviation in subject no. 7 is 41 with a value of Ua 2.21. From the measurement results, the average error value generated by the module is very small with a maximum error value of 0.51%. Still at the maximum allowable error threshold so that it can be declared fit for use.

Meanwhile, performance measurements for respiratory rate and body temperature are described in Tables 2 and 3.

From the data, In Table 2 it is shown that the measurements were carried out on 10 subjects with each measurement 6 times. The subject's average breathing was 19 BrPM. The highest standard deviation in subject no. 6 is 2.5 with a value of Ua 1.02. From the measurement results, the average error value generated by the module is

**Table 1** Results of testing the performance of telemedicine heart rate parameters (BPM)

| Subject | Mean (BPM) | SD (BPM) | Ua (BPM) | Error (%) |
|---|---|---|---|---|
| 1 | 77.66 | 1.63 | 0.66 | 0.432 |
| 2 | 69.66 | 1.63 | 0.66 | 0.480 |
| 3 | 98.33 | 1.5 | 0.61 | 0.505 |
| 4 | 89.83 | 1.47 | 0.60 | 0.559 |
| 5 | 98.16 | 1.47 | 0.60 | 0.511 |
| 6 | 79.5 | 5.04 | 2.06 | 0.625 |
| 7 | 87.83 | 5.41 | 2.21 | 0.566 |
| 8 | 81 | 3.22 | 1.31 | 0.613 |
| 9 | 85.83 | 3.06 | 1.24 | 0.389 |
| 10 | 98.16 | 1.47 | 0.60 | 0.511 |

**Table 2** Results of testing the performance of telemedicine respiratory rate parameters (BrPM)

| Subject | Mean (BrPM) | SD (BrPM) | Ua (BrPM) | Error (%) |
|---|---|---|---|---|
| 1 | 19 | 1.78 | 0.73 | 4.58 |
| 2 | 20.66 | 1.21 | 0.49 | 3.12 |
| 3 | 20.83 | 0.75 | 0.30 | 3.10 |
| 4 | 19.33 | 1.03 | 0.42 | 3.33 |
| 5 | 19 | 2 | 0.81 | 3.63 |
| 6 | 19.33 | 2.5 | 1.02 | 3.57 |
| 7 | 20 | 2.19 | 0.89 | 3.22 |
| 8 | 19.5 | 2.42 | 0.99 | 4.87 |
| 9 | 19.33 | 1.03 | 0.42 | 3.33 |
| 10 | 19 | 2 | 0.81 | 3.63 |

**Table 3** The results of testing the performance of telemedicine temperature parameters (°C)

| Subject | Mean (°C) | SD (°C) | Ua (°C) | Error (°C) |
|---|---|---|---|---|
| 1 | 35.06 | 0,23 | 0.09 | 0.3 |
| 2 | 34.25 | 0.13 | 0.05 | 0.35 |
| 3 | 35.83 | 0.28 | 0.11 | 0.43 |
| 4 | 36.06 | 0.16 | 0.06 | 0.31 |
| 5 | 34.3 | 0.16 | 0.06 | 0.3 |
| 6 | 35.06 | 0.23 | 0.09 | 0.3 |
| 7 | 34.25 | 0.13 | 0.05 | 0.35 |
| 8 | 35.83 | 0.28 | 0.11 | 0.43 |
| 9 | 36.06 | 0.16 | 0.06 | 0.31 |
| 10 | 34.3 | 0.16 | 0.06 | 0.3 |

very small with a maximum error value of 0.62%. Still at the maximum allowable error thresh-old so that it can be declared fit for use. It is still at the maximum allowable error threshold.

From the data, In Table 3 it is shown that the measurements were carried out on 10 subjects with each measurement 6 times. The subject's average breathing was 35 °C. The highest standard deviation in subject no. 9 is 0.16 with a value of Ua 0.06. From the measurement results, the average error value generated by the module is very small with a maximum error value of 0.31 °C. Still at the maximum allowable error thresh-old so that it can be declared fit for use. It is still at the maximum allowable error threshold.

## 3.2 *Statistical Analysis*

Statistical analysis was used to see if there was a significant difference between the messages sent on the android system and the data display on the tool module. The statistical results shown in Table 4 illustrate the T-test for the BPM parameter, Respiratory rate, Temperature Parameter.

The data in Table 4 shows the statistical analysis value of the T-test equal variance on the BPM parameter measuring the standard error value is 0.8036, then the P-value = 0.19335 (P-value > 0.05) and the result of sig is no. While the results of the T-test

**Table 4** T-Test results statistical analysis

| | Std err | p-value | Sig |
|---|---|---|---|
| BPM parameter | 0.8036 | 0.19335 | No |
| Respiratory rate | 0.9789 | 0.31388 | No |
| Temperature parameter | 0.8036 | 0.19335 | No |

respiratory rate at standard error obtained an error value of 0.9789, obtained P-value = 0.31388 (P-value > 0.05) and the result of sig is no. The value of statistical analysis T-test equal variance at temperature standard error value of 0.8036, then obtained P-value = 0.194318 (P-value > 0.05) and the result of sig is no.

## 4 Discussion

From the results of the analysis of the calculation of the BPM measurement data, the maximum error value generated is 0.62% in the 6th sample measurement and the resulting minimum error value is 0.38% in the 9th sample measurement. the entire sample BPM measurement is 0.49%. Thus the error value is still within the allowable tolerance limit of 5%. So that the BPM parameter is declared suitable for use. While the results of the analysis of the calculation of respiratory rate measurement data, the maximum error value generated is 4.8% in the 8th sample measurement and the resulting minimum error value is 3.1% in the 3rd sample measurement. The average error value of all measurements Respiration of the sample is 3.5%. Thus the error value is still within the allowable tolerance limit of 10%. So that the respiratory rate parameter is declared suitable for use. For body temperature parameters, the results of the analysis are obtained with the maximum error value generated is 0.43 and the resulting minimum error value is 0.3 °C. The average error value of all sample measurements is 0.33 °C. Thus the error value is still within the allowable tolerance limit of 1 degree Celsius. So that the temperature parameter is declared fit for use. While the statistical analysis calculations were still within the tolerance range specified. The results of the T-Test statistic of BPM parameters test obtained P-value = 0.19335 this value indicates that the alpha value is more than 0.05, then this indicates that there is no significant difference between the two groups. The results of the T-Test statistic of Respiratory rate parameters test obtained P-value = 0.31388, and the results of the T-Test statistic of temperature parameters test obtained P-value = 0.194318 this value indicates that the alpha value is more than 0.05, then this indicates that there is no significant difference between the two groups. Allowed and there is no significant difference between the data sent via android and the data received so that it is declared suitable for medical use with an average value (P-value > 0.05).

Pu Zhang et al. mobile phone system implemented as part of telemedicine [17]. The remote monitoring system uses a Java-enabled 3G Mobile Phone with Java jiggles installed on the mobile phone, this system is very helpful for doctors in monitoring the patient's condition but the time it takes to start the application is quite long and the ECG signal image sent sometimes disappears because other than that mode can't be used globally. In the research of Abi Zeid Daou et al. [21] Vital sign monitoring has also been made with an Android application with a Bluetooth connection to send/receive data between platforms and Android. This system is quite good with an accuracy value of 95%. However, in this study there is no data storage if it is off-line and the power consumption is too high.

The weakness in this study is that there is no data stored in the database so that if there is a decrease in power on the smartphone, the previously sent data cannot be read. The results obtained from this study can be implemented for diagnostic purposes and this tool is feasible to use. It is also useful for monitoring the condition of patients in the isolation room/ICU to reduce the risk of transmission to medical personnel in hospitals.

## 5 Conclusion

In this study, a Vital Sign Monitor Based On telemedicine Via Android has been created. The results of this study indicate that the average value of the vital sign monitor base on telemedicine performance test via android is (P-value >0.05). The performance of sending vital sign data via android on the BPM measurement obtained an error value of 0.62%, for the measurement of the respiratory rate an error value of 4.87% was obtained and the temperature measurement obtained an error value of 0.43 °C. This shows that this design is suitable for telemedicine systems because there is no significant difference. This system can be developed for further research by adding measurement parameters according to standard tools used in the medical world and adding a patient database storage system.

## References

1. Brekke IJ, Puntervoll LH, Pedersen PB, Kellett J, Brabrand M (2019) The value of vital sign trends in predicting and monitoring clinical deterioration: a systematic review. PLoS ONE 14(1):1–13
2. Prasath JS, Need II, Wireless OF (2013) Wireless monitoring of heart rate using microcontroller. 2(2):214–219
3. Kellett J, Sebat F (2017) Make vital signs great again—a call for action. Eur J Intern Med 45:13–19
4. Gajbhiye AM, Pawar AC, Majramkar AM, Kendre SS (2016) Wireless ICU surveillance system using ARM7. 2(11):667–673
5. Field MJ (1996) A telecommunications: *telemedicine*. Committee on evaluating clinical applications of telemedicine, institute of medicine. ISBN: 0-309-55312-1
6. Abo-Zahhad M, Ahmed SM, Elnahas O (2014) A wireless emergency telemedicine system for patients monitoring and diagnosis. Int J Telemed Appl
7. Shivakumar NS, Sasikala M (2014) Design of vital sign monitor based on wireless sensor networks and telemedicine technology. Proceeding IEEE Int Conf Green Comput Commun Electr Eng ICGCCEE 2014 (3)
8. Fan Y, Xu P, Jin H, Ma J, Qin L (2019) Vital sign measurement in telemedicine rehabilitation based on intelligent wearable medical devices. IEEE Access 7:54819–54823
9. Firmansyah RA (2019) Monitoring heart rate and temperature based on internet of things. 1(2):1–7
10. Sarath S, George ARS (2018) Tele-health monitoring system. (3):101–104
11. Abdul-Jabbar HM, Abed JK (2020) Real time pacemaker patient monitoring system based on internet of things. IOP Conf Ser Mater Sci Eng 745(1):28–30

12. Rahman A, Rahman T, Ghani NH, Hossain S, Uddin J (2019) IoT based patient monitoring system using ECG sensor. 1st International conference robotics electrical signal processing techniques. ICREST 2019. pp 378–382
13. S. P. O. Parameter (2019) Central monitor based on personal computer using single wireless receiver. 1(1):45–49
14. Fanani A, Irianto BG, Pudji A (2019) Central monitor based on personal computer using single wireless receiver. Indones J Electron Electromed Eng Med Informa 1(1):45–49
15. Shelar M (2013) Wireless patient health monitoring system. 62(6):2–6
16. Pattichis CS, Kyriacou E, Voskarides S, Pattichis MS, Istepanian R, Schizas CN (2002) Wireless telemedicine systems: an overview. IEEE Antennas Propag Mag 44(2):143–153
17. Zhang P, Kogure Y, Matsuoka H, Akutagawa M, Kinouchi Y, Zhang Q (2007) A remote patient monitoring system using a java-enabled 3G mobile phone. Annu Int Conf IEEE Eng Med Biol—Proc 3713–3716
18. Digarse PW, Patil SL (2017) Arduino UNO and GSM based wireless health monitoring system for patients. Proc 2017 Int Conf Intell Comput Control Syst ICICCS 2017, vol 2018-Janua. pp 583–588
19. Hai VD, Hung PM, Trung LHP, Hung DV, Thuan ND, Dang Hung P (2017) Design of software for wireless central patient monitoring system. Proceedings KICS-IEEE international conference information communication with Samsung LTE 5G special work. ICIC 2017. pp 214–217
20. Megalingam RK, Kaimal DM, Ramesh MV (2012) Efficient patient monitoring for multiple patients using WSN. Proceedings 2012 international conference advances mobile networks, communications its applied MNCApps 2012. pp 87–90
21. Abi Zeid Daou R, Aad E, Nakhle F, Hayek A, Börcsök J (2015) Patient vital signs monitoring via android application. 2015 international conference advance biomedical engineering ICABME 2015, no. 9. pp 166–169
22. Maghfiroh AM, et al (2021) State-of-the-art method to detect R-peak on electrocardiogram signal: a review. (10):321–329
23. Lei R, Ling BW, Feng P, Chen J (2020) Estimation of heart rate and respiratory rate from PPG signal using complementary ensemble independent component analysis and non-negative
24. Askarian B, Jung K, Chong JW (2019) Monitoring of heart rate from photoplethysmographic signals using a Samsung Galaxy Note8 in underwater environments. Sensors (Switzerland) 19(13)
25. Das S, Pal S, Mitra M (2016) Real time heart rate detection from PPG signal in noisy environment. pp 70–73
26. Duvernoy J (2015) Guidance on the computation of calibration uncertainties. World Meteorol Organ (119)

# Image Classification for Egg Incubator Using Transfer Learning VGG16 and InceptionV3

**Apri Junaidi, Faisal Dharma Adhinata, Ade Rahmat Iskandar, and Jerry Lasama**

**Abstract** Image classification can be used in a variety of fields, including chicken farming, where it can be used to monitor incubator conditions by capturing the image in the machine and then using transfer learning to classify the image in the incubator. This study has a problem with obtaining the highest accuracy while also reducing overfitting in the model, to obtain classification results with the expected accuracy, this study employs three algorithms: VGG16, InceptionV3, and Deep Learning. Each algorithm will be tested on a dataset comprised of three classes: egg, chick, and hatched egg. There are 1470 images in the chick class, 1719 images in the egg class, and 1715 images in the hatched egg class. In the training and validation processes, researchers also do some data preprocessing, such as augmentation for data adjustment. The accuracy of each algorithm was determined in this study; VGG16 had an accuracy of 0.90, while InceptionV3 had an accuracy of 0.97. Deep Learning has chosen the model with the highest accuracy out of the two that were created. The accuracy of this Deep Learning model is 0.8125. This research is dealing with the issue of overfitting as it develops the Deep Learning architecture. However, it can be reduced by adding several Dropout layers to the Deep Learning architecture. Observations made during the research that each algorithm has a different level of accuracy because the architecture of each algorithm is different, even though researchers use the same dataset and testing environment. Transfer Learning using VGG16 and InceptionV3 has an accuracy of more than 90% in this study. Based on the study's findings, it is possible to conclude that using transfer learning and adding a dropout layer can produce high accuracy while reducing overfitting.

**Keywords** Image classification · Deep learning · Transfer learning · Egg incubator

A. Junaidi (✉) · F. D. Adhinata · J. Lasama
Institut Teknologi Telkom Purwokerto, Jl. DI Panjaitan No. 128, Purwokerto 53147, Indonesia
e-mail: apri@ittelkom-pwt.ac.id

A. R. Iskandar
Akademi Telkom Jakarta, Jalan Daan Mogot KM.11, RT.1/RW.4, Kedaung Kali Angke, Cengkareng, Kota Jakarta Barat, DKI Jakarta 11710, Indonesia



T. Triwiyanto et al. (eds.), *Proceedings of the 2nd International Conference on Electronics, Biomedical Engineering, and Health Informatics*, Lecture Notes in Electrical Engineering 898, https://doi.org/10.1007/978-981-19-1804-9_7

## 1 Introduction

Image classification is an exciting research topic today [1], and it can cover many fields of science, including agriculture, animal husbandry, medical images [2, 3], biology [4, 5], physics, sugar production [6] and many others. Image classification is one of the artificial intelligence methods used to quickly detect an image [7, 8] based on input from training data, which is then processed in some algorithm with classification output from several images. This study is about hatching chicken eggs; hatching the chicken produces a variety of images that can be studied using image classification.

Broiler meat is an inexpensive and easily accessible source of animal protein. With such a low price, this was predicted which demand for broiler chicken may continue to rise [9]. Incubating directly with the mother or using modern equipment such as an egg incubator is how most breeders hatch poultry. Egg incubation is a technology that allows breeders to produce chicks from eggs through the use of engineering techniques [10], Egg incubation is more efficient than mother hatching [11].

So far, only the temperature and humidity of the air in the incubator have been monitored during the hatching process. Image classification can help farmers monitor the progress of the environment in the incubator during the incubation process by categorizing the images in the incubator. Several research teams have used image classification in the agricultural production, such as the Convolutional Neural Network for Industrial Egg Classification, to classify the types of eggs Good Egg, Poor Growth Egg, Wind Egg, Dead Egg, Unusual Air-Chamber Egg, and Reversed Egg, and this study resulted in classification accuracy of 92.3% [12]. Deep learning-based classification method for hatching eggs [13]. The training method that combines the pre-trained network and multi-layer network features outperforms the canonical network in terms of accuracy. The experiment is carried out on 5-day hatching eggs in a specific period with an obsolete feature that is extremely difficult to extract. The hatching eggs are classified into three types: fertile eggs, dead eggs, and infertile eggs. The final accuracy in this study is 99.5% [14].

Several researchers have also investigated transfer learning in various image classifications, such as the Indian Food Image Classification with Transfer Learning study, for training and validating, an Indian food dataset of 20 classes with 500 images in each class is used. IncceptionV3, VGG16, VGG19, and ResNet are the models used. Following testing, it was discovered that Google InceptionV3 outperformed other models, with an accuracy of 87.9% and a loss rate of 0.5893 [15].

UNESCO has designated batik as one of Indonesia's cultural heritages. It has a distinct pattern associated with the Indonesian region. Because Indonesia is made up of different cultures, a cultural preservation system is required. To address these issues, this study proposes a deep learning method for classifying the various types of batik. The VGG16 architecture with Random Forest as a classifier was used in this study. The results show that precision, recall, F-score, and accuracy are all greater than 97% [16]

Another study used deep learning image classification in environmental protection to solve the identification and classification of domestic waste using the VGG16 convolutional neural network model. Finally, this project categorizes household waste into recyclable waste, hazardous waste, kitchen waste, and other waste. After actual testing, the waste classification system based on the VGG16 network proposed in this paper has a correct classification rate of 75.6%, which meets the needs of daily use [17].

The project Classification of Chicken Meat Freshness Using Convolutional Neural Network Algorithms uses image classification to classify the identification of chicken meat freshness using a convolutional neural network algorithm. The dataset used by the researcher was a broiler chicken breast image dataset. In this study, two types of chicken meat were used: fresh and rotten. Furthermore, the researchers created their own CNN architecture called Ayam6Net, which has an accuracy of 92.9% [17].

Image classification is widely used in several research fields [18], as evidenced by the numerous studies that have been submitted. Several Convolutional Neural Network (CNN) architectures are used in this image classification, and many also use Transfer Learning. This study proposes the use of a design convolutional neural network to achieve the best accuracy results, as well as a transfer learning model that employs pre-trained models VGG16 and InceptionV3, so the research question formulated for this study is how to achieve the best accuracy in classifying images of chicken eggs in an incubator environment? Overfitting is a common problem encountered while developing the CNN model [19, 20], so several approaches are required to overcome overfitting and improve accuracy.

Previous research did not explain how to reduce overfitting in a model; previous research focused on achieving accuracy; therefore, the improvement in this research is in addition to achieving accuracy, but also on how to reduce overfitting in datasets created from scratch using transfer learning and deep learning.

According to several references, adding a dropout layer to the CNN architecture is one way to reduce overfitting. Dropout is a powerful technique that can be used in machine learning or deep learning to improve the generalization error of large neural networks, such as overfitting [21]. At the start of each training iteration, dropout maps with the same neuron size in each layer were randomly initialized to mark the active or inactive status of the associated neurons. During the training iteration, the off-state neurons are removed from the network [22], consists of setting the output of each hidden neuron to zero with a probability of 0.5 [23].

## 2 Method

This research was conducted in two stages. The first stage was to build a deep learning model using CNN, as shown in Fig. 1, and the second stage was to create a model using pre-trained models, namely VGG16 and InceptionV3. Several stages are carried out, beginning with the dataset collector and ending with preprocessing. The image

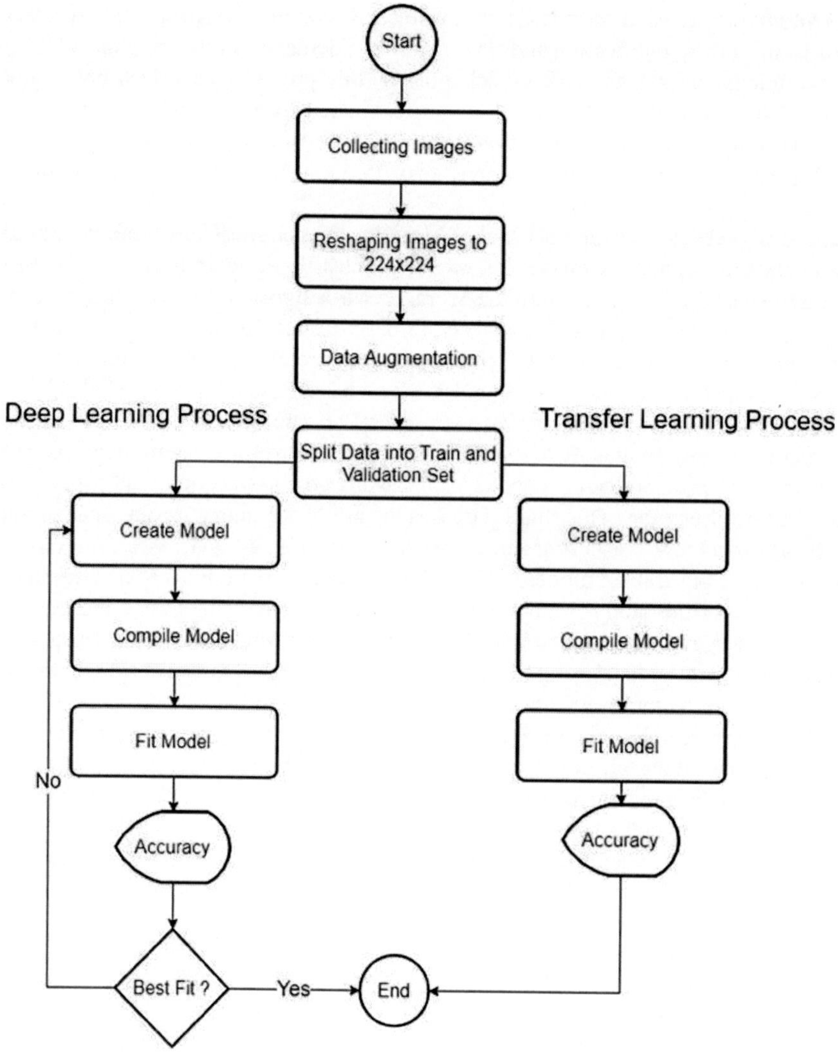


**Fig. 1** Research method

reshape process is standardized to 224 × 224, then continued with augmentation data, training data creation, and data validation.

For the deep learning stage, the process begins with model creation, model compile, and model fit, so that accuracy results are obtained. To obtain the best accuracy results, the model must be accurate while also avoiding overfitting problems. If overfitting occurs, the process loops back to the model creation stage. The deep learning process is complete when accuracy is obtained and there are no overfitting issues.

For the transfer learning stage, after the preprocessing process begins with model creation, model compilation, and model fit, so that accuracy results are obtained, for transfer learning, in general, always get the best accuracy and good accuracy validation, so that there is no overfitting in data processing for this research, It is due to the fact that transfer learning techniques attempt to transfer knowledge from previous tasks to a target task when the latter has less high-quality training data [24]. As a result, once high accuracy is obtained, the process is complete.

## 2.1 Dataset

The dataset used in this study is a picture of chicks, eggs, and hatching eggs, some of which were taken from Google Images, but others were taken with the researcher's cellphone camera by taking photos of chicks, eggs, and observing and recording videos of the hatching process of chicks, videos of which can be found on the researcher's YouTube channel https://www.youtube.com/watch?v=3QHepqR8XfA.

Following the image collection process, the image augmentation process is carried out with the following number of images for each class: There are 1470 images of chicks in total. The total number of egg images is 1719. There are 1715 hatching images in total.

Figure 2 illustrates an image for the dataset in which a represents the chick class, b represents the egg class, and c represents the hatching egg class. Researchers use 80% for training data and 20% for data validation in the distribution of training data and data validation. Based on the amount of data, 3924 images for training with three classes and 980 images for data validation with three classes.

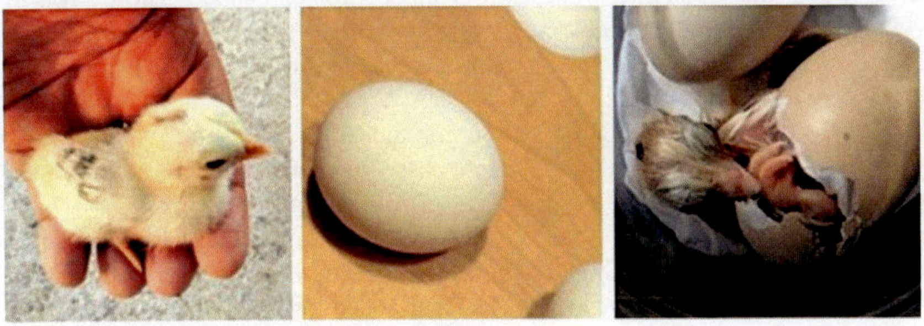

a b c

**Fig. 2** Dataset classes **a**: chick, **b**: egg, **c**: hatching egg

**Table 1** First model

| Layer | Output shape | Param |
|---|---|---|
| conv2d_12 (Conv2D) | (None, 222, 222, 16) | 448 |
| dropout_5 (Dropout) | (None, 222, 222, 16) | 0 |
| max_pooling2d_12 (MaxPooling2D) | (None, 111, 111, 16) | 0 |
| conv2d_13 (Conv2D) | (None, 109, 109, 32) | 4640 |
| dropout_6 (Dropout) | (None, 109, 109, 32) | 0 |
| max_pooling2d_13 (MaxPooling2D) | (None, 54, 54, 32) | 0 |
| conv2d_14 (Conv2D) | (None, 52, 52, 64) | 18,496 |
| dropout_7 (Dropout) | (None, 52, 52, 64) | 0 |
| max_pooling2d_14 (MaxPooling2D) | (None, 26, 26, 64) | 0 |
| conv2d_15 (Conv2D) | (None, 24, 24, 128) | 73,856 |
| max_pooling2d_15 (MaxPooling2D) | (None, 12, 12, 128) | 0 |
| flatten_3 (Flatten) | (None, 18,432) | 0 |
| dense_3 (Dense) | (None, 3) | 55,299 |
| Total params: 152,739 | | |
| Trainable params: 152,739 | | |
| Non-trainable params: 0 | | |

## 2.2 Proposed Model

In this study, the researcher proposes four models for obtaining accuracy, two of which are deep learning models and two of which are transfer learning models. CNN customized with an architectural arrangement similar to Table 1 is used by researchers for deep learning.

By overfitting the resulting model, the first model has an accuracy of 0.6312%. When a model fails to generalize well from observed data to invisible data, it is said to be overfitting [25].

To avoid overfitting, the researcher created a second model architecture (Table 2) with a nearly identical architectural model to the first. However, after the flatten layer in the second architecture, the researcher added a dropout layer with a value of 0.5. This architectural layer configuration can reduce overfitting while increasing accuracy to 0.8125%.

With the architecture depicted in Table 1, it is possible to reduce overfitting in the model depicted in Table 2.

Figures 3 and 4 demonstrate that improving the structure of the deep learning architecture reduces overfitting. On second models, the researcher added a dropout layer with a value of 0.5.

**Table 2** Second model

| Layer | Output shape | Param |
|---|---|---|
| conv2d_4 (Conv2D) | (None, 222, 222, 16) | 448 |
| dropout_1 (Dropout) | (None, 222, 222, 16) | 0 |
| max_pooling2d_4 (MaxPooling2D) | (None, 111, 111, 16) | 0 |
| conv2d_5 (Conv2D) | (None, 109, 109, 32) | 4640 |
| max_pooling2d_5 (MaxPooling2D) | (None, 54, 54, 32) | 0 |
| conv2d_6 (Conv2D) | (None, 52, 52, 64) | 18,496 |
| max_pooling2d_6 (MaxPooling2D) | (None, 26, 26, 64) | 0 |
| conv2d_7 (Conv2D) | (None, 24, 24, 128) | 73,856 |
| max_pooling2d_7 (MaxPooling2D) | (None, 12, 12, 128) | 0 |
| flatten_1 (Flatten) | (None, 18,432) | 0 |
| dropout_2 (Dropout) | (None, 18,432) | 0 |
| dense_1 (Dense) | (None, 3) | 55,299 |
| Total params: 152,739 | | |
| Trainable params: 152,739 | | |
| Non-trainable params: 0 | | |

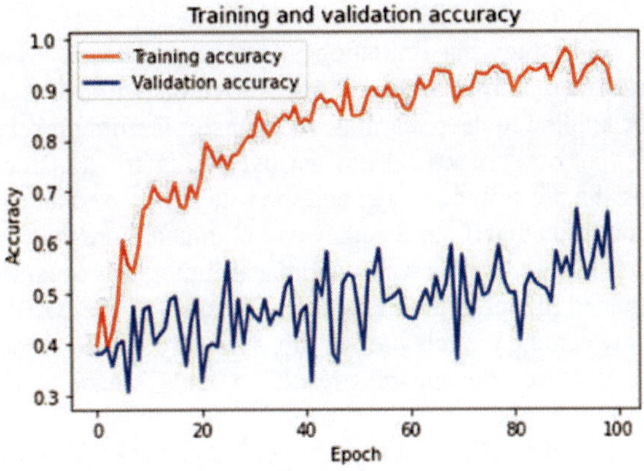


**Fig. 3** Overfitting on first model

## 3 Result and Discussion

In several previous studies, such as the Indian Food Image Classification with Transfer Learning study, this study resulted in an accuracy of 87.9%, research conducted by Rajayogi et al. [9], identification and classification of domestic waste

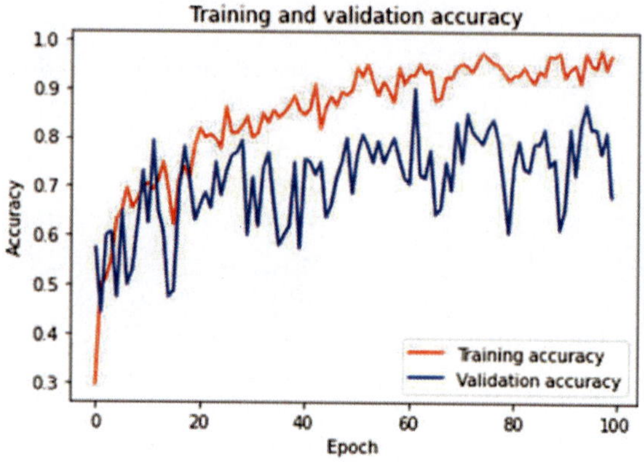


**Fig. 4** Reduce overfitting in second model

using the VGG16 convolutional neural network model. This paper has a correct classification rate of 75.6% [11].

Based on the findings of these two previous studies, there are some similarities in terms of using transfer learning but different accuracy results, as shown in Table 1. For researchers using VGG19, to see differences and increasing accuracy results in the current study also using InceptionV3. VGG16 has an accuracy quality of 0.90, while InceptionV3 has an accuracy quality of 0.97.

In addition to transfer learning, this study used deep learning to form two models, the first of which produced an accuracy of 0.6312 and the second of which produced an accuracy of 0.8125.

This study has limitations, namely on datasets created from scratch; it does not use datasets from online dataset providers with some preprocessing so that they can be applied to deep learning and transfer learning research.

The researcher did not get overfitting for transfer learning because the model used a pre-trained model and the researcher used an early stopping scheme with the condition that if the accuracy was obtained more than 90%, the training on the model was stopped in this study, and the accuracy was obtained more than 90% for the pre-trained model in the first epoch of training. The results of the accuracy comparison between the models used in this study are shown in Table 3.

Based on the accuracy results in Table 3, each model can be described as shown in Fig. 5.

Based on Fig. 5, it is possible to conclude that transfer learning with pre-trained models VGG16 and InceptionV3 achieves the highest accuracy. The first and second models were created using CNN and the architectural arrangement shown in Figs. 4 and 5.

**Table 3** Model comparison

| Deep learning | | Transfer learning | |
|---|---|---|---|
| First model | Second model | VGG16 model | InceptionV3 |
| Epoch: 100 | Epoch: 100 | Epoch: 100 | Epoch: 100 |
| Input: 224 × 224 × 3 | Input: 224 × 224 × 3 | Input: 224 × 224 × 3 | Input: 224 × 224 × 3 |
| Dropout: Yes, 3 layers | Dropout: Yes, 2 layers | Dropout: No | Dropout: No |
| Validation split: 0.2 | Validation split: 0.2 | Validation split: 0.2 | Validation split: 0.2 |
| Overfitting: Yes | Overfitting: Reduce | Overfitting: No | Overfitting: No |
| Accuracy: 0.6312 | Accuracy: 0.8125 | Accuracy: 0.90 | Accuracy: 0.97 |

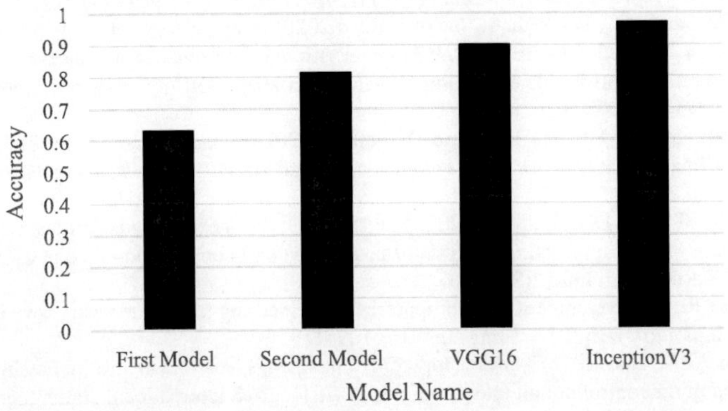


**Fig. 5** Comparison of accuracy for each model created

## 4 Conclusion

Testing under the same data conditions in each class, the number of epochs, and validation split based on the accuracy results recorded in Table 1, it can be seen that the deep learning model produces lower accuracy than the transfer learning model, and based on research on CNN characteristics, overfitting is always the result. However, it can be reduced by incorporating multiple dropout layers into the CNN architecture. This study demonstrates that transfer learning is more effective in image classification in the egg incubator environment. Future research could use transfer learning models or simply increase the number of images in the dataset. The dataset in this study can be trained with ensemble learning for research results that provide the most recent contributions.

## References


1. Bilbao I, Bilbao J (2019) Overfitting problem and the over-training in the era of data: particularly for artificial neural networks. Proceedings—2019 IEEE 9th international conference intelligence computer informatics system ICICIS 2019, no. Icicis. pp 173–177
2. Thanh HT, Yen PH, Ngoc TB (March 2021) Pneumonia classification in X-ray images using artificial intelligence technology. In Proceedings of 2020 applying new technology in green buildings, ATiGB 2020. pp 25–30. https://doi.org/10.1109/ATiGB50996.2021.9423017
3. Truong TD, Pham HTT (2020) Breast cancer histopathological image classification utilizing convolutional neural network. IFMBE Proc 69:531–536. https://doi.org/10.1007/978-981-13-5859-3_92
4. Zhang J, Xia Y, Xie Y, Fulham M, Feng DD (2018) Classification of medical images in the biomedical literature by jointly using deep and handcrafted visual features. IEEE J Biomed Heal Inf 22(5):1521–1530. https://doi.org/10.1109/JBHI.2017.2775662
5. Liu J et al (2018) Applications of deep learning to MRI Images: a survey. Big Data Min Anal 1(1):1–18. https://doi.org/10.26599/BDMA.2018.9020001
6. Chayatummagoon S, Chongstitvatana P (Jan 2021) Image classification of sugar crystal with deep learning. In: KST 2021–2021 13th international conference knowledge and smart technology. pp 118–122. https://doi.org/10.1109/KST51265.2021.9415841
7. Tiwari V, Pandey C, Dwivedi A, Yadav V (Dec 2020) Image classification using deep neural network. In: Proceedings—IEEE 2020 2nd international conference on advances in computing, communication control and networking, ICACCCN 2020. pp 730–733. https://doi.org/10.1109/ICACCCN51052.2020.9362804
8. Joshi SR, Headley DB, Ho KC, Paré D, Nair SS (2019) Classification of brainwaves using convolutional neural network. Eur Signal Process Conf 2019(2). https://doi.org/10.23919/EUSIPCO.2019.8902952
9. Wibowo KC, Putri DS, Hidayat S (2020) Pedaging Di Indonesia Dalam Rangka Mewujudkan Ketahanan Pangan forecasting analysis of production and consumption of Ras Chicken meat in. Maj Teknol Agro Ind 12(2):58–65
10. Aru OE (2017) Development of a computerized engineering technique to improve incubation system in poultry farms. J Sci Eng Res 4(6):109–119
11. Sanjaya WSM, et al (2018) The development of quail eggs smart incubator for hatching system based on microcontroller and internet of things (IoT). 2018 international conference information communication technology. ICOIACT 2018, vol 2018-Janua, pp 407–411. https://doi.org/10.1109/ICOIACT.2018.8350682.
12. Shimizu R, Yanagawa S, Shimizu T, Hamada M, Kuroda T (2018) Convolutional neural network for industrial egg classification. Processing—international society design conference 2017, ISOCC 2017. pp 67–68. https://doi.org/10.1109/ISOCC.2017.8368830
13. Geng L, Liu H, Xiao Z, Yan T, Zhang F, Li Y (2020) Hatching egg classification based on CNN with channel weighting and joint supervision. Multimed Tools Appl 79(21–22):14389–14404. https://doi.org/10.1007/s11042-018-6784-9
14. Geng L, Yan T, Xiao Z, Xi J, Li Y (2018) Hatching eggs classification based on deep learning. Multimed Tools Appl 77(17):22071–22082. https://doi.org/10.1007/s11042-017-5333-2
15. Rajayogi JR, Manjunath G, Shobha G (2019) Indian food image classification with transfer learning, CSITSS 2019–2019 4th international conference computer system information technology sustainable solution processing, vol 4. pp 1–4. https://doi.org/10.1109/CSITSS47250.2019.9031051
16. Arsa DMS, Susila AANH (2019) VGG16 in Batik classification based on random forest. Proceedings 2019 international conference information management technology. ICIMTech, vol 1, no. August. pp 295–299. https://doi.org/10.1109/ICIMTech.2019.8843844
17. Wang H (2020) Garbage recognition and classification system based on convolutional neural network vgg16. Proceedings—2020 3rd international conference advances electronics materials computer software engineering. AEMCSE 2020, pp 252–255. https://doi.org/10.1109/AEMCSE50948.2020.00061

18. Vo AT, Tran HS, Le TH (Jan 2017) Advertisement image classification using convolutional neural network. Proceedings—2017 9th international conference knowledge system engineering KSE 2017, vol 2017. pp 197–202. https://doi.org/10.1109/KSE.2017.8119458
19. Li H, Li J, Guan X, Liang B, Lai Y, Luo X (2019) Research on overfitting of deep learning. Proceeding—2019 15th International conference computer intelligence security CIS 2019. pp 78–81. https://doi.org/10.1109/CIS.2019.00025
20. Hinton GE, Srivastava N, Krizhevsky A, Sutskever I, Salakhutdinov RR (2012) Improving neural networks by preventing co-adaptation of feature detectors. pp. 1–18, [Online]. Available: http://arxiv.org/abs/1207.0580
21. Dahl G, Sainath T, Hinton G (2013) Improving deep neural netowrks for larfe vocabulary continuous speech recognition (LVCSR) using recitified linear units and dropout, department of computer science , university of Toronto, Acoust. Speech signal processing (ICASSP), 2013 IEEE international conference. pp 8609–8613, [Online]. Available: https://ieeexplore.ieee.org/abstract/document/6639346/
22. Q. Li, W. Cai, X. Wang, Y. Zhou, D. D. Feng, and M. Chen (Dec 2014) Medical image classification with convolutional neural network. 2014 13th international conference control automation robotics vision, ICARCV 2014, vol 2014. pp 844–848. https://doi.org/10.1109/ICARCV.2014.7064414
23. Zhang Y, Gao J, Zhou H (2020) Breeds classification with deep convolutional neural network. ACM international conference proceeding series. pp 145–151. https://doi.org/10.1145/3383972.3383975
24. Pan SJ, Yang Q (2010) A survey on transfer learning. IEEE Trans Knowl Data Eng 22(10):1345–1359. https://doi.org/10.1109/TKDE.2009.191
25. Ying X (2019) An overview of overfitting and its solutions. J Phys Conf Ser 1168(2). https://doi.org/10.1088/1742-6596/1168/2/022022

# Method for Obtain Peak Amplitude Value on Discrete Electrocardiogram

**Sabar Setiawidayat and Aviv Yuniar Rahman**

**Abstract** The main results of cardiac examination using an electrocardiograph are to obtain the morphology of the heart's electrical waves and the amplitude value of the P, QRS and T waves. The peak amplitude value is associated with hypertrophy, coronary, ischemia, and myocardial infarct disease. The fact is that the results of the examination only provide information for the peak value of R only. This limited information causes manual calculations to be carried out using small boxes on ecg paper. This study proposes a method to obtain peak amplitude values. The application of the voltage threshold on the discrete lead II electrocardiogram will obtain peak R values. Obtaining the R-R duration will obtain cycle duration, peak P, peak Q, peak S and peak T in each cycle. The results of the study on 10 discrete ecg samples from CVCU RSSA Malang showed that each sample had a peak R value in each cycle along with its peak PQST value. When the peak amplitude value is obtained, manual calculations are no longer needed so that the time for interpretation and diagnosis can be faster.

**Keywords** Peak amplitude · R-R duration · Discrete · Electrocardiogram

## 1 Introduction

The results of non-invasive cardiac examinations using an electrocardiograph are generally presented on a monitor screen or printed on ecg paper [1], both examination 1 lead (for monitoring), 3 leads (for vectorcardiogram, standard Einthoven) and 12 leads (for standard clinical) [2]. The results of the examination consist of the morphology of the cardiogram waves and information on the duration and amplitude values [3]. Wave morphology is presented in two dimensions, namely voltage amplitude (mV) against time function (ms) [4]. Morphology is needed to see the waveform in each lead, while the magnitude information is needed to find out the number or

S. Setiawidayat (✉) · A. Y. Rahman
Widyagama University of Malang, Malang, Indonesia
e-mail: sabarset@widyagama.ac.id



T. Triwiyanto et al. (eds.), *Proceedings of the 2nd International Conference on Electronics, Biomedical Engineering, and Health Informatics*, Lecture Notes in Electrical Engineering 898, https://doi.org/10.1007/978-981-19-1804-9_8

duration value and the amplitude value of the morphology [5]. This amount of information is very important to predict the patient's heart condition whether it is within the limits of normal or abnormal conditions.

In fact, the information on this quantity is very limited, presented both on the monitor screen and on the ecg paper, so because of the importance of this value, the value that has not been informed will be calculated manually by doctors using small boxes on the ecg paper or using a ruler. This manual calculation takes time to look at morphology in order to obtain the appropriate value. Regarding the progressive nature of heart disease, the results of the examination must be fast and correct so that the results of the diagnosis are right on target. Progressive disease is a disease that is a race against time, meaning that if the diagnosis is not immediately carried out in patients with heart disease, it can lead to an increase in the stage, or even the patient's life.

It is known that the heart can contract (beat) periodically because of the depolarization of the atrial and ventricular muscle cells [6]. The occurrence of depolarization is caused by the propagation of impulses propagated by the Sino Atria (SA node) autonomic, periodic, automatically [7]. Each periodization of this beat is often referred to as a cardiac cycle, which includes atrial depolarization, ventricular depolarization and ventricular repolarization [8].

Einthoven as the inventor of the Electrocardiogram, named atrial depolarization as the P wave, ventricular depolarization as the QRS wave and ventricular repolarization as the T wave [4]. Each wave has a wave peak, namely the P peak for the P wave, the R peak for the QRS wave and the T peak for the T wave [9].

Figure 1 Illustrate the normal clinical features of the electrocardiogram. In the Figure, a 1 cycle electrocardiogram under normal conditions is presented on an ecg paper, as a guide for manual calculations. It appears that in 1 cycle there are 5 peak amplitudes (P, QRS, S, T), 2 segments (PR, ST) and 4 intervals (PR, QRS, ST, QT). Each box has an area of 1 $mm^2$, where vertically measuring 0.1 mV for voltage amplitude and horizontally measuring 40 ms for duration [10].

Table 1 shows the limiting information for amplitude and duration values for normal heart conditions. It appears that for the maximum amplitude under normal conditions, the peak P value is 0.2 mV (0.15 mV + 0.05 mV), the peak R value is 2.0 mV (1.5 mV + 0.5 mV) and the peak T value is 0.5 mV (0.3 mV + 0.2 mV). The duration of the P wave is 130 ms (110 ms + 20 ms), the duration of the PQ/PR interval is 200 ms (160 ms + 40 ms), the duration of the QRS wave is 120 ms (100 ms + 20 ms) and the duration of the QT interval is 440 ms. (400 ms + 40 ms).

Figure 2 shows an example of an electrocardiogram from a standard clinic electrocardiograph examination. In the picture there is information on one R peak value, which is 1.6 mV, QRS wave duration is 94 ms, QT interval duration is 428 ms, PR interval duration is 166 ms, P wave duration is 118 ms, R-R duration is 1274 ms. It seems that the information provided is more related to the duration (interval), while the information related to the amplitude is very minimal. Due to this limited information, doctors perform manual calculations for other peak amplitude values using small boxes of ecg paper or a ruler.

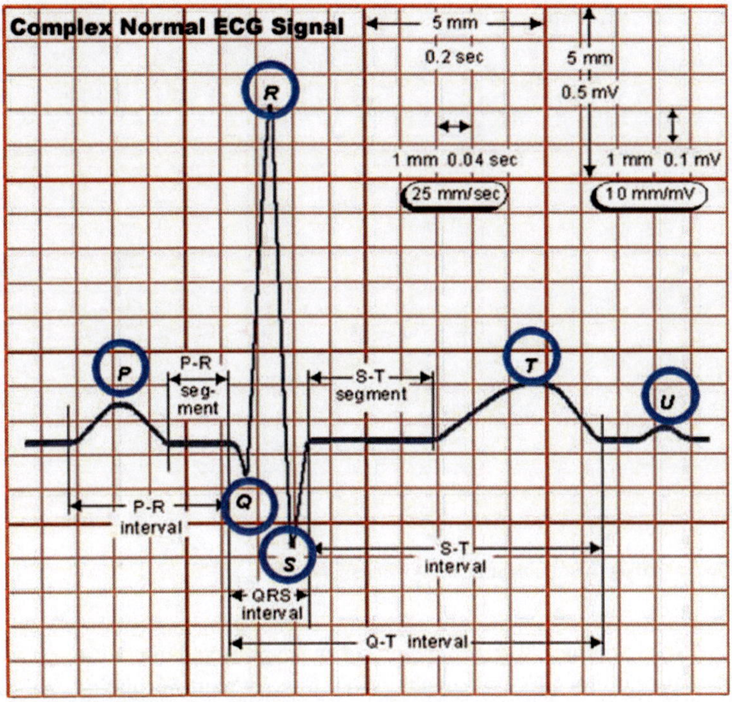


**Fig. 1** Illustrates the normal clinical features of the electrocardiogram

**Table 1** Limit values for normal heart conditions [10]

| Feature | Normal value | Normal limit |
|---|---|---|
| P width | 110 ms | ±20 ms |
| PQ/PR interval | 160 ms | ±40 ms |
| QRS width | 100 ms | ±20 ms |
| QT interval | 400 ms | ±40 ms |
| P amplitude | 0.15 mV | ±0.05 mV |
| QRS height | 1.5 mV | ±0.5 mV |
| ST level | 0 mV | ±0.1 mV |
| T amplitude | 0.3 mV | ±0.2 mV |

Several researchers who have conducted research related to the identification of peak amplitudes include [11] using the High Order Statistical Algorithm to obtain an accurate R peak at a sampling frequency of 1 kHz. [12] QRS detection for Telehealth ECG recording with the UNSW algorithm and comparing it with the Pan-Tompkins (PT) and Gutiérrez-Rivas algorithms [13]. Efficiency QRS complex Detection related to accuracy and computation time of the MIT-BIH Arrhythmia database, using the Moving Windows Integrator (MWI) Optimization to produce faster durations

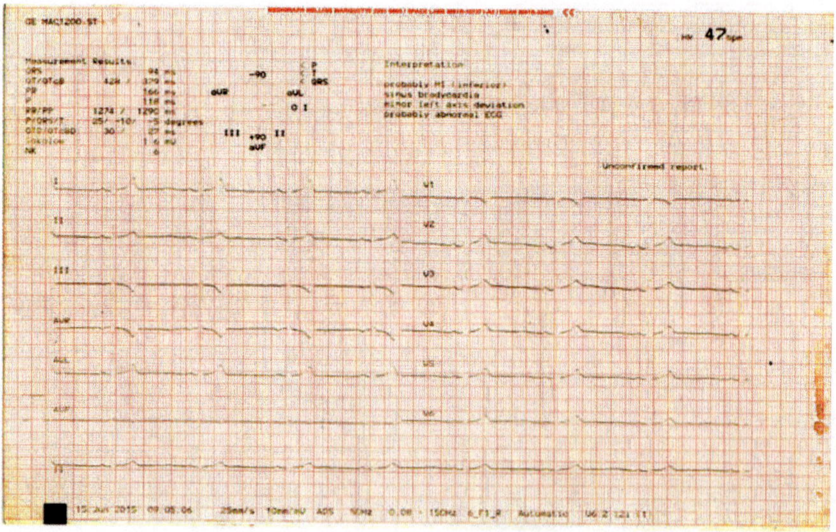

**Fig. 2** Electrocardiogram examination results standard clinic

with maintained accuracy. Ref. [14] proposed an adaptive and time-efficient R-peak detection algorithm for ECG processing. First, wavelet multi-resolution analysis to improve the representation of the ECG signal. Second, change the large negative R-peak to positive-peak. Third, a first-order forward differential approach to find the R-peak. Ref. [15] proposed software to be able to represent 12-lead cardiogram from discrete ecg data using PQRST algorithm. Ref. [16] propose a data filtering method to obtain peak amplitude in each cycle. Ref. [17] proposed a correlated peak amplitude for normal and abnormal conditions using correlation analysis. Ref. [18] propose additional information in the results of cardiac examinations using an electrocardiograph. Ref. [19] proposed a method for detecting the amplitude and duration of QRS waves. Ref. [20] proposed a new approach to detect QRS complexes based on automata to deterministic with the addition of some constraints. Ref. [21] proposed a demo of the ECG denoising algorithm based on the self-convolution window (SCW) called the Hamming self-convolution window, using the MIT-BIH arrhythmia database. Ref. [22] introduced the method of phasor transformation, as well as rules for extracting morphological features of heart rate during physiological and pathological conditions for the detection of P waves. The limitations of the database led the authors to use the MIT-BIH Arrhythmia Database. Ref. [23] proposed feature extraction using Burg's method of autoregressive (AR) modeling and Hilbert's transform for the detection of R-peaks in efficient automated ECG signals using the MIT-BIH Arrhythmia Database. Ref. [24] Propose an algorithmic method for marking R-wave peaks using a database from PhysioNet. Ref. [25] proposed Identification Of ECG Signal By Using Backpropagation Neural Network.

Based on the research that has been done by these researchers, the authors conclude that the results of cardiac examinations to obtain the peak amplitude value in each cycle using a discrete electrocardiogram have not been carried out. The difficulties faced by researchers are ideas and methods to obtain peak amplitude values and how to obtain discrete electrocardiogram sample data. On that basis, the authors propose a method to obtain the peak amplitude in each cycle using a discrete electrocardiogram (ecg discrete). Discrete ecg sample files for research can be obtained from the physiobank databases physionet [26], but the author chose the file from the cardiovascular care unit (CVCU) Saiful Anwar Hospital (RSSA) Malang because it was sampled at a frequency of 250 Hz. Availability of discrete ecg sample files as a result of examination of patients with normal conditions, arrhythmias, and hyperthophy, the authors chose normal condition sample files because they are easy to observe and study. These files were generated from an examination using a discrete 12 lead electrocardiograph (ecgd), which was calibrated with a standard clinic electrocardiograph (ecgs) of the Fukuda Denshi brand [27].

## 2 Methodology

The data used in this study are discrete electrocardiogram data text files, namely amplitude (mV) as an integer function (N). Discrete data is a continuous analog signal that is sampled at a certain frequency using an Analog to Digital converter (ADC) device [28]. Table 2 shows discrete 12 lead data from sampling at a frequency of 250 Hz during a 10 s examination that the author got from the Cardiovascular care unit (CVCU) RSSA Malang Sampling at a frequency of 250 Hz is defined as the amount of data collected in 1 s as many as 250 samples, so for examination for 10 s there are 2500 sample data, where each integer represents a duration of 4 ms [29].

The data processing is carried out in three stages, namely the stage of determining the peak R value for each cycle, the stage of determining the duration of the cycle, and the stage of determining the peak value of PQST. Figure 3 shows the three-stage flow diagram and Fig. 4 illustrates the Voltage threshold, dR and Position peak P, Q, S, T determination.

### *2.1 Determination of Peak R Value in Each Cycle*

In this stage the amplitude value of 0.6 mV is the threshold for the peak area of R lead II. This value has taken into account the Pmax value and Tmax value for abnormal conditions as well as the minimum limit for the peak R value. Grouping of value data is carried out if there are more than 1 peak R values with a duration of 4 ms, which is then filtered by the one with the highest value maximum. One maximum value in each group is the peak value of R which represents each cycle. Determination of the

**Table 2** Data sample ecg discrete 12 lead

| Integer (N) | Lead (mV) | | | | | | | | | | | |
|---|---|---|---|---|---|---|---|---|---|---|---|---|
| | I | II | III | aVR | aVL | aVF | V1 | V2 | V3 | V4 | V5 | V6 |
| 1 | −0.199 | −0.382 | −0.183 | 0.291 | −0.008 | −0.282 | 0.004 | −0.141 | −0.323 | −0.293 | 0.059 | 0.029 |
| 2 | −0.211 | −0.386 | −0.175 | 0.298 | −0.018 | −0.280 | 0.006 | −0.146 | −0.327 | −0.296 | 0.055 | 0.027 |
| 3 | −0.225 | −0.395 | −0.170 | 0.310 | −0.028 | −0.282 | 0.006 | −0.150 | −0.329 | −0.295 | 0.055 | 0.026 |
| 4 | −0.238 | −0.405 | −0.167 | 0.321 | −0.036 | −0.286 | 0.002 | −0.157 | −0.333 | −0.293 | 0.057 | 0.025 |
| 5 | −0.246 | −0.411 | −0.165 | 0.328 | −0.041 | −0.288 | −0.004 | −0.166 | −0.339 | −0.292 | 0.059 | 0.025 |
| 6 | −0.247 | −0.414 | −0.167 | 0.330 | −0.040 | −0.290 | −0.007 | −0.175 | −0.344 | −0.293 | 0.062 | 0.025 |
| 7 | −0.242 | −0.415 | −0.174 | 0.328 | −0.034 | −0.294 | −0.009 | −0.183 | −0.349 | −0.297 | 0.064 | 0.027 |
| 8 | −0.233 | −0.419 | −0.187 | 0.326 | −0.023 | −0.303 | −0.008 | −0.187 | −0.353 | −0.301 | 0.065 | 0.029 |
| 9 | −0.226 | −0.425 | −0.200 | 0.325 | −0.013 | −0.312 | −0.008 | −0.190 | −0.357 | −0.306 | 0.063 | 0.033 |
| 10 | −0.226 | −0.432 | −0.206 | 0.329 | −0.010 | −0.319 | −0.010 | −0.195 | −0.365 | −0.314 | 0.059 | 0.035 |
| 11 | −0.231 | −0.435 | −0.204 | 0.333 | −0.014 | −0.320 | −0.017 | −0.204 | −0.376 | −0.324 | 0.053 | 0.033 |
| 12 | −0.234 | −0.428 | −0.195 | 0.331 | −0.019 | −0.312 | −0.027 | −0.215 | −0.389 | −0.333 | 0.047 | 0.029 |
| 13 | −0.232 | −0.415 | −0.183 | 0.324 | −0.025 | −0.299 | −0.033 | −0.222 | −0.396 | −0.336 | 0.044 | 0.024 |
| ‘’ | ‘’ | ‘’ | ‘’ | ‘’ | ‘’ | ‘’ | ‘’ | ‘’ | ‘’ | ‘’ | ‘’ | ‘’ |
| 2500 | −0.231 | −0.348 | −0.116 | 0.290 | −0.058 | −0.232 | 0.095 | −0.118 | −0.227 | −0.204 | −0.131 | −0.105 |

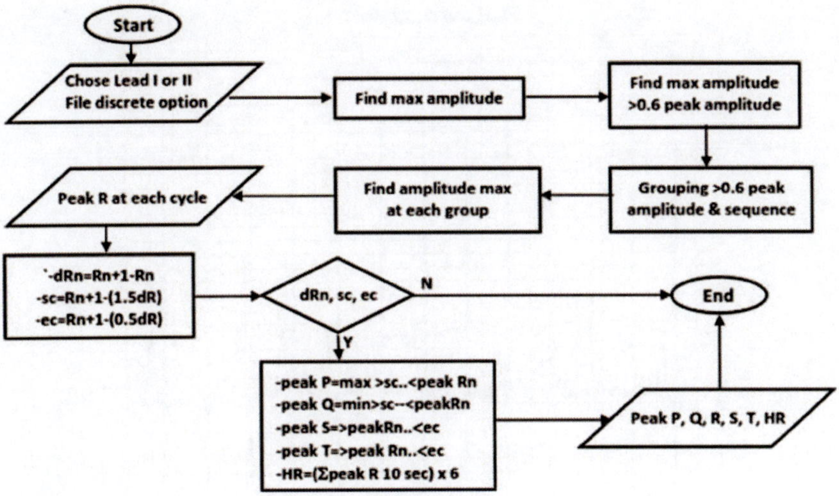


**Fig. 3** Flowchart of finding peak amplitude and heart rate

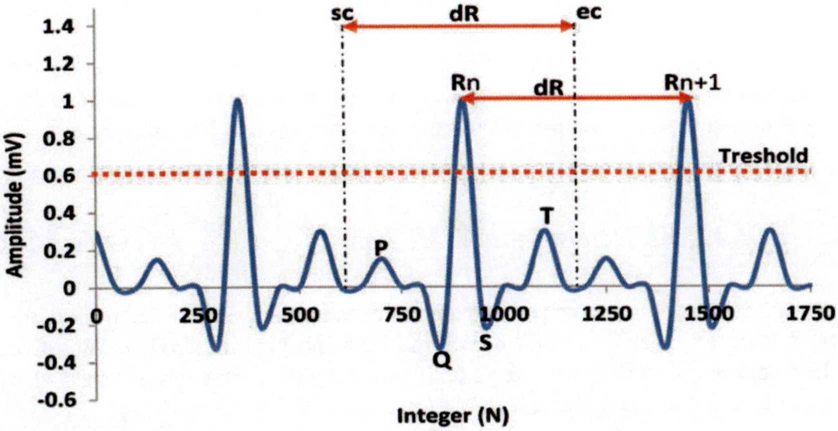


**Fig. 4** Voltage threshold, dR and position peak P, Q, S, T determination

threshold to obtain the peak R value is illustrated in Fig. 4. After obtaining the peak R value, the duration between peak R and the next peak R is dR.

## 2.2 *Method of Determining Cycle Duration*

Determination of the cycle is to determine the position of the beginning and end of the wave in 1 period. In each cycle, the beginning of the wave is the position of the

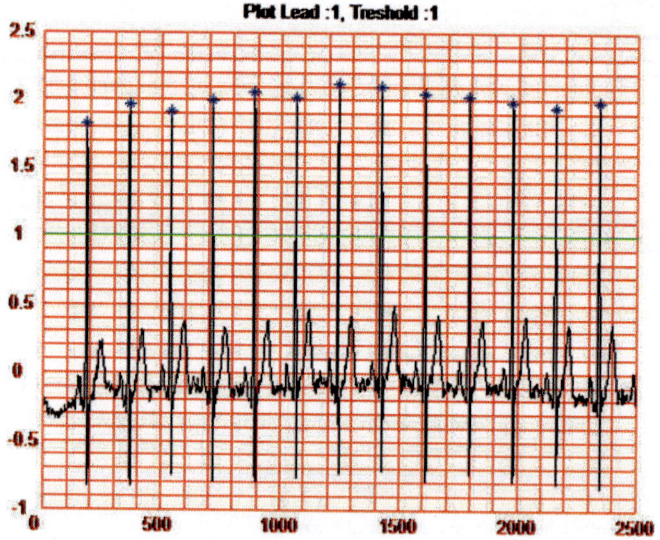


**Fig. 5** Masd-250-1 lead I record cardiogram presentation

starting point (sc, start cycle) and the end of the wave is the position of the end point (ec, end cycle), obtained by moving forward dR by 0.5 dR from the peak of R so that the position of the start of the cycle and the end of the cycle is Nsc and Nec.

### 2.3 *PQST Peak Determination Method*

The maximum and minimum positive amplitude values between sc and peak R are peak P values and peak Q values, while the maximum positive and maximum negative values between peak R and ec are peak S values and peak T values. Figure 5 also shows the initial position (sc) and end of wave (ec).

## 3 Result and Discussion

Sample data used in this study is secondary data, namely 10 samples of text electrocardiogram data from CVCU Saiful Anwar Hospital (RSSA) Malang with an examination time of 10 s. The sample data are records masd-250-1, masd-250-2, masd-250-3, masd-250-4, masd-250-5, masd-250-6, masd-250-7, masd-250-8, masd-250-9, masd-250-10.

Figure 5 shows the cardiogram of the MATLAB program for the sample masd-250-1 lead I at a threshold of 1 mV, while Fig. 6 shows the morphological cardiogram

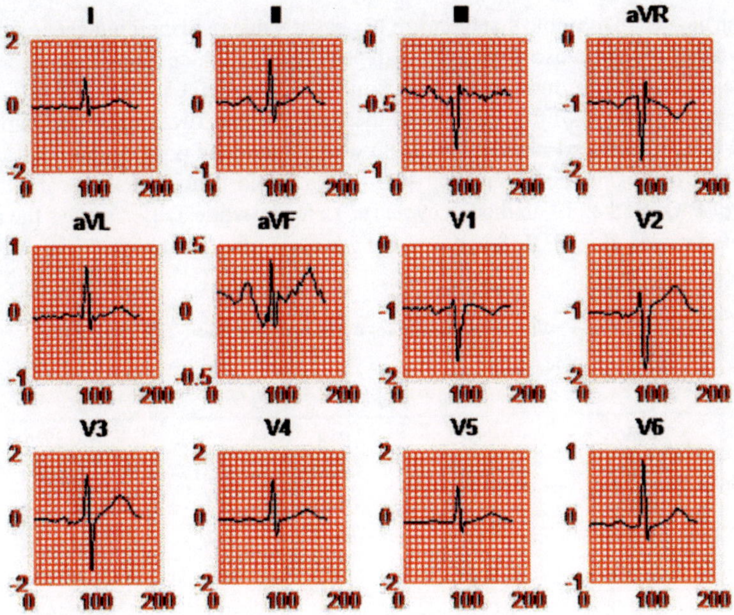


**Fig. 6** The morphology of each lead wave at the 5th masd-250-1 record

of 12 leads in the 5th cycle for the sample masd-250-1.

Table 3 shows the peak R value, the integer position of the peak R value (N), the initial position (Nsc) and the end of the wave (Nec) in each cycle.

**Table 3** The number of masd-250-1 cycle records is based on the peak R on the 1.0 mV threshold

| Cycle | N | Peak R | dR | Nsc | Nec |
|---|---|---|---|---|---|
| 1 | 184 | 1.816 | 179 | 95 | 274 |
| 2 | 363 | 1.960 | 176 | 275 | 451 |
| 3 | 539 | 1.907 | 173 | 453 | 626 |
| 4 | 712 | 1.998 | 175 | 635 | 800 |
| 5 | 887 | 2.059 | 175 | 800 | 975 |
| 6 | 1062 | 2.015 | 178 | 973 | 1151 |
| 7 | 1240 | 2.119 | 181 | 1150 | 1331 |
| 8 | 1421 | 2.092 | 185 | 1329 | 1514 |
| 9 | 1606 | 2.043 | 184 | 1514 | 1698 |
| 10 | 1790 | 2.026 | 185 | 1698 | 1883 |
| 11 | 1975 | 1.987 | 183 | 1884 | 2067 |
| 12 | 2158 | 1.939 | 184 | 2066 | 2250 |
| 13 | 2342 | 1.963 | −2342 | 3513 | 1171 |

It can be seen in the table that there are 13 peak R values and their integer positions, but dR is negative because there is no 14th peak R and its integer position. The peak R value is obtained from the maximum value in each group of amplitude values. N is the integer position of the presence of the peak R value. dR is the duration of the peak R (Rn) to the next peak R (Rn + 1) while Nsc is the position of the starting point of the cycle obtained from NRn + 1 − NRn. Table 4 shows the peak amplitude values of P, Q, R, S and T in the 5th cycle for 12 leads, while Table 5 shows the peak amplitude values of P, Q, R, S and T in the 5th cycle for all samples.

**Table 4** The peak PQRST value for each lead for cycle 5.sample masd-250-1

| Lead | Peak amplitude (mV) | | | | |
|---|---|---|---|---|---|
| | P | Q | R | S | T |
| I | 0.0366 | −0.2556 | 2.059 | −0.7993 | 0.3911 |
| II | 0.2351 | −0.1507 | 1.327 | −0.5174 | 0.4930 |
| III | 0.1985 | 0.1049 | −0.674 | 0.2819 | 0.1019 |
| aVR | −0.1358 | 0.2032 | 1.367 | 0.6584 | −0.4420 |
| aVL | −0.0609 | −0.1803 | −1.722 | −0.5406 | 0.1446 |
| aVF | 0.2168 | −0.0229 | 0.376 | −0.1178 | 0.2975 |
| V1 | −0.0833 | 0.2163 | 0.319 | −0.5319 | −0.1232 |
| V2 | −0.0945 | 0.0440 | 0.509 | −1.5206 | 0.6092 |
| V3 | 0.0178 | −0.0090 | 1.333 | −1.5931 | 0.6239 |
| V4 | −0.1033 | −0.1889 | 2.817 | −1.4838 | 0.4942 |
| V5 | −0.2919 | −0.4168 | 2.364 | −1.2162 | 0.2272 |
| V6 | −0.1234 | −0.3006 | 1.706 | −0.7413 | 0.1949 |

**Table 5** The value of peak amplitude lead II in cycle 5 for the RSSA sample

| Sample | Peak P | Peak Q | Peak R | Peak S | Peak T |
|---|---|---|---|---|---|
| Masd-250-1 | 0.225 | −0.176 | 1.385 | −0.517 | 0.451 |
| Masd-250-2 | 0.092 | −0.140 | 1.987 | −0.240 | 0.205 |
| Masd-250-3 | 0.032 | −0.145 | 1.715 | −0.245 | 0.386 |
| Masd-250-4 | 0.073 | −0.075 | 1.162 | −0.482 | 0.421 |
| Masd-250-5 | 0.078 | −0.154 | 1.348 | −0.717 | 0.290 |
| Masd-250-6 | −0.054 | −0.148 | 1.122 | −0.257 | 0.510 |
| Masd-250-7 | 0.015 | −0.176 | 0.842 | −0.129 | 0.216 |
| Masd-250-8 | 0.114 | −0.554 | 2.209 | −0.561 | 0.273 |
| Masd-250-9 | 0.001 | −0.099 | 0.408 | −0.708 | 0.251 |
| Masd-250-10 | 0.067 | −0.199 | 0.811 | −0.439 | 0.268 |

## 4 Conclusion

The proposed method can be used to obtain the peak amplitude R and R-R duration (dR) in each cycle. The obtained cycle duration (dR), the minimum value between the initial position of the cycle (Nsc) to the peak R position is the peak Q value, while the minimum value between the peak R position and the end position of the cycle (Nec) is the peak S value. maximum amplitude between the initial position of the cycle to the peak position of Q, while the peak value of T is obtained from the maximum amplitude value between the position of peak S to the position of the end of the cycle (Nec). Obtaining peak amplitude values in each cycle, it is possible no longer needed manual calculations using boxes on ecg paper so that interpretation time and diagnosis time can be faster.

This study still has shortcomings, namely (i) not using discrete ecg samples for abnormal heart conditions, therefore this research can be continued for conditions such as arrhythmia, coronary, ischemia, myocardial infarction, with a larger number of samples, (ii) the proposed method not tested using discrete ecg data from Physionet, including discrete ecg samples with varying sampling frequency.

## References


1. Chia B (2000) Cninical electrocardiography, 3rd edn. World Scientific, New Jersey
2. De Luna AB (2012) Clinical electrocardiography, a textbook, 4th edn. Barcelona, Spain: Wiley-Blackwell
3. Setiawidayat S, Rahman AY (Nov 2018) New method for obtaining peak value R and the duration of each cycle of electrocardiogram. In: 2018 international conference on sustainable information engineering and technology (SIET). Malang, Indonesia, pp 77–81. https://doi.org/10.1109/SIET.2018.8693151
4. Guyton AC, Hall JE (2006) Textbook of medical physiology, 11th edn. Elsevier Saundes, Mississippi
5. Setiawidayat S, Sakti S, Sargowo D (2016) Determining the ECG 1 cycle wave using discrete data. J Theor Appl Inf Technol 88(1):8
6. Goldberger AL (2006) Clinical electrocardiography, 7th edn. Mosby, Elsevier
7. John RH (2003) The ECG in practice, 4th edn. Churchill Livingstone An imprint of Elsevier Science Limited, Notingham UK
8. Iaizzo PA (2005) Handbook of cardiac anatomy, physiology, and devices, ANSI Z39.48-1984 (American National Standards Institute). Totowa, New Jersey 07512: © 2005 Humana Press Inc.
9. Natale A (2007) Handbook of cardiac electrophysiology. Informa healtcare UK Ltd
10. Clifford GD, Azuaje F, McSharry PE (2006) Advanced methods and tools for ECG data analysis. Artech House, Boston-London
11. Bhatti AT, Kim JH (Sep 2015) R-peak detection in ECG signal compression for heartbeat rate patients at 1 kHz using high order statistic algorithm. J Multidiciplinary Eng Sci Technol JMEST 2(9):7
12. Khamis H, Weiss R, Xie Y, Chang CW, Lovell NH, Redmond SJ (2016) QRS detection algorithm for telehealth electrocardiogram recordings. IEEE Trans Biomed Eng 63(7):1377–1388. https://doi.org/10.1109/TBME.2016.2549060

13. Amri MF, Rizqyawan MI, Turnip A (Oct 2016) ECG signal processing using offline-wavelet transform method based on ECG-IoT device. In: 2016 3rd international conference on information technology, computer, and electrical engineering (ICITACEE). pp 1–6. https://doi.org/10.1109/ICITACEE.2016.7892404
14. Qin Q, Li J, Yue Y, Liu C (2017) An adaptive and time-efficient ECG R-peak detection algorithm. J Healthc Eng 2017:1–14. https://doi.org/10.1155/2017/5980541
15. Setiawidayat S (Sep 2017) Software design for the representation of parameter values of electrocardiogram 12-lead, 4th international conference advance molecular bioscience biomedical engineering ICAMBBE. vol 4. p 6
16. Setiawidayat S, Iman Putri S (Oct 2016) Filtering data Diskrit Elektrokardiogram untuk penentuan PQRST dalam satu Siklus, Sentia 2016-Politek. Negeri Malang. vol 8. p 8
17. Setiawidayat S (2021) Correlation of peak amplitude ECG between leads based on the condition of the heart. Clin Med 08(02):11
18. Setiawidayat S (2020) Improved Information on heart examination results uses a 12-lead discrete electrocardiograph. Eur J Electr Eng Comput Sci 4(1):8
19. Setiawidayat S, Rahman AY, Hidayati R (2020) Deteksi Puncak Amplitudo dan Durasi Gelombang QRS Elektrokardiogram Menggunakan discrete data. J Rekayasa Sist Teknol Inf RESTI, 4(3):9. https://doi.org/10.29207/resti.v4i3.1658
20. Hamdi S, Ben Abdallah A, Bedoui MH (Dec 2017) Real time QRS complex detection using DFA and regular grammar. Biomed Eng OnLine 16(1). https://doi.org/10.1186/s12938-017-0322-2
21. Kaur H, Rajni R (2017) Electrocardiogram signal analysis for R-peak detection and denoising with hybrid linearization and principal component analysis. Turk J Electr Eng Comput Sci 13. https://doi.org/10.3906/elk-1604-84
22. Maršánová L, Němcová A, Smíšek R, Vítek M, Smital L (2019) Advanced P wave detection in ecg signals during pathology: evaluation in different arrhythmia contexts. Sci Rep 9(1):19053. https://doi.org/10.1038/s41598-019-55323-3
23. Gupta V, Mittal M (2020) Efficient R-peak detection in electrocardiogram signal based on features extracted using hilbert transform and burg method. J Inst Eng India Ser B 101(1):23–34. https://doi.org/10.1007/s40031-020-00423-2
24. Yu Q, Liu A, Liu T, Mao Y, Chen W, Liu H (2019) ECG R-wave peaks marking with simultaneously recorded continuous blood pressure. PLoS ONE 14(3):e0214443. https://doi.org/10.1371/journal.pone.0214443
25. Fahira Adriati S, Setiawidayat S, Rofii F (June. 2021) Identification Of ECG signal by using backpropagation neural network. J Phys Conf Ser 1908(1):012014. https://doi.org/10.1088/1742-6596/1908/1/012014
26. Physionet M-B. http://www.physionet.org/physiobank/database/mitdb. https://archive.physionet.org/cgi-bin/atm/ATM
27. Setiawidayat S (2019) Komparasi Hasil Pemeriksaan Jantung antara perangkat ECGs dan ECGd menggunakan Uji Mann-Whitney. Conference innovation applied science technology ciastech-2019, vol 2. p 8
28. Webster JG (2010) Medical instrumentation, application and design, 4th edn. Wiley Inc., Wisconsin-Madison
29. Prutchi D, Norris M (2005) Design and development of medical electronic instrumentation, vol 1. Wiley Inc., New Jersey

# Design and Implementation of Urine Glucose Measurements Based on Color Density

**Dian Neipa Purnamasari, Miftachul Ulum, Riza Alfita, Haryanto, Rika Rokhana, and Hendhi Hermawan**

**Abstract** Increasing community routines lead to lifestyle changes such as the selection of fast food for time efficiency. Fast food is synonymous with non-nutritional foods (only a small amount of nutrients) that have a high content of sugars, calories, salts, and additives to increase the risk of various diseases. Too high sugar content in the body can cause the risk of diabetes, the risk of heart disease, obesity, etc. This paper describes the design of a system of measuring urine glucose based on color density. The addition of a standard solution of glucose in urine is used to determine urine glucose levels through urine color. Discoloration of urine is detected using the TCS3200 color sensor connected to the microcontroller. The color readings will be matched with the RGB color interpretation that best suits the standard urine color in the laboratory. Based on the results of system testing, two of the five tested patients had the same glucose levels between the laboratory results and the proposed system. However, on the urine color reading, the two patients had different results, namely orange and cloudy yellow. In conclusion, the difference in color between the two patients was due to the limited range of yellow readings on the sensor, but this did not affect the determination of glucose levels in the urine. The proposed system cannot replace the results of laboratory tests, but can be used as a tool for the early detection of glucose levels in urine at a faster time.

**Keywords** Urine · Glucose level · Color density

D. N. Purnamasari (✉) · M. Ulum · R. Alfita · Haryanto
Universitas Trunojoyo Madura, Jawa Timur, Indonesia
e-mail: dian.neipa@trunojoyo.ac.id

R. Rokhana · H. Hermawan
Politeknik Elektronika Negeri Surabaya, Surabaya, Indonesia



T. Triwiyanto et al. (eds.), *Proceedings of the 2nd International Conference on Electronics, Biomedical Engineering, and Health Informatics*, Lecture Notes in Electrical Engineering 898, https://doi.org/10.1007/978-981-19-1804-9_9

# 1 Introduction

In the normal condition of the human body, urine does not contain glucose as there are organs in charge to absorb glucose and return it to circulation. The presence of glucose in the urine can indicate several diseases, including diabetes, kidney, etc. Generally, to detect diabetes, blood glucose tests are used, but urine tests can also be used to indicate or monitor the presence of glucose in the body. The urine method has the advantage of being painless and less expensive for diabetics. The International Diabetes Federation (IDF) organization estimates that in 2019, there are 463 million people in the world suffering from diabetes and this number is predicted to continue to increase to reach 700 million people in 2045. Indonesia, which belongs to the Southeast Asia region is ranked 7th with the highest number of sufferers, so it can be estimated magnitude of Indonesia's contribution to diabetes cases in Southeast Asia [1].

Several studies discuss the level of glucose in the urine [2–25]. There are several ways to determine the presence of glucose in the urine, one of which is using a substance in the reagent which will change its nature and color when reduced by glucose. A urine glucose test can be performed using a reduction reaction with Fehling's solution, Benedict's, and Clinitest. While the other method uses an enzymatic reaction with the dipstick method [14]. Fadhilah and Vanawati in their research compared the reaction of glucose reduction in urine between the Benedict method heated by Fire Methylation with 100° water bath [15]. The results obtained two methods do not affect the presence or absence of glucose content in the urine, but the method used affects the time of the process. Sufia and Fikri in their research compared differences in urine glucose levels, using several methods by adding vitamin C [16]. The result is the addition of vitamin C to the test solution, causing discoloration and positive glucose results in the urine. Some factors that can affect the results of glucose levels in the urine include the influence of drugs, stress conditions, cigarettes, heavy bags before the examination, and non-sugar substances that can reduce such as formaldehyde [17]. Ghosh et al., their research discussing how to provide an automated system that can help diabetic patients in controlling blood sugar [18]. The proposed system uses image processing and fuzzy methods. The results obtained the accuracy of the proposed system reached 96.93% to assist diabetic patients in controlling and monitoring sugar levels in the body. Ahada et al. in their research proposed a tool to measure urine color using the TCS3200 color sensor [19]. The method used to detect urine color is Artificial Neural Network. This is done to facilitate the detection of urine color without the need for laboratory testing. The proposed system uses a TCS3200 sensor, Arduino Uno, Relay, urine container, and an electric stove. The results obtained are the proposed system can detect blood sugar levels in the urine with a success percentage of 90%. Listyalina et al. in their research proposed a new method for analyzing urine color changes using the reaction of Benedict's solution [20]. The interpretation of the urine color used takes into account the intensity of the RGB color. To get the reaction of Benedict's solution, the authors' heat enters the urine that has been given Benedict's solution into boiling water for 5 min, then the solution is shaken to get the color of the urine. The results of color readings were matched with glucose levels in standard laboratory tests, and it was found that out of 10 urine sample tests used had the same results as glucose levels in laboratory tests. Rahmat et al., proposed a urine color strip reading system using a scanner [21]. The method used is Euclidean Distance, Otsu, and RGB Color Extraction. This method is used to match the color of urine with a standard reference urine examination. The results obtained are the higher the resolution of the scanner used, the higher the accuracy of the urine color reading. Lidia et al. proposed computer-based diabetes, detection, and monitoring system [22]. Detection of diabetes is proposed using urine strips. The results of the urine strip reading will be detected using a color sensor that is adjusted to RGB color. The proposed system uses a fuzzy method to group RGB colors. The results obtained are that there are significant differences between the proposed system and laboratory testing. Ghosh et al. proposed an automated urine blood sugar estimation in a toilet system [23]. Urine color estimation uses fuzzy logic obtained from research data sets. The results obtained are that the proposed system can control high blood sugar levels through regular urine monitoring. Gahan et al., proposed a portable tool for early detection of chronic kidney disease using urine strips, TCS3200, and a microcontroller [24]. The proposed system detects color changes to detect albumin in the urine. The colors detected are green and yellow which indicate the presence or absence of albumin in the urine. The proposed study is a urine glucose level detection system adapted from the research of Ahada, et al. [19] and Listyalina, et al. [20]. In previous studies using manual heating by heating on an electric stove until it changes color or heating in boiling water and then shaking until it changes color. Furthermore, this study also uses the same comparison technique as the study [20] by validating the results using standard laboratory testing.

In this paper, we propose a tool to detect glucose in the urine based on urine color. Glucose in urine can be determined by adding Benedict's solution to change the nature and color of urine. The reduction method is done by heating the urine that has been given Benedict's solution using Peltier. Changes in urine color are detected using a color sensor and the results are sent to a smartphone via Bluetooth. The advantage of the proposed tool is that it is easy to carry, does not depend on the intensity of the room light because the color sensor has a LED, and this tool can provide information from the results of urine color readings. The urine color results obtained are in the form of RGB colors which are arranged in such a way as to approach the actual urine color.

## 2 Materials and Method

This section describes the planning steps along with making a system consisting of hardware design and software design. The hardware components consist of a microcontroller, color sensor, Peltier, temperature sensor, Bluetooth, and LCD. While software design consists of designing a user interface using a smartphone. The block diagram of the proposed system configuration is shown in Fig. 1.

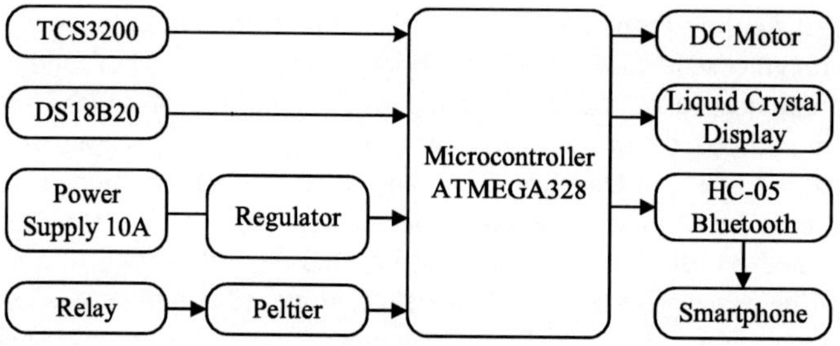


**Fig. 1** Block diagram of the proposed system

Figure 1 presents the overall system for making a urine glucose level, detection device using urine color readings. The microcontroller is the unit that controls the entire system functions to process data received from the color sensor (TCS3200) and temperature sensor (DS18B20). Data from the temperature sensor will affect whether or not the DC motor and Peltier are active. The DC motor is used as a stirrer head in the solution stirrer to be tested, while the Peltier is used as a solution heater. DC motor and Peltier stop working when the temperature is 40 °C. There is a change in the color of the urine that is captured by the color sensor. The results of the data obtained from the color sensor are the red, green, and blue values that will be sent and displayed on the LCD and the android application. Data communication between the microcontroller and android is done using Bluetooth. In the android application, the color results obtained will be interpreted according to the color of urine in a standard laboratory. To validate the tested urine data, before starting the test, the urine sample will be divided into two samples, namely as urine samples for the proposed device, and sent to the laboratory to be tested with a standard urine examination process.

## 2.1 *Hardware Design and Manufacture*

The design and manufacture of hardware describe the minimum system design and color sensor design. In this research the micro-controller used is ATMega328. While the color sensor used is TCS3200.

**Minimum System Design and Manufacturing**

This research requires 19 I/O pins which are realized using the AT-Mega328 which has 29 I/O pins. To make a microcontroller chip can work, a minimum circuit is needed. In making a minimum system, several supporting circuits are needed, including a reset circuit, an oscillator circuit, and a regulator circuit.

The microcontroller chip requires a reset to return the chip to its original state. In the reset circuit that was made, a 10 k resistor was added to limit the current flowing in the circuit. The input voltage required for this reset circuit is 5 V according to the minimum required input voltage of the system. In the minimum system circuit, an

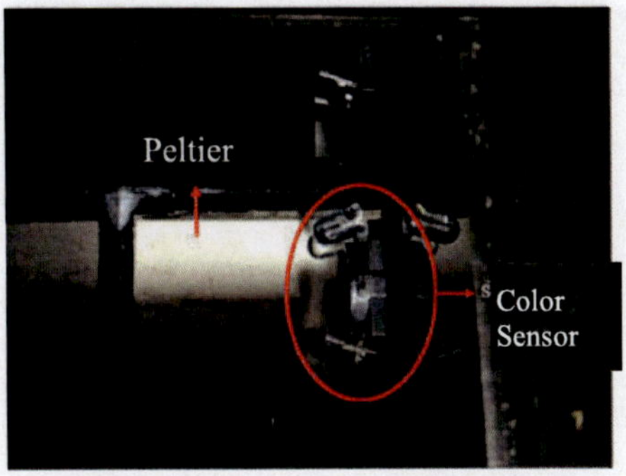


**Fig. 2** Color sensor placement

oscillator circuit is needed to generate a frequency in the microcontroller. Determination of the capacitor used is adjusted to the oscillator operating mode at the minimum system. The design of the regulator is required to change the input voltage according to the minimum required voltage of the system. In this research, the regulator circuit made is a 5 V regulator using a linear regulator such as the LM7805.

**Color Sensor Design TCS3200**

The TCS3200 color sensor has a photodetector array. The filters of each color are evenly distributed throughout the array to eliminate locations between colors. Internal to an oscillator device that produces a square wave output of a frequency proportional to the intensity of the selected color. In this research, the color sensor was placed on the side of the test glass. This is because the distance of the color sensor used is 1 cm to get maximum results. The placement of the color sensor is shown in Fig. 2.

## 2.2 *Software Design and Development*

In the android application that was made, Bluetooth was used as a data transmission medium. The first thing to do is to turn on Bluetooth to start pairing with the detector. After successfully activated, the information received will be matched with the information that has been stored in the application. Then the results will be displayed on the user's android screen. The information displayed on the android application is information on urine color, glucose levels, and status in the form of diabetes or not. The flow diagram of the system work program for the android application is shown in Fig. 3.

In the android application made 7 layers have different functions. The first layer is used as a splash screen, which is the first display that appears before the main menu of the application. This layer has a delay of 1 s before entering the next layer. Next, after the splash screen layer, a second layer will appear where this layer will ask for permission to activate Bluetooth on Android first. Next, the blank space displays the menu buttons of the paired devices. That button serves to display Bluetooth that has

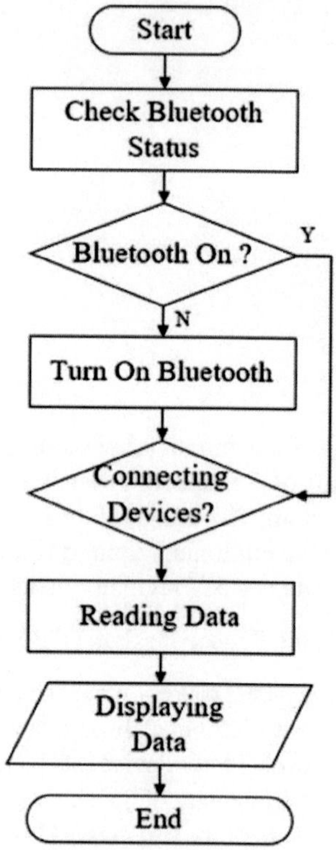


**Fig. 3** Program design on android

been connected to Android. To enter the next layer, select Bluetooth HC-05. This is because this application is designed only for data exchange in Bluetooth HC-05 which has SPP 00,001,101-0000-1000-8000-00805F9B34FB. SPP on Bluetooth is a Serial Port Protocol that functions to convert serial ports to Bluetooth. If the Bluetooth HC-05 is connected, a message will appear in the form of the words "Connected", otherwise if the Bluetooth is pressed instead of the Bluetooth HC-05, the message "Connection Failed" will appear. Is it a Bluetooth SPP? Try again.". Once connected, the main menu of the program will appear. The main menu display in the application is shown in Fig. 4.

Figure 4 shows that this layer has 4 buttons each connected to another layer. Like the Back button, this button serves to return to the second layer to disconnect the Bluetooth connection with Android. While the other three buttons will connect to the next layer that contains information related to diabetes mellitus such as the effects of diabetes, how to avoid diabetes, and how to regulate the state of the body when you have diabetes mellitus. The last layer is the layer that contains information about the detected urine color. There is a color sequence that indicates a person has diabetes or not. The color of this urine can be influenced by the food consumed every day. So this color is just a tool.

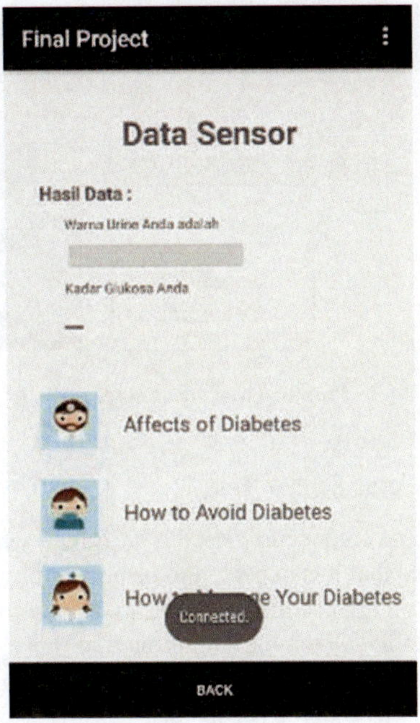


**Fig. 4** Main menu display when connected by bluetooth

## 3 Result

This section discusses the testing of the proposed system. The purpose of this test and analysis is to determine the success of all the tools and programs that have been designed. Testing is carried out on each part first, then each part is tested as a whole. After the testing and data collection process, the next step is to analyze the test results. The reference used in the analysis process is the data obtained during the planning process and also the data from the theoretical analysis.

### *3.1 Hardware Testing*

In this research, a series of hardware and software used in the system has been created. The following are the results of the hardware that has been made to support the performance of the system. The hardware circuit that has been made in this final project consists of a minimum ATMega328 system, a DS18B20 circuit, and a Peltier circuit. In addition, additional equipment is needed to support the performance of this system, including color sensors, temperature sensors, DC motors, and 12 V 10 A switching supplies. The results of the hardware configuration that have been made are shown in Fig. 5.

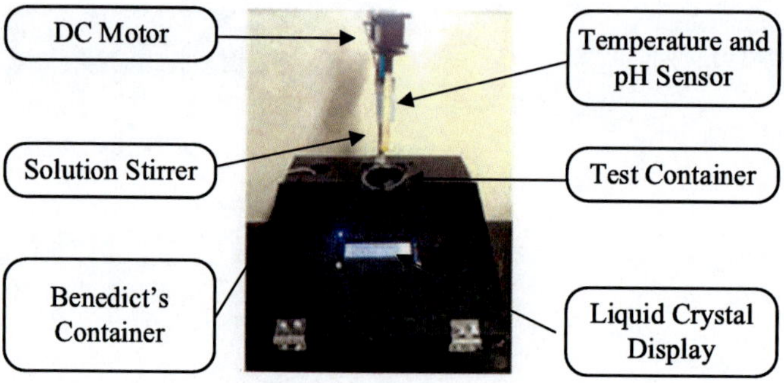


**Fig. 5** Proposed tool creation results

## Color Sensor Test

The color sensor used is TCS3200 which in this research is used to detect urine color so that it is expected to be able to indicate the presence of glucose. The test this time did not use urine but used several other color solutions that matched the urine color table. Given the importance of this tool, it is necessary to test. The schematic of the TCS3200 color sensor test circuit can be seen in Fig. 6.

The color sensor test is carried out according to the scheme in Fig. 6. Before starting the test, we prepared four colored liquids as in Fig. 7. Then, the color sensor is pointed at each colored liquid. The distance between the sensor and the object is ±1.5 cm. The results of the sensor readings will be compared with the colors that appear on the android application.

From the test results, it can be seen that four-color samples were used, namely red, orange, yellow, and green. For each color that has been tested, the color of the test results corresponds to the color received on android. So, it can be said that the color sensor used can detect the color of the liquid very well. The results of color sensor test can be seen in Fig. 8.

**Fig. 6** TCS3200 color sensor testing circuit scheme

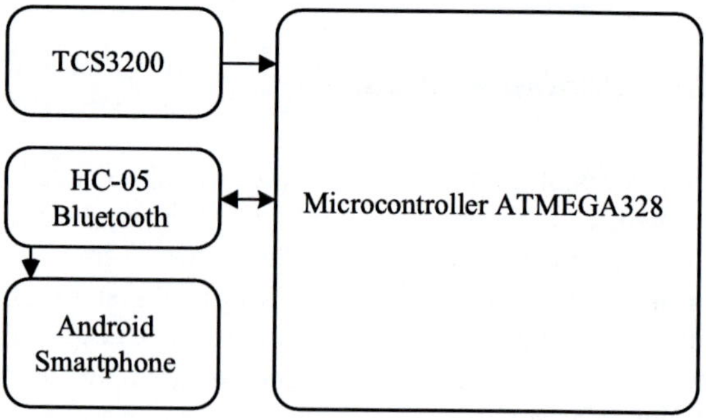

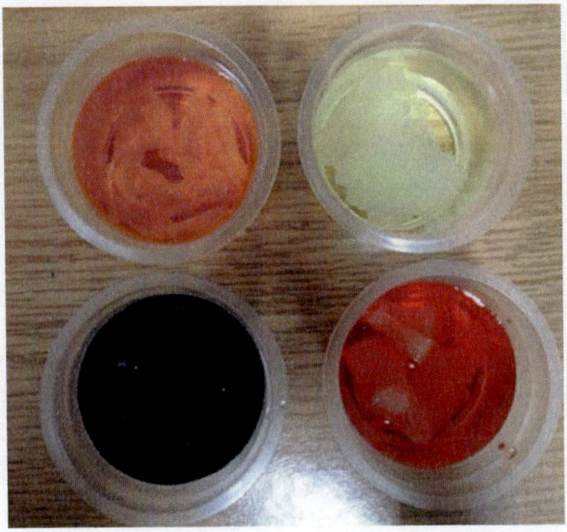

Fig. 7 Colored liquid

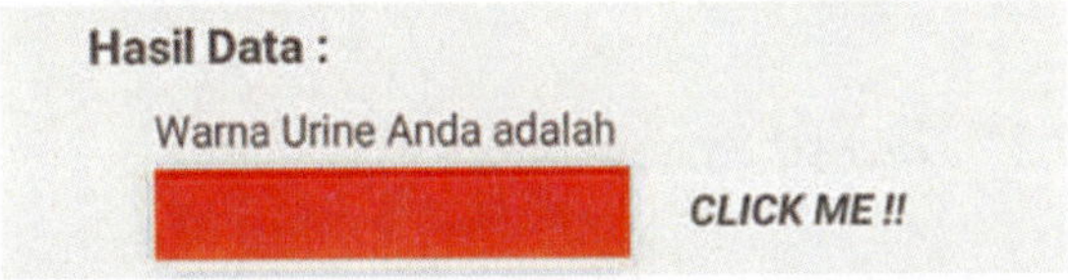


Fig. 8 Red color reading results on android apps

## Urine Color Test

In this test, the TCS3200 color sensor was used to determine the level of precision of the sensor on the color gradation of urine, especially yellow and orange. Given the importance of this tool, it is necessary to test. Based on the results of the urine color test, measurement values are obtained as in Table 1. In Table 1, it can be seen that the color of urine used is the color of urine in general. Clear urine and light yellow urine are urine conditions when the user consumes too much water so that the

Table 1 Urine color test results

| Color | Reading results on android | |
|---|---|---|
| | Color | Glucose level |
| Clear | White | Negative |
| Light yellow | Yellow | Negative |
| Yellow | Yellow | Negative |
| Cloudy yellow | Orange | Positive (+2) |
| Light orange | Orange | Positive (+2) |
| Orange | Orange | Positive (+2) |
| Cloudy orange | Red | Positive (+3) |

**Table 2** Overall system test results

| Name | Color | | Glucose level | |
|---|---|---|---|---|
| | Color | Lab | Tool | Lab |
| Patient 1 | Yellow | Clear yellow | Negative | Negative |
| Patient 2 | Yellow | Clear yellow | Negative | Negative |
| Patient 3 | Yellow | Clear yellow | Negative | Negative |
| Patient 4 | Orange | Cloudy yellow | Positive (+2) | Positive (+2) |
| Patient 5 | Orange | Cloudy yellow | Positive (+2) | Positive (+2) |

urine produced has a lot of water content. Yellow urine is the color of normal urine in general. While other urine colors are the color of urine when the user consumes too little water. The condition of urine turning cloudy yellow to orange can also be caused by the user taking drugs so that for the accuracy of decision making, further examination can be carried out in the laboratory. In the test results, it was found that the color sensor used can distinguish the color of urine for people with diabetes mellitus with the color classification in Table 1.

### 3.2 *Overall System Test*

Based on the testing of the entire system that has been made, the test results data are shown in Table 2. The test results above indicate that the results of the tools in this research were compared with the data from the results of tests in the laboratory. The parameters used in testing the whole system are color parameters and glucose levels. While the parameter used to decide whether there is an indication of diabetes or not in this research is glucose levels, so if the user has a positive glucose level, it can be interpreted that the user indicates diabetes mellitus.

Based on the test results of the entire system, the comparison of color readings and glucose levels in five patients tested was by laboratory tests. Two of the five patients tested indicated diabetes mellitus. Based on the laboratory results, it was found that the two patients had a positive glucose level (+2) with a cloudy yellow urine color, but from the system test results, the urine color reading was orange. This color difference is due to the limited range of yellow readings on the sensor, but this does not affect the determination of glucose levels in urine.

## 4 Discussion

In this work, we propose the design of a urine glucose level measurement tool based on urine color. One way to determine the presence of glucose in the urine is to add Benedict's solution to a urine sample. The addition of Benedict's solution to the urine sample is done manually. The design of the proposed tool has a Peltier component as a solution heater and a DC motor as a solution stirrer (solution homogenization) that can work simultaneously. When the device is activated, the Peltier component and DC motor will be active. The Peltier will heat the urine solution until the solution temperature reaches 40 °C and the DC motor will continue to stir the urine solution. Both components will stop working when the temperature sensor reading is more than 40 °C. This is because, in the process of heating the solution, a temperature of 40 °C is required for the sample being tested for the reduction process to occur [25]. Furthermore, color detection is carried out using a TCS3200 color sensor. The results of reading color data in the form of red, green, and blue values will be sent to the smartphone to be converted into urine colors according to standard laboratory references. The colors that system can get are white, yellow, orange, and red. While the urine color reference in standard laboratories are clear, light yellow, yellow, cloudy yellow, orange, cloudy orange, and red. The color of clear urine is interpreted as white in the proposed tool, this is because the TCS3200 color sensor has a super bright LED which is used to read the light intensity value. The urine color which is light yellow and yellow in the proposed device is interpreted to be yellow. The cloudy yellow and orange colors in the proposed tool are interpreted as orange. The cloudy orange and red colors in the proposed tool are interpreted as red. However, our proposed device design has limitations on urine color readings.

The proposed study refers to previous studies [19, 20] which discussed the measurement of glucose levels in urine using a color sensor. In previous studies, to obtain urine glucose levels, Benedict's solution was needed for the reduction process. Urine samples that have been dropped with Benedict's solution are heated in boiling water until a color change occurs. A change in the color of urine indicates that the urine contains glucose. Research [19] heated urine manually using an electric stove until it changed color, while research [20] heated urine in boiling water, and then the solution was shaken until it changed color. In the proposed study, we overcome this problem by making a device that can heat and stir the solution simultaneously until a color change occurs. After the urine sample changes color, the urine color will be detected using a color sensor and generate red, green, and blue (RGB) values. In previous studies, after obtaining the urine RGB value, the value was processed using the Artificial Neural Network method to facilitate detection and reduce testing in standard laboratories [19]. In the proposed study, the results of reading color data will be converted to RGB colors that match the color of urine in a standard laboratory. We validated the test data using urine testing in a standard laboratory as was done in previous studies [20]. This is done so that we can find out whether the research conducted is following the results of urine examination in a standard laboratory. The proposed system cannot replace the results of laboratory tests, but can be used as a tool for the early detection of glucose levels in urine at a faster time.

# 5 Conclusion

In this paper, we propose a tool to detect glucose in the urine based on urine color. Glucose in urine can be determined by adding Benedict's solution to change the nature and color of urine. The test results from the whole system show that the proposed system can detect differences in urine color and glucose levels in users. There is a color difference between the results of the system and the results of the lab test, but it does not affect the determination of glucose levels. This difference is due to the limited range of yellow readings on the sensor. In future work, the determination of diabetes can be developed to determine the level of diabetes, can add other parameters to better support the indications of diabetes mellitus, and the heater can be replaced with more energy-efficient components.

# References


1. International Diabetes Federation: IDF Diabetes Atlas, 9th edn. Brussels, Belgium: International Diabetes Federation (2019)
2. Wang L, Deng Y, Zhai Y et al (2019) Impact of blood glucose levels on the accuracy of urinary N-acety-β-D-glucosaminidase for acute kidney injury detection in critically ill adults: a multicenter, prospective, observational study. BMC Nephrol 20:186
3. Chen J, Guo H, Yuan S et al (2019) Efficacy of urinary glucose for diabetes screening: a reconsideration. Acta Diabetol 56:45–53
4. Robinson S, Dhanlaksmi N (2017) Photonic crystal-based biosensor for the detection of glucose concentration in urine. Photonic Sens 7:11–19
5. Qin Y, Zhang S, Cui S et al (2021) High urinary excretion rate of glucose attenuates serum uric acid level in type 2 diabetes with normal renal function. J Endocrinol Invest 44:1981–1988
6. Radhakumary C, Sreenivasan K (2011) Naked eye detection of glucose in urine using glucose oxidase immobilized gold nanoparticles. Anal Chem 83(7):2829–2833
7. Su L, Feng J, Zhou X, Ren C, Li H, Chen X (2012) Colorimetric detection of urine glucose-based ZnFe2O4 magnetic nanoparticles. Anal Chem 84(13):5753–5758
8. Karim MN, Anderson SR, Singh S, Ramanathan R, Bansal V (2018) Nanostructured silver fabric as a free-standing NanoZyme for colorimetric detection of glucose in urine. Biosens Bioelectron 110:8–15
9. Stefan-van Staden RI, Popa-Tudor I, Ionescu-Tirgoviste C, Stoica RA, Magerusan L (2019) Molecular enantiorecognition of D-and L-glucose in urine and whole blood samples. J Electrochem Soc 166(9):B3109
10. Sharma P, Sharan P (2014) Design of photonic crystal-based biosensor for detection of glucose concentration in urine. IEEE Sens J 15(2):1035–1042
11. Zhang Z, Chen Z, Cheng F, Zhang Y, Chen L (2017) Highly sensitive on-site detection of glucose in human urine with naked eye based on enzymatic-like reaction mediated etching of gold nanorods. Biosens Bioelectron 89:932–936
12. Gu X, Wang H, Schultz ZD, Camden JP (2016) Sensing glucose in urine and serum and hydrogen peroxide in living cells by use of a novel boronate nanoprobe based on surface-enhanced Raman spectroscopy. Anal Chem 88(14):7191–7197
13. Zhang X, Sucre-Rosales E, Byram A, Hernandez FE, Chen G (2020) ultrasensitive visual detection of glucose in urine based on the iodide-promoted etching of gold bipyramids. ACS Appl Mater Interf 12(44):49502–49509
14. Zamanzad B (2009) Accuracy of dipstick urinalysis as a screening method for detection of glucose, protein, nitrites, and blood. East Mediterr Health J 15(5):1323–328

15. Fadhilah F, Vanawati N (2019) Comparison of glucose reduction in urine using benedict method heated by methylated flame with 100 °C waterbath. Indonesia J Med Lab Sci Technol 1(2):44–51
16. Sufia F, Fikri Z (2018) Pengaruh Glukosa Urine Metode Benedict, Fehling dan Stick Setelah Ditambahkan Vitamin C Dosis Tinggi/1000 mg. Jurnal Analis Medika Bio Sains 5(2):2–6
17. Nadeak FDP, Riyanto RL (2019) Determination of urine glucose levels laboratory of Sari Mutiara Hospital Medan. Jurnal Ilmiah Biologi UMA (JIBIOMA) 1(2):53–57
18. Ghosh P, Bhattacarjee D, Nasipuri M, Basu DK (2010) Round-the-clock urine sugar monitoring system for diabetic patients, Department of Computer Science and Engineering - RCC Institute of Information Technology dan Jadavpur University, India
19. Ahada L, Subur J, Taufiqurrohman M (2019) Alat Ukur Kadar Gula Darah Non-Invasive Dalam Urin Menggunakan TCS3200 Metode Artificial Neural Network. SinarFe7 2(1):69–72
20. Listyalina L, Dharmawan DA, Utari EL (2020) Identifying glucose levels in human urine via red green blue color compositions analysis. J Electric Technol UMY (JET-UMY) 4(1)
21. Rahmat RF, Royananda MA, Muchtar R, Taqiuddin S, Adnan R, Anugrahwaty R (2018) Budi-arto: automated color classification of urine dipstick image in urine examination. J Phys Conf Ser 978:012008
22. Lidia F, Setiawidayat S, Effendy DU (2018) Rancang Bangun Sistem Pendeteksi dan Pemantauan Rekam Medis Penyakit Diabetes Secara Non-Invasive Berbasis Komputer. Jurnal Widya Teknika 26(2):170–181
23. Ghosh P, Bhattacharjee D, Nasipuri M (2019) Intelligent toilet system for non-invasive estimation of blood-sugar level from urine. IRBM
24. Gahan BG, Sumir RM, Thomas N, Umesh P, Priyanka L, Rahul U, Chaturvedi J, D'Souza R, Tauheed A (2019) A portable color sensor based urine analysis system to detect chronic kidney disease. In: International conference on communication systems and networks (COMSNETS)
25. Firmansyah R, Mawardi H, Riandi MU (2009) Mudah dan Aktif Belajar Biologi 2. Pusat Perbukuan, Departemen Pendidikan Nasional, Jakarta

# Pressure Wave Measurement of Clay Conditioned Using an Ultrasonic Signal with Non-destructive Testing (NDT) Methods

**Lusiana and Triwiyanto Triwiyanto**

**Abstract** Every material has its characteristics, if we want to know its characteristics, we usually do mechanical testing. Mechanical testing is usually a destructive test. The purpose of this research is to measure the pressure wave of clay conditioned with the help of an ultrasonic signal. The contribution of this research is to propose a method of measuring the wave propagation of clay by the Non-Destructive Test (NDT) technique using low-cost ultrasonic sensors. The proposed method is to create a system to generate a signal using 40 kHz ultrasonic sensors functioned as a transmitter and receiver with a variance of three samples of clay conditioned. The length of sample 1 is 2.8 cm, sample 2 is 2.9 cm, and sample 3 is 3 cm. This research, using an ultrasonic echo signal to calculate the time interval (t) of the echo signal that can be represented by the value of the velocity of pressure wave (Vp). From the experimental results, the value of sample 1 are $t = 62.77 \times 10^{-6}$ s and $Vp = 916.47$ m/s, sample 2 are $t = 75.27 \times 10^{-6}$ s and $Vp = 870.09$ m/s, sample 3 are $t = 65.5 \times 10^{-6}$ s and $Vp = 800.08$ m/s. The value of the velocity pressure wave shown that the shortest length of the sample also has a higher Vp. The implication of this research is to find other ultrasonic sensors for getting more good results to measuring the propagation velocity in material.

**Keywords** Pressure wave · Ultrasonic · NDT · Low-cost

## 1 Introduction

Material has properties that characterize it. The mechanical properties of the material are one of the most important factors. To obtain the mechanical properties of the material, mechanical testing is usually carried out. Mechanical testing is basically a destructive test, namely by applying pressure to the material being tested until the material is destroyed. The NDT technique has been widely used to test several materials, including testing on concrete. Using the same technique, namely NDT,

Lusiana (✉) · T. Triwiyanto
Poltekkes Kemenkes Surabaya, Jl. Pucang Jajar Tengah No. 56, Surabaya, Indonesia
e-mail: lusiana.tekmed@poltekkesdepkes-sby.ac.id



T. Triwiyanto et al. (eds.), *Proceedings of the 2nd International Conference on Electronics, Biomedical Engineering, and Health Informatics*, Lecture Notes in Electrical Engineering 898, https://doi.org/10.1007/978-981-19-1804-9_10

the authors conducted research with a different material, namely clay, in which this test used an ultrasonic sensor to determine the characteristics of the clay. Non-Destructive Test (NDT) is an evaluation of the physical properties of the object without destroying the function of the object being tested. In NDT, testing using ultrasonic waves is more popularly used because the test is considered safe for use on various types of object materials and can reach the internal objects being tested [1]. The mechanical properties of a material determine its manufacturability, performance and longevity. This means that knowledge of mechanical properties is very important for the physical and mechanical characterization of composite materials [2]. In its application in the industrial world, the main problem is how measurements can be made without touching the object. Ultrasonic sensors are the main key to answer these problems. Many examples are found in the engineering world. One of them is non-destructive testing materials. The ultrasonic sensor uses TOF (Time of Flight) method which refers to the time taken for a pulse to travel from the transmitter to an observed object and back to the receiver [3, 4]. Ultrasound positioning for use indoors thought of as time-of-flight (TOF) measurement [5]. The mechanical properties of a material are to determine its manufacturability, performance and service life. This means that mechanical properties is very important for the physical and mechanical characterization of composite materials [2]. Rojek et al. found that the best method for measuring elasticity is the ultrasonic method. In this ultrasonic pulse echo testing technique using the piezoelectric effect. Where a high-voltage electric pulse (less than 20 ns and an amplitude of 100–200 V) excites the piezoelectric crystal to produce ultrasonic waves on the specimen surface. Then the wave travels through the specimen, so that the transducer reflects ultrasound waves from the side opposite the specimen [6]. The Pulse echo ultrasonic method can easily find defects in homogeneous materials. In this method, the matter of great concern is the transit time of waves and energy loss due to attenuation and scattering of waves [7]. Sound waves or ultrasonic waves correspond to the mechanical and elastic energy in the form of particle motion. The motion transmitted from atom to atom is referred to as a transient wave. These waves are propagated in a gas, liquid or solid environment over a conditioned distance [8]. The concept of ideal elastic material deforms in proportion to the applied load and recovers instantaneously both to its original dimensions and its original state (no damage) when the load is removed. So an ideal elastic wave is a mechanical disturbance that propagates through a material causing oscillations of the particles of that material about their equilibrium positions but no other change [9].

There are clear implications for the interpretation of seismic waves traveling through the Earth and other planetary-sized bodies [10]. If an anisotropic stress is applied to a material (e.g., a simple tension), ultrasonic waves are found to travel at different speeds depending on whether they are propagating parallel or perpendicular to the applied stress [11]. This 'acoustoelastic' effect can be used to measure the so-called third order elastic constants [12].

As the dimensions of geological objects may be many orders of magnitude larger than typical laboratory specimens, elastic wave sources of high energy are usually required to obtain information about them. For this reason, the structure of solid planetary bodies, such as the Earth and Moon, was historically largely determined by examination of the propagation of waves generated by earthquakes, nuclear explosions, and artificial or meteoritic impact [13]. Speed of sound are essential for characterizing reference materials used in ultrasonic applications [14]. For ultrasound, the acoustic properties such as characteristic acoustic impedance, attenuation and speed of sound are essential [15] Evaluation of mechanical properties using ultrasound is based on several common assumptions. Under the assumptions of homogeneity, isotropy and linear elasticity, longitudinal wave sound speed, c, is related to the Young's modulus [16]. The speed of propagation of sound waves in the material changes according to the type of material characteristics. Due to this behavior, information about the structure in the material can be obtained. A high rate of sound transmission means less pores and thus higher power. As the pulse is transferred to the material by the transducer, it undergoes multiple reflections. A complex stress wave system was developed which includes longitudinal waves (pressure waves) propagating through the material. The following is the pulse of velocity equation for pressure waves (Vp) Eq. (1)

$$Vp = \frac{L}{t} \tag{1}$$

Where V indicate the velocity in m/s, L indicate the lengths of the clay in meters, and t indicate the time in seconds. The Ultrasonic Testing (UT) evaluation system consists of a series of transmitters and receivers, transducers, and display devices. Based on the information carried by the signal, the location of the crack, the size of the defect, its orientation other characteristics can be determined [17]. The advantages of ultrasonic testing include scanning speed, good resolution, flaw detection capability, and the ability to use in the field. Disadvantages include difficulty in setup, requiring skill to scan parts accurately, and ensuring accurate testing of the sample being tested.

In 1999, C. M. Aracne-Ruddle et al. conducted a study entitled Ultrasonic Velocities in Unconsolidated Sand/Clay Mixtures at Low Pressures [18]. The methodology in this study is to use the theory of Primary wave (PW) and Secondary wave (SW) wave propagation given by Clewell and Simon [19] with the wave propagation velocity formulation to determine the elasticity property of the medium, which is given in the following equation [20]. The experiments carried out in this study using a Function generator to generate a signal of 500 V, T1 (transmitter) ultrasonic waves to T2 (Receiver). Then T2 converts ultrasonic waves into electric waves. Oscilloscope 1 (plotted excitation signal) is sent to T1 via Channel 1, which is then received by T2 on Channel 2. On channel 2 of this oscilloscope, compressive waves and shear waves can be observed. Oscilloscope 2 serves to collect data which is then processed using LabView on MAC. In 2005, Saad A. Abo-Qudais conducted a research entitled effect of concrete mixing parameters on propagation of ultrasonic waves [21]. This research was conducted to evaluate the effect of concrete aggregate gradation, water-cement ratio, and curing time on UPV (ultrasonic pulse velocity). The ultrasonic equipment used in this study is a portable ultrasonic non-destructive digital indicating tester (PUNDIT) with a generator having an amplitude of 500 V producing a wave of 54 kHz. Ultrasonic measurements were carried out at 3, 7, 28, and 90 days after placing the concrete. The results of the analysis show that the larger the size of the aggregate used in the manufacture of Portland cement concrete, the higher the ultrasonic wave velocity measured. In 2006 Laux et al. conducted a study entitled Ultra-sonic investigation of ceramic clay membranes [16]. Whose research uses the longitudinal ultrasonic velocity assessment method, in which this method includes several measurements, namely reflection mode, volume fraction of porosity, and global longitudinal attenuation evaluation. Reflection mode measures ultrasound echo reflected.

Recently, a study for measuring the mechanical properties using portable ultrasonic non-destructive digital indicating tester (PUNDIT) has been developed. In 2011, Sedat KURUGÖL. Doing research the title is Correlation of Ultrasound Pulse Velocity with Pozzolanic Activity and Mechanical Properties in Lime-Calcined Clay Mortar [22]. In their research they use 3 kinds of clay, calcined in 4 different temperatures (the process of heating an object to a high temperature, but still below the melting point to remove volatile content). Their using PUNDIT and hydraulic test to measure mechanical properties. The result from the measurement Compressive strength, Flexural strength, and Splitting strength. In 2013, Bogas and others doing research the title is Compressive strength evaluation of structural lightweight concrete by non-destructive ultrasonic pulse velocity method [23]. This research is measuring the strength of many kinds of concrete using non-destructive ultrasonic pulse velocity methods. This research uses about 84 compositions of many kinds of samples, which were tested between 3 and 180 days for compressive strengths ranging from 30 to 80 MPa. This study examines the relationship between Ultrasonic Pulse Velocity and compressive strength, while also predicting the compressive strength of concrete by using a non-destructive ultrasonic pulse Velocity test. The equipment used in this research is PUNDIT (portable ultrasonic non-destructive digital indicating tester). In 2015, España et al. conducted a study entitled Ultrasonic sensor for industrial inspection based on acoustic impedance [24]. This study discusses ultrasonic inspection using the panniel method, which in this panniel method analyzes the properties of the inspected acoustic impedance sample to identify defects. In 2017, Wiciak et al. conducted a study entitled Sensor and dimensions effects in ultrasonic pulse velocity measurements in mortar specimens [25]. This study uses the methodology that the condition of concrete greatly affects the quality of the design, manufacture and application of loads to structures, loading characteristics, poor environment, or aging. Conditions to the sensation of concrete are used for safety in buildings. In this study, researchers used a non-destructive testing technique using a UPV (ultrasonic Pulse Velocity) tool with a longitudinal wave propagation (P-wave) methodology on the material (Vp).

The speed of sound does not vary significantly with respect to the variations in the temperature. However, the reflecting surface and the medium of transmission of the sound waves affect its performance notably [26].

Based on previous research, which has explained how elastic propagates on the earth's surface [13] where the wave propagation moves continuously oscillating/pressure wave (PW) which is the initial idea in creating the measurement method in this study. Wave propagation is one of the important things in the characteristics of matter [14]. Where in this study, using the non-destructive ultrasonic test method (NDT) [18–25] in measuring the conditioned clay but with using a low-cost ultrasonic sensor by utilizing the time (TOF) [3, 4] in the wave propagation. Therefore, the purpose of this study to propose a method of measuring the wave propagation to determine the characteristics of clay by Non-Destructive Test (NDT) technique using low-cost ultrasonic sensors. Finding the wave velocity P (pressure wave) is the final goal of this research, which focuses on the characterization of clay conditioned, using the NDT (Non-Destructive Test) method. The contribution of this study using low-cost ultrasonic sensors for measuring the propagation wave from the clay conditioned to determine the characteristics of the clay with the technique of Non-Destructive Test (NDT) using an ultrasonic sensor. This measurement, the nature or character of the clay can be known so that it can help modeling soil properties.

## 2 Materials and Method

### 2.1 *Clay Conditioned*

The samples used for pressure wave measurements are clay conditioned 1, 2, and 3. Clay conditioned 1 is shown in Fig. 1a, has the characteristics of physical length 2.8 cm and diameter 3.5 cm, and has a density of 1856.97573 g/m$^3$. It has a smoother texture, is less dry, and has a slightly darker color. Clay conditioned 2 is shown in Fig. 1b, has a physical characteristic of 2.9 cm in length and 3.5 cm in diameter, and has a density of 1792,94,208 g/m$^3$.

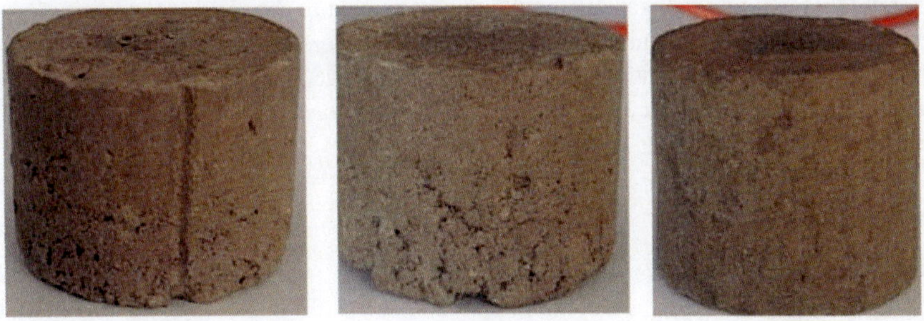

(a) (b) (c)

**Fig. 1** Clay conditioned **a** sample 1, **b** sample 2, **c** sample 3

**Table 1** Characteristics of clay samples

| Clay sample | Length (cm) | Diameter (cm) | Density (g/m$^3$) |
|---|---|---|---|
| 1 | 2.8 | 3.5 | 1856.97573 |
| 2 | 2.9 | 3.5 | 1792,94,208 |
| 3 | 3 | 3 | 1663.85025 |

It has a coarser texture and is very dry compared to the other 2 samples and has a slightly lighter color. Clay conditioned 3 is shown in Fig. 1c, has a physical characteristic of 3 cm in length and 3.5 cm in diameter and has a density of 1663.85025 g/m$^3$. It has the smoothest and wetter texture among the other 2 Clay conditioned and has the darkest color among the other 2 Clay conditioned. The initial hypothesis in measuring pressure waves is that the value of the wave propagation velocity on the material (Vp) has a value range between 1100 and 2500 m/s.

## 2.2 Dataset Description

Characteristics of 3 samples in this research were used are conditioned lay samples. This clay consists of a composition of sand, clay, silt, and gravel which are then compacted. The conditioned state here is that we have to make the clay sample to be tested. The mechanism for making the clay sample is by determining/planning the density of the material to be remolded, then checking the dry density of the material, the last one being remolded dry soil added with water and printed to the density that has been set/planned (Table 1).

## 2.3 Data Acquisition

System of this research shown in Fig. 2 This system used a *function generator* GW instek GFG-3015 to generate a signal that will be sent to the UST (converting electrical signals into mechanical signals). Also, an agilent technologies MSO6054A oscilloscope is used which are connected to the UST (Ultrasonic Transmitter) and USR (Ultrasonic Receiver) sections. This oscilloscope is also used to record ultrasonic signals obtained from the two sensors.

## 2.4 Data Collection

Figure 3 showing the proposed method of measurement tested clay conditioned sample. This proposed method of measurement is for collect the data in this research. This proposed method using 2 kinds of ultrasonic sensors with 40 kHz. One of the

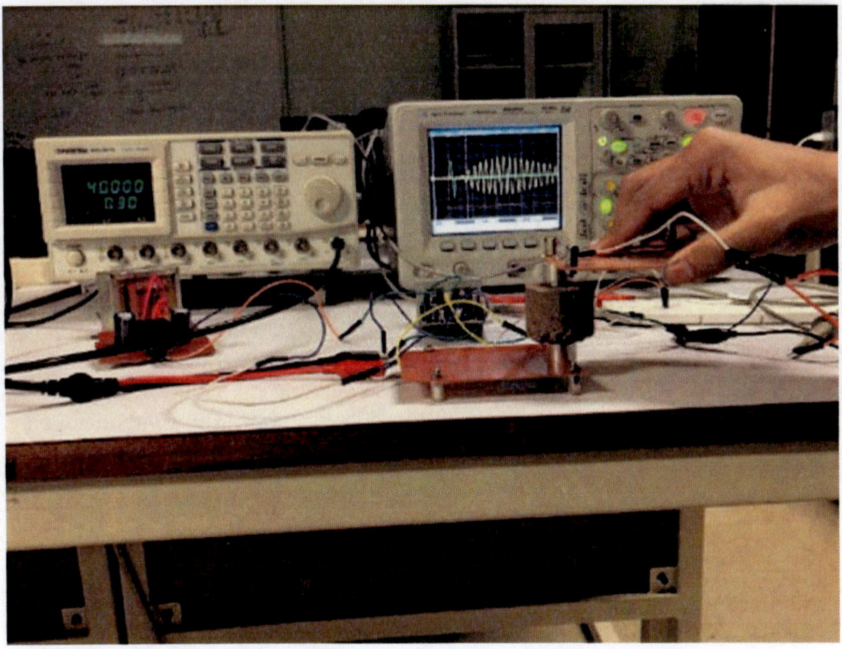

**Fig. 2** System of the proposed method

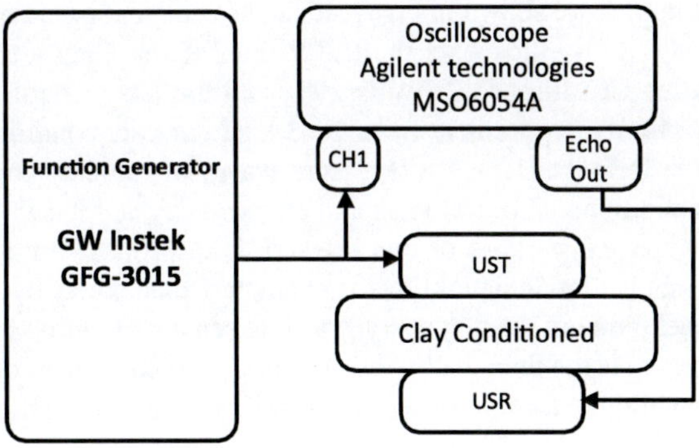


**Fig. 3** Block diagram of the proposed method

ultrasonic sensors is a transmitter (UST) and the other one a receiver (USR). UST transmitted the ultrasonic signal to the clay conditioned sample. Then the signal that penetrates the clay sample is received by the ultrasonic receiver (USR).

**Table 2** Analysis of measurement data

| Clay sample | Length (cm) | Travel time (s) | Pressure wave velocity/Vp (m/s) |
|---|---|---|---|
| 1 | 2.8 | 32 | 875 |
| 2 | 2.9 | 29 | 1000 |
| 3 | 3 | 33 | 909.09 |

### 2.5 Data Analysis

Based on Table 2, it can be explained that the size of the conditioned clay sample used as the test sample in this study did not affect the travel time obtained based on the sound wave propagation of the conditioned clay sample. The conditioned clay sample number 2 which has a length of 2.9 cm and a density of 1792,94,208 g/$m^3$ produces the highest sound speed of 1000 m/s.

## 3 Result

Pressure wave measurement uses two ultrasonic sensors (UST and USR) which are placed above and below the test sample as shown in Fig. 3.

The measurement results of pressure wave (PW) using an oscilloscope on all test samples are shown in Fig. 4. It can be seen that based on the results of measurement with an oscilloscope, the travel time of the Clay Conditioned 1 PW is 32 s, the Clay Conditioned 2 PW is 29 s, and the Clay Conditioned 3 PW is 33 s. Results of time measurement from the 3 kinds of clay conditioned are then calculated into the formula (1.1). Vp (Pressure wave) of the clay conditioned 1 is 875 m/s, clay conditioned 2 is 1000 m/s and clay conditioned 3 is 909.09 m/s Fig. 5.

As the purpose of this research is to propose a method of measuring the wave propagation to determine the characteristics of clay by Non-Destructive Test (NDT) technique using low-cost ultrasonic sensors. Finding the wave velocity P (pressure wave) is the final goal of this research, which focuses on the characterization of clay conditioned, using the NDT (Non-Destructive Test) method as shown in Figs. 1 and 3.

## 4 Discussion

After getting the value of travel time, then the researcher calculates the value of the pressure wave propagation speed (Vp). This Vp value represents the value of the speed of sound wave propagation in the material with the implementation of Eq. (1). Clay conditioned 1 with a sample length of 2.8 cm and a density of 1856.97573 g/$m^3$

**Fig. 4** Pressure wave measurement method

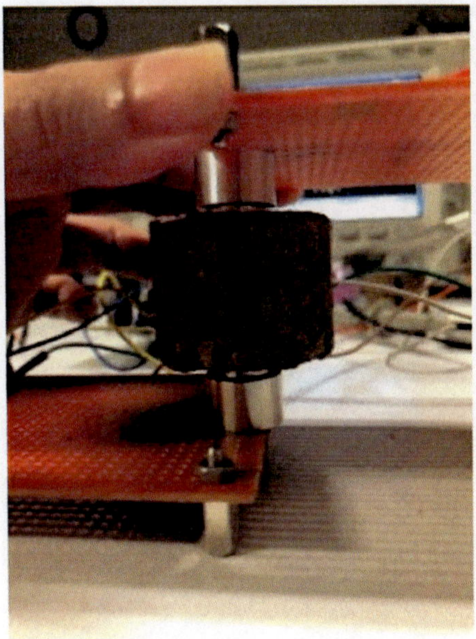

has a Vp (PW) value of 875 m/s, Clay conditioned 2 with a sample length of 2.9 cm and a density of 1792,94,208 g/m3 has a Vp (PW) value. of 1000 m/s, Sample 3 with a sample length of 3 cm and a density of 1663.85025 g/m3 has a Vp (PW) value of 909.09 m/s. It can be seen that clay conditioned 2 has the highest pressure wave propagation velocity (Vp) in the material among the other test samples 909.09 m/s.

Comparing from the previous research [4–6] we can propose a method with the different sensors (low cost sensors) to finding the Vp of each sample. Limitation from this research is to find the velocity of pressure wave (Vp) as we know the goals from this research That focusing with NDT method with clay conditioned samples. The implication of this research is to find other ultrasonic sensors (more robbust of ultrasonic sensors) for getting more good results to measuring the propagation velocity in material.

## 5 Conclusion

The purpose of this research is to propose a method as we seen in Fig. 3 and measuring the wave propagation as we seen in Fig. 4 to determine the characteristics of clay (we can see it by the ultrasonic signal that can produce by each clay conditioned samples) by Non-Destructive Test (NDT) technique using low-cost ultrasonic sensors as we seen in Fig. 3 especially the placing of the sensors. The results of the characterization of the Clay conditioned informed that the density value and the length of the material were not directly proportional to the magnitude of the wave propagation velocity in

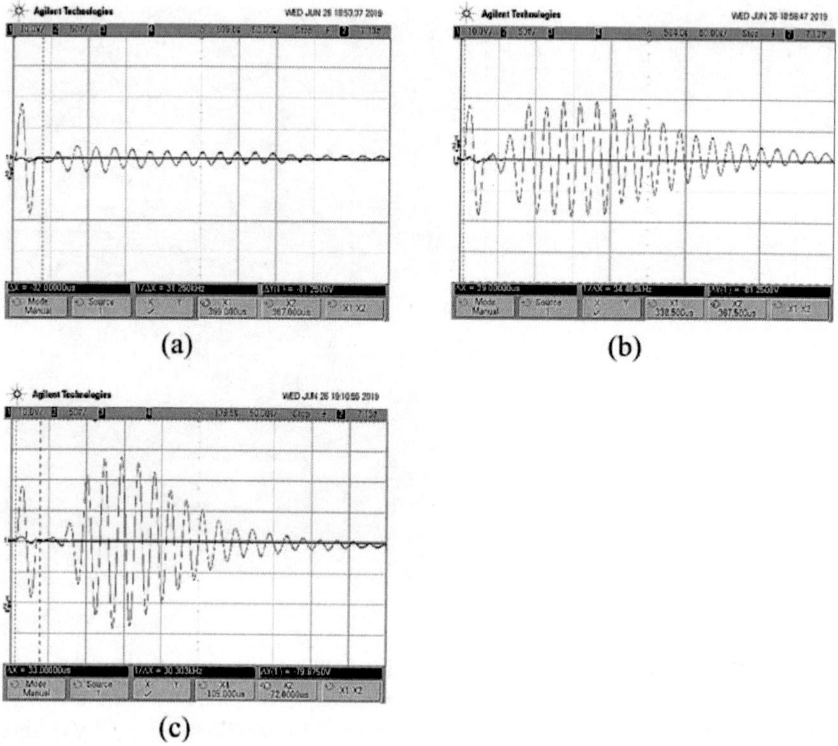


**Fig. 5** PW measurement using oscilloscope **a** clay conditioned 1, **b** clay conditioned 2, **c** clay conditioned 3

the material (Vp). This kind of ultrasonic sensor has a slight weakness especially in penetrating the depth of the material. The implication of this research is to find other ultrasonic sensors for getting more good results to measuring the propagation velocity in material. Future work for this research is to measure the secondary wave (SW) after we can find the value of primary wave/pressure wave velocity (Vp).

## References

1. Reinhold Ludwig DR (1989) A non-destructive ultrasonic imaging system. IEEE Trans Instrum Meas 38(I)
2. Šturm R, Grimberg R, Savin A, Grum J (2015) Destructive and non-destructive evaluations of the effect of moisture absorption on the mechanical properties of polyester-based composites. Compos Part B Eng 71:10–16
3. Holm S (2000) P32-ultrasound_positioning, p DA972-99 IF-24221_373_p32-ultrasound_positionin

4. Paredes JA, Álvarez FJ, Aguilera T, Villadangos JM (2018) 3D Indoor positioning of UAVs with spread spectrum ultrasound and time-of-flight cameras. Sens (Switz) 18(1):1–15
5. Wong GSK, Embleton TFW (1985) Variation of the speed of sound in air with humidity and temperature 5:1710–1712
6. Gholizadeh S (2016) A review of non-destructive testing methods of composite materials. Procedia Struct Integr 1:50–57
7. Wang M, Zheng D, Xu Y (2019) A new method for liquid film thickness measurement based on ultrasonic echo resonance technique in gas-liquid flow. Meas J Int Meas Confed 146:447–457
8. Hildebrand BP et al (1972) Acoustics 3.1
9. Walley SM, Field JE (2016) Elastic wave propagation in materials. Ref Modul Mater Sci Mater Eng 0–8
10. Duffy TS, Ahrens TJ (1992) Sound velocities at high pressure and temperature and their geophysical implications. J Geophys Res 97(B4):4503–4520. https://doi.org/10.1029/91JB02650
11. Toupin RA, Bernstein B (1961) Sound waves in deformed perfectly elastic materials. Acoustoelastic effect R. J Acoust Soc Am 33:2
12. Hughes DS, Kelly JL (1953) Second-order elastic deformation of solids. Phys Rev 92(5):1145–1149. https://doi.org/10.1103/PhysRev.92.1145
13. Wang Y, Guo J (2004) Modified Kolsky model for seismic attenuation and dispersion. J Geophys Eng 1(3):187–196. https://doi.org/10.1088/1742-2132/1/3/003
14. Maia TQS, Alvarenga AV, Souza RM, Costa-Félix RPB (2021) Feasibility of reference material certification for speed of sound and attenuation coefficient based on standard tissue-mimicking material. Ultrasound Med Biol 47(7):1904–1919. https://doi.org/10.1016/j.ultrasmedbio.2021.03.015
15. Sjöstrand S et al (2020) Tuning viscoelasticity with minor changes in speed of sound in an ultrasound phantom material. Ultrasound Med Biol 46(8):2070–2078. https://doi.org/10.1016/j.ultrasmedbio.2020.03.028
16. Laux D, Ferrandis JY, Bentama J, Rguiti M (2006) Ultrasonic investigation of ceramic clay membranes. Appl Clay Sci 32(1–2):82–86. https://doi.org/10.1016/j.clay.2005.09.001
17. Lu Y (2010) Non-destructive evaluation on concrete materials and structures using cement-based piezoelectric sensor
18. Weidinger DM, Zhao H, Kwok AOL, Kang X, Ge L (2020) Small strain moduli of compacted silt by ultrasonic pulse velocity measurements. Mar Georesour Geotechnol. 38(10):1257–1264. https://doi.org/10.1080/1064119X.2019.1657209
19. Clewell DH, Simon RF (1950) Seismic wave propagation. Geophys 15(1):50–60. https://doi.org/10.1190/1.1437577
20. Lama VSVRD (1978) Lama Vutukuri.pdf in handbook on mechanical properties of rocks, p 3
21. Abo-Qudais SA (2005) Effect of concrete mixing parameters on propagation of ultrasonic waves. Constr Build Mater 19(4):257–263. https://doi.org/10.1016/j.conbuildmat.2004.07.022
22. Kurugöl S (2012) Correlation of ultrasound pulse velocity with pozzolanic activity and mechanical properties in lime-calcined clay mortars. Gazi Univ J Sci 25(1):219–233
23. Bogas JA, Gomes MG, Gomes A (2013) Compressive strength evaluation of structural lightweight concrete by non-destructive ultrasonic pulse velocity method. Ultrasonics 53(5):962–972. https://doi.org/10.1016/j.ultras.2012.12.012
24. España JJG, Builes JAJ, Tabares AFJ (2015) Ultrasonic sensor for industrial inspection based on the acoustic impedance. In: 20th Symp Signal Process Images Comput Vis STSIVA 2015—Conference Proceedings, pp. 1–6. https://doi.org/10.1109/STSIVA.2015.7330435.
25. Wiciak P, Cascante G, Polak MA (2017) Sensor and dimensions effects in ultrasonic pulse velocity measurements in mortar specimens. Procedia Eng. 193(519):409–416. https://doi.org/10.1016/j.proeng.2017.06.231
26. Kundu S, Acharya US, Mukherjee S (2019) In: Proceedings of 2019 4th international conference on informatics and computing ICIC. 602:331–341

# Deep Learning Approach in Hand Motion Recognition Using Electromyography Signal: A Review

**Triwiyanto Triwiyanto, Triana Rahmawati, Andjar Pudji, M. Ridha Mak'ruf, and Syaifudin**

**Abstract** Electromyography (EMG) signals have very high complexity and random characteristics. EMG signals are widely used in the process of controlling rehabilitation engineering devices. Exploration of the right feature extraction must be carried out to produce a good classifier model accuracy. However, this requires a fairly long time consumption. Recently, the Deep learning classifier has grown rapidly, including its use in hand gesture recognition through EMG signal patterns. The selection of a deep learning classifier using a suitable algorithm will produce good accuracy. The purpose of this study is to review articles related to the development of deep learning, especially to recognize the pattern of human hand gestures using EMG signal. The steps taken were exploring articles from various database sources such as pubMed, ScienceDirect, and IEEE Xplore using the keywords EMG, deep learning, and hand gesture for articles published in the last ten years, 2010–2021. The results of the bibliometric analysis using VOSviewer showed that there are three clusters associated with these keywords, namely EMG, deep learning, and male/female. Furthermore, mostly, authors used raw EMG signals as input for deep learning CNN. In addition to using raw EMG signals, some authors used spectrograms and continuous wavelet transforms of EMG signals.

**Keywords** EMG · Deep learning · CNN · Hand gesture

## 1 Introduction

Electromyography (EMG) is one of the bio-electrical signals generated by our bodies when the limbs (upper or lower limb) perform an activity or movement [1, 2]. EMG signal activity can be used for various purposes, including detecting the position of the human limb, measuring the speed of movement for the upper or lower limb, detecting muscle fatigue, and recognizing hand gestures [2–5]. In addition, EMG signals can also be used for medical examinations, including muscle spasms and injury [6].

T. Triwiyanto (✉) · T. Rahmawati · A. Pudji · M. R. Mak'ruf · Syaifudin
Poltekkes Kemenkes Surabaya, Jl. Pucang Jajar Tengah No. 56, Surabaya 60282, Indonesia
e-mail: triwi@poltekkesdepkes-sby.ac.id



T. Triwiyanto et al. (eds.), *Proceedings of the 2nd International Conference on Electronics, Biomedical Engineering, and Health Informatics*, Lecture Notes in Electrical Engineering 898, https://doi.org/10.1007/978-981-19-1804-9_11

In the field of medical rehabilitation, EMG signals are widely used for equipment monitoring and control purposes [2]. Furthermore, the application of bionic prosthetic hands, upper and lower limb exoskeletons also often uses EMG signals as control [7–9]. However, the basic problem in using EMG signals is that there are many variables that must be considered, including the condition of the subject, the location of the electrode installation, the level of muscle fatigue, environmental noise, and changes in the EMG signal that depend on time [10, 11]. Since the EMG signal has a random and stochastic nature, it is impossible to predict the consistency of the signal that will be issued when the muscle contracts [12]. This is because when the EMG signal is tapped on the surface of the skin, thousands of muscle fibers actually contribute to the muscle electrical signal, thus forming a random EMG signal [13]. However, it can be ascertained that the amplitude of the EMG signal is almost related to the strength of muscle contraction given during static testing of upper or lower limb movements but is not linear. To solve the problem of random characteristics of the EMG signal, and the non-linearity of the EMG signal, some researchers used machine learning to recognize each movement pattern generated.

Various kinds of machine learning have been developed by researchers for general purpose applications such as in medical [14–16], industry [17, 18], and education [19]. Furthermore, some machine learnings were applied to recognize EMG signal-based hand gestures, among others, artificial neural network (ANN) [20, 21], support vector machine (SVM) [14, 22, 23], and linear discriminant analysis (LDA) [24, 25]. In general, the process of recognizing hand gestures through EMG signals consists of data acquisition, segmentation, feature extraction, and classifier, as shown in Fig. 1.

EMG signals are tapped on the part to be studied; for example, when we are going to develop a prosthetic hand with a basic open and close movement pattern, the muscles to be tapped are the flexor carpi radialis longus and extensor carpi. In offline mode, the recorded EMG signal (EMG dataset) is then segmented into several parts. In general, the segmentation width used is 100–200 ms to maintain the control process in real-time [2, 26]. Feature extraction is a process to get the dominant features in hand gesture pattern recognition. The feature extraction stage can use time, frequency, and time–frequency domains. In general, for real-time development, time-domain features are mostly used to process EMG signal extraction. The feature extraction or feature engineering stage in the conventional classifier generally requires quite a lot of effort when choosing the right feature to produce high accuracy, namely through the exploration process and the combination of features. Therefore, in the

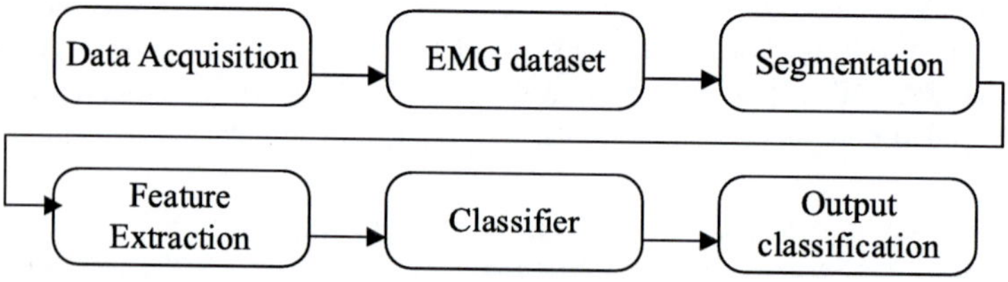


**Fig. 1** Standard procedure for hand motion classification using EMG signal

next development, researchers develop a feature that can recognize or learn during the training process, which is called feature learning. Feature learning will simplify the pattern recognition process by eliminating the feature extraction stage. Feature learning that uses the CNN algorithm in several layers is hereinafter referred to as deep learning. In the development of an exoskeleton or prosthetic hand, a simple architecture is important because it will result in fast computation time. Therefore, the purpose of this study is to review articles related to deep learning and pattern recognition using EMG signals. This is to produce a recommendation of the best architectural model to recognize EMG signal patterns for the purposes of designing rehabilitation equipment.

## 2 Deep Learning Method

Feature learning performs EMG signal extraction through the convolution process, which is between the signal and the kernel. The kernel is a matrix, in this case a 1-dimensional matrix, which functions to detect dominant features. The 1-dimensional convolution process is shown in Fig. 2a. During the convolution process, the kernel is multiplied by the signal successively up to the 5th column and accumulated so that the final result is a $5 \times 1$ feature map. In order to reduce the dimension of the feature map, the max-pooling algorithm can be applied in this case, as shown in Fig. 2b. In contrast to the convolution process, in the max-pooling process, for each mapped matrix, the highest value will be chosen so that a smaller feature map will be produced.

Research related to machine learning has grown so rapidly using both supervised and non-supervised learning models [27]. The use of machine learning with a supervised model is mostly applied to the development of EMG signal pattern recognition to recognize hand gestures. Machine learning with conventional methods consists

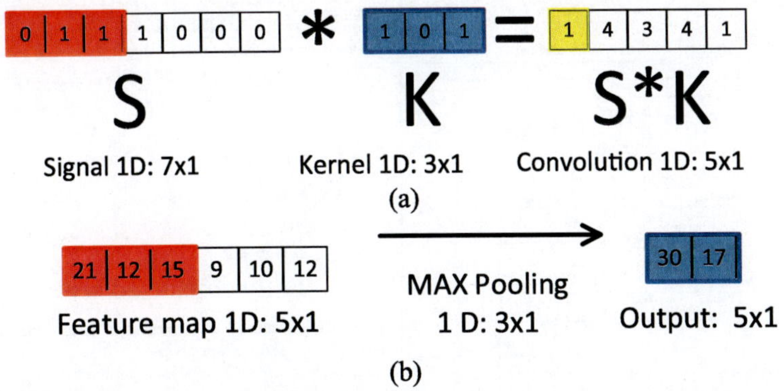


**Fig. 2** A simple example of **a** one-dimensional convolution, **b** one-dimensional max pooling

of segmentation, feature extraction, and classifier [28]. However, determining the suitable feature extraction takes a long time because it requires exploration and a combination of features. Machine learning with feature learning will have additional value if it can be combined to reduce the exploration time to determine the feature extraction model used. Deep learning is machine learning that combines the conventional multi-layer neural network and the convolution layer on the front, hereinafter referred to as deep learning with the convolution neural network (CNN) algorithm [29, 30]. The convolution layer can replace the role of the feature extraction stage so that this layer can be referred to as feature learning. Feature learning will study the pattern recognition process during the training stage.

One example of applying deep learning with the CNN algorithm to recognize hand gesture patterns based on EMG signals is shown in Fig. 3. It can be seen that the model is composed of a combination of convolution and multi-layer perceptron processes. Overall the classifier model shown in Fig. 3 consists of eight layers, three convolution layers, one max-pooling layer, one flattened layer, two hidden layers, and one output layer.

One example of applying deep learning with the CNN algorithm to recognize hand gesture patterns based on EMG signals is shown in Fig. 3. It can be seen that the model is composed of a combination of convolution and multi-layer perceptron processes. Overall the classifier model shown in Fig. 3 consists of 8 layers, three convolution layers, one max pooling layer, one flattened layer, two hidden layers, and one output layer.

In the case of EMG signal pattern recognition to recognize hand gestures, as shown in Fig. 3, the classifier model gets three channels of EMG signal input. Each EMG signal from the three channels is segmented with a window width of 200 samples. After the segmentation process, 800 EMG signal segments are generated for each channel. The EMG signal on each channel is convoluted with a 1-dimensional kernel

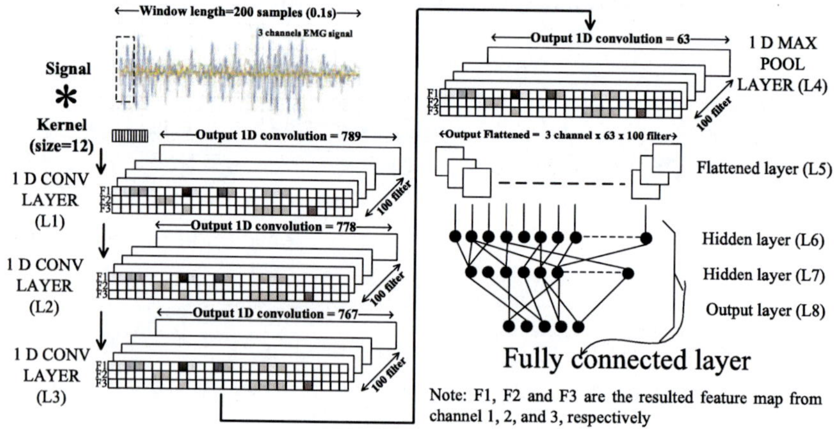


**Fig. 3** Structure of hand gesture recognition using convolution neural network

(size = 12). In this model, the number of feature maps (filters) planned for each convolution and max-pooling layer is 100. As shown in Fig. 3, in each convolution stage, the width of the feature map is reduced. In layer 4, the max-pooling layer, the 1-dimensional feature map matrix is reduced to $63 \times 1$. At this stage, the max-pooling layer is used to reduce the dimension of the feature map resulting from the previous convolution layer while producing an average for the previous layer. The final part of the convolution and max-pooling process is flattening, which is the result of the max-pooling of 3 EMG signal channels being made into a single 1-dimensional matrix. The next stage of the CNN deep learning model is a fully connected layer, which consists of several hidden layers and one output layer, as is the process for conventional multi-layer perceptrons. The number of hidden nodes is adjusted to the complexity of the signal pattern to be recognized. Furthermore, the number of output nodes depends on the number of classes that the machine learning model will recognize. The deep learning model with the CNN algorithm has advantages in terms of feature learning, namely reducing the feature extraction stage. However, the weakness of the CNN deep learning model is that the learning time required is relatively long compared to conventional machine learning models. This is because, there is a convolution process in the CNN deep learning model, namely, multiplication and addition for each signal matrix and kernel. Therefore, in this paper, we will review the advantages and disadvantages of using deep learning to recognize EMG signal patterns.

## 3 Material and Method

In this review article, we focused on a deep learning-based method to map the application of machine learning in recognizing EMG signal patterns to classify hand gestures. Articles were obtained from various available databases, including the IEEE explore, PubMed, and Science Direct databases. The articles collected are in the past ten years, namely, from 2010 (January) to 2021 (July), as shown in Fig. 4. After applying the selection criteria, the number of articles which discussed EMG signal pattern recognition using deep learning specifically recognizing hand movement patterns is twelve articles from 150 articles.

### *3.1 Keyword Analysis*

Bibliometrics was used to map the articles related to the keywords used to prepare this review paper. The analysis tool used in this study is VOSviewer, an application that can map the relationship between one reference and other references in a network (Fig. 5). The main keywords used in this review paper are EMG and deep learning. Furthermore, the inclusion criteria used are all hand gestures related to hand movements.

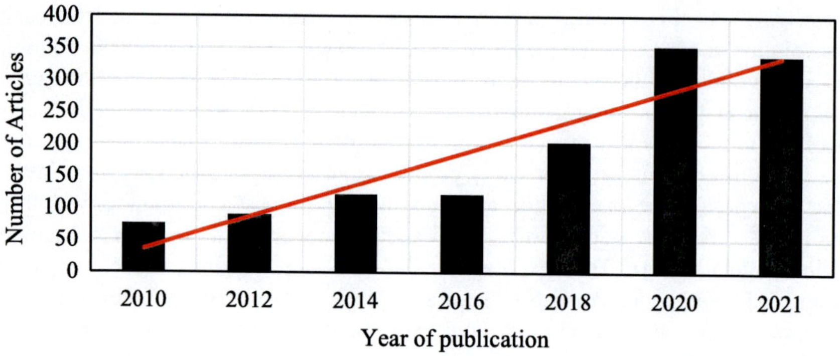


**Fig. 4** The trend line number of articles published in 2010–2021 for EMG, deep learning, and hand recognition

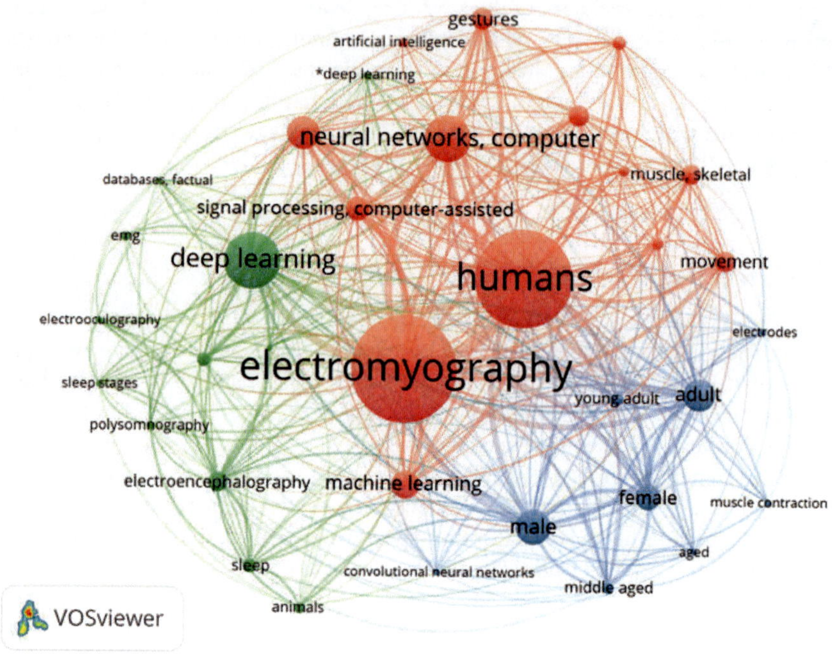


**Fig. 5** The bibliographic analysis of EMG using keyword of EMG, deep learning, hand motion

In addition, in the bibliometric analysis, exclusion criteria are facial motion, speech recognition, lower limb, and multimodal gestures with other bio-electric signals. The results of the analysis using VOSviewer showed that there are three clusters related to these keywords, namely cluster one, which shows the most prominent map (shown in red) among the other two clusters (Fig. 5).

**Table 1** The keyword clustering result using VOSviewer

| Cluster | Keyword | Color |
|---|---|---|
| 1 | Artificial intelligence, artificial limbs, electromyography, gesture, hand, human, machine learning, movement, muscle, skeletal, neural network, computer, pattern recognition, automation, signal processing, support vector machine | Red |
| 2 | Deep learning, animals, database, electrocardiography, Electroencephalography, EMG, polysomnography, sleep, sleep stage, wearable electronics devices | Blue |
| 3 | Adult, aged, convolution neural network, electrodes, female, male, middle aged, muscle contraction, young adult | Green |

In this cluster, electromyography is mostly associated with humans because the use of EMG signals is widely used for human support or rehabilitation tools [31]. The most frequently encountered keywords for this cluster are artificial intelligence, artificial limbs, gesture, hand, machine learning, and others. The second cluster is deep learning which deals more with various applications related to various signals, including EMG, electro-oculography, polysomnography, and sleep monitoring. The third cluster is related to rehabilitation tools that can support human life. Details of the nodes that connect each cluster can be seen in Table 1.

## 3.2 Results

Hand gestures can be identified through EMG signal pattern recognition. The electrodes can be tapped in the upper arm area just below the elbow crest [1, 32]. Several muscle groups that became the object of research were the extensor carpi radialis longus and the flexor carpi ulnaris [1]. The electrode installation is in a bipolar mode, i.e., two muscle-leading electrodes and one ground electrode [33]. The number of electrodes leads that are often used to recognize hand gestures is 2–10 pairs, with the number of classes in the range of 2–18 classes. The summary of the researchers who applied deep learning with convolution neural network method in solving the case of EMG signal pattern recognition to classify hand gestures is shown in Table 2. In this series, we only took articles sourced from journals with complete documentation such as public datasets, number of leads, and a clear proposed method.

Based on Table 2, it appears that the CNN input used in this study is the raw EMG signal, spectrogram, or CWT. Several researchers used raw EMG as CNN input, this is because deep learning architecture in this case is simpler and does not require pre-processing [35–37, 39, 40, 42, 45]. Cote-Allard compared CNN input using raw, spectrogram, or CWT. The performance obtained is that CNN using input from CWT produced better accuracy than using raw and spectrogram [34].

**Table 2** Summary of deep learning application using EMG signal for hand gesture recognition

| Author | Application | DL algorithm | Dataset | Results |
|---|---|---|---|---|
| Cote-Allard et al. [34] | 7 hand gestures recognition | Transfer learning with three modality inputs: raw EMG, spectrogram and CWT | 36 able-body, and Ninapro dataset | Accuracy is 98.31 and 68.98% for CWT and raw input, respectively |
| Triwiyanto et al. [35] | 10 hand gestures recognition | CNN using raw EMG data | Rami khushaba repository | Accuracy ranged between 77 and 93% |
| Atzori et al. [36] | 50 hand movements | CNN using raw EMG data | Ninapro dataset 1, 2 and 3 | CNN accuracy datasets 1: 66.59%, datasets 2: 60.27%, datasets 3: 38.9% (amputee) |
| Laezaa [37] | 40 hand movements | CNN, RNN, and CNN + RNN using raw EMG data | Ninapro dataset 7 | CNN = 89.01% RNN = 91.81% CNN + RNN = 90.43% |
| Xia et al. [38] | Detecting limb motion | CNN + RNN using CWT as EMG feature | 8 healthy subjects | RCNN = 90.3% |
| Shioji et al. [39] | Personal ID by recording hand open | CNN using raw EMG signal | 8 healthy subjects | CNN = 94.9% |
| Park et al. [40] | 6 hand movements | CNN using raw EMG signal | Ninapro | CNN = 90% |
| Geng et al [41] | 8 hand gestures | CNN using image EMG | 52 gesture Ninapro and 27 gestures | 89.3% for single frame EMG, 99% for 40 images EMG |
| Yu et al. [42] | 27 hand gestures | CNN using 8 channel × 16 electrodes | 23 healthy subjects | Maximum accuracy 95% |
| Cote-allard et al. [43] | To guide 6 DOF robotic arm using 7 hand gestures | CNN using myo-armband, spectrogram, 8 channels | 18 healthy subjects | 97.9% real-time |
| Zhai et al. [44] | 50 hand gestures | CNN using EMG spectrogram | Ninapro DB2 and DB3 | Intact subject 88.42%, amputee 73.31% |
| Hartwell et al. [45] | 14 hand gestures | Compact CNN using myo-armband and wireless electrodes | 10 healthy subjects | 84.2% |

## 4 Discussion

Based on the summary of studies related to deep learning in recognizing hand movement, as shown in Table 2, this shows that deep learning using CNN produces better accuracy than other classifiers. In these studies, support vector machine (SVM), k-nearest neighborhood (KNN), and linear discriminant analysis (LDA) are commonly used as comparisons. Based on this description, it appears that the use of CNN is still a very promising pattern recognition method.

In the process of reviewing the article, we found that most of the researchers used the Ninapro public dataset and others measured the EMG signal directly to the subject. The use of the Ninapro dataset is preferred because there are various types of electrodes, including wireless electrodes (Trigno electrode) and Myo-armband (8 channel dry electrodes wireless). Furthermore, several researchers used high-density electrodes in the process of recording EMG signals with an $8 \times 16$ electrode matrix [46, 47]. Several researchers tested the proposed method using an intact body (healthy subject) and amputee person to see the difference in the performance of the proposed classifier. Mostly, from the results of the article review, it was found that the performance of the classifier applied to the EMG signal from the amputee experienced a decrease in the accuracy. This is because, functionally, the muscles associated with hand gestures do not work normally. Generally, the researchers targeted three basic movements, namely basic finger movements, basic wrist movements (flexion, extension, pronation, supination, adduction, and abduction), and basic functional movements (hook grasp, ring grasp, tripod grasp, large grasp, small diameter grasp, etc.).

Deep learning using the CNN algorithm has advantages in terms of feature learning at the convolution stage because it can replace the role of the feature extraction process in conventional classifier models. Based on the literature survey, some researchers use raw EMG signals as direct CNN input (75%), but some other researchers still use feature extraction processes such as spectrograms and continuous wavelet transform (CWT) EMG signals (25%). As done by Alard et al., the results of the CNN classifier accuracy comparing the use of input directly from the raw EMG signal and after going through the CWT process are 68.98 and 98.31%, respectively [34]. In the CNN algorithm, several researchers proposed a one-dimensional (1D) convolution process between the signal and the kernel [35–37, 39, 40, 42, 43, 45]. Meanwhile, several other researchers applied the CNN two-dimensional (2D) convolution algorithm between the signal and the kernel. In this case, some EMG channels are assumed to be a two-dimensional (2D) image, as well as the kernel used is a two-dimensional kernel [41]. To improve the accuracy of the classifier, some researchers combined the CNN deep learning algorithm with other algorithms, for example, the recurrent neural network (RNN), but the resulting accuracy showed a significant difference in accuracy [37].

Deep learning using the convolution neural network algorithm is still a trend for researchers in developing pattern recognition for EMG signal patterns, especially recognizing hand gestures. The convolution process between the signal and the kernel is a process of multiplication and accumulation of addition so that it requires a long training process when compared to the conventional classifier, which uses the feature extraction stage [35]. Furthermore, the length of the training process in deep learning with the CNN algorithm is also determined by the configuration of the proposed model, namely how many convolution layers and how many hidden layers are used in the final stage (fully connected layers). Furthermore, the development of deep learning with the CNN algorithm can be investigated, especially in reducing the number of convolution layers so that the resulting training process can run faster.

The real implication of the deep learning classifier model with the CNN algorithm is the implementation of the system in embedded systems so that the system can recognize EMG signal patterns from various parameters without a calibration process and without exploration to determine the right feature extraction for certain parameter conditions. Furthermore, the deep learning classifier with the CNN algorithm can be applied to a wide variety of applications related to medical rehabilitation engineering, for example, prosthetic hand design, upper and lower limb exoskeletons, and wheelchair electronics.

## 5 Conclusion

The purpose of this paper is to review papers related to the topic of machine learning, especially deep learning on the introduction of EMG signal patterns to hand gestures. The results of the review paper show that mostly authors use raw EMG signals as input to the CNN model using the 1D convolution process. Furthermore, in addition to using raw EMG signals, several other researchers use CNN input that has been processed using the spectrogram method and continuous wavelet transform with the aim of increasing the accuracy of the model. The use of raw EMG input for deep learning CNN has advantages in terms of a simpler architecture and faster computation time compared to using spectrogram or CWT input. The author used more public datasets sourced from Ninapro datasets in addition to primary data from intact and amputee subjects. In the future, a review of the application of deep learning in rehabilitation equipment can be carried out so that readers get accurate recommendations before conducting research.

## References


1. Martini FH, Nath JL, Barholomew EF (2012) Fundamental of anatomy and physiology, 9th edn. Pearson education, Boston
2. Asghari Oskoei M, Hu H (2007) Myoelectric control systems—a survey. Biomed Signal Process Control 2(4):275–294
3. Jones CL, Wang F, Morrison R, Sarkar N, Kamper DG (2014) Design and development of the cable actuated finger exoskeleton for hand rehabilitation following stroke. IEEE/ASME Trans Mechatron 19(1):131–140

4. Choi C, Kim J (2007) A real-time EMG-based assistive computer interface for the upper limb disabled. In: 2007 IEEE 10th international conference rehabilitation robot ICORR'07, pp 459–462
5. Triwiyanto T, Oyas W, Hanung AN, Herianto H (2018) Adaptive threshold to compensate the effect of muscle fatigue on elbow-joint angle estimation based on electromyography. J Mech Eng Sci 12(3):3786–3796
6. Zhang Q, Hayashibe M, Fraisse P, Guiraud D (2011) FES-induced torque prediction with evoked emg sensing for muscle fatigue tracking. IEEE/ASME Trans Mechatron 16(5):816–826
7. Bandou Y, Fukuda O, Okumura H, Arai K, Bu N (2018) Development of a prosthetic hand control system based on general object recognition analysis of recognition accuracy during approach phase. In: ICIIBMS 2017—2nd international conference intelligent informatics and biomedical science, pp 110–114
8. Noce E et al (2019) EMG and ENG-envelope pattern recognition for prosthetic hand control. J Neurosci Methods 311:38–46
9. Atique MDM, Rabbani SE (2018) A cost-effective myoelectric prosthetic hand. J Prosthet Orthot 30(4):231–235
10. Basmajian JV, De Luca CJ (1985) Chapter 8 muscle fatigue and time-dependent parameters of the surface EMG signal. Muscles alive their functions revealed by electromyography, Williams & Wilkins Baltimore, pp 201–222
11. Basmajian JV, De Luca CJ (1985) Chapter1: introduction. Muscles alive their functions revealed by electromyography, pp 1–18
12. De Luca CJ (1997) The use of surface electromyography in biomechanics. J Appl Biomech 13(2):135–163
13. Basmajian J, De Luca CJ (1985) Description and analysis of the EMG signal. Muscles alive their functions revealed by electromyography, pp 65–100
14. Assegie TA (2021) Support vector machine and k-nearest neighbor based liver disease classification model. Indones J Electron Electromed Eng Med Inform 3(1):9–14
15. Mishra S (2021) Malaria parasite detection using efficient neural ensembles. J Electron Electromed Eng Med Inform 3(3):119–133
16. Kirana AP, Bhawiyuga A (2021) Novel coronavirus pandemic in Indonesia: cases overview and daily data time series using naïve forecast method. Indones J Electron Electromed Eng Med Inform 3(1):1–8
17. Yunardi RT, Apsari R, Yasin M (2020) Comparison of machine learning algorithm for urine glucose level classification using side—polished fiber sensor. J Electron Electromed Eng Med inform 2(2):33–39
18. Kareem SW, Askar S, Hawezi RS, Qadir GA (2021) A comparative evaluation of swarm intelligence algorithm optimization: a review. J Electron Electromed Eng Med Inform 3(3):111–118
19. Dietterich TG (2009) Machine learning in ecosystem informatics and sustainability
20. Ahsan M (2011) Electromyography (EMG) signal based hand gesture recognition using artificial neural network (ANN). Mechatronics (ICOM), pp 17–19
21. Ahsan MR, Ibrahimy MI, Khalifa OO (2012) A step towards the development of VHDL model for ANN based EMG signal classifier. In: 2012 international conference on informatics, electronics and vision (ICIEV), pp 542–547
22. Xing K, Yang P, Huang J, Wang Y, Zhu Q (2014) A real-time EMG pattern recognition method for virtual myoelectric hand control. Neurocomput 136:345–355
23. Ishikawa K, Toda M, Sakurazawa S, Akita J, Kondo K, Nakamura Y (2010) Finger motion classification using surface-electromyogram signals. In: Proceeding—9th IEEE/ACIS international conference computer and information science ICIS, pp 37–42
24. Bhattacharya A, Sarkar A, Basak P (2017) Time domain multi-feature extraction and classification of human hand movements using surface EMG. In: 2017 4th international conference on advance computing communication system (ICACCS), pp 1–5
25. Raurale SA (2014) Acquisition and processing real-time EMG signals for prosthesis active hand movements. In: 2014 international conference on green computing communication and electrical engineering (ICGCCEE), pp 1–6

26. Phinyomark A, Phukpattaranont P, Limsakul C (2012) Feature reduction and selection for EMG signal classification. Expert Syst Appl 39(8):7420–7431
27. Mcclure N (2017) TensorFlow machine learning cookbook. PACKT publishing Ltd., Birmingham UK
28. Triwiyanto O, Wahyunggoro H, Nugroho A, Herianto (2017) An investigation into time domain features of surface electromyography to estimate the elbow joint angle. Adv Electr Electron Eng 15(3):448–458
29. Epelbaum T (2017) Deep learning: technical introduction, pp 1–106 arXiv:1709.01412
30. Ieracitano C, Mammone N, Bramanti A, Hussain A, Morabito FC (2019) A convolutional neural network approach for classification of dementia stages based on 2D-spectral representation of EEG recordings. Neurocomput 323:96–107
31. Vaca Benitez LM, Tabie M, Will N, Schmidt S, Jordan M, Kirchner EA (2013) Exoskeleton technology in rehabilitation: towards an EMG-based orthosis system for upper limb neuromotor rehabilitation. J Robot
32. Konrad P (2005) The ABC of EMG a practical introduction to kinesiological electromyography
33. Basmajian JVV, De Luca CJ (1985) Chapter 2 apparatus, detection, and recording, muscles alive their function revealed by electromyography 2:19–65
34. Cote-Allard U, Fall CL, Drouin A, Campeau-lecours A (2019) Deep learning for electromyographic hand gesture signal classification using transfer learning. Trans Neural Syst Rehabil Eng 4320:1–11
35. Triwiyanto T, Pawana IPA, Purnomo MH (2020) An improved performance of deep learning based on convolution neural network to classify the hand motion by evaluating hyper parameter. IEEE Trans Neural Syst Rehabil Eng 28(7):1678–1688
36. Atzori M, Cognolato M, Müller H (2016) Deep learning with convolutional neural networks applied to electromyography data: a resource for the classification of movements for prosthetic hands. Front Neurorobot 10:1–10
37. Laezza R (2018) Deep neural networks for myoelectric pattern recognition an implementation for multifunctional control. Chalmers University of Technology, Gothenburg, Sweden
38. Xia P (2017) EMG-based estimation of limb movement using deep learning with recurrent convolutional neural networks. Artif Organs
39. Shioji R, Ito S, Ito M, Fukumi M (2017) Personal authentication based on wrist EMG analysis by a convolutional neural network. In: Proceedings of the 5th IIAE international conference on intelligent systems and image processing, pp 12–18
40. Park K, Lee S (2016) Movement intention decoding based on deep learning for multiuser myoelectric interfaces. In: 2016 4th international winter conference on brain-computer interface (BCI), pp 7–8
41. Geng W, Du Y, Jin W, Wei W, Hu Y, Li J (2016) Gesture recognition by instantaneous surface EMG images. Sci Rep 6–13
42. Du Y, Jin W, Wei W, Hu Y, Geng W (2017) Surface EMG-based inter-session gesture recognition enhanced by deep domain adaptation. Sensors 17:6–9
43. Côté-Allard U, Fall CL, Gigu P (2016) A convolutional neural network for robotic arm guidance using sEMG based. In: International conference on intelligent robots and systems, 2017
44. Zhai X, Jelfs B, Chan RHM, Tin C (2017) Self-recalibrating surface EMG pattern recognition for neuroprosthesis control based on convolutional neural network. Front Neurosci 11:1–11
45. Hartwell A, Kadirkamanathan V, Anderson SR (2018) Compact deep neural networks for computationally efficient gesture classification from electromyography signals. In: 2018 7th IEEE international conference on biomedical robotics and biomechatronics (biorob)
46. Rantalainen T, Kłodowski A, Piitulainen H (2012) Effect of innervation zones in estimating biceps brachii force-EMG relationship during isometric contraction. J Electromyogr Kinesiol 22(1):80–87
47. Staudenmann D, Roeleveld K, Stegeman DF, van Dieen JH (2010) Methodological aspects of SEMG recordings for force estimation—a tutorial and review. J Electromyogr Kinesiol 20(3):375–387

# Battery Charger Design in a Renewable Energy Portable Power Plant Based on Arduino Uno R3

**Anggara Trisna Nugraha, Dwi Sasmita Aji Pambudi, Agung Prasetyo Utomo, and Dadang Priyambodo**

**Abstract** Indonesia is a tropical country that has two seasons, namely the dry season and the rainy season. This makes the earth receive solar power of 1.74 × 1017 Watts every day of which 1–2% is converted into wind energy. According to BPPT in 2018, from the availability of wind energy of 9.29 GW, only 0.0005 GW was used. In addition, Indonesia, which is located in the tropics with high average rainfall (2000–3000 mm/year), provides a large enough potential for air energy. With high rainfall, Indonesia has water energy potential of 75.67 GW and only 4.2 GW has been utilized. According to BPPT, in 2018 coal reserves will be exhausted within 68 years. To overcome this problem, the government is currently doing energy reading which aims to utilize renewable energy that exists in nature. One of the important components in this power plant is the battery which functions as storage where after the battery needs to be recharged. Inappropriate battery recharging process can cause battery performance degradation. This can be overcome by creating a charging battery that can maintain its voltage level. This is done to maintain battery performance and extend battery life. To maintain the output voltage level on the charge controller, a PI control is used. From the tests that have been carried out, it is found that the efficiency of this buck converter system is 85.60–95.7% with an error percentage of 1.373%. From the data obtained, it can be said that the charge controller can work well. So from this research is expected to extend the life and maintain battery performance.

**Keywords** Battery charger · Renewable energy · Portable power plant

## 1 Introduction

Indonesia is located on the equator which is the trajectory of air movement due to the difference in air pressure in the two hemispheres, known as the monsoon wind. The phenomenon of monsoon winds which is then supported by the location of Indonesia's territory which is on the equator and geographical conditions consisting

A. T. Nugraha (✉) · D. S. A. Pambudi · A. P. Utomo · D. Priyambodo
Politeknik Perkapalan Negeri Surabaya, Sukolilo, Surabaya 60111, Indonesia
e-mail: anggaranugraha@ppns.ac.id



T. Triwiyanto et al. (eds.), *Proceedings of the 2nd International Conference on Electronics, Biomedical Engineering, and Health Informatics*, Lecture Notes in Electrical Engineering 898, https://doi.org/10.1007/978-981-19-1804-9_12

of 70% of the water area causes Indonesia to have large wind energy [1]. In addition, this earth receives a power of 1.74 × 1017 W. About 1–2% of the energy is converted into wind energy [2]. Thus, wind energy is 50–100 times greater than the energy converted into biomass by all plants on earth [3]. According to BPPT 2018, the potential for wind energy in Indonesia is 9.29 GW but its utilization is only around 0.0005 GW. In addition, Indonesia, which is located in the tropics with high average rainfall (2000–3000 mm/year) provides a large potential for water energy. With this high rainfall, Indonesia has a water energy potential of 75.67 GW and only 4.2 GW has been utilized [4].

With the increase in the electrification ratio in 2025, the demand for electricity is certain to increase 7 times in the next 30 years [5]. Currently, power plants that have COD (Commercial Operation Date) only operate around 4% (±1.5GW) [6]. Under these conditions, a program to increase the availability of electrical energy is expected to be achieved in 2026 [7]. In 2025 fossil energy will still be the main energy source with a percentage of 58% [8]. According to BPPT 2018, coal reserves will run out in 68 years. One of the largest electricity users in Indonesia is the household sector. During January–July 2020, the largest electricity consumption from the household sector was 42.25% or reached 47.5 TWh [9].

One way that can be done is by utilizing renewable energy which is so abundantly available in nature [10]. In a study conducted by Jamal in 2020 on the angle of the vertical wind turbine blades with 4 angle variations with the aim of knowing the most efficient angle position. From the research conducted, it was found that the highest power coefficient that can be produced by wind turbines is in wind turbine research with a pitch angle of 45° Cp max 7.39% with a tsr of 0.422. From this research, the conclusion is based on the value of Cp and tsr. Furthermore, the most important component in a hybrid generator is the battery [11]. Where after use, the battery needs to be recharged [12].

The process of charging the battery with an inappropriate voltage level will reduce the lifetime of the battery. In a previous study conducted by Robiansyah in 2019, research was carried out on charger controllers through the use of a buck converter circuit which aims to design a charge controller for the use of electrical energy on a small scale. Where from the research conducted, it was found that the output voltage value of the charger controller was a maximum of 13.5 V with a maximum current output of 3 A.

For this reason, this study was conducted to determine the vertical wind turbine from the side of the power output produced. For this reason, PI control was used in this study so that the output voltage of the buck converter can be adjusted according to battery needs. In this study, the voltage level of 14.4 V was used in the design of the charge controller system. This aims to maintain performance and maintain the life time of the battery. So that the battery lifetime will last a long time and the battery performance will not decrease.

## 2 Method and Results

The main purpose of this research is to make a charge controller that can control the output of the power plant automatically. There are many charger controllers on the market. However, of the many charger controllers sold in the market, the charger controller is used to control the output of solar panels [13]. The charger controller used in the output of water and wind turbines is still very expensive. In addition, the charger controller used in the turbine also does not have an interface [14]. So this will make it difficult for users to monitor the input and output of the charger controller system itself. In addition, it is also very rare to find a charger controller that can be used to do a hybrid so that the price itself soars high enough for a PWM-class charger controller [15].

From these problems, a charger controller was designed that can be used to control input from solar panels, wind turbines and floating turbines and can also be used for hybrids of the three. Below is a flow diagram of the work system of the charger controller that will be made (Fig. 1).

From the flow diagram, it can be seen that the output from the turbine and solar panels will go to the buck controller and previously the voltage and current values will be measured by a voltage sensor and a current sensor with type INA219. Everywhere this voltage sensor utilizes the working principle of a voltage divider circuit and the current sensor used uses I2C communication. After the output of this generator is measured, it will then enter the buck converter circuit and will be processed so that the output of the buck converter is 14.4 V which will be used to charge the battery. before the output of the buck converter enters the battery, the voltage sensor and current sensor must first measure it. In this circuit, a cut off relay circuit is also added which is useful for disconnecting charging when the battery is fully charged. This buck converter uses the PI control method which is useful for adjusting the duty cycle so that the output issued by the buck converter can be as desired.

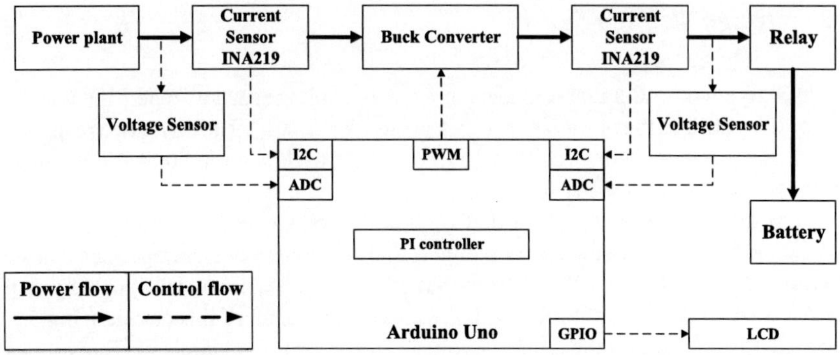


**Fig. 1** The architectural design

## 2.1 Tool and Materials

In this research, several sensor modules and a microcontroller are used which have technical specifications as below. The first is the INA219 current sensor which is a current sensor used for DC electric current. The INA219 sensor can be used to measure the voltage, current and power of a circuit. In operation, an I2C connection is used so that 16 sensor units can be used simultaneously. In addition, this sensor has an accuracy of 0.5%. This sensor uses the SOT23-8 and SOIC-8 packages and is also equipped with a filtering option and also with a calibration register.

While in this study using an Arduino Uno R3 microcontroller board with the following specifications.

The microcontroller used in this study has dimensions of 68.6 × 53.4 mm with a weight of 25 g using an Atmega328P IC with an operating voltage of 5 V but a voltage of 7–12 V can be used because this microcontroller uses a regulator IC so that it can reduce the voltage entered in the jack. Power in this microcontroller. This microcontroller has 14 digital pins where there are 6 pins that can be used as PWM outputs. In addition, this microcontroller also has 6 analog pins. This microcontroller has a memory capacity of 32 kb of which 0.5 kb is used as a bootloader and there is also 2 kb of SRAM and 1 kb of EEPROM.

Data from the measurement of the voltage sensor and current sensor will be displayed on a 16 × 2 LCD with the following specifications. The LCD used consists of 16 columns and 2 rows, besides that this LCD is also equipped with a backlight. Regarding the display of the LCD itself has 192 characters stored. In operation, it can be addressed in 4-bit and 8-bit modes. And lastly there is also a programmable character generator. In this study also used two voltage sensors where the voltage sensor used applies the principle of voltage divider where the voltage sensor design process can be seen in Sect. 2.2.

## 2.2 Design Voltage Sensor

In the charger controller that is made, there are two voltage sensors where the voltage sensor used utilizes the principle of a voltage divider circuit by utilizing two resistors. Figure 2 is the equivalent circuit [16] of the voltage divider circuit that will be made (Fig. 2).

From the picture, it is known that to make a voltage sensor, two resistors are needed. Where in this study it is planned that the maximum voltage that can be measured by this circuit is 25 V. The output of this circuit will go to the analog pin of the Arduino Uno microcontroller with the maximum output of this circuit being 5 V because it is adjusted to the working voltage of the Arduino Uno [17]. The voltage that enters the analog pin of the microcontroller will then be processed into 8-bit data using an ADC (analog to digital converter). To find the value of the resistor to be used, the calculation is carried out as follow; $R_2 = 10\ k\Omega$, $V_{in} = 25$ V, and $V_{out}$

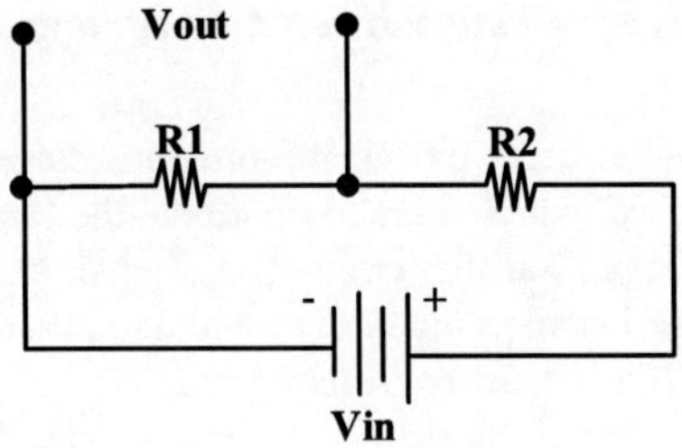


**Fig. 2** Equivalent circuit of voltage sensor

= 5 V. To find $R_1$, it can be calculated using Eq. (1):

$$V_{out} = \frac{R_1}{R_1 + R_2} \times V_{in}[18] \quad (1)$$

For this reason, the resistor values used are 10 and 2.5 kΩ.

After completing the calculation of the value of the resistor used, it is continued with the sensor calibration stage. It is intended that the output of this voltage sensor has a small error percentage value. This stage begins by measuring the resistance values of the two resistors.

From the measurements that have been made, it is known that the resistance value of the input voltage sensor is R1 of 2.482 kΩ and R2 of 9.88 kΩ. While the output voltage sensor is R1 of 2.488 kΩ and R2 of 9.90 kΩ. After that the resistance value obtained will be used in making a program list using the Arduino IDE application by utilizing the voltage divider formula and the resistance value that has been obtained.

The calibration process of the voltage sensor was carried out at the Elka Power Laboratory of the Surabaya State Shipping Polytechnic on the date of June 25th 2021. The calibration process is carried out using a power supply and also a load in the form of a potential which aims to change the resistance value of the load so that the measured voltage value will also vary.

After getting the ADC value from the process of measuring the varying current values displayed by the serial monitor from the Arduino IDE, then the output value of the voltage sensor and the measurement value using a multimeter is carried out using Excel to make it easier to make linear graphs and take trendline data so that as a reference to the formula used will be used as a standard value for measuring DC current at the input and output of the buck converter circuit [18]. The following is the voltage sensor calibration measurement data.

The calibration data is used to find a calibration equation that aims to improve sensor performance in measuring quantities in the system that is made [19].

## 2.3 Design Buck Converter

After carrying out the previous stage, namely calibrating the sensors that will be used, which aims to minimize the error value generated in testing the tool, then the buck controller circuit is designed. In this buck converter circuit, several sensors will be installed including a voltage sensor (using the voltage divider principle) and an INA219 current sensor [20].

From the data collection, the input voltage (Vin) is 18 V, the frequency (fs) is 0.98 kHz, and the ripple voltage (Vs) is 2 V. So that the quantities used in the components of the buck converter can be calculated as shown in Eq. (20) with minimum inductor value:

$$Lmin = \frac{(1 - D)R}{2fs}[22] \quad (2)$$

where Lmin indicates the minimum value of the inductor used, D is the duty cycle value, R is the resistor value and Fs is the PWM frequency. The minimum capacitor value can be calculated based on Eq. (3):

$$C = \frac{D(1 - D)V_{in}}{8Lf^2\Delta Vc}[23] \quad (3)$$

where C indicates the minimum value of the capacitor used, D is the duty cycle value, Vin is the input voltage and Vc is the capacitor voltage.

From the above calculations, it can be seen that the buck converter circuit to be made is as follows [21]. In the switching circuit, a MOSFET of type irf460 is used with the help of an NPN transistor as an intermediary for the Arduino PWM and the input voltage. In the transistor circuit also used two resistors with a size of 10 and 1 k. The use of this resistor is intended to prevent a short with ground [22]. Likewise with the input from the collector pin everywhere when the leg is not given a resistor, there will be a short between the collector transistor leg, the MOSFET gate leg and the ground of the buck converter circuit. For that given a resistor with a size of 10 k.

When the PWM value is one, the current from the collector leg will flow towards the emitter leg so that the MOSFET will be energized which causes the gate to open resulting in a closed circuit position and current from the source will be continued to the inductor [23]. Conversely, when the gate leg is not energized, the current from the drain leg will not be forwarded to the inductor (Fig. 3).

The picture is a circuit that has been made with proteus 8 professional by utilizing the arduino uno microcontroller as a trigger on the mosfet [24].

Furthermore, calculations are carried out on the quantities used in the PI control, where it is known that:

From the experiments conducted, data obtained in the form of steady state time (*TS*) of 0.06 *s*, in addition to the steady state voltage (*YSS*) of 14.26 *V*, and the target voltage (*XSS*) of 14.4 V.

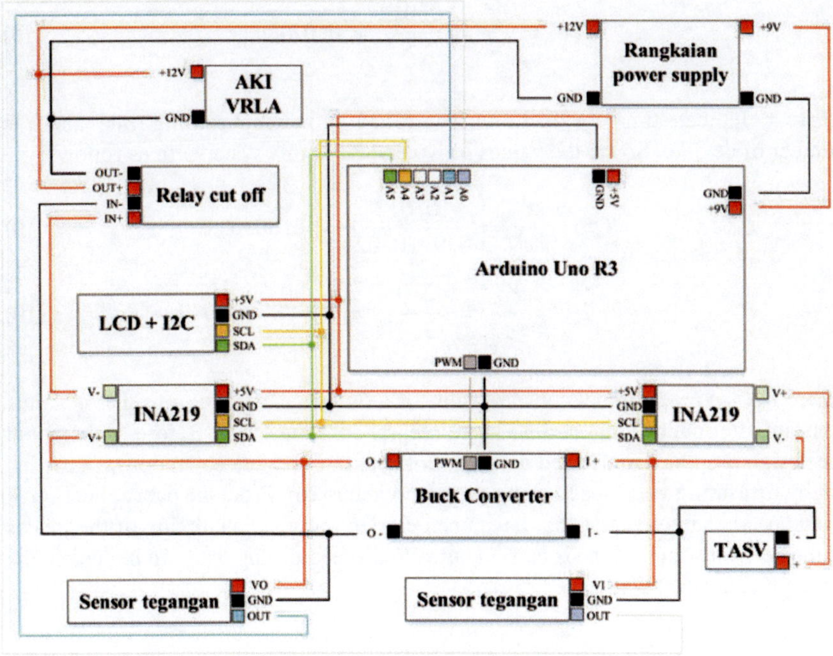


**Fig. 3** Circuit of buck converter in Porteus 8 Profesional

$$K = \frac{Y_{SS}}{X_{SS}}[25] \quad (4)$$

where K is the gain, Yss is the crest of the wave, and Xss is the setpoint. Next is the determination of the value of the time constant (τ) [25]

$$t_s = 5\tau \quad (5)$$

where is the time constant, ts is the settling time. Next, calculate the value of ts*:

$$t_s{}^* = 5\tau \quad (6)$$

$$t_s{}^* = \frac{1}{n^*} x t_s \quad (7)$$

where ts* is the settling time after being controlled, ts is the settling time before being controlled. So:

$$\tau^* = \frac{t_s{}^*}{n} = \frac{0,012}{5} = 0,024 \tag{8}$$

where $\tau^*$ indicate time constant after controlled $t_s{}^*$ indicate settling time, and n is number of devider. So for the values of Kp and Ki in this system are as follows:

$$Kp = \frac{\tau}{k\tau^*} = \frac{0,012}{0,99x0,024} = 0,5050 \tag{9}$$

$$Ki = \frac{Kp}{\tau} = \frac{42,087}{13,378} = 42,087 \tag{10}$$

where Kp is a proportional constant value, is a time constant, k is a gain, * is a time constant after controlling, and Ki is an integral constant value. Before carrying out the design process, wind speed data was collected where data collection was carried out by measuring wind speed using an anemometer [26]. From the data collection of wind speed characteristics that have been carried out, the calculation of the blades of the vertical wind turbine is carried out. Wind speed testing data can be seen in the research results section.

## 2.4 Design of Vertical Axis Turbine

After getting data on wind speed characteristics testing where the data obtained is from wind speed testing on the Kenjeran beach which has been chosen to be the place for this research. Where the wind speed test is carried out using an anemometer to measure wind speed. From the measurements made, it was found that the average wind speed was 4.66 m/s. The next step is to design a vertical wind turbine blade. The first design stage is done by calculating the total area of the turbine blades (the area of the tube blanket).

$$P = Cpr\frac{1}{2}\rho Av^3 \tag{11}$$

where P is power (Watts), Cpr is Rotor Power Coefficient (0.3), ρ is viscosity of air, A is total area of all blades ($m^2$), v is wind speed (m/s)

$$A = \frac{2P}{Cpr\rho v^3} \tag{12}$$

where A indicate area, P indicate power, ρ indicate viscosity and v indicate velocity.

The average turbine Cpr value is 0.158, so:

$$= \frac{2x15}{0,158 \times 40,75 \times 4,66} \tag{13}$$

$$= 1.9538m^2 \tag{14}$$

From the calculations that have been made, it is found that the total number of turbine blades is 3 $m^2$. After that proceed with determining the size of each blade. In this study, a vertical axis wind turbine with 3 blades was used.

$$A = K \times L \tag{15}$$

where A is area of the entire blade ($m^2$), L is blade length (m), K is circumference of circle/width of blade (m),

$$K = \frac{A}{L} \tag{16}$$

After obtaining the length and width of the blade, the next calculation will be on the length of the bowstring of the blade. This is used to find out how big the curvature of the blade is. This calculation technique is carried out by using the formula for a triangle in a circle with the shape of an equilateral triangle.

$$D = \frac{K}{\pi} \tag{17}$$

After that, the length of the bowstring for each blade is determined. This is done to determine the curvature of the turbine blades that are designed.

$$\mathrm{r} = \frac{a \times b \times c}{4 \times Labc} \tag{18}$$

$$7.07 = \frac{a \times b \times c}{4 \times \frac{1}{2} \times a \times a\sqrt{2}} \tag{19}$$

Because a = b = c, so:

$$7.07 = \frac{a}{2x\sqrt{2}} \tag{20}$$

The following is a detailed size of the turbine that has been carried out in the design process (Fig. 4).

After that, this wind turbine will be given four support legs which are useful for maximizing the wind speed that hits this vertical wind turbine. This is because the higher the position, the greater the wind speed in that place. This phenomenon is because the higher a place is, the smaller the resistance value that is subjected to

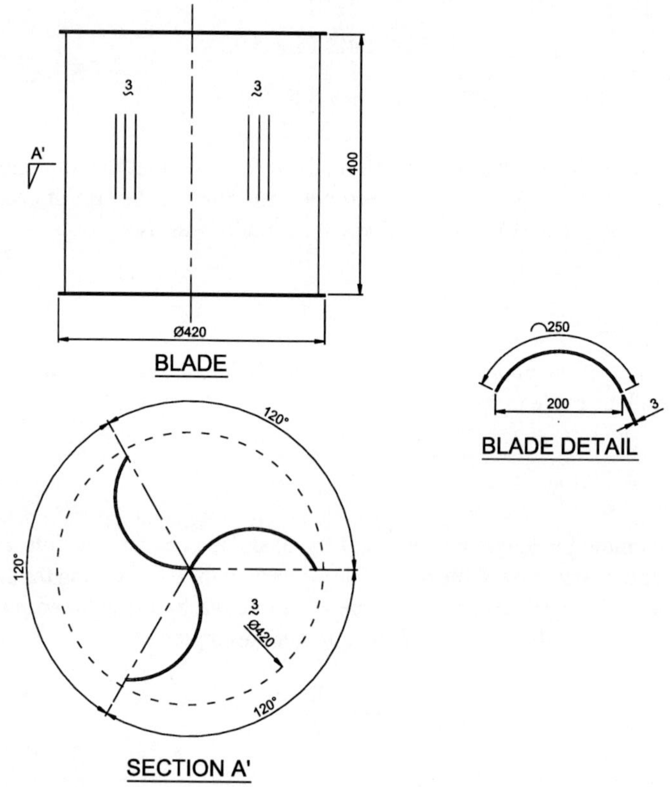


**Fig. 4** Details of vertical turbine size

the wind. The length of the legs of the turbine is planned as long as 3 m which is composed of two L irons which are cut into two parts.

## 2.5 *Result*

The tests were carried out with the outputs of wind turbines, floating turbines and solar panels. The first test was carried out on solar panels, where the aim of knowing the maximum power that can be produced by solar panels. The test was carried out at 9:00 to 15:00 WIB. The test is carried out using a DC lamp load and measured using a multimeter to determine the amount of voltage and current output from the solar panel. The data can be seen in the Table 1 (Table 2).

From the tests that have been carried out, a graph can be shown in Fig. 5. The next test is testing the power output of the floating turbine. This test is conducted to

**Table 1** Solar cells testing

| Time | Voltage (V) | Current (A) | Power (W) | Temperature (°C) |
|---|---|---|---|---|
| 9:00 | 18,79 | 2652 | 49,831 | 49 |
| 10:00 | 18,75 | 2837 | 53,194 | 54 |
| 11:00 | 18,44 | 2787 | 51,392 | 56 |
| 12:00 | 18,5 | 2607 | 48,230 | 62 |
| 13:00 | 18,12 | 2787 | 50,500 | 58 |
| 14:00 | 18,36 | 2787 | 51,169 | 59 |
| 15:00 | 18,59 | 2612 | 48,557 | 58 |
| Average | 18,507 | 2724 | 50,410 | 56.57 |

**Table 2** Floating turbine test

| Num | V river's flow 0.42 m/s | |
|---|---|---|
| | Voltage (V) | Current (A) |
| 1 | 18,660 | 2570 |
| 2 | 18,610 | 2480 |
| 3 | 19,900 | 2470 |
| 4 | 18,864 | 2550 |
| Average | 19,009 | 2518 |
| Power (W) | 47,854 | |

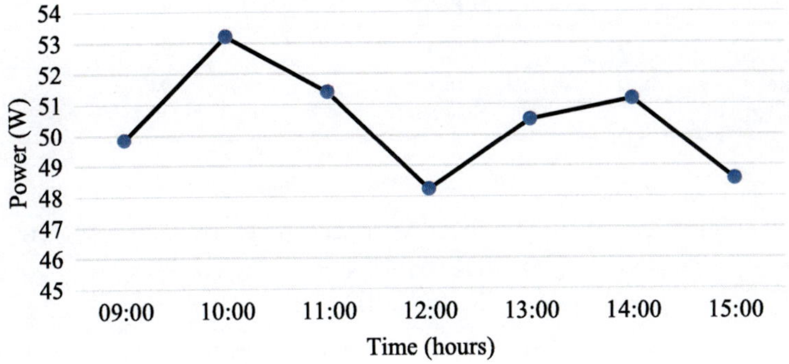


**Fig. 5** Graph of solar cells testing

determine the power generated by the turbine to hydro energy. The data can be seen in Table 4.

From the tests that have been carried out, a graph can be shown in Fig. 6. Next is testing of vertical wind turbines where this test aims to determine the amount of electrical power produced by wind energy with a power plant prototype. The test was carried out with 4 variations of speed. The test result data can be seen in the Table 3.

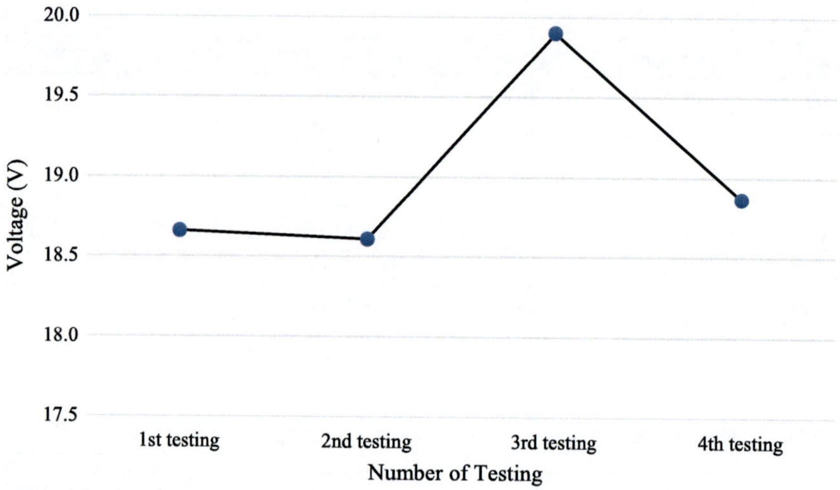


**Fig. 6** Graph of floating turbine test

**Table 3** Wind turbine testing

| Variation of wind speed | Test variables | |
|---|---|---|
| | Voltage (V) | Current (A) |
| 4 | 18.1 | 2.93 |
| 5 | 18.3 | 3.1 |
| 4,5 | 18.2 | 3.08 |
| 4.3 | 18.4 | 2.98 |
| Average | 18.250 | 3.023 |
| Power (W) | 49.05 | |

**Table 4** Buck converter testing

| Duty Cycle (%) | Vin (V) | Iin (A) | Vout (V) | Iout (A) | Pin (W) | Pout (W) | Eff (%) |
|---|---|---|---|---|---|---|---|
| 77,664 | 18,580 | 2607 | 14,430 | 3037 | 48,438 | 43,824 | 90,474 |
| 77,853 | 18,540 | 2792 | 14,434 | 3222 | 51,764 | 46,506 | 89,844 |
| 79,057 | 18,230 | 2742 | 14,412 | 3172 | 49,987 | 45,715 | 91,454 |
| 77,637 | 18,450 | 2525 | 14,324 | 2955 | 46,586 | 42,327 | 90,858 |
| 79,152 | 18,400 | 2435 | 14,564 | 2865 | 44,804 | 41,726 | 93,130 |
| 72,296 | 19,690 | 2425 | 14,235 | 2855 | 47,748 | 40,641 | 85,115 |
| 77,790 | 18,654 | 2505 | 14,511 | 2935 | 46,728 | 42,590 | 91,144 |
| 77,233 | 18,290 | 2562 | 14,126 | 2992 | 46,859 | 42,265 | 90,196 |
| 79,978 | 17,910 | 2742 | 14,324 | 3172 | 49,109 | 45,436 | 92,520 |
| 80,242 | 18,150 | 2742 | 14,564 | 3172 | 49,767 | 46,197 | 92,826 |
| 81,502 | 18,380 | 2567 | 14,980 | 2997 | 47,181 | 44,895 | 95,154 |

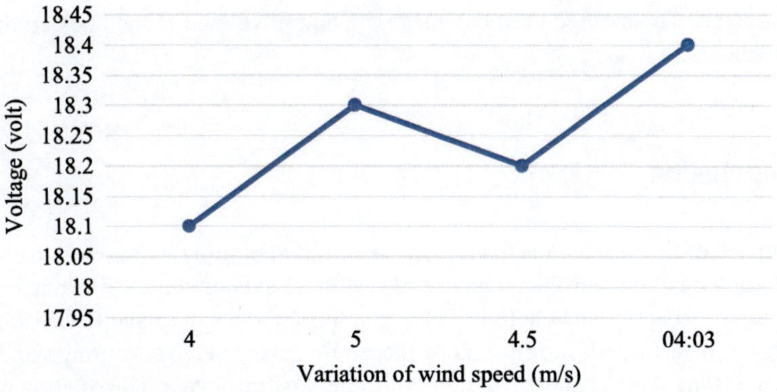


**Fig. 7** Graph of wind turbine test

From the tests that have been carried out, a graph can be shown as Fig. 7. The next test is a test of the buck converter where the input of the buck converter is obtained from the output of the hybrid power plant. Furthermore, the output of the buck converter is adjusted so that the output of the buck converter is 14.4 V which is then used to charge the battery which can be used for electrical loads. In Table 1 is a test data from the buck converter (Table 4).

## 3 Discussion

From the research that has been done, it is found that the power generated from this prototype design is 95.47–101.62 W. In addition to the buck converter test, it is found that the efficiency value of the buck converter is 85.115–95.154%. From the research conducted, it was found that the output voltage value of the charge controller is stable where the largest error value from the output voltage value is 0.972%. As for the output current from the buck converter, it has a value greater than the amount of the input current where in the buck converter test with the PI method it was found that the average value of the output current was 16.84 mA, while the average input current was 15.73 mA. From the research that has been done, it can be seen that the use of PI control can make the output voltage and buck converter stable, which is different from previous research conducted by Robiansyah where the output voltage in this study still has oscillations [10]. The tool that has been made has a limit, namely the maximum input voltage that can be controlled is 25 V, where when the voltage exceeds 25 V passes through this charge controller, the voltage sensor circuit in it will burn because it does not match the planning calculations that have been done previously. In addition, if the voltage is more than 25 V it will make the voltage that goes to the Arduino pin exceed 5 V which makes over voltage which can damage the

Arduino itself. The method used can make the output voltage of the buck converter more stable.

## 4 Conclusion

The purpose of this research is to support the program of utilizing renewable energy by making a charge controller. The use of a vertical axis on the turbine makes this design easier to apply anywhere because this turbine does not have to be directed towards the wind, so this turbine can be placed in a place that has varying wind and water directions. This is known as a portable and flexible device. The rotation of the generator increases with the difference in gear ratios. With the higher the intensity of sunlight, the higher the voltage and current generated and vice versa. The power generated from the design of this prototype is 95.47–101.62 W. From the tests that have been done, it is found that the efficiency of this buck converter system is 85.60–95.7% so that this buck converter is expected to extend the lifetime and maintain battery performance. Further research can be carried out on the manufacture of windings in the inductor and the effect of the cross-sectional area used in it.

## References


1. Floyd TL (2012) Electronic devices (electron flow version). Prentice Hall, New Jersey
2. Gautam AR, Deshpande DM, Suresh A, Mittal A (2013) A double input DC to DC BuckBoost converter for low voltage fotovoltaic/wind systems. Int J ChemTech Res 5:1018–1020
3. Gurav R (2017) Paper of implementation of MPPT charge control based BuckBost converter. Maharasta, India
4. Nugraha AT, Priyambodo D Design of pond water turbidity monitoring system in arduino-based catfish cultivation to support sustainable development goals 2030 No. 9 industry, innovation, and infrastructure. J Electron Electromed Eng Med Inform 2.3:119–124
5. Nugraha AT, Priyambodo D (2021) Design of a monitoring system for hydroganics based on Arduino Uno R3 to realize sustainable development goals number 2 zero hunger. J Electron Electromed Eng Med Inform 3.1:50–56
6. Pikatan S (1999) Conversion of wind energy. Department of Mathematics and Natural Sciences, University of Surabaya, Surabaya
7. Priyambodo D (2020) Prototype hybrid power plant of solar panel and vertical wind turbine as a provider of alternative electrical energy at Kenjeran Beach Surabaya. J Electron Electromed Eng Med Inform 2(3):108–113
8. Dutta A (2012) Design of an arduino based MPPT solar charger controller. Brac University, Bangladesh
9. Rahman S (2012) Design of a charge controller circuit with MPPT for photovoltaic system. Brac University, Bangladesh
10. Rashid MH Power electronics circuits, device and applications. Prentice Hall, New Jersey
11. Kastha D, Bose BK (1994) Fault mode single-phase operation of a variable frequency induction motor drive and improvement of pulsating torque characteristics. IEEE Trans Industr Electron 41(4):426–433
12. Kazimierczuk MK (2015) Pulse-width modulated DCDC power converter. Wiley Inc., USA

13. Priyambodo D (2020) Design and build a photovoltaic and vertical Savonious turbine power plant as an alternative power supply to help save energy in skyscrapers. J Electron Electromed Eng Med Inform 2(3):57–63
14. Qazi S (2017) Standalone photovoltaik (pv) systems for disaster relief and remote areas. Elsevier, United State
15. Tong CW (1997) The design and testing of a wind turbine for Malaysian wind condition, thesis, UTM
16. Rashid MH (2015) Alternative energy in power electronics. Elsevier, USA
17. Umanand L (2007) Non-conventional energy systems. Indian Institute of Science Bangalore, Bangalore
18. Feigenspan J (2011) Program comprehension of feature-oriented software development. In: International conference on software engineering
19. Kadry S (2011) A new proposed technique to improve software regression testing cost. Int J Secur Appl 5(3)
20. Kumar S, Sugandha Chakraverti SC, Agarwal, Chakraverti AK (2012) Modified COCOMO model for maintenance cost estimation of real time system software. Int J Res Eng Appl Sci 2(3)
21. Kelly T, Buckley J (2009) Cognitive levels and software maintenance sub-tasks, PPIG—Limerick
22. Nallusamy S, Ibrahim S, Mahrin MN (2011) A software redocumentation proses using ontology based approach in software maintenance. Int J Inf Electron Eng 1(2)
23. Dimitrakis P (2017) Charge-trapping non-volatile memories. Springer International Publishing, London
24. Istepanian R (2001) In digital controller implementation and fragility. Springer, London, p 87
25. Meza GR (2017) Controller tuning with evolutionary multiobjective optimization. Springer International Publishing, Switzerland
26. Sathyajith M (2006) Wind energy. In R. A. Fundamentals. Springer, Berlin, Heidelberg
27. Storey MA (2006) Theories, tools and research methods in program comprehension: past, present and future. Springer, https://doi.org/10.1007/s11219-006-9216-4

# The Auxiliary Engine Lubricating Oil Pressure Monitoring System Based on Modbus Communication

**Anggara Trisna Nugraha, Ruddianto, Mahasin Maulana Ahmad, Dwi Sasmita Aji Pambudi, Agung Prasetyo Utomo, Mayda Zita Aliem Tiwana, and Alwy Muhammad Ravi**

**Abstract** The problem with lubricating oil that often arises is low engine oil pressure. If the operator is not aware of the condition and the handling is too late, it can cause damage to the machine components. With the availability of a reliable alarm monitoring system, handling problems that endanger the engine will be quickly resolved and increase safety on board. This research aims to create a reliable and efficient alarm monitoring system to make it easier for operators to monitor the condition of the auxiliary engine. This research uses an experimental method with a new alarm monitoring system architecture and fault diagnosis algorithms through the auxiliary engine lubricating oil pressure transmitter in marine vessel Meratus Benoa. Tests show that the system can generate alarms with a time delay less then one second since the abnormal condition appears. The results indicate that the system is reliable in real-time monitoring and efficient processing time in abnormal machine conditions. This reliable and efficient alarm monitoring system can be a solution and a basis for research on ship alarm monitoring systems.

**Keywords** Auxiliary engine · Lubricating oil · The alarm monitoring system · Modbus RTU

## 1 Introduction

Lubricating oil has an essential role in diesel generators [1, 2]. The function of this lubricating oil is to reduce the friction and wear of the two metal surfaces of the engine [3–5]. It is necessary to lubricate the engine bearings, crankshaft, turbocharger, and other moving parts [6, 7]. Each diesel generator has a separate, independent engine lubricating oil system [8]. The problem with lubricating oil that often arises is low oil pressure for the engine. If the operator does not know the condition and the handling is too late, damage to machine components can occur [9, 10]. Thus, an efficient

A. T. Nugraha (✉) · Ruddianto · M. M. Ahmad · D. S. A. Pambudi · A. P. Utomo · M. Z. A. Tiwana · A. M. Ravi
Politeknik Perkapalan Negeri Surabaya, Sukolilo, Surabaya 60111, Indonesia
e-mail: anggaranugraha@ppns.ac.id



T. Triwiyanto et al. (eds.), *Proceedings of the 2nd International Conference on Electronics, Biomedical Engineering, and Health Informatics*, Lecture Notes in Electrical Engineering 898, https://doi.org/10.1007/978-981-19-1804-9_13

and reliable lubricating oil pressure monitoring system is vital to maintaining the lubricating oil pressure in auxiliary engine components [11, 12].

Many studies have researched engine parameters. In [13], Zhu researched sensors to measure oils properties, such as wear, debris, water, viscosity, aeration, soot, corrosion, and Sulfur content. Zhukov dedicates the manufacture of a universal monitoring system for marine diesel engines in [14]. His research provides details on the existing monitoring component. The discussion details are the various parameters, measurement methods from existing sensing tools, and measuring instruments on monitored machines.

Zaghloul [15] provides a practical design of an alarm monitoring system that uses a Supervisory Control and Data Acquisition (SCADA). In the planned design, the alarm monitoring system can access the entire status of the ship's engine parameters and display it on the human–machine interface (HMI). Gan et al. [16] made a simulator alarm monitoring system that can monitor and simulate real-time. Complex engine room simulation models and object-oriented programming are using Visual Studio and C# language. The journal Lee [17] discusses the alarm process scheme for fault detection algorithms determined based on the basic design requirements of the alarm monitoring system. Wang et al. in [18] discuss the solution to the communication problem uses the CAN bus and RS485 communication.

From previous studies, they still provide complex and expensive solutions. Zhu [13] only discusses the principles of the sensors used in the lubricating oil monitoring system without discussing the monitoring process of the readings of these sensors. Zhukov [14] only focuses on existing instruments and the concept of planning a universal monitoring system and has no detailed discussion of the architecture system. Zaghloul [15] discusses the architectural design of the alarm monitoring system and ignores the fault detection algorithm for alarm activation. While, the simulator made by Gan et al. [16] is suitable for training activities but too complex to be implemented in a practical system.

This study aims to provide a cheap and straightforward solution to an alarm monitoring system. Using the Outseal PLC and Logic Panel Autonics, the technical designs, including fault diagnosis algorithms, can be featured in reliable, efficient, and effective real-time online monitoring. This prototype was built based on the basic design requirements described in [17] and the communication method adopted from the Modbus RS485 protocol interface in [18]. The only parameter observed is the auxiliary engine lubricating oil pressure. With the Autonics Logic Panel as a monitoring center that displays parameter information, this research makes it easier for operators to monitor the condition of the auxiliary engine.

## 2 System Method

This research aims to develop an inexpensive, reliable, and efficient alarm monitoring system to monitor auxiliary engine lubricating oil pressure. Figure 1 shows the architectural design. The sensor is a pressure transmitter on the field device to

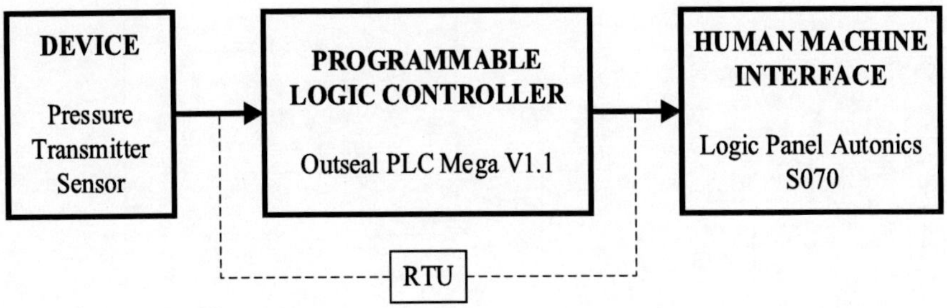


**Fig. 1** The architectural design

send data to the PLC. Furthermore, the data from the field device read by the PLC is send to the human–machine interface via Modbus RTU communication. However, to make this system an alarm monitoring system, an algorithm for determining fault conditions must be determined first [19].

Through Outseal studio, an efficient determination algorithm generates an alarm when an abnormal condition occurs. In this case, the alarm monitoring system created can fulfill two objectives: the analog monitoring function and fault diagnosis. With the equipment and design considerations used, the alarm monitoring system made is affordable and reliable. In addition, the use of the RS485 Modbus protocol interface for communication between the PLC and the human–machine interface provides an efficient solution for operators because it has a communication distance of 1200 m with a speed of 200 Kb/s [20]. Thus, the operator can monitor the engine from the engine control room.

## 2.1 *Layout Lubricating Oil System*

The lubricating oil system of the diesel generator is stored. It supplies the necessary clean lubricating oil to the engine bearings, crankshaft, turbocharger, and other engine moving parts to operate the diesel generator. The design provides adequate lubrication and cooling for the various moving parts of the engine to prevent friction in the engine from resulting in wear [8]. The diesel generator lubricating oil system is shown schematically in Fig. 2.

Figure 2 shows valve arrangements to provide component isolation capabilities in the event of system leakage. The system consists of an engine-driven lube oil pump, oil cooler, several temperature controls valves, an electric motor-driven pre-lube pump, oil heater, several heat exchangers, strainers, filters, piping, valves, makeup tank, controls, and instrumentation [21].

Engine from the crankcase through the filter drives the pump to push the lubricating oil, preventing foreign matter from entering and damaging the pipes. The engine-driven pump delivers lubricating oil under pressure required by the engine [22]. An oil temperature control valve supplies oil to the engine or the lubrication

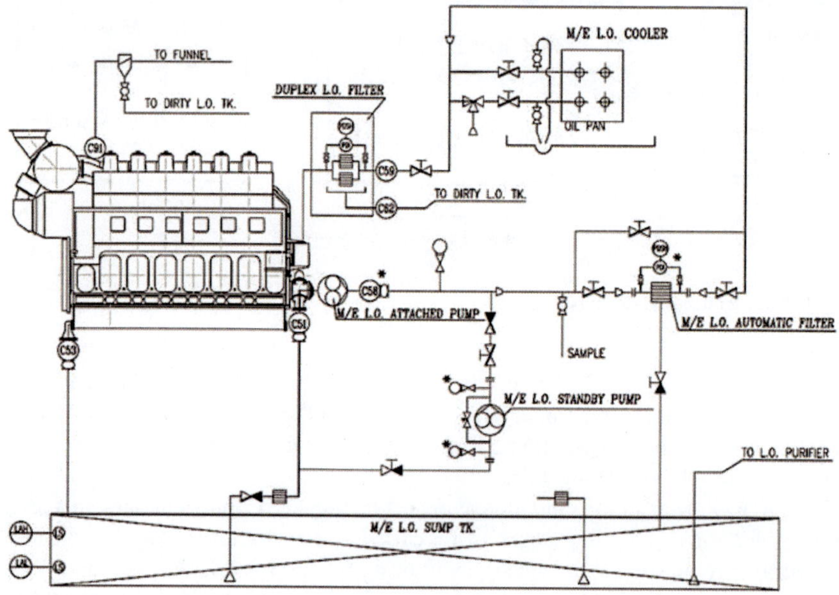


**Fig. 2** Lubricating oil system diagram in the diesel generator

oil heat exchanger in a motor-operated three-way valve. The lubrication oil heat exchanger has the task of cooling the lubricating oil system flowing in the engine. It has a temperature that matches the lube oil temperature specifications when the engine operates and maintains the oil temperature when it is not operating [23]. All lube oil that has flowed into the engine will flow into the lube oil sump tank. This sump tank has filled and drains connections to obtain a lube oil sample for lube oil analysis [24].

## 2.2 *Design Base of Alarm System*

This paper provides a design method of alarm monitoring in real-time using Outseal PLC Mega V1.1 and Logic Panel Autonics S070. PLC Outseal Mega V1.1 is the PLC used in this study. However, other types of PLCs can use the approach used in this study. This PLC Outseal Mega V1.1 works on 24VDC voltage and has two analog input ports to accept 0–5 V voltage or 4-20 mA current. The communication facility between devices owned by this PLC is through the RS485 Modbus communication protocol [25].

However, this study also uses HMI, the Logic Panel Autonics S070. Logic Panel operates at 24 VDC. Apart from being a display, this device has an internal PLC,

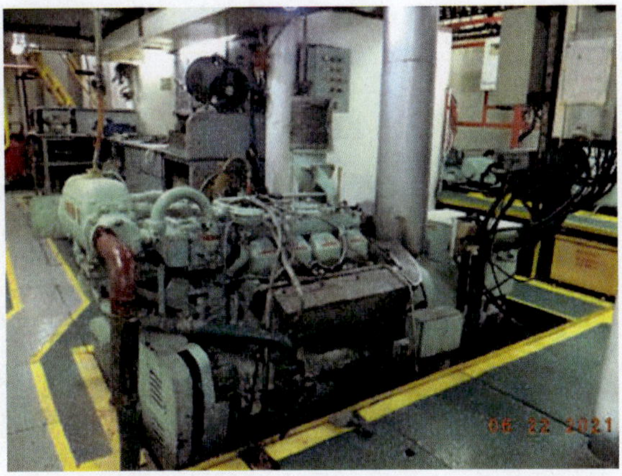


**Fig. 3** The auxiliary engine of MV Meratus Benoa

which provides digital input/output. In addition, data processing becomes slow if this device works as a PLC and a display.

HMI and PLC communicate via Modbus RTU RS485 protocol. PLC Outseal still cannot do online monitoring and Modbus communication simultaneously. Thus, HMI performs simulation functions in real-time. The communication between PLC Outseal and PC is only for sending program and PC to PLC or PC fetching program from PLC via USB port [26].

The object of this research is the auxiliary engine of MV Meratus Benoa, as shown in Fig. 3. Thus, the ship's battery is functions as a 24 V PLC supply voltage provider. This PLC can be expanded with other Outseal PLCs to increase the number of I/O. Two analog input ports are available on one Outseal Mega V1.1 PLC module, namely A1 and A2. Data retrieval in this study utilizes MV Meratus Benoa auxiliary engine oil pressure data. Furthermore, the PLC analog input port will receive oil pressure data from the pressure transmitter.

## 2.3 *Analog Monitoring Function*

Pressure transmitter and PLC connection are via PLC analog port. Each Outseal PLC Mega V1.1 module has two analog input ports, namely A1 and A2. Each port is capable of accepting 0–5 V or 0–20 mA input with an integer range of 0–1023. PLC Outseal can do the current reading of 0–20 mA by adding a shunt resistor of 250 Ω. The only one analog input port is used in this study, namely A1, as shown in Fig. 4. The pressure transmitter used has an output range of 4–20 mA, which is equivalent to 0–1 Mpa or 0–10 bar. So, to ensure the safety of PLC, the value converter used is 4–20 mA to 0–5 V.

The primary purpose of this alarm monitoring function is to maximize operator visibility regarding the lubricating oil auxiliary engine parameters. Logic Panel S070

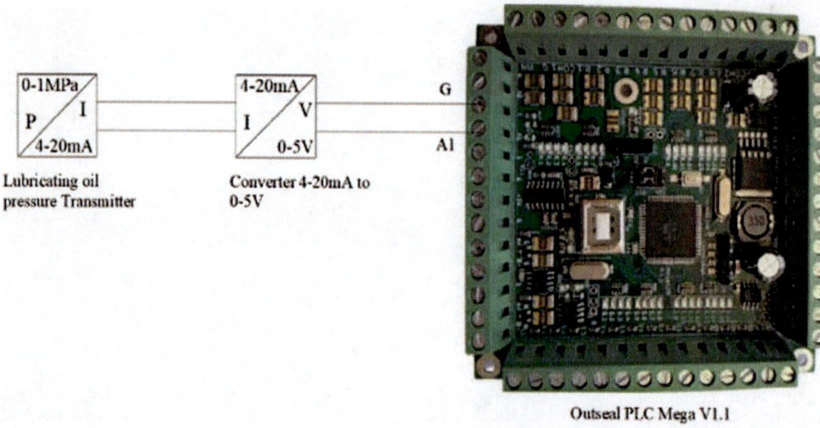


**Fig. 4** Analog input port A1

displays PLC analog input signals in bar charts and numbers with units (bars) equivalent to actual oil pressure. The alarm activation limit is set through the program on the PLC to prevent changes made by irresponsible parties.

## 2.4 *Fault Diagnosis Algorithm*

There are three steps in diagnosing abnormal conditions in an alarm monitoring system: fault detection, caution, and recovery [27]. This diagnostic step involves monitoring the system, the timing of the abnormal condition, and identifying the fault that occurred. The approach taken is to analyze the difference between sensor readings and the expected results. So, the abnormal conditions will be detected if there is a difference between the actual and expected value. Once an abnormal condition is detected, an alarm must be activated to alert the operator. The human–machine interface will also display the type and time of the error. Figure 5 shows the flowchart illustrating this error algorithm.

## 2.5 *Programming Alarm Lubricating Oil Pressure*

As a lubricating oil pressure sensor, a pressure transmitter sends a current of 4–20 mA to the PLC. The PLC reads this pressure value as an integer value which requires a conversion process to get the real value pressure. The PLC's internal A/D converter, the SCALE function, is used to get the real value pressure from the pressure transmitter. Figure 6, line 0, displays a ladder diagram for converting the integer value to the actual pressure value. The input data received by A1 is an integer

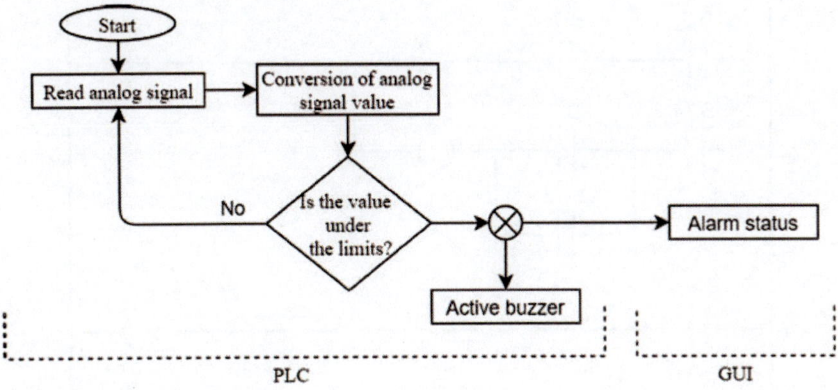


**Fig. 5** Fault diagnosis algorithm

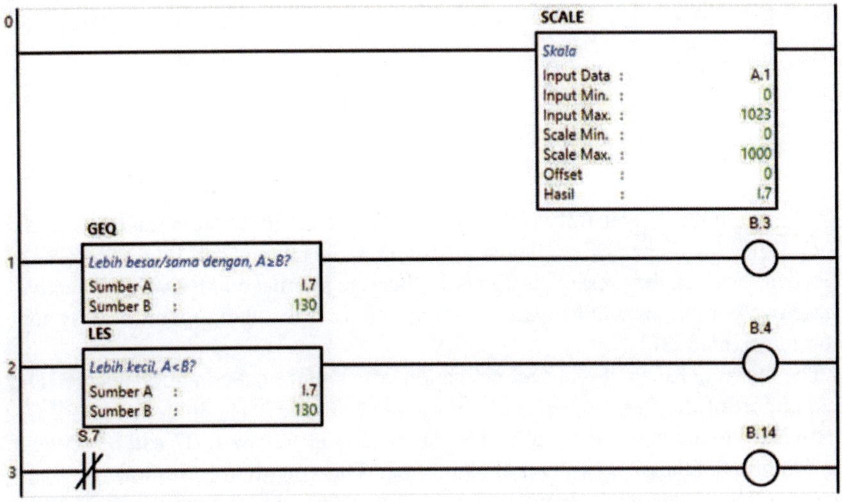


**Fig. 6** Ladder diagram for A/D converter

value of 1023. The value is on a scale of 1000 to get a more accurate reading value by obtaining a four-digit number. Then the Logic Panel will process this value. The value displayed in the Logic Panel is 10 bar, with two numbers after the comma as the actual pressure value.

This program using the GEQ and LES functions due to the lubricating oil pressure should not be lower than 0.12–0.15 MPa or 1.2–1.5 bar [28], are used, as shown in Fig. 6. When the oil pressure is below that standard, a warning alarm will fire [29]. In this study, the low-pressure limit value used is 1.3 bar. The GEQ function is to get the logic TRUE or FALSE from the internal coil B3. When the oil pressure is above 1.3 bar, the internal coil B3 will be active, and if the oil pressure value is below

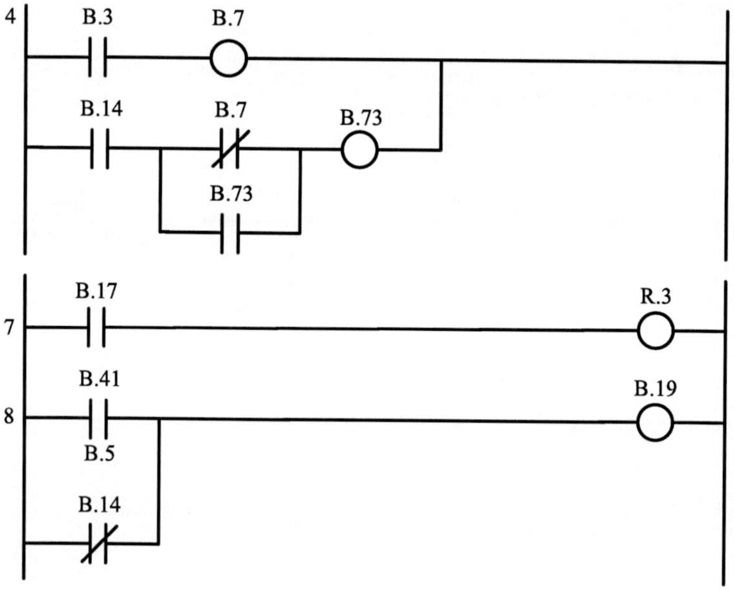


**Fig. 7** Ladder diagram alarm lubricating oil pressure

1.3 bar, the internal coil B3 will be inactive. The LES function is the opposite of GEQ. When the oil pressure is below 1.3 bar, then the internal coil B4 will be active. Meanwhile, when the pressure is above 1.3 bar, the internal coil B4 will be inactive. These two conditions will activate other conditions in the alarm monitoring system program created [30].

The alarm consists of a buzzer activation when abnormal conditions occur. The Output port of the PLC connects the buzzer and the PLC. The initialization of the alarm is triggered by the internal coil B7 shown in Fig. 7, row 4. B7 will be active if the condition of the oil pressure is above 1.3 bar. This condition corresponds to line 1 in Fig. 6. The alarm will be logically FALSE when this condition occurs because the lubricating oil low alarm contact condition is Normally Closed (NC). The alarm will be TRUE when coil B7 is not active, as indicated by the active buzzer. Push Button Buzzer STOP is available to deactivate the buzzer when an alarm condition occurs. Switch S7, in Fig. 6, line 3, is used as a push-button STOP which will deactivate the buzzer when an abnormal condition occurs. HMI will display the alarm list because of the Internal coil B73. This internal coil is the interlock of the alarm list.

## 2.6 Interface Design

GP Editor is the default software from Logic Panel Autonics to design the interface. The interface consists of three sections: analog parameters, alarm lists, and indicators

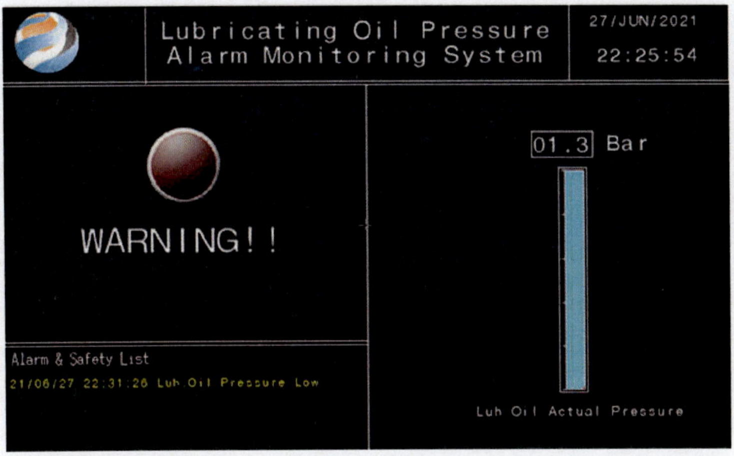


**Fig. 8** HMI interface design

in Fig. 8. Setting update data parameter reading is done every 100mS. The displayed data format has been set with an unsigned data type to display the positive value of the lubricating oil pressure. The alarm indicator is also displayed in the Logic Panel with the indicator light flashing. At the same time, WARNING appears to give operators clearer visibility that an abnormal condition has occurred.

### 2.7 *Data Analysis*

The data from prototype testing using tabulation by presenting data in tabular form. Representation of test results using graphs to see the performance of the prototype. Data analysis used descriptive analysis to explore new information from the graph of the test results. This new information is in the form of conformity of the prototype performance with the system design.

## 3 Results

The testing is on the MV Meratus Benoa auxiliary engine. The marine diesel engine type is HND MWM Series 234. The operating range of the generator is 1500 rpm, the working frequency is 50 Hz, and the working voltage is 400 V. Table 1 shows the test results. The test starts when the engine is not operating. At first, the oil pressure is 0 bar when the engine is not operating. Then, the oil pressure will rise significantly up to 6 bar, so it takes much pressure to drain the oil into the engine. Along with the increase in RPM until the idle RPM condition or engine working speed is reached,

**Table 1** Oil pressure data

| Trial order | Engine speed (Rpm) | Oil pressure (bar) | Alarm condition |
|---|---|---|---|
| 1 | 0 | 0 | Active |
| 2 | 500 | 6 | Inactive |
| 3 | 800 | 5.57 | Inactive |
| 4 | 1000 | 5.55 | Inactive |
| 5 | 1200 | 5.34 | Inactive |
| 6 | 1300 | 5.34 | Inactive |
| 7 | 1370 | 5.34 | Inactive |
| 8 | 1400 | 5.3 | Inactive |
| 9 | 1500 | 5.2 | Inactive |
| 10 | 1515 | 5.2 | Inactive |

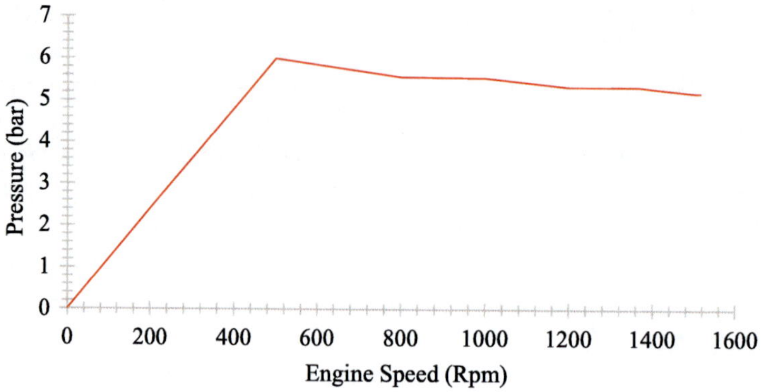


**Fig. 9** Changes in oil pressure and engine speed

the oil pressure gradually decreases to 5.2 bar due to the decrease in the viscosity of the noble oil and the increase in oil temperature. Figure 9 shows the representation of the increase in lubricating oil pressure.

## 4 Discussions

Testing the alarm monitoring system aims to determine the system's response when the limit pressure value is under the setting value. At first, the prototype read the pressure of lubricating oil in 0 bar. This condition indicates that the oil pressure does not meet the standard limit of the system, i.e., the oil pressure must be above 1.3 bar. Due to the condition, the alarm goes on, and the buzzer is active. The active alarm, when the oil pressure is below the limit value, which is 1.3 bar, proves that the alarm monitoring system can effectively warn the operator if the oil pressure is abnormal. Thus, by activating the alarm, the alarm monitoring function of this system has fulfilled its purpose.

The basic design requirements used in this study met several requirements in [17] of them: the alarm provides alerting, informing, guiding, and confirming to assist the operator to take the necessary action to preserve normal operating conditions; the system processes fault algorithms and displays alarms for optimizing the use of the man–machine interface; and the system has a segmented and distributed architecture to localize any failures and real-time processing of data.

Using Outseal PLC, programming this system is more accessible than research by [16], which tends to be complex and requires expensive allocation of costs. Monitoring engine conditions is also made easier with the Autonics S070 Logic Panel interface. Not only does it provide an interface design [15] or details of existing alarms on the engine [14], but this prototype also provides system design, interface design, and fault diagnosis algorithms. By adopting Modbus RS485 communication from [18], the alarm monitoring system is working smoothly according to its function.

This research still has many shortcomings. Monitoring given is still limited to lubricating oil pressure. In addition, alerting is still limited to low lubricating oil pressure errors. There is no reliability test on the ship in sailing conditions and extreme conditions. Error determining algorithms still tend to be simple and still not suitable for complex systems. However, with these shortcomings, the prototype is reliable and efficient for berthing ships. So, it can be easier for the operator to monitor the condition of the auxiliary engine lubricating oil pressure directly and in real-time. Also, this research can be a solution and a basis for research on ship alarm monitoring systems.

## 5 Conclusions

This study provides a design of an effective alarm monitoring system for monitoring lubricating oil pressure. This Design method of the alarm monitoring system uses the PLC and Logic Panel S070 based on Modbus RTU communication. The design of the auxiliary engine lubricating oil pressure monitoring system tests a pressure transmitter installed on the auxiliary engine MV Meratus Benoa. The test results show that the prototype can provide an alarm signal effectively by the initial purpose of making this system.

The test results also show that the system is cheap, reliable, and efficient to warn the operators because it clearly shows faults in the machine. Even so, this alarm monitoring system still requires further research by adding other parameters to the ship's auxiliary engine. The addition of parameters will also be very useful in developing the function of the auxiliary engine lubricating oil alarm monitoring system. So that when the engine condition is still not on, the monitoring alarm system does not detect any errors as occurred during the data collection process in this study. In future research, testing and analysis can be carried out on lubricating oil and become more complex with other parameters and fault diagnosis algorithms.

## References


1. Wang J, Wang Z, Gu F, Ma X, Fei J, Cao Y (2020) An investigation into the sensor placement of a marine engine lubrication system for condition monitoring. In: Advances in asset management and condition monitoring, vol 166, pp 573–582. Springer, Cham. https://doi.org/10.1007/978-3-030-57745-2_48
2. Zhu J, Yoon JM, He D, Qu Y, Bechloefer E (2013) Lubrication oil condition monitoring and remaining useful life prediction with particle filtering. Int J Prognost Health Manage 1–15
3. Hermawan A, Rahardja IB, Syam MY, Sukismo H (2019) Analysis of viscosity of lubricating oil on generator machine working hours at KP. Macan Tutul 4203. J Appl Sci Adv Technol 1(3):69–74
4. Stevens P (1988) Oil and gas dictionary, Palgrave Macmillan UK
5. Koppad D, Paramanandham N (2020) Non-destructive testing for cracks in concrete. Adv Commun Syst Netw Lecture Notes Electric Eng 656
6. Allal AA, Melhaoui Y, Kamil A, Mansouri K, Youssfi M (2020) Ship main engine lubricating oil system's reliability analysis by using Bayesian network approach. Int J Eng Res Afr 48:108–125
7. Elsevier, Sealing technology developed to meet demands of unconventional wells in the oil and gas sector, Sealing Technology, pp 1–14, April 2018
8. Okrent D (1987) The safety goals of the U.S. Nuclear Regulatory Commission, Science, vol 236, no 4799, pp 296–300
9. Council International Des Machines a Combustion, Guidlines for Diesel Engines Lubrication, French: CIMAC Working Group (2004)
10. Dionysious K, Bolbot V, Theotokatos G (2021) A functional model-based approach for ship systems safety and reliability analysis: application to a cruise ship lubricating oil system. J Eng Maritime Environ 1–17
11. Wu S, Chen X, Chen H, Lu J (2020) Intelligent fire early warning and monitoring system for ship bridge based on WSN. Int J Sci 7(08):248–255
12. Falces DB, Barrena JLL, Arraiza AL, Menendez J (2017) Monitoring of fuel oil process of marine diesel engine. Appl Thermal Eng 517–526
13. Zhu X, Zhong C, Zhe J (2017) Lubricating oil condition sensors for online machine health monitoring. Tribiol Int 109:473–484
14. Zhukov V, Butsanets A, Sherban S, Igonin V (2020) Monitoring system of ship power plants during operation. Adv Intell Syst Comput 419–428
15. Zaghloul MS (2014) Online ship control system using supervisory control and data acquisition (SCADA). Int J COmput Sci Appl 3(1):6–10
16. Gan H, Ren G, Zhang J (2011) A novel marine engine room monitoring and alarm system integrated simulation. In: International conference on electronic & mechanical engineering and information technology, pp 2226–2229
17. Lee CK, Shin JH, Koo IS, Park JK (1997) A basic design of alarm system for the future nuclear power plants in Korea, Taejon, Korea
18. Wang CS, Xiao HR, Pan WG, Han YZ (2011) Design of monitoring and alarm system for the ship engine room. Adv Mater Res 268–270
19. Alvarez GP (2020) Real-time fault detection and diagnosis using intelligent monitoring and supervision systems, fault detection, diagnosis and prognosis. IntechOpen
20. Hung PD, Chin VV, Chinh NT, Tung TD (2020) A flexible platform for industrial applications based on RS485 networks. J Commun 15(3):245–255
21. United States Nuclear Regulatory Commision (NRC), Emergency Diesel Generator Lubricating Oil System Functional Arrangement, United States Nuclear Regulatory Commision (NRC) (2013)

22. Rostek E, Babiak M, Wroblewski E (2017) The influence of oil pressure in the engine lubrication system on friction losses, TRANSCOM 2017. In: International scientific conference on sustainable, modern and safe transport, pp 771–776
23. James NO, Ishiodu AA, Odokwo VE (2016) Design and construction of a tube type lubricating oil heat exchanger. Int J Eng Adv Technol Stud 4(3):1–17
24. Allal AA, Melhaoui Y, Kamil A, Mansouri K, Youssfi M (2020) Ship main engine lubricating oil system's reliability analysis BU using Bayesian network approach. Int J Eng Res Afr 48(1663–4144):108–125
25. Seneviratne P Building Arduino PLCs, Building Arduino PLCs, pp 127–138, 29 May 2017
26. Bidyanath K (2021) A survey on open-source SCADA for industrial automation using raspberry Pi. In: Trends in wireless communication and information security, vol 740, pp 19–26. Lecture Notes in Electrical Engineering
27. Jones & Bartlett Learning (2019) Fundamentals of automotive maintenance and light repair. In: Engine repair, pp 1572–1581. Jones & Bartlett Learning
28. Zou C, Huang S, Yu J (2012) Research on Cam & Tappet friction test method for anti-wear performance evaluation of engine oil. In: Proceedings of the FISITA 2012 world automotive congress, china, lecture notes in electrical engineering, pp 533–534
29. Henan Diesel Engine Group Co, LTD (1998) MWM Marine Diesel Generator Set Operation Manual, China: Henan Diesel Engine Group Co, Ltd Research Institute of Technical Center
30. Autonics Corporation, LP-S070 User Manual, 2020. Online. Available: https://www.autonics.com/service/data/view/6/216776. Accessed 03 Dec 2021

# Global Positioning System Data Processing Improvement for Blind Tracker Device Based Using Moving Average Filter

**Sevia Indah Purnama, Mas Aly Afandi, and Egya Vernando Purba**

**Abstract** Assistive technology in medical devices to aid visual impairments are providing an increasing trend in research and development. An important problem that can occur in blind people is misread user location. This condition makes trouble while families with visual impairments wants to find them. Tracking device for blind people is widely used to track blind people position. The tracking device uses a global positioning system to track position. The quality of the global positioning system in both hardware and software is very important to this tool. This research aims to improve the data processing in global positioning system by implementing a moving average filter. Moving average filter is a filter that commonly implementing to reduce noise from outlier data. Moving average filter can be implemented to reduce the impact of misreading location. Data research shows that moving average filter gives improvement while tracking route. Tracking route while using moving average filter also gives more accurate route. Blind tracker device in this research has been done and can be used to track blind people. Moving average filter reduce error reading position 3.73 m in tenting one and 1.35 m in testing 2. Future work can be adding moving average filter in FPGA technology to minimize the device.

**Keywords** Global positioning system · Assistive technology · Tracker device · Data processing

S. I. Purnama (✉)
Department of Biomedical Engineering, Institut Teknologi Telkom Purwokerto, Purwokerto, Indonesia
e-mail: sevia@ittelkom-pwt.ac.id

M. A. Afandi · E. V. Purba
Department of Telecommunication Engineering, Institut Teknologi Telkom Purwokerto, Purwokerto, Indonesia

 
T. Triwiyanto et al. (eds.), *Proceedings of the 2nd International Conference on Electronics, Biomedical Engineering, and Health Informatics*, Lecture Notes in Electrical Engineering 898, https://doi.org/10.1007/978-981-19-1804-9_14

# 1 Introduction

Human life development technology rapidly changes by technological updates in various fields such as education, medical, agriculture and many more. The development medical fields in technology that assist human with disabilities called assistive technology [1, 2]. Assistive technology had various range include assist for bind or low vision people [3]. According to estimates from the Ministry of Health Republic of Indonesia, the number of blind people in Indonesia is 1.5% of the total population. If the current population of Indonesia is approximately 250 million, it means that at least currently there are 3,750,000 people who are blind, blind or have low vision. This is not a small number, according to the 2010 population census, the school-age population is 40% of the total population. This means, 40% of the 3,750,000 visually impaired in Indonesia are visually impaired of school age 6–18 years [4]. Along with the ever-changing and varied technology, many assistive devices or tools have been developed to assist blind people to improve their activities [5, 6]. Some make tools such as sticks, shoes, sandals, and others. Some use the same tools but have different advantages and various components. Assistive devices for the visually impaired still have many opportunities to be developed to be better [7, 8]. The most important part for developing blind tracker device is Global Positioning System (GPS) [9]. GPS is a satellite-based navigation system consisting of at least 24 satellites. Each satellite transmits a unique signal and orbital parameters that allow the GPS device to decode and calculate the satellite exact location. GPS consists of three parts, namely the space segment (outer space) the ground segment (earth) and the user segment (users). The GPS receiver uses this information and trilateration to calculate user exact location. Basically, GPS receiver measures the distance to each satellite by the amount of time it takes to receive the transmitted signal. By measuring the distance from a few more satellites, the receiver can determine user position and display it. GPS can calculate other information, such as speed, bearing, track, trip distance, distance to destination. GPS device can be found in many devices such as cellphone and smartwatch. Some of them use dedicated GPS that cannot be modified. Blind tracker device cannot use this kind of GPS. Blind tracker device must be use GPS component that can be modified. Modified GPS is needed because cellphone and smartwatch is expensive. Besides, cellphone and smartwatch are not made for tracking people. Blind tracker device needs some kind of standalone GPS. In many cases standalone GPS gives misread location. This condition can be occurred because of outlier data or wrong location read. Filtering method for GPS data processing improvement such as Kalman Filter [9, 10]. Another improvement also has done using gaussian process regression [11, 12]. Signal processing can be implemented to avoid this case. Signal processing method that can be used to improve misread standalone GPS is moving average filter. Research shows that moving average filter is a filter that can be used to minimize impact of outlier data. This research is aim to develop blind tracker monitoring system. Blind tracker device output is location data and visualize location data Google Maps. Improvement location reading trough GPS also has been done in this research. Moving average filter is implementing in blind tracker device development. Research experiment for blind tracking device consists of location reading, tracker reading, and measuring signal quality. Data testing shows moving average filter increasing accuracy for location reading in blind tracker device.

## 2 Material and Method

Blind tracker device arranged by 2 major system which is hardware system and software system. Hardware system consist of microcontroller, GPS, GPS antenna, and battery. Microcontroller that used to develop blind tracker device is ATMega 328. Blind tracker device use standalone GPS built in SIM 7000E and antenna GNSS (Global Navigation Satellite System) Glonass.

### *2.1 Data Acquisition*

Figure 1 shows how blind tracker hardware was built for this research. This hardware is quite simple and small. Blind tracker device dimension is 15 cm × 7 cm × 7 cm. Blind tracker device can be used as a belt for blind people. The output data is longitude and latitude for read location. Longitude and latitude data can be visualize using google maps to compare the actual location and reading location. Blind tracker device not only record location but also signal strength. Signal strength data is CSQ (Cell Signal Quality) and RSSI (Receive Signal Strength Indicator). To read longitude, latitude, CSQ, and RSSI need software configuration. This role has been done by software system. System software programmed using Arduino IDE (Integrated

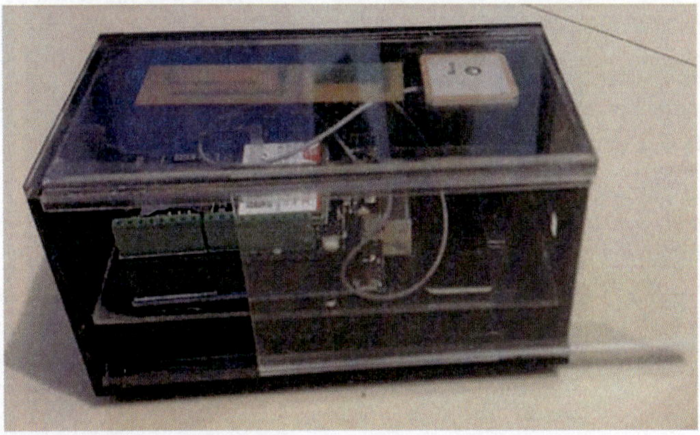

**Fig. 1** Blind tracker hardware data acquisition

Development Environment). Blind tracker software arranged by activating GPS, read location data, and read signal strength. This software configuration is used to obtain data without optimization. This device is used for data acquisition for this research.

### 2.2 Data Processing

The aim of this research also improves GPS reading location. To optimize location reading needed some filter to process longitude and latitude data in GPS standalone device. Moving Average Filter can be used to optimize standalone GPS device for blind tracker device. Moving average filter is a filter that commonly used to reduce noise from sensor such as temperature sensor, humidity sensor, velocity sensor, and many more [13–18]. Moving average filter can be defined as a low pass filter with finite impulse response [19–21]. Moving average filter has characteristic that can be eliminate outlier data [22, 23]. In many case, standalone GPS hardware can gives outlier location. Outlier location gives misread location. This condition must be avoided in tracker device. Moving average filter is implemented to reduce possibility of misread location. Moving average filter formula can be defined with

$$y(i) = \frac{1}{M} \sum_{j=0}^{M-1} x(i - j). \tag{1}$$

Equation 1 shows that output moving average filter y(i) can be obtain by summing input x in interval (i − j). When i means newest data divided with M. Variable M in moving average filter equation is an any number called window. High window gives robustness to deal with outlier but slower the output calculation [24, 24]. Lower window gives fast output calculation but reduce response to deal with outlier. Moving average window for data tracking is 3. This value based on requirement for faster data process while tracking (Fig. 2).

### 2.3 Data Collection

Figure 3 shows data tracking collection process. Scenario 1 is used to get data tracking without moving average filter. Scenario 2 is used to get data tracking with moving average window. This research used 3 locations to get data tracking. Data tracking from scenario 1 and scenario 2 will be compared trough Google Maps. Visualization in Google Maps is needed to see the effect of moving average filter to blind tracker device. Comparing visualization data trough scenario 1 and scenario 2 will confirm how optimize blind tracker device with using moving average filter. Tracking data will show blind tracker device performance. Tracking data will represent tracking route while blind tracker device is used.

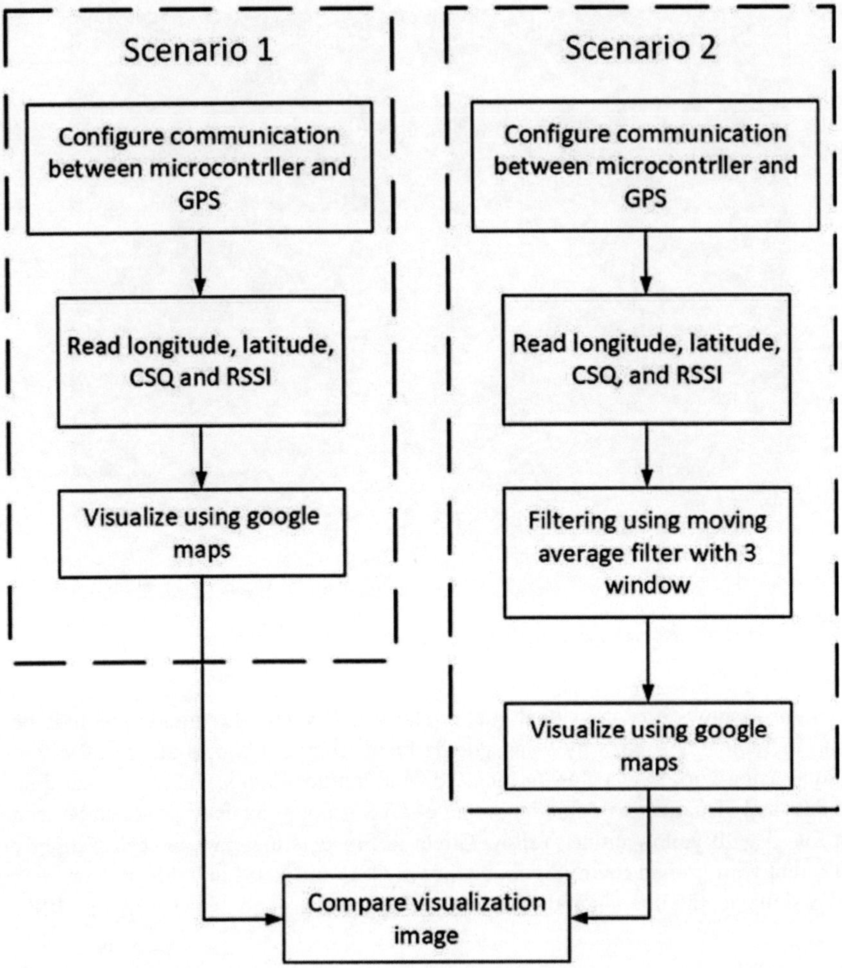


**Fig. 2** Data collection scenario

## 3 Result

This research retrieval data location and signal quality. Data tracking will be retrieving while the device is used with moving. Data tracking use 2 different places. Signal quality data consist of CSQ and RSSI when measuring location. Signal quality is important factor for GPS location reading. Bad signal quality in GPS can cause outlier data location. This research uses 10 data to measure longitude, latitude, CSQ, and RSSI in each places respectively. Longitude and latitude data will be visualized in to location using google maps.

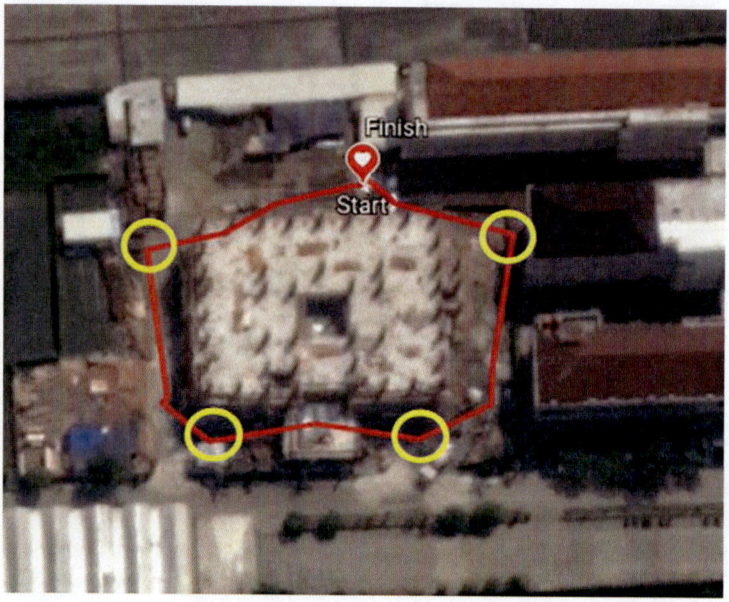


**Fig. 3** Google maps visualization data test 1 without moving average filter

Table 1 shows how the signal quality and location data. Longitude and latitude data in Table 1 visualize by using google maps. Figure 4 shows the visualization output using google maps using longitude and latitude data in Table 1. According to data and visualization data, the output of GPS is not good enough. It can be seen in Fig. 3 with yellow circle. Yellow Circle in Fig. 3 is location point that slightly different with tracing route. Signal quality in CSQ and RSSI in Table 1 shows that GPS signal to satellite is good. The CSQ value range around 26–31 dBm and RSSI

**Table 1** Data retrieval in places 1 before implementing moving average filter

| No | CSQ (dBm) | RSSI (dBm) | Latitude | Longitude | Annotation |
|---|---|---|---|---|---|
| 1 | 29 | −55 | −7.43455076 | 109.25177764 | Good signal quality |
| 2 | 29 | −55 | −7.43455171 | 109.25176239 | Good signal quality |
| 3 | 26 | −61 | −7.43455266 | 109.25176239 | Good signal quality |
| 4 | 26 | −61 | −7.43455266 | 109.25176239 | Good signal quality |
| 5 | 26 | −61 | −7.43458175 | 109.25165557 | Good signal quality |
| 6 | 30 | −53 | −7.43462705 | 109.25158691 | Good signal quality |
| 7 | 31 | −51 | −7.43465423 | 109.25148010 | Good signal quality |
| 8 | 30 | −53 | −7.43486499 | 109.25151824 | Good signal quality |
| 9 | 31 | −51 | −7.43487310 | 109.25151062 | Good signal quality |
| 10 | 28 | −57 | −7.43492555 | 109.25157928 | Good signal quality |

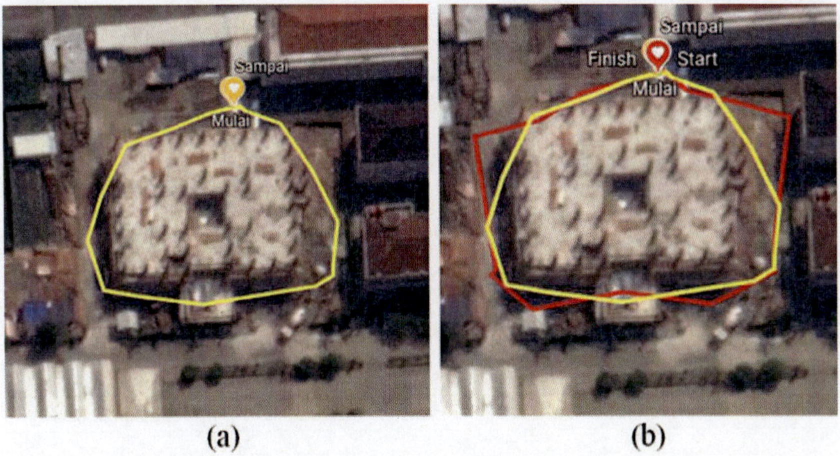


**Fig. 4** **a** Google maps visualization data with moving average filter, **b** comparison google maps visualization data between tracking with moving average filter and without moving average filter

value range around (−61) to (−51). It can be representing the weather while this data taken. Good signal quality means the device is good.

Table 2 shows how the signal quality and location data in device 2 with moving average filter. Longitude and latitude data in Table 1 visualize by using google maps. Figure 4a. shows the visualization output using google maps using longitude and latitude data in Table 1. Figure 4b show comparation data tracking visualization. The data shows that tracking with moving average filter is smoother than without moving average filter. The Yellow line is more representative the tracking route. Tracking system using moving average filter is more tighten than without moving average filter. Signal quality in CSQ and RSSI in Table 2. shows that GPS signal to satellite is good. The CSQ value range around 23–30 dBm and RSSI value range around

**Table 2** Data retrieval in places1 with moving average filter

| No | CSQ (dBm) | RSSI (dBm) | Latitude | Longitude | Annotation |
|---|---|---|---|---|---|
| 1 | 28 | −57 | −7.43455171 | 109.2517675 | Good signal quality |
| 2 | 25 | −63 | −7.434552343 | 109.2517624 | Good signal quality |
| 3 | 30 | −53 | −7.434562357 | 109.2517268 | Good signal quality |
| 4 | 30 | −53 | −7.434587153 | 109.2516683 | Good signal quality |
| 5 | 27 | −59 | −7.43462101 | 109.2515742 | Good signal quality |
| 6 | 27 | −59 | −7.434715423 | 109.2515284 | Good signal quality |
| 7 | 24 | −65 | −7.43479744 | 109.251503 | Good signal quality |
| 8 | 24 | −65 | −7.43488788 | 109.251536 | Good signal quality |
| 9 | 27 | −59 | −7.434897893 | 109.2516047 | Good signal quality |
| 10 | 23 | −73 | −7.434910767 | 109.2517242 | Good signal quality |

**Table 3** Data retrieval in test 2 before implementing moving average filter

| No | CSQ (dBm) | RSSI (dBm) | Latitude | Longitude | Annotation |
|---|---|---|---|---|---|
| 1 | 27 | −59 | −7.42522144 | 109.23079681 | Good signal quality |
| 2 | 27 | −59 | −7.42518186 | 109.23071289 | Good signal quality |
| 3 | 27 | −59 | −7.42521762 | 109.23061370 | Good signal quality |
| 4 | 31 | −51 | −7.42497491 | 109.23062133 | Good signal quality |
| 5 | 31 | −51 | −7.42497348 | 109.23062896 | Good signal quality |
| 6 | 31 | −51 | −7.42499971 | 109.23062133 | Good signal quality |
| 7 | 31 | −51 | −7.42503786 | 109.23050689 | Good signal quality |
| 8 | 31 | −51 | −7.42497825 | 109.23033905 | Good signal quality |
| 9 | 31 | −51 | −7.42492008 | 109.23017120 | Good signal quality |
| 10 | 31 | −51 | −7.42491197 | 109.23002624 | Good signal quality |

(−73) to (−53). It can be representing the weather while this data taken. Comparing Tables 1 and 2, the data shows that moving average filter reduce error 3.73 m.

Table 3 shows how the signal quality and location data. Longitude and latitude data in Table 3 visualize by using google maps. Figure 5 shows the visualization output using google maps using longitude and latitude data in Table 3. According to data and visualization data, the output of GPS is not good enough. It can be seen in Fig. 3 with yellow circle. Yellow Circle in Fig. 3 is location point that slightly different with tracing route. Signal quality in CSQ and RSSI in Table 1 shows that GPS signal to satellite is good. The CSQ value range around 27–31 dBm and RSSI value range around (−59) to (−51). It can be representing the weather while this data taken. Good signal quality means the device is good.

Table 4 shows how the signal quality and location data in device 2 with moving average filter. Longitude and latitude data in Table 4 visualize by using google maps. Figure 6a. shows the visualization output using google maps using longitude and latitude data in Table 4. Figure 6b show comparation data tracking visualization. According to data and visualization data shows that tracking with moving average filter is smoother than without moving average filter. The Yellow line is more representative the tracking route. Tracking system using moving average filter is more tighten than without moving average filter. Signal quality in CSQ and RSSI in Table 4 shows that GPS signal to satellite is good. The CSQ value range around 23–30 dBm and RSSI value range around (−73) to (−53). It can be representing the weather while this data taken.

According to data from Tables 1, 2, 3, and 4 shows that moving average filter gives improvement for reading route and location. Device with moving average filter gives representative route while tracking. Testing read location also has been done. This research uses 2 locations to test reading location using blind tracker device. Location testing scenario has been explained in Fig. 2. Distance between real location that obtain from cellphone and location reading. Comparing Tables 3 and 4, the data shows that moving average filter reduce error 1.35 m.

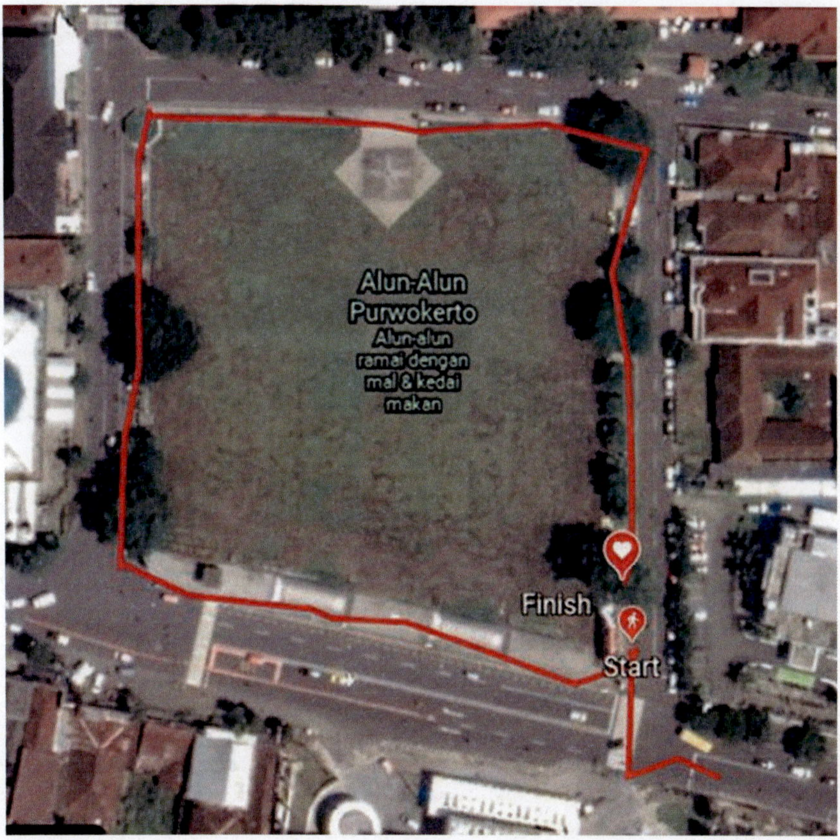


**Fig. 5** Google maps visualization data test 2 without moving average filter

**Table 4** Data retrieval in places 2 with moving average filter

| No | CSQ (dBm) | RSSI (dBm) | Latitude | Longitude | Annotation |
|---|---|---|---|---|---|
| 1 | 31 | −51 | −7.425206973 | 109.2307078 | Good signal quality |
| 2 | 31 | −51 | −7.425124797 | 109.2306493 | Good signal quality |
| 3 | 31 | −51 | −7.425055337 | 109.2306213 | Good signal quality |
| 4 | 31 | −51 | −7.4249827 | 109.2306239 | Good signal quality |
| 5 | 31 | −51 | −7.425003683 | 109.2305857 | Good signal quality |
| 6 | 31 | −51 | −7.425005273 | 109.2304891 | Good signal quality |
| 7 | 31 | −51 | −7.42497873 | 109.2303391 | Good signal quality |
| 8 | 31 | −51 | −7.424936767 | 109.2301788 | Good signal quality |
| 9 | 28 | −57 | −7.424908157 | 109.2300593 | Good signal quality |
| 10 | 31 | −51 | −7.424899413 | 109.2299957 | Good signal quality |

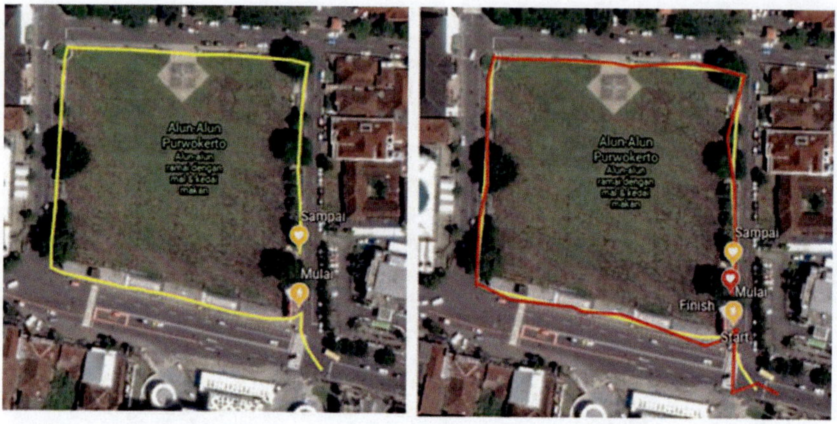


(a) (b)

**Fig. 6** **a** Google maps visualization data test 2 with moving average filter, **b** comparison google maps visualization data between tracking with moving average filter and without moving average filter

## 4 Discussion

According data retrieval using blind tracker device shows that moving average filter improve the accuracy of location reading. Comparing with another research, moving average is more simple, faster data processing, and improve accuracy. The limitation in moving average filter is the quality of GPS device itself. If the GPS has low quality and many outlier position data than moving average filter also give wrong data position. This data processing can be implemented in low specification device like microcontroller and still gives improvement data reading.

## 5 Conclusion

The aim of this research is to improve accuracy in position data reading for blind tracker devices. This research conclude that blind tracker device works well. Blind tracker device can be used to track user route. GPS in SIM 7000E get good satellite signal while CSQ value around 23–31 and RSSI value around (−73) to (−51). Moving average filter gives improvement for location reading. Data position error is reduced by 3.73 m while testing in places 1 and reduced by 1.35 m while testing in places 2. Comparing data GPS between device without moving average filter and with moving average filter can be seen by google maps visualization. According to google maps visualization implementing moving average filter more representative the track route. Data research prove that blind tracker device can be used to track blind people. For the future work can be done by embedding moving average filter in FPGA device so the device will be very compact and small.

## References

1. Andrich R (2020) Towards a global information network on assistive technology. In: 2020 international conference on assistive and rehabilitation technologies (iCareTech), pp 1–4
2. Benssassi EM, Gomez J, Boyd LE, Hayes GR, Ye J (2018) Wearable assistive technologies for autism: opportunities and challenges. IEEE Pervasive Comput 17(2):11–21
3. Mulfari D, Celesti A, Fazio M, Villari M, Puliafito A (2016) Using google cloud vision in assistive technology scenarios. In: 2016 IEEE symposium on computers and communication (ISCC), pp 214–219
4. Kurniasih N (2014) Situasi Penyandang Disabilitas. Ministry of Health Republic of Indonesia, Jakarta, p 56
5. Pawluk DTV, Adams RJ, Kitada R (2015) Designing haptic assistive technology for individuals who are blind or visually impaired. IEEE Trans Haptics 8(3):258–278
6. Noman M, Shehieb W, Sharif T (2019) Assistive technology for integrating the visually-impaired in mainstream education and society. In: 2019 advances in science and engineering technology international conferences (ASET), pp 1–5
7. Ai J et al (2020) Wearable visually assistive device for blind people to appreciate real-world scene and screen image. In: 2020 IEEE international conference on visual communications and image processing (VCIP), p 258
8. Roseli NHM, Aziz N, Mutalib AA (2010) The enhancement of assistive courseware for visually impaired learners. In: 2010 international symposium on information technology, vol 1, pp 1–6
9. Kumar Dabbakuti JRK, Kowshik Chandu Y, Sai Koushik Reddy A, Prabu AV (2021) Retrieve, processing and analysis of global positioning system derived ionospheric total electron content using IGS products BT. Adv Electrical Comput Technol 719–726
10. Singh A, Sonal (2016) An improvement over Kalman filter for GPS tracking. in: 2016 3rd international conference on computing for sustainable global development (INDIACom), pp 923–927
11. Kumalasari IN, Zainudin V, Pratiarso A (2020) An implementation of accuracy improvement for low-cost GPS tracking using Kalman Filter with Raspberry Pi. In: 2020 international electronics symposium (IES), pp 123–130
12. Ye W, Wang B, Liu Y, Gu B, Chen H (2020) Deep Gaussian process regression for performance improvement of POS during GPS outages. IEEE Access 8:117483–117492
13. Boloix-Tortosa R, Murillo-Fuentes JJ, Payán-Somet FJ, Pérez-Cruz F (2018) Complex Gaussian processes for regression. IEEE Trans Neural Netw Learn Syst 29(11):5499–5511
14. Afandi MA, Nurandi S, Enriko IKA (2021) Automated air conditioner controller and monitoring based on internet of things. Indones J Electron Instrum Syst 11(1):83–92
15. Safaei Pirooz AA, Flay RGJ, Minola L, Azorin-Molina C, Chen D (2020) Effects of sensor response and moving average filter duration on maximum wind gust measurements. J Wind Eng Ind Aerodyn 206:104354
16. Alvarez-Ramirez J, Rodriguez E, Carlos Echeverría J Detrending fluctuation analysis based on moving average filtering. Phys A Stat Mech Appl 354
17. Redhyka GG, Setiawan D, Soetraprawata D (2015) Embedded sensor fusion and moving-average filter for inertial measurement unit (IMU) on the microcontroller-based stabilized platform. In: 2015 international conference on automation, cognitive science, optics, micro electro-mechanical system, and information technology (ICACOMIT), pp 72–77
18. Li H, Zhang X, Xu C, Hong J (2020) Sensorless control of IPMSM using moving-average-filter based PLL on HF pulsating signal injection method. IEEE Trans Energy Convers 35(1):43–52

19. Jain A, Rajpourhit BS (2015) Analysis and design of adaptive moving average filters based low-gain PLL for grid connected solar power converters. In: 2015 IEEE power & energy society general meeting, pp 1–5
20. Lyons RG (2010) Understanding digital signal processing, 3rd edn. Prentice Hall, Boston
21. Haque ME, Khan MNS, Sheikh MRI (2015) Smoothing control of wind farm output fluctuations by proposed low pass filter, and moving averages. In: 2015 international conference on electrical & electronic engineering (ICEEE), pp 121–124
22. Loukas A, Simonetto A, Leus G (2015) Distributed autoregressive moving average graph filters. IEEE Signal Process Lett 22(11):1931–1935
23. Smith SW (1999) The scientist and engineer's guide to digital signal processing, 2nd edn. California Technical Publishing, California
24. Serheiev-Horchynskyi O (2019) Analysis of frequency characteristics of simple moving average digital filtering system. In: 2019 IEEE international scientific-practical conference problems of infocommunications, science and technology (PIC S&T), pp 97–100
25. Liu J, Isufi E, Leus G (2019) Filter design for autoregressive moving average graph filters. IEEE Trans Signal Inf Process Netw 5(1):47–60

# Real-Time Masked Face Recognition Using FaceNet and Supervised Machine Learning

**Faisal Dharma Adhinata, Nia Annisa Ferani Tanjung, Widi Widayat, Gracia Rizka Pasfica, and Fadlan Raka Satura**

**Abstract** The coronavirus pandemic has led to the implementation of health protocols such as the use of masks worldwide. Without exception, work activities also require the wearing of masks. This condition makes it difficult to recognize an individual's identity because the mask covers half of the face, especially when the employee is present. The attendance system recognizes a face without a mask more accurately, in contrast, a masked face makes identity recognition inaccurate. Therefore, this study proposes a combination of facial feature extraction using FaceNet and several classification methods. The three supervised machine learning methods were evaluated, namely multiclass Support Vector Machine (SVM), K-Nearest Neighbor, and Random Forest. Furthermore, the masked face recognition system was evaluated using real-time video data to assess the accuracy and processing time of the video frame. The accuracy result on real-time video data using a combination of FaceNet with K-NN, multiclass SVM, or Random Forest of 96.03%, 96.15%, and 54.04% are obtained respectively and in processing time per frame of 0.056 s, 0.055 s, and 0.061 are obtained respectively. The results show that the combination of the FaceNet feature extraction method with multiclass SVM produces the best accuracy and data processing speed. In other words, this combination can reach 18 fps at real-time video processing. Based on these results, the proposed combined method is suitable for real-time masked face recognition. This study provides an overview of the masked face recognition method so that it can be a reference for the contactless attendance system in this pandemic era.

**Keywords** Coronavirus pandemic · FaceNet · Masked face recognition · Multiclass SVM · Real-time

---

F. D. Adhinata (✉) · N. A. F. Tanjung · G. R. Pasfica · F. R. Satura
Department of Software Engineering, Faculty of Informatics, Institut Teknologi Telkom Purwokerto, Purwokerto, Indonesia
e-mail: faisal@ittelkom-pwt.ac.id

W. Widayat
Department of Informatics Engineering, Faculty of Informatics, Institut Teknologi Telkom Purwokerto, Purwokerto, Indonesia

 
T. Triwiyanto et al. (eds.), *Proceedings of the 2nd International Conference on Electronics, Biomedical Engineering, and Health Informatics*, Lecture Notes in Electrical Engineering 898, https://doi.org/10.1007/978-981-19-1804-9_15

## 1 Introduction

The coronavirus pandemic has led to the implementation of health protocols worldwide, such as the use of masks. This is important to suppress the escalation of the virus which spreads through direct contact with sufferers or indirectly by touching infected surface areas [1]. Furthermore, in the workplace, attendance activities are usually carried out using fingerprints. This condition promotes the spread of coronavirus via indirect contact. Meanwhile, one of the safe attendance systems is the use of facial biometric data [2, 3]. The human face generally consists of two eyes, as well as the area above and below the nose [4]. An individual is usually recognized through facial features such as shape, hair, nose, mouth, eyes, and eyebrows. However, the use of masks makes the area under the nose covered, therefore, special techniques are needed for masked face recognition at segmentation, facial feature extraction, and classification stages.

Masked face recognition has recently become a new case study due to the difficulties associated with identifying faces covered with masks [5]. Aswal et al. [6], using a combination of RetinaFace and VGGFace2 for the masked face identification process, produced an accuracy of 94.5% but failed to run on real-time data. Therefore, a variety of other methods is needed to accurately run in real-time. The first stage of masked face recognition is segmentation for face detection. This process captures the entire face area from hair to chin, meanwhile, various types of mask motifs used need to be ignored, thereby limiting the segmentation process of the facial area to the upper part of the nose. Therefore, the facial features used in this study are the area above the nose which includes hair, eyes, and eyebrows.

The next step is the main stage of masked face recognition, namely feature extraction, and classification of identities based on facial features. One technique that is often used to extract facial image features is the deep convolutional neural network [7]. FaceNet uses a deep convolutional neural network to extract facial features, It maps each face image to a Euclidean space in which the distances between faces are proportional to the similarity [8]. Furthermore, several studies have used FaceNet for facial data classification [9–11]. Zhao et al. [9] used this technique for recognition at low resolution and obtained an accuracy value of 100% on the identities of 21 people. Also, Pranoto and Kusumawardani [10] used FaceNet for a student attendance system and produced an accuracy above 95%. This technique is not only used for identity recognition, but also to recognize facial expressions [11]. A previous study produced an accuracy of 94.68% and recognized three facial expressions, namely focused, unfocused, and fatigue. Therefore, this study aims to use FaceNet for facial feature extraction. The key to the accuracy of masked face recognition is the classification stage. Several supervised machine learning techniques have been used in masked face recognition studies. The Random Forest was used to classify 40 people's identities with an accuracy of 97.17% [12]. Furthermore, the K-Nearest Neighbor produced an accuracy of 81% with a value of K = 1 [13]. The multiclass SVM was also applied to face recognition systems and produced an accuracy of 86.76% [14]. Therefore, this study analyzed the combination of FaceNet feature extraction with K-Nearest

Neighbor, multiclass SVM, or Random Forest methods. In addition, the processing speed of real-time video data and its accuracy were also evaluated.

This paper is organized as follows. In Sect. 2, the design of the proposed system contains a flowchart and an explanation of the methods. Section 3 contains experiments at the training stage, which are used for testing using real-time video data, and ends with a discussion related to previous research. Section 4 contains conclusions from the results of masked face recognition research.

## 2 Materials and Method

The masked face recognition system consists of training and testing stages using real-time video. Figure 1 shows the proposed system architecture. Figure 1 shows that the training phase begins with the acquisition of facial data and the respective identity. Furthermore, the facial data used is a cropped face in the area above the nose, the face area was then resized to match the size of the pre-trained FaceNet model. The pre-processing stage results were stored in an array form and further

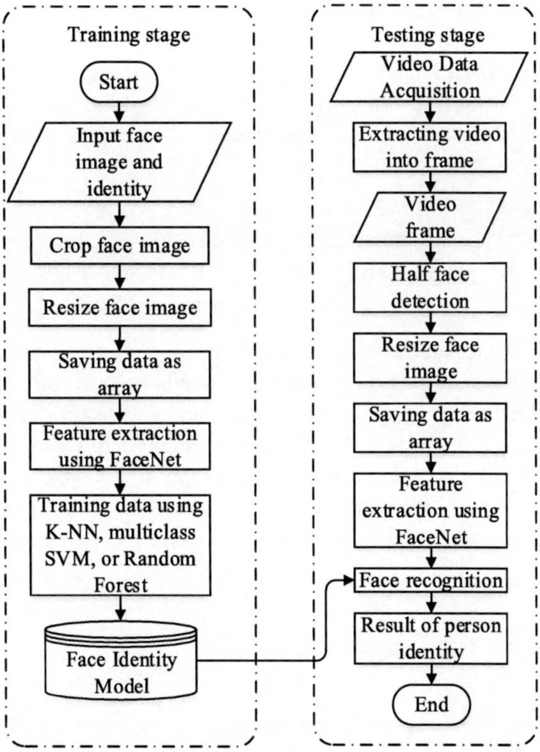


**Fig. 1** The proposed system of real-time masked face recognition

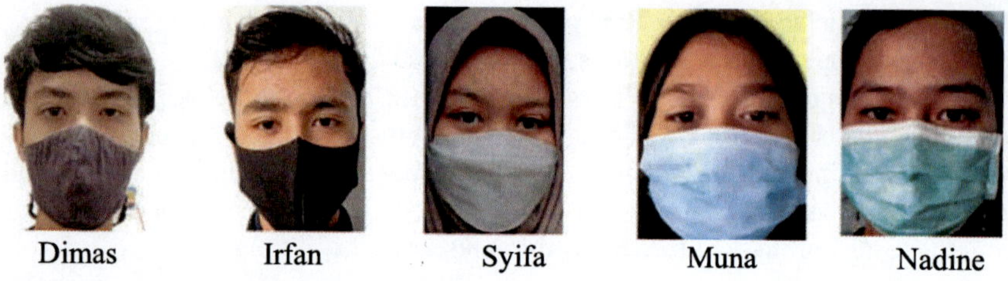


**Fig. 2** Example of training data and its identity

extracted using FaceNet's facial features. The facial feature extraction results were trained in the form of a model using several supervised machine learning methods, namely K-NN, multiclass SVM, or Random Forest. Moreover, the parameters of each supervised learning method were then evaluated to obtain the best value for training and testing accuracy. The best facial identity model results were stored for use in the testing phase with real-time video data.

In the testing stage, real-time video data were used to test the speed of the proposed system in processing each video frame. The video data was first extracted into video frames, while the frame obtained was segmented to obtain the face area above the nose. Furthermore, the obtained facial area was also resized for feature extraction processing and the results were stored in an array. The testing phase feature extraction also used FaceNet, while the results were matched with the facial identity model. The output of this system is a face bounding box that contains the identity of the person, meanwhile, the accuracy and video data processing speed in real-time were evaluated.

### *2.1 Data Acquisition*

The masked face recognition system uses an image as training data and real-time video as testing data. The training data used include 24 identities, with each identity totaling 10 images, 8 as training, and 2 as testing data. Meanwhile, the subject data used in this study varied in age, ranging from 3 to 41 years old. This age variation is such that the research results apply to all ages. Furthermore, for real-time video data, a 2 MP camera with 15 fps was used. The faces used were all towards the front of the camera. Figure 2 shows an example of training data used in this study.

### *2.2 Data Segmentation*

The facial segmentation results contained masks with various motifs, therefore, the detected face was cropped only on the face, namely the area above the nose. Figure 3

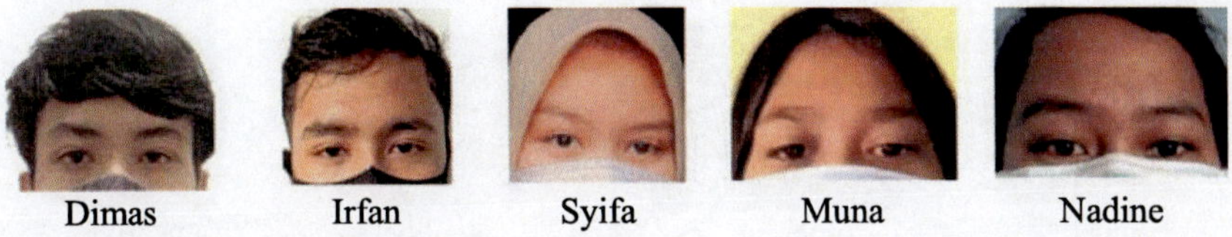


**Fig. 3** Face segmentation results

shows an example of cropped training data. Furthermore, the segmented facial data were then resized to 160 × 160. This is to adjust the size of the pre-trained FaceNet model at the feature extraction stage. The resize results were stored in the form of an array and processed in the feature extraction stage.

## 2.3 *Feature Extraction Using FaceNet*

FaceNet is a face recognition system developed in 2015 by Google researchers which obtained leading results based on a variety of benchmark datasets [8]. It achieved state-of-the-art accuracy by combining deep convolutional networks and triplet loss. Figure 4 shows the feature extraction of the FaceNet pre-trained model using the Triplet Loss function. Furthermore, FaceNet has a significant advantage over previous systems because it learns the mapping from the photos and generates embeddings without relying on a bottleneck layer for recognition or verification. Following the creation of the embeddings, all subsequent actions such as recognition or verification are carried out using domain-specific standard methods, with the newly formed embeddings serving as the feature vector. The network is trained such that the squared L2 distance between embeddings is proportional to the degree of similarity between faces. In addition, scaled and altered images are used for training as well as severely cropped images around the facial area.

The triplet loss function is used to encode the faces of three images namely an anchor, a positive, and a negative image. It is believed that vectors with the same identity get increasingly similar (have a lower distance), meanwhile, vectors

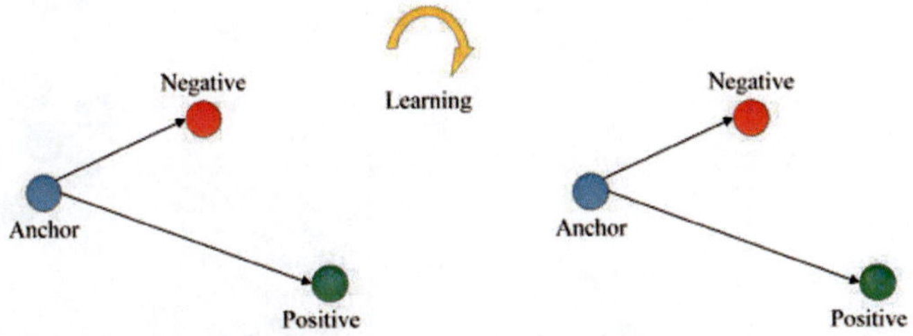


**Fig. 4** The triplet loss function [6]

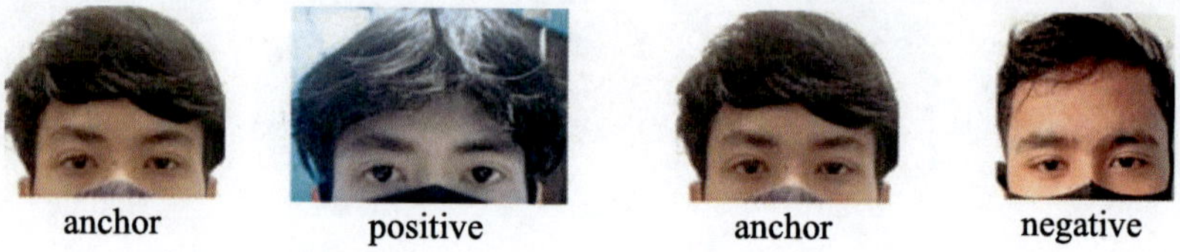


**Fig. 5** The illustration of triplet loss function

with different identities become less similar (have a more significant distance) [15]. Figure 5 shows that the anchor and positive images belong to the same person, while the negative image belongs to another individual. The focus on training a model to generate embeddings directly, rather than via an intermediate layer was significantly emphasized in this study.

## 2.4 *Classification Using Supervised Machine Learning*

Supervised Learning is a process of grouping data based on a label. In this study, the image data were grouped based on the respective identity. The label used is the identity of each person, meanwhile, the classification stage used the three classifier methods, namely K-Nearest Neighbor, SVM multiclass, and Random Forest.

**K-Nearest Neighbor**

The K-Nearest Neighbor (KNN) method of data classification is utilized for face recognition [16, 17]. Each pixel in the face conveys a different piece of information, therefore, face identity was detected based on each pixel classification. The face was selected by the most common class. Figure 6 shows the illustration of K-NN in this study.

**Fig. 6** The illustration of K-NN

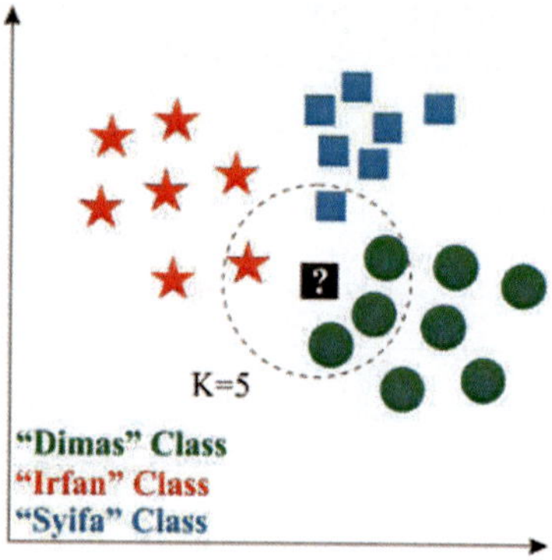

The training data consist of vectors in a multidimensional feature space, each data with a label. In the training stage, the feature vectors and class labels associated with the training samples are stored. Meanwhile, in the classification stage, *K* is a user-defined, and an unlabeled vector (test face image) and is classified by assigning the label that appears most frequently among the *K* training samples closest to that particular test face. A test image is recognized by connecting it with the label of the nearest face in the training set, allowing for the calculation of the distance between both points [18]. The most common search technique is via the use of the Euclidean and Manhattan distance formulas demonstrated in Eqs. 1 and 2.

$$d(x, y) = \sqrt{\sum_{i=1}^{n} (x_i - y_i)^2} \tag{1}$$

$$d(x, y) = \sum_{i=1}^{n} |x_i - y_i| \tag{2}$$

In this study, two distance algorithms were tested, namely Euclidean and Manhattan distance. Furthermore, the value of K in each distance algorithm was also evaluated.

**Multiclass SVM**

Support Vector Machines (SVM) [19] are a type of machine learning technique invented by Vapnik and colleagues [20]. The earliest methods of implementing SVM to solve multiclass classification problems are the One-vs-Rest (OvR) SVM algorithms [21]. In the OvR stage, SVM was trained for each class k that is an expert at classifying k (one) versus non-k (the rest), hence, a binary classifier was created for each k class. Figure 7 shows the illustration of multiclass SVM in this study.

The model formed was indicated with the blue color as the positive class, while the white color is negative. Furthermore, the maximum value of each class comparison is calculated in the prediction process. The inputs for the model formation are 24 class labels (person identities) and image features on each label, meanwhile, experiments

**Fig. 7** The illustration of SVM multiclass

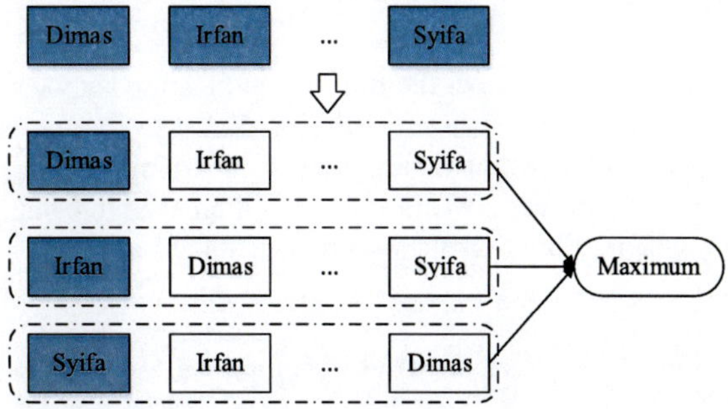

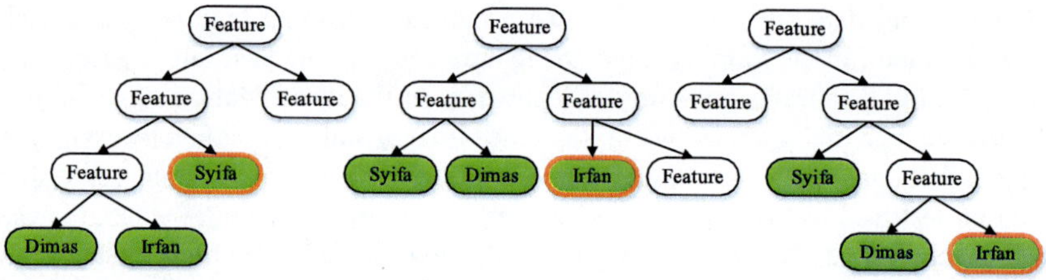


**Fig. 8** The illustration of random forest

were carried out using three multiclass SVM kernels, namely sigmoid, polynomial, and linear.

**Random Forest**

Random forest [22] is a widely known technique for developing predictive models for classification and regulation [23]. The random forest algorithm is used to construct a randomized decision tree. Furthermore, this algorithm frequently produces excellent predictors for each iteration. This method aims to create numerous predictors before aggregating the diverse predictions rather than acquiring an optimum technique at once. The features were then used to categorize or regress a sample of qualitative and/or quantitative variables. Figure 8 illustrates the Random Forest categorization results.

Random forest classification is accomplished using training sample data and then creating a tree. The classification is based on the most decisions observed from the constructed trees. Meanwhile, the construction of trees uses randomly chosen variables and then classifies all the trees produced [24]. For instance, a Random Forest contains three decision trees, when the classification results from two trees are "Irfan" and one tree is "Syifa", then the most votes are used, namely "Irfan" class. In the classification stage using the random forest method, the criterion parameter and the number of trees were evaluated.

## 2.5 System Evaluation

The accuracy value at the training and testing stages was measured as well as data processing speed using real-time video. The Python language library, scikit-learn was used to measure the accuracy of the training phase, meanwhile, the metric used was accuracy_score. This value was then used to calculate the correct prediction of the system. Equation 3 shows the accuracy formula.

$$Accuracy\left(y, y'\right) = \frac{1}{n_{samples}} \sum_{i=0}^{n_{samples}-1} 1(y_i' = y_i) \tag{3}$$

where $y_i'$ is the predicted value of the $i$-th sample and $y_i$ is the actual value, then the fraction of true predictions is $n_{samples}$. To determine the accuracy value at the testing stage, the correct rate (CR) value was calculated by dividing the number of correct video frame data (C) by the total number of frames used for testing (A). The correct rate equation is shown in Formula 4 [25].

$$CR = \frac{C}{A} \tag{4}$$

Meanwhile, the computer configuration used to run the program significantly affects the speed of real-time video data processing. Therefore, a desktop computer configuration with an Intel Core i3-9100F CPU @ 3.60 GHz and 8192 MB DDR4 RAM was used to train face data. The operating system is Windows 10 Pro 64-bit. In addition, a 2.0 MP camera with 15 fps was also used.

## 3 Result and Discussion

The masked face recognition system uses the accuracy and speed of video processing to measure the system's robustness. This study has several experiments at the face data training stage using the K-NN, SVM multiclass, and Random Forest methods. Then the best results from each training process will be used for testing on real-time video data.

### *3.1 Training Face Data Using K-NN*

The masked face identities were classified via the K-NN method by calculating the closest distance using the Manhattan and Euclidean distance algorithms. The result was used to compare the similarity of the test and training feature database. Figure 9 shows the experimental results of variations in the value of K for each K-NN distance algorithm.

The experiment on the K-NN method used an odd K value because the number of classes studied was even, namely 24. Furthermore, the results showed that the K value had a significant effect on training and testing accuracy. The best results were obtained using the value of K = 1, meaning that only one nearest neighbor is needed to classify people's identities. The image used as input for training data makes the features obtained very close to each identity. Therefore, higher K values decrease accuracy as shown in Fig. 9. Moreover, based on the variation of the distance algorithm, the use of Manhattan and Euclidean distance does not significantly affect the accuracy results. Therefore, the value of K = 1 with the Euclidean distance algorithm was used as the test in real-time video data.

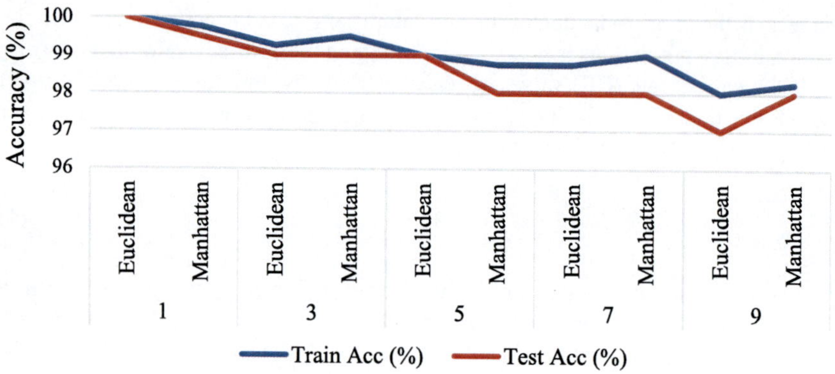


**Fig. 9** The graph of classification result using K-NN method

## 3.2 *Training Face Data Using Multiclass SVM*

The multiclass SVM algorithms kernel is a collection of mathematical functions. It transforms input data into the desired format. Meanwhile, the model output is poor when the transformation is incorrect. Different SVM algorithms use various kernel functions. In this study, three experiments were conducted with the sigmoid, linear, and polynomial kernels to classify masked facial identities. Figure 10 shows the results of kernel variations using multiclass SVM.

In the learning process using SVM multiclass, image features were transformed into feature space using a kernel trick. The best results were obtained using a polynomial kernel with 100% training and testing accuracy. Furthermore, the image training data used produced numerous and scattered features, which were difficult to separate using straight-line kernels such as sigmoid and linear. However, the polynomial kernel was able to separate the scattered identity classes. Therefore, testing on real-time video was carried out via a multiclass SVM with a polynomial kernel.

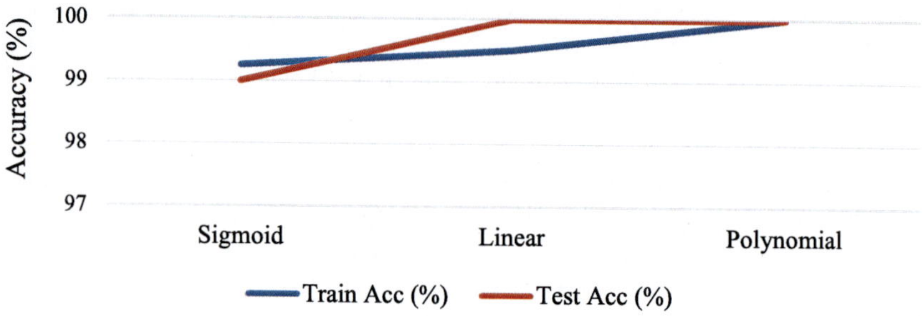


**Fig. 10** The graph of classification result using multiclass SVM method

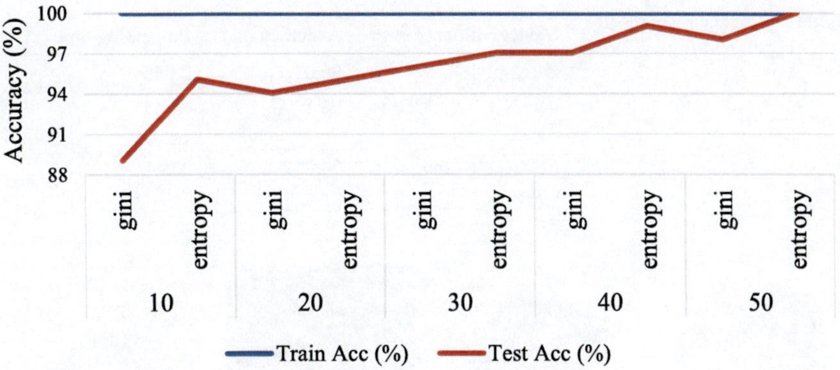


**Fig. 11** The graph of classification result using random forest method

## 3.3 *Training Face Data Using Random Forest*

The classification of masked face identity using random forest produced several decision trees which were used for making predictions. From all the decision trees obtained, voting was carried out to produce the final prediction. Furthermore, an experiment was conducted on the effect of the criterion parameters and number of trees on accuracy results. Figure 11 shows the experimental results of variations in the number of trees for each criterion function.

The experimental training data using random forest obtained accuracy values in variations of the criterion and number of tree parameters. However, for 10 trees, the accuracy value obtained was overfitting, where the test accuracy was smaller than the training. Although the training time was shorter, 0.1051 and 0.4268 s for 10 and 50 trees respectively, overfitting indicates that the model built is not good. The results showed that the use of criterion and 50 trees produced a training and testing accuracy of 100%. Therefore, the model with these results was used for testing the real-time video data.

## 3.4 *Testing Using Real-Time Video Data*

The real-time video was used for testing data, meanwhile, the camera resolution used was Full HD (1920 × 1080). Furthermore, the best model from the classification results was obtained using K-NN, multiclass SVM, and Random Forest. Then, accuracy was evaluated by observing the face in the video frames detected whether the identity is true or false based on Eq. 4. Moreover, the video data processing speed was evaluated by calculating the average of all detected frames. Table 1 shows the results of accuracy and speed using real-time video data.

**Table 1** The accuracy result of testing on real-time video data

| Model building | Accuracy (%) | Processing time (s) |
|---|---|---|
| FaceNet + K-NN | 96.03 | 0.056 |
| FaceNet + multiclass SVM | 96.15 | 0.055 |
| FaceNet + random forest | 54.04 | 0.061 |

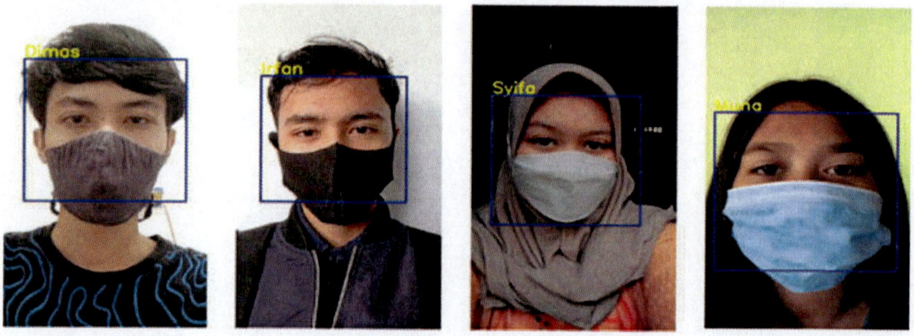


**Fig. 12** The result of real-time video data testing

Based on Table 1, the combination of FaceNet with Multiclass SVM produced the best results with an accuracy of 96.15%. These results are not significantly different from the combination of FaceNet with K-NN. However, in terms of processing speed, FaceNet and Multiclass SVM combination was the fastest, with 0.055 s or 18 fps. Therefore, this combination runs in real-time and is entirely accurate. An example of test results using video data is shown in Fig. 12.

## 3.5 *Discussion*

The experimental results of three supervised learning methods show that the parameters of the K-NN, multiclass SVM, and Random Forest methods significantly affect accuracy. In the K-NN method, the K value significantly influenced the accuracy as shown in Fig. 9. In addition, the type of kernel used also affects the accuracy. Meanwhile, in the Random Forest method, the criterion parameter and the number of trees significantly affect the accuracy. The best results were obtained using FaceNet with multiclass SVM and a polynomial kernel. This result was better than the previous study [6], with an elevated accuracy from 94.5 to 96.15% and run in real-time at 18 fps. These results can be used as a reference regarding a safer contactless attendance system during the pandemic era. The world community has started using special techniques to break the spread of the coronavirus, one of which is the development of a contactless masked face recognition method.

There were certain limitations in this study particularly when the hairstyle and face expression are changed. Therefore, the shape of the hair was not changed and used normal expression during the experiments. Future studies are recommended to use a combination of other feature extraction techniques to increase the accuracy of results.

## 4 Conclusion

The coronavirus pandemic health protocol requires the use of face masks when performing daily activities worldwide. This condition makes face recognition inaccurate because the face is partially covered. Furthermore, the combination of deep learning methods used in previous studies produced quite a good accuracy but failed to run in real-time data. Therefore, we propose combining pre-trained models and supervised learning classification methods in a masked face recognition system. The combination of FaceNet and multiclass SVM methods used in this study increased the accuracy by 1.65% (from 94.5 to 96.15%) and run in real-time at 18 fps. These results prove that the system built has good accuracy and is relatively fast in processing real-time data. Future research can use a feature extraction algorithm that can extract the changing features of the human hair so that the results are more accurate for masked face recognition.

**Acknowledgements** Thanks to LPPM Institut Teknologi Telkom Purwokerto through the Internal Research Grant for funding in the publication process of this journal.

## References

1. Leung NHL (2021) Transmissibility and transmission of respiratory viruses. Nat Rev Microbiol 19:528–545
2. Li L, Mu X, Li S, Peng H (2020) A review of face recognition technology. IEEE Access 8:139110–139120
3. Sunaryono D, Siswantoro J, Anggoro R (2021) An android based course attendance system using face recognition. J King Saud Univ Comput Inf Sci 33(3):304–312
4. Logan AJ, Gordon GE, Loffler G (2017) Contributions of individual face features to face discrimination. Vision Res 137:29–39
5. Li Y, Guo K, Lu Y, Liu L (2021) Cropping and attention based approach for masked face recognition. Appl Intell 51(5):3012–3025
6. Aswal V, Tupe O, Shaikh S, Charniya NN (2020) Single camera masked face identification. In: Proceedings—19th IEEE international conference on machine learning and applications. IEEE, pp 57–60
7. Maity S, Das P, Jha KK, Dutta HS (2021) Face mask detection using deep learning. Appl Artif Intell Mach Learn 495–509
8. Schroff F, Kalenichenko D, Philbin J (2015) FaceNet: A unified embedding for face recognition and clustering. In: 2015 IEEE conference on computer vision and pattern recognition (CVPR). IEEE, pp 815–823

9. Zhao Y, Yu AP, Xu DT (2020) Person recognition based on facenet under simulated prosthetic vision. J Phys Conf Ser 1437(1)
10. Pranoto H, Kusumawardani O (2021) Real-time triplet loss embedding face recognition for authentication student attendance records system framework. JOIV Int J Inform Vis 5(2)
11. Adhinata FD (2021) Fatigue detection on face image using Facenet algorithm and K-nearest neighbor classifier. J Inf Syst Eng Bus Intell 7(1):22–30
12. Kremic E, Subasi A (2016) Performance of random forest and SVM in face recognition. Int Arab J Inf Technol 13(2):287–293
13. Wirdiani NKA, Hridayami P, Widiari NPA, Rismawan KD, Candradinata PB, Jayantha IPD (2019) Face identification based on K-nearest neighbor. Sci J Inform 6(2):150–159
14. Arafah M, Achmad A, Indrabayu, Areni IS (2019). Face recognition system using Viola Jones, histograms of oriented gradients and multi-class support vector machine. J Phys Conf Ser 1341(4)
15. Goel R, Mehmood I, Ugail H (2021) A study of deep learning-based face recognition models for sibling identification. Sensors 21(15)
16. Setiawan E, Muttaqin A (2015) Implementation of K-nearest neightbors face recognition on low-power processor. TELKOMNIKA (Telecommunication Computing Electronics and Control) 13(3)
17. Septiana N, Suciati N (2020) Combination of fast hybrid classification and K value optimization in K-NN for video face recognition. Register Jurnal Ilmiah Teknologi Sistem Informasi 6(1):65–73
18. Beli ILK, Guo C (2017) Enhancing face identification using local binary patterns and K-nearest neighbors. J Imag 3(3)
19. Bhardwaj A, Srivastava P (2021) A machine learning approach to sentiment analysis on web based feedback. Appl Artif Intell Mach Learn 127–139
20. Boser BE, Guyon IM, Vapnik VN A training algorithm for optimal margin classifiers. In: Proceedings of the 5th annual ACM workshop on computational learning theory, pp 144–152
21. Duan KB, Rajapakse JC, Nguyen MN (2007) One-versus-one and one-versus-all multiclass SVM-RFE for gene selection in cancer classification. Lect Notes Comput Sci 4447:47–56
22. Feroz N, Ahad MA, Doja F (2021) Machine learning techniques for improved breast cancer detection and prognosis—a comparative analysis. In: Applications of artificial intelligence and machine learning, pp 441–455
23. Tyralis H, Papacharalampous G, Langousis A (2019) A Brief review of random forests for water scientists and practitioners and their recent history in water resources. Water 11(5)
24. Zhai Y, Zheng X (2018) Random forest based traffic classification method in SDN. In: 2018 international conference on cloud computing, big data and blockchain (ICCBB), pp 1–5
25. Zeng XD, Chao S, Wong F (2010) Optimization of bagging classifiers based on SBCB algorithm. In: 2010 international conference on machine learning and cybernetics, vol 1, pp 262–267

# Emerging Potential on Laser Engraving Method in Fabricating Mold for Microfluidic Technology

**Muhammad Yusro**

**Abstract** The microfluidic device needs multi-step fabrication, and this process relatively takes time because it requires meticulous treatment. This approach, using laser engraving, reduces the conventional mold fabrication step which is created by soft lithography in the cleanroom. For biomedical research purposes, a certain dimension of the microfluidic design needs to be achieved. Meanwhile, different material needs different variable setting in laser engraving. This article's research objectives are seeking the optimum variable to achieve targeted dimension and investigating the influenced parameters lead to better understand the laser engraving fabrication process. The Poly (methyl methacrylate) (PMMA) sheets had been engraved to a particular dimension refers to the mold design that uses in the microfluidic device. The result showed that parameters meet the desired dimension found at values: 1000 for resolution, 95 for power, 500 for frequency, and 60 for speed. It can be noted that these adjusted parameters were performed for a single passage. Moreover, these influenced parameters also had been investigated to see their effect related to the engraving result. The result showed that the speed was the most significant parameter meanwhile the frequency has a stagnant value in the laser engraving process. This study also observed that higher resolution could smoother the rough surface. This study emerges the potential of laser engraving as rapid prototyping machinery for microfluidic technology.

**Keywords** Laser engraving · Microfluidic · Mold

## 1 Introduction

Microfluidic technology has been widely used in biomedical engineering research. This approach has advantageous characteristics to be applied in cell modeling

M. Yusro (✉)
Biomedical Engineering Study Program, Faculty of Telecommunication and Electrical Engineering, Institut Teknologi Telkom Purwokerto, Jalan D.I. Panjaitan 128, Purwokerto, Indonesia
e-mail: yusro@ittelkom-pwt.ac.id



T. Triwiyanto et al. (eds.), *Proceedings of the 2nd International Conference on Electronics, Biomedical Engineering, and Health Informatics*, Lecture Notes in Electrical Engineering 898, https://doi.org/10.1007/978-981-19-1804-9_16

(in vitro) that requires modulation of a signaling molecule to mimics living system [1]. Microfluidic technology has advantages in biomedical research because it has control regarding the environment, manipulates the molecules as the signals, provides three-dimensional interaction, and offers time-lapse imaging [1, 2]. It has been reported that microfluidic device assists in biology and medical research such as real-time PCR sample preparation [3, 4], human organ-on-chip [5], pathogen nucleic acids analysis in infectious diseases [6, 7], early detection for prostate cancer [8], protease activity for endometriosis [9], and genetically targeted isolation and cultivation of microorganisms [10].

A conventionally microfluidic device that is used in biomedical research is fabricated in the cleanroom and takes the punctilious steps. It has been reported the protocol to a fabricated microfluidic device for biomedical application in cleanroom using soft lithography [11]. That method has multi-steps to create Polydimethylsiloxane (PDMS) chip which in the next step will integrate with the coverslip using plasma etching. The reported step, initiated by applying a SU8 photoresist on the silicon wafer, after that, covering the transparency mask and exposure it to the ultraviolet. Following the step, the developing pattern will appear in silicon waver, PDMS will be utilized in the next step to be cured and then to be detached. At the end of the process, a PDMS chip has been created with a customized structure including reservoir, channel, and the inlet of injection.

Laser engraving is the technology to be used in rapid prototyping and can reduce the thickness of material in microns range [12], detailed on the final product [12], software-controlled [13], and engraving the different materials such as metallic [13, 14], wood, polymeric, ceramic [15]. The laser engraving method has the potential to create the mold that could be used in a microfluidic device in biomedical research. This method can reduce the time fabrication, chemical waste, and has great precision.

The scientific paper related to the fabrication of the microfluidic device using laser engraving for biomedical purposes has been reported. It has been informed that laser engraving could make microfabricated polyester conical microwells for cell culture applications [16]. Another paper has been also described that a microfluidic device can be used as a proper device to study bacterial taxis, drug testing, and biofilm formation [17]. It indicates that laser engraving has the potential to be used for biomedical research purposes.

The main task of the laser engraving experiment is to analyze the physical properties of laser engraving by optimizing its parameters [18]. This study has the requirement to obtain the optimized parameters to build a customized microfluidic chip that is matched biomedical research requirements. Laser engraving can create certain dimensions. Nonetheless, this method needs to be optimized because the different material has different properties that influenced the result. By investigating the role and effect of the variables, laser engraving can fabricate the mold as a template of PDMS chip including targeted dimension. The main advantage of using this approach is to tackle one of the challenges that conventional microfluidic fabrication which has a lengthy fabrication process. This research is imposed to fill the gap by assessing the laser engraving process by investigating the parameters toward dimension to emerge its potential in fabricating microfluidic devices. However, the article that discussion regarding mold fabrication using this method has not been reported yet. It is shown in Table 1 regarding the scientific article and their main objective research compared to this report.

**Table 1** The articles of laser engraving for microfluidic fabrication

| References | Research objectives | Result | Material |
|---|---|---|---|
| [19] | Fabricating and modifying PMMA microfluidic devices containing PDMS valves and pumps | Design, fabrication, characterization, and application of pneumatic microvalves and micropumps based on PMMA | PMMA PDMS |
| [20] | Creating rapid fabrication of miniaturized structures microfluidic device | A valid alternative to produce microchannels | PMMA |
| [21] | Emerging cost-effective biocompatible fluidics in minutes from design to final integration with optical biochips | Microfluidic channels laser-cut in thin double-sided tapes | ARcare®: polyester double-sided pressure-sensitive |
| [22] | Describing the effects of different modes and engraving parameters on the dimensions of microfluidic structures | Microchip electrophoretic devices | PMMA |
| [23] | Engraving glass-based capillary electrophoresis devices | Glass microchip | Microscope glass slides |
| [24] | Creating a low entry barrier for the rapid prototyping of thermoplastic microfluidics | H-filter and T-junction droplet generator | PMMA |
| [15] | Finding out the significant process parameters using Taguchi and ANOVA Methods | Parameter effect on surface roughness and engraving depth | PMMA |
| This article | Reaching certain dimensions and investigate parameters (Resolution, speed, passage, power, frequency) | Customized Microfluidic Mold | PMMA |

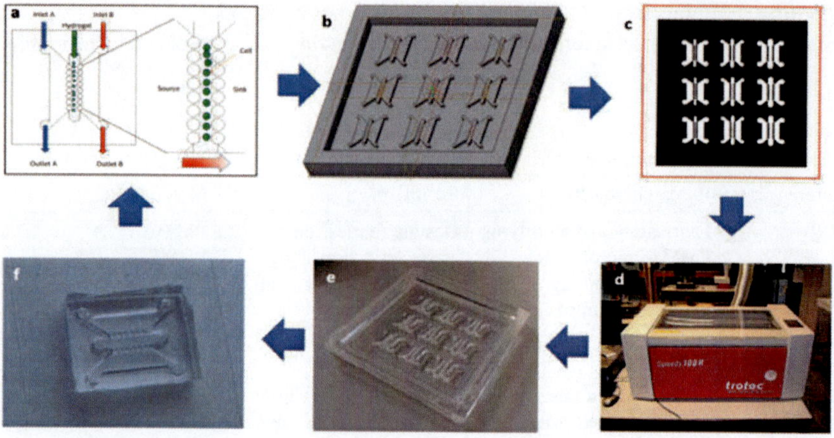


**Fig. 1** The illustration shows the rapid prototyping sections in this research

## 2 Methods

The main objective of the research is to study the potential laser engraving to be used in fabricating microfluidic device's mold. This study has three big steps: (1) Designing a microfluidic chip negative as a mold (2) Investigating laser parameters during the fabrication process (3) Evaluating the result concerning dimension requirement.

### *2.1 Designing Microfluidic Mold*

The customized microfluidic design in this study was inspired by a chip that is widely utilized to culture multiple cell types in hydrogel [11] and provides gradient concentration in the cell chamber [1, 2]. The key concept regarding this pattern is illustrated in Fig. 1a. The architectural structure of the design is required to be constructed. The figures such as channel, inlet, outlet, sink, and source molecule gradient and pillars need to meet certain dimensions to meet the function. This design has been drawn using Inkscape software.

### *2.2 Investigating Fabrication Processes*

Laser engraving machine Trotec Speedy 100R will be employed as the main tool to conducts this experiment. Laser engraving has variables that must be adjusted to obtain a certain dimension. In this report, five variable which is: (a) Resolution defines how many dots can be lined up in an inch without overlapping measuring in dots/inch (DPI). (b) Passage determines the number of engraving or cutting passes. (c) Power describes the output power of the laser. (d) The frequency parameter is decisive and is given in Hz (Hertz). It specifies the number of laser pulses per second. (e) Speed describes the movement of the laser head. Fast speeds lead to short exposure times, slow speeds lead to long exposure times. Every measurement in this experiment was taken three times for data replication. The material that was used in this experiment was 5 mm thickness of Polymethyl methacrylate (PMMA) sheets that were purchased at FABLAB (Leuven, Belgium).

### 2.3 *Pursuing Chip Requirement*

Generally, a microfluidic chip is constructed by two main compartments. On the top, there is a main building based on PDMS (Sylgard 184 Silicon Elastomer) and the coverslip functioned as a base at the bottom. The main building is constructed from fabricated mold. The liquid PDMS was poured into the template. The main building can be detached from the mold after it is placed in the oven for two hours.

It has been shown in Fig. 1 the fabrication of a microfluidic chip consists of multiple steps. It can be divided into six steps which are: (a) Designing of microfluidic structure refers to the model which used an in vitro method. This architecture consists of two chambers as the wings functioned as a source and sink regarding the diffusion process of molecules acting as a signal (b) Iterating design was made by a computer-aided drawing (CAD). (c) transforming design to be used in laser engraving (top view) (d) Using the laser engraving machine as a main tool of the research. This machine has the variables that need to be optimized to reach the targeted result. (e) Establishing mold for constructed microfluidic chip, and (f) Assembling microfluidic structure and coverslip to be applied in biomedical research.

## 3 Result

### 3.1 *Microfluidic Mold Based on PMMA Successfully Fabricated*

As mentioned in the introduction that the microfluidic design has a specific dimension to fit the requirement in biomedical research and experiment. It could be seen in Fig. 2a. that some features and detailed dimensions have been drawing by computer-aided drawing. In Fig. 2b. this design was transformed into top view and given unique colors so that laser engraving could remove the material layer by layer based on them. In this research, black color was chosen to mark the features. The laser removed the

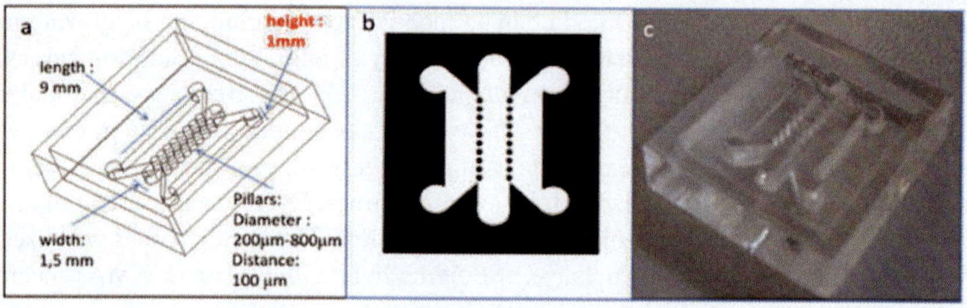


**Fig. 2** **a** Rapid prototyping design drawn by computer-aided design. **b** Top view of mold; black area indicates the region that will be removed layer by layer. **c** The PMMA mold fabricated by laser engraving process

black area of Poly (methyl methacrylate) (PMMA) material, and the result will be a mold (Fig. 2c) that will be used to cast the main part.

## *3.2 Influenced Parameter in Laser Engraving Has Been Investigated*

The optimizing parameter is compulsory to reach the targeted dimension. Every parameter has its characteristic related to the engraving result. In Fig. 3, five parameters have been investigated to see their trend and effect. Three variables which are resolution, passage, and power reported that had a positive trend. This means if the value of those parameters becomes higher, more depth will be achieved. On the other hand, the speed has been noted in a negative trend, the faster speed is applied, the less depth will be attained. Meanwhile, the frequency was observed that there is no correlation regarding the depth.

To study the comparison between the variables, each parameter has been compared in one graph. Figure 3f showed that speed has the strongest penetration compared to the others. The penetration expresses how much depth the layer was removed. By modulating the value of this parameter, the layers could be removed until 3 mm. The highest range was also observed in this parameter. The interesting result comes from the passage and frequency. The passage has the lowest effect regarding penetration. It means that it is not necessary to increase the passage because it only has a little effect on the depth. This is a good sign because it can reduce the time process. Frequency was performed as the weakest parameter related to the range. It means that whatever the number that is given in the fabrication process. The result is remaining the has the same number. It was also expressed in Fig. 3d. The investigated parameters have been summarized in Table 2 to make it easier to see the result.

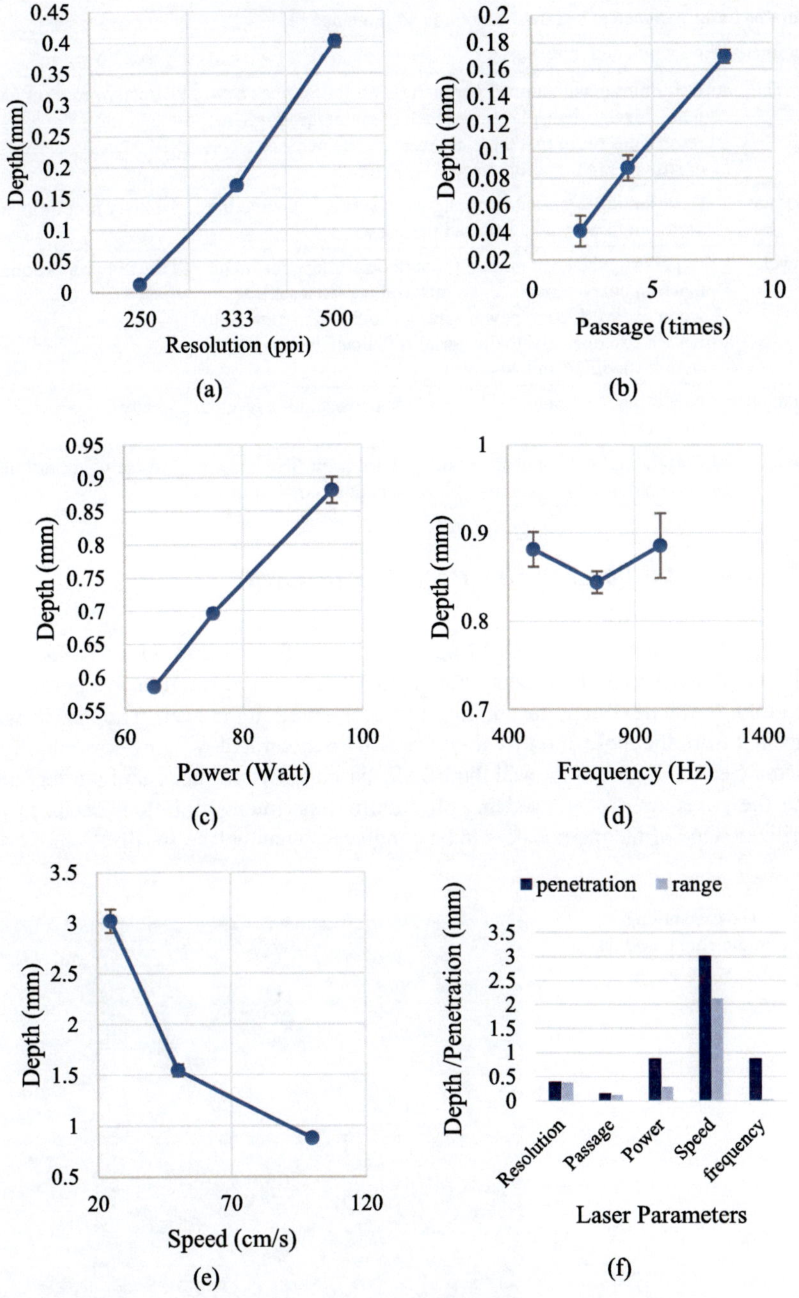


**Fig. 3** The Influence parameters on laser engraving method versus depth **a** resolution, **b** passage, **c** power, **d** frequency, and **e** speed. The illustration related to their penetration and range to the depth is expressed in (**f**)

Table 2 Laser parameters and their function and influence [25]

| Parameters | Function and influence | VS depth |
|---|---|---|
| Resolution | Determining with a pixel per inch (PPI). It describes how many pixels are displayed per inch of an image. Higher resolutions mean that there are more pixels per inch creating a high-quality image | Directly proportional |
| Passage | Determining the number of engravings. It is related to the stress imposed on the material per pass | Directly proportional |
| Power | Expressing the laser output. It could be set depends on the material characteristic. If the material is robust such as wood or PMMA, the power setting should be in high value. On the other hand, if the material is delicate like paper, the setting should be in low power | Directly proportional |
| Frequency | Indicating the number of laser pulses per second is given in Hz (Hertz) | Steady |
| Speed | Correlating to the movement of the laser head. The faster it moves; the shorter material has been exposed by laser | Inversely proportional |

## *3.3 Microfluidic Chip Has Been Constructed*

Microfluidic chip-based on PDMS needs to integrate coverslip with PDMS main building. After the mold has been fabricated, PDMS mixed solution was poured on the mold. In the next step, the solution has been cured in the oven. The PDMS was detached from the mold and this structure will be integrated with the coverslip by a plasma cleaner. Figure 4 showed the PDMS-based structure successfully integrated with the coverslip. To be used in cell culture experiments, this tool needs to be sterilized. One of the methods could be conducted by autoclave sterilization.

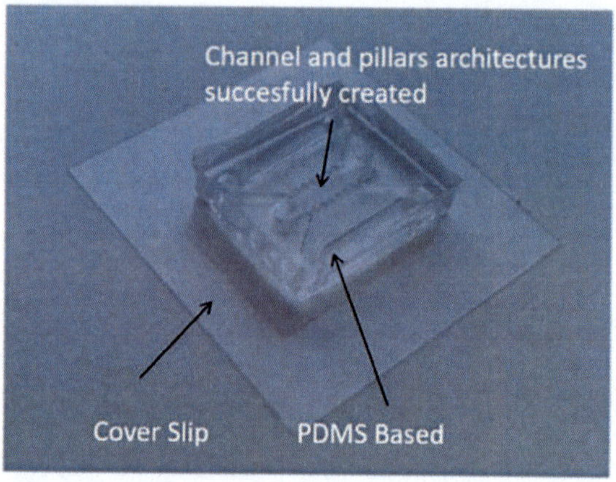


**Fig. 4** The assembling microfluidic chip based on PDMS

## 4 Discussion

This article is imposed to reach a certain dimension and investigate parameters (resolution, speed, passage, power, frequency). The goal of this article is to pursue a customized microfluidic mold that could help the fabrication of microfluidic technologies. It can be seen from the result that microfluidic mold based PMMA is successfully engraved with a certain dimension. The dimension could be achieved by modulating the influenced parameter. In this article, the optimized parameters that have been found to obtain specific dimension of the feature. It should be noted that the optimized parameter sets the passage parameter in a single passage. This procedure could reduce the time of processing. Table 2 provides the formula to attain the structure in this experiment. Regarding the study of influenced parameters related to specific material, this investigation also could be a reference for the fabrication process using laser engraving especially using PMMA material (Table 3).

Compared to the previous works [15], instead of using speed and power as the main parameter, this research suggests that resolution could by the main role to get the smoothest result. It also has been mentioned that. the slower the speed of most materials, it has the better the effect for the resulting engraving [18]. So that, even though the speed is the most influential effect based on the data result, the resolution comes as the chosen one to get the better result. Based on the experiment, the higher PPI has been applied to the process, the smoother surface is observed in the mold. An illustration about PPI and its influenced related to smoothness could be seen in Fig. 5. This is the reason why the protocol suggested the highest number of resolutions which was 1000 PPI.

It should be noted that the purpose of this article is to make a mold and it is not a direct microfluidic chip fabrication. This protocol needs to move to the next step for creating a PDMS part for establishing the complete microfluidic chip. From this perspective, making mold is not time efficient. However, this approach chooses to keep the PDMS as a part that directly contacted to cell or living environment. It is because that the material must be highly biocompatible. Furthermore, the engraving process by a laser to PMMA material produced debris which could damage the cell environment. So that this method only makes the mold as the solution to reduce the initial step in fabricating microfluidic technologies, not the direct fabrication. Even though this method is only reducing the initial part of fabrication. By using laser

**Table 3** The adjusted value of parameters to obtain specific features

| Parameter | Height |
|---|---|
| Resolution (ppi) | 1000 |
| Power (W) | 95 |
| Passage (times) | 1 |
| Frequency (Hz) | 500 |
| Speed (cm/s) | 60 |
| Mean + STD (mm) | 1.05 + 0.08 |

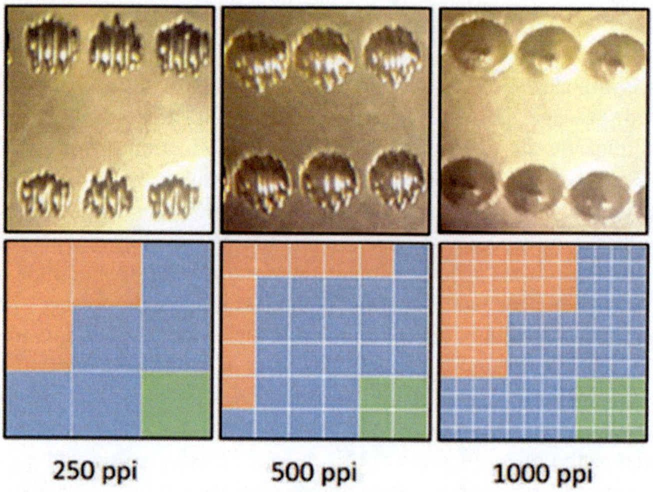


**Fig. 5** The resolution affects the smoothness of the engraving result

engraving, the mold fabrication process does not need to go to the cleanroom to create a mold and use a chemical compound that produces waste. The customized design of mold is made by drawing software. It also becomes the advantages regarding the requirement for biomedical purposes could be provided by changing the architecture of the mold.

## 5 Conclusion

Emerging potential on laser engraving in fabricating a mold for microfluidic technologies means to assess the feasibility of this approach to reach certain dimensions that meet the biomedical environment requirement by microfluidic technologies. Moreover, this method also investigates the effect of parameters and ensembles them to reach the structures. Based on the result and analysis, the microfluidic mold could be fabricated using the laser engraving method and meet the dimension requirement founding at values: 1000 for resolution, 95 for power, 500 for frequency, and 60 for speed. It can be noted that these adjusted parameters were performed for a single passage for reducing time for production. The investigated parameters of laser engraving namely speed, resolution, power, passage, and speed affected the result (depth). Speed was noted as the most significant parameter among the others. Meanwhile, resolution plays as the parameter that could smoother the engraved result. The microfluidic device based on PDMS could be fabricated by pouring the PDMS into the fabricated mold and detached to integrate with the coverslip constructing the complete microfluidic chip. Future research could be the cell culture experiment conducted in this chip to strengthen the proof that this new approach has potential in biomedical research.

## References


1. Zervantonakis IK, Kothapalli CR, Chung S, Sudo R, Kamm RD (2011) Microfluidic devices for studying heterotypic cell-cell interactions and tissue specimen cultures under controlled microenvironments. Biomicrofluidics 5(1)
2. Chung S, Sudo R, Vickerman V, Zervantonakis IK, Kamm RD (2010) Microfluidic platforms for studies of angiogenesis, cell migration, and cell-cell interactions: sixth international bio-fluid mechanics symposium and workshop March 28–30, 2008 Pasadena, California. Ann Biomed Eng 38(3):1164–1177
3. Barlocchi UMG, Villa FF (2012) Microfluidic system for real time PCR sample preparation. Lect Notes Electr Eng 109 LNEE:257–260
4. Caputo D et al (2014) Thermally actuated microfluidic system for polymerase chain reaction applications D. Lect Notes Electr Eng 268 LNEE:313–316
5. Lucia Giampetruzzi LF, Barca A, De Pascali C, Capone S, Verri T, Siciliano P (2019) Human organ-on-a-chip: around the intestine bends, pp 135–140
6. Emanuele Luigi Sciuto SC A Novel lab-on-disk system for pathogen nucleic acids analysis in infectious diseases, pp 135–140
7. Emanuele Luigi Sciuto SC (1997) Abstract: innovative lab-on-disk technology for rapid and integrated analysis of pathogen nucleic acids Emanuele, pp 1–398
8. Najeeb SP, Chavali M (2014) Nano-based PSA biosensors: an early detection technique of prostate cancer. J Biomimetics Biomater Biomed Eng 20:87–98
9. Chen CH et al (2013) Multiplexed protease activity assay for low-volume clinical samples using droplet-based microfluidics and its application to endometriosis. J Am Chem Soc 135(5):1645–1648
10. Ma L et al (2014) Gene-targeted microfluidic cultivation validated by isolation of a gut bacterium listed in human microbiome project's most wanted taxa. Proc Natl Acad Sci USA 111(27):9768–9773
11. Shin Y et al (2012) Microfluidic assay for simultaneous culture of multiple cell types on surfaces or within hydrogels. Nat Protoc 7(7):1247–1259
12. Agalianos F, Patelis S, Kyratsis P, Maravelakis E, Vasarmidis E, Antoniadis A (2011) Industrial applications of laser engraving : influence of the process parameters on machined surface quality. Machine 1242–1245
13. Balchev I, Atanasov A, Lengerov A, Lazov L (1859) Investigation of the influence of the scanning speed and step in laser marking and engraving of aluminum. J Phys Conf Ser 1:2021
14. Bin Haron MNF, Romlay FRBM (2019) Parametric study of laser engraving process of AISI 304 stainless steel by utilizing fiber laser system. IOP Conf Ser Mater Sci Eng 469(1)
15. Imran HJ, Hubeatir KA, Al-Khafaji MM (2021) $CO_2$ laser micro-engraving of PMMA complemented by Taguchi and ANOVA methods. J Phys Conf Ser 1795(1)
16. Sheean (2013) Microfabricated polyester conical microwells for cell culture applications. Lab Chip 23(1):1–7
17. Pérez-Rodríguez S, García-Aznar JM, Gonzalo-Asensio J (2021) Microfluidic devices for studying bacterial taxis, drug testing and biofilm formation. Microb Biotechnol
18. Xie L, Chen X, Yan H, Xie H, Lin Z (2020) Experimental research on the technical parameters of laser engraving. J Phys Conf Ser 1646(1)
19. Zhang W et al (2009) PMMA/PDMS valves and pumps for disposable microfluidics. Lab Chip 9(21):3088–3094
20. Romoli L, Tantussi G, Dini G (2011) Experimental approach to the laser machining of PMMA substrates for the fabrication of microfluidic devices. Opt Lasers Eng 49(3):419–427

21. Patko D, Mártonfalvi Z, Kovacs B, Vonderviszt F, Kellermayer M, Horvath R (2014) Microfluidic channels laser-cut in thin double-sided tapes: cost-effective biocompatible fluidics in minutes from design to final integration with optical biochips. Sens Actuators B Chem 196:352–356
22. Garcia CD, Gabriel EFM, Coltro WKT (2020) Fast and versatile fabrication of PMMA microchip electrophoretic devices by laser engraving. In: 18th international conference on miniaturized systems and chemical life science MicroTAS 2014, vol. 35, no 16, pp 1725–1727
23. da Costa ET, Santos MFS, Jiao H, do Lago CL, Gutz IGR, Garcia CD (2016) Fast production of microfluidic devices by CO2 laser engraving of wax-coated glass slides. Electrophoresis 37(12):1691–1695
24. Matellan C, Del Río Hernández AE (2018) Cost-effective rapid prototyping and assembly of poly(methyl methacrylate) microfluidic devices. Sci Rep 8(1):1–13
25. Trotec: What do the laser parameters mean? Optimal laser parameters for laser engraving and laser cutting for CO2 laser applications (2021). www.troteclaser.com. [Online]. Available: https://www.troteclaser.com/en-ms/knowledge/tips-for-laser-users/laser-parameters-definition/. Accessed on 26 Sept 2021

# Application of Denoising Weighted Bilateral Filter and Curvelet Transform on Brain MR Imaging of Non-cooperative Patients

**Fani Susanto, Arga Pratama Rahardian, Hernastiti Sedya Utami, Lutfiana Desy Saputri, Kusnanto Mukti Wibowo, and Anita Nur Mayani**

**Abstract** The use of a volume phase array type coil in the brain magnetic resonance imaging (MRI) examination of non-cooperative patients is associated with image noise arising from random electrical fluctuations in the body and causing it to not reflect the true pixel intensity value. Therefore noise reduction is needed in medical image processing. This research to apply denoising weighted bilateral filter and curvelet transform (WBFCT) on T2 weighted turbo spin echo (TSE) brain MRI images in non-cooperative patients. The aim of this research is to determine the differences in information on MRI brain images of T2 TSE sequences in non-cooperative patients between before and after the application of denoising WBFCT. This experimental research was carried out on MRI brain images of T2 TSE sequences in 19 non-cooperative patients. Then proceed with the application of denoising WBFCT on the image. Image assessment using 3 radiologists with data analysis using statistical processing and image post processing. The result shows that information on the brain MRI image of the T2 TSE sequence experienced differences in image information between before and after the application of denoising WBFCT (p-value <0.001), with an average mean square error (MSE) and peak signal-to-noise ratio (PSNR) of 387.995 and 70.5369 dB, where the image after denoising WBFCT had the most optimal image information. Finally, by denoising WBFCT can optimally produce information on MRI brain images of T2 TSE sequences in axial sections in non-cooperative patients.

**Keywords** Denoising · WBFCT · MRI brain · T2 TSE brain · Non-cooperative patients

---

F. Susanto (✉) · A. P. Rahardian · H. S. Utami · L. D. Saputri
Department of Radiologic Imaging Technology, Universitas Muhammadiyah Purwokerto, Purwokerto 53182, Banyumas, Indonesia
e-mail: fanisusanto@ump.ac.id

K. M. Wibowo
Department of Electromedical Engineering, Universitas Muhammadiyah Purwokerto, Purwokerto 53182, Banyumas, Indonesia

A. N. Mayani
Department of Radiology, STIKES Guna Bangsa Yogyakarta, 55283 Yogyakarta, Indonesia



T. Triwiyanto et al. (eds.), *Proceedings of the 2nd International Conference on Electronics, Biomedical Engineering, and Health Informatics*, Lecture Notes in Electrical Engineering 898, https://doi.org/10.1007/978-981-19-1804-9_17

# 1 Introduction

MRI radiodiagnostic examination produces images of sections of the human body using a magnetic field without the use of X-rays. MRI is able to produce images with optimal spatial resolution, good contrast between tissues, without ionizing radiation and can produce images with various sections (multiplanar), namely axial, coronal and sagittal sections without first image reconstruction1. MRI examination is now a routine examination in large hospitals. In principle, almost all organs of the body can be examined with an MRI. The MRI examination is 90% done on the brain and vertebrae organs while the remaining 10% is for examination of other organs [1–4].

MRI examination becomes a challenge in itself when patients are found with non-cooperative conditions. Radiographers are required to be able to produce optimal images, including in the MRI brain examination. MRI brain examination in non-cooperative patients is attempted to be carried out as quickly as possible with optimal results without being disturbed by noise or artifacts due to patient movement. Therefore, it is necessary to modify the examination protocol to minimize the occurrence of miss diagnostic information on MRI brain examination with non-cooperative patients [5].

In MRI brain examination, one of the pulse sequences used is TSE with T2 weighting [6]. According to Bitar et al., the T1 weighting shows a good anatomical image, while the T2 weighting has the advantage that it can reveal existing abnormalities, because many soft tissues included in the pathological process have a higher water content than normal conditions and the fluid will appear bright on the weighting. T2. T2 weighting is commonly used with TSE sequences. The TSE enters the spin echo sequence with multiple 1800 refocused radio frequency (RF) pulses after one 900 pulse to produce a sequence of echo [7]. According to Westbrook, TSE sequences are widely used for T2-weighted images because the scan time obtained is short and the use of TSE sequences will increase the signal to noise ratio (SNR) value.

MRI brain examination uses a volume phased array coil which is commonly used in parallel imaging techniques. This coil uses data from multiple coils or channels arranged around the scanning area to either reduce scan time or increase resolution [6]. In general, in most MRI applications, the coils associated with image noise are dominated by "body noise", which arises from random electrical fluctuations in the body. Noise in MRI images occurs during acquisition, storage and transmission and is based on the number of coils in the imaging system [8–10]. The appearance of noise in the form of stripes, spots, black and white in the MRI image causes the contrast to decrease. In addition, noise also causes the pixel intensity value to not reflect the actual pixel intensity value [8, 9] and noise can interfere with the visual quality of the resulting MRI image. Therefore noise reduction or denoising is needed in medical image processing [9–14].

Image denoising has an important role in processing MRI images before they are analyzed by a radiologist. The denoising process aims to obtain a more detailed MRI image and remove noise contained in the MRI image while retaining important information [14]. Routray et al. [15], developed a new denoising technique by combining bilateral filter and curvelet transform techniques. This technique is called WBFCT. The WBFCT technique preserves edges and textures based on a combination, which decomposes the noisy image into low and high frequency portions using a weighted bilateral filter and high frequency sections processed with hard shrinkage curvelets. The WBFCT technique has the advantage of being able to maintain the texture of the curvelet transformation. This WBFCT technique also outperforms other image denoising methods with high peak signal to noise ratio (PSNR) parameter values.

Routray et al. [15] conducted a study by applying the WBFCT de-noising technique to digital images with the result that there are differences in image information using the WBFCT denoising compared to other denoising techniques seen from the PSNR alues. However, the research carried out has not been tested into medical images. Meanwhile, Javaid [16] conducted research by applying Denoising Cuckoo's Search with a Curvelet trans-form to remove noise and amplify medical images without reducing information and as a result, Denoising Cuckoo's Search with Curvelet transform was better at eliminating impulse, gaussian and speckle noise. However, from these previous studies, it has not been used in medical imaging such as MRI images, especially in non-cooperative patients. This encourages the need for research to obtain optimal images on MRI images by applying denoising techniques.

This study aims to apply the WBFCT denoising technique to medical images, namely the T2 TSE MRI brain image in non-cooperative patients and to compare before and after the application of WBFCT denoising to the medical image. This is important considering that non-cooperative patients are very susceptible to suboptimal image results due to the appearance of movement artifacts and noise. This WBFCT denoising technique needs to be applied in medical images such as T2 TSE MRI brain images, especially in non-cooperative patients to improve the quality of the resulting MRI images.

## 2 Literature Review

The WBFCT denoising technique combines a weighted bilateral filter with a curvelet transform. The weighted bilateral filter decomposes the image input noise into low-frequency and high-frequency parts. After decomposition, most of the image information is stored in the low frequency while the edge and texture details are contained in the high frequency image. The purpose of this technique is to filter noise and geometric details with pixel averages so that image details at high frequencies are maintained. Then the high frequency part is processed using hard shrinkage curvelets to maintain the essential geometric components and estimate the detail of the image. In the end, the detail of the image is added with the low frequency portion and produces an image with reduced noise with more detailed geomteric (edges/textures) [15].

Measurement of denoising image processing performance is carried out with 2 (two) types of measurements to evaluate WBFCT performance by looking at error sensitivity and image quality assessment. The most widely used measure of error sensitivity is to calculate the value of MSE, SNR and PSNR. MSE is calculated by averaging the squared intensity of the original image (input) and the resulting image pixels (output). MSE is the average squared error value between the original image and the manipulated image. MSE has no units. SNR and PSNR are very useful in measuring image contrast but PSNR is useful when dealing with contrast adjustments in the desired region. SNR is defined poorly for homogeneous images, so for evaluation of image construction the PSNR value is more recommended [11].

PSNR includes parameters that are used as indicators to measure the similarity of the noise-contaminated image with the original image or compare the results of denoise image processing with the initial image or original image. PSNR is the ratio between the maximum value of the measured signal and the amount of noise that affects the signal. To determine PSNR, first determine the MSE value with the unit of PSNR is decibels (dB) [17, 18].

The MSE parameter indicates that the more similar the two images are, the MSE value of the MSE value is closer to zero, the smaller the MSE, the better the quality of the reconstructed image. While on the PSNR parameter, two images are said to have a low level of similarity if the PSNR value is below the value of 30 dB. PSNR values falling below 30 dB indicate relatively low quality, where distortion due to insertion is evident. However, high image quality is at a value of 40 dB and above [19].

## 3 Material and Method

### *3.1 Study Design*

This study is a pre-experimental pre-post test design.

### *3.2 Patients*

The study used 16 MR brain patients aged 18–60 years with pathology and in a non-cooperative patients consisting of 10 women and 6 men with a normal body mass index (18.5–24.9 kg/m$^2$) and willing to be the sample of this study at Premier Bintaro Hospital. Exclusion criteria consisted of patients have claustrophobia and some contraindications to MRI examination such as pacemakers and non-MRI compatible metallic implants.

**Table 1** Parameters of MR brain sequence T2 TSE axial slices

| Parameter | T2 TSE brain axial |
|---|---|
| Time recovery (TR)<br>Time echo (TE) | 4034 ms<br>100 ms |
| Slice thickness | 5 mm |
| Number of excitation (NEX | 3 |
| Number of slice | 20 |
| Field of view (FOV) | 230 |
| Matrix | 328 × 20 |
| Parallel imaging | SENSE |

## *3.3 MR Imaging Protocol*

The examination was carried out using a Philips 1.5 T MR scan tool with the routine MR brain protocol. Researchers used images from only one sequence in the study, namely T2 TSE sequence images of axial slices on MR brain examination. The inspection parameters for the sequence follows the Table 1.

## *3.4 Image Analysis*

Assessment of MR brain images of T2 TSE sequences in axial sections in non-cooperative patients between before and after the application of denoising WBFCT was carried out qualitatively and quantitatively.

**Qualitative Image Assessment**

Qualitative assessment was carried out using visual grading from 3 radiology specialists with more than 5 years of experience in MRI services. Visual grading was carried out on the anatomy of the cerebral cortex, basal ganglia, thalamus, pons and cerebellum. Visual grading assessment uses 3 rating scales follow Table 2.

**Quantitative Image Assessment**

Quantitative image assessment using the calculation of the mean square error (MSE) and peak signal to noise ratio (PSNR) obtained from the MR brain image sequence

**Table 2** Visual grading assesment [20, 21]

| Score | Name | Description |
|---|---|---|
| 1 | Poor | No visible anatomy, no clear boundaries and cannot be analyzed |
| 2 | Enough | The anatomy is quite visible, the boundaries are quite clear and can be analyzed |
| 3 | Good | Visible anatomy, well defined and easy to analyze |

TSE axial cut between before and after the application of the WBFCT denoising technique.

### 3.5 Statistical Analysis

Statistical analysis of the results of the T2 TSE axial section of MR brain image assessment in non-cooperative patients qualitatively using SPSS with Cohen's Kappa test ($K < 0.20$ bad agreement, 0.21–0.40 fair agreement; 0.41–0.60 moderate agreement; 0.61–0.80 good agreement; and 0.81–1.00 perfect agree-ment) [22, 23] and then continued by using the Wilcoxon test. The Wilcoxon test was carried out both for the overall anatomy and for each anatomical criterion to obtain which image was the most optimal between the MR brain images before or after the application of WBFCT denoising.

## 4 Results

The results of the MR brain image assessment are shown from the results of the Friedman Test, qualitative image analysis through image assessment with visual grading by a radiology doctor and quantitatively shown from the results of calculating the MSE and PSNR values.

### 4.1 Qualitative Analysis

Assessment of information on MR brain image sequences T2 TSE axial slices in non-cooperative patients between before and after the application of qualitative denoising WBFCT was carried out using visual grading and the Wilcoxon test results were obtained follows the Table 3.

From Table 2, the results of the Wilcoxon test above, show that both overall and for each anatomical criterion of the cerebral cortex, basal ganglia, thalamus, pons and thalamus, have an average p-value $<0.05$, which means that at MR image of brain T2 TSE sequence axial sections of non-cooperative patients showed differences in all anatomical criteria evaluated between before and after the application of denoising WBFCT.

The significant difference between the two images occurred because in the MR brain image before the application of WBFCT denoising, there was no image processing after the examination was completed. This of course results in the resulting image still containing noise (see Fig. 1). MRI examination in non-cooperative patients is also a challenge for radiographers to be able to produce optimal image quality without the emergence of artifacts and noise. Due to this, patients who cannot stay still

**Table 3** Wilcoxon test results for each anatomical criterion of MR brain image sequence T2 TSE axial slices in non-cooperative patients between before and after applying of denoising WBFCT

| Anatomy | WBFCT | Mean rank | Each anatomical criteria | Overall |
|---|---|---|---|---|
| Cortex cerebri | Before | 1.78 | 0.039 | <0.001 |
| | After | 2.16 | | |
| Basal ganglia | Before | 1.84 | 0.047 | |
| | After | 2.13 | | |
| Thalamus | Before | 1.38 | <0.001 | |
| | After | 2.34 | | |
| Pons | Before | 1.75 | 0.049 | |
| | After | 2.13 | | |
| Cerebellum | Before | 2.06 | 0.018 | |
| | After | 2.25 | | |

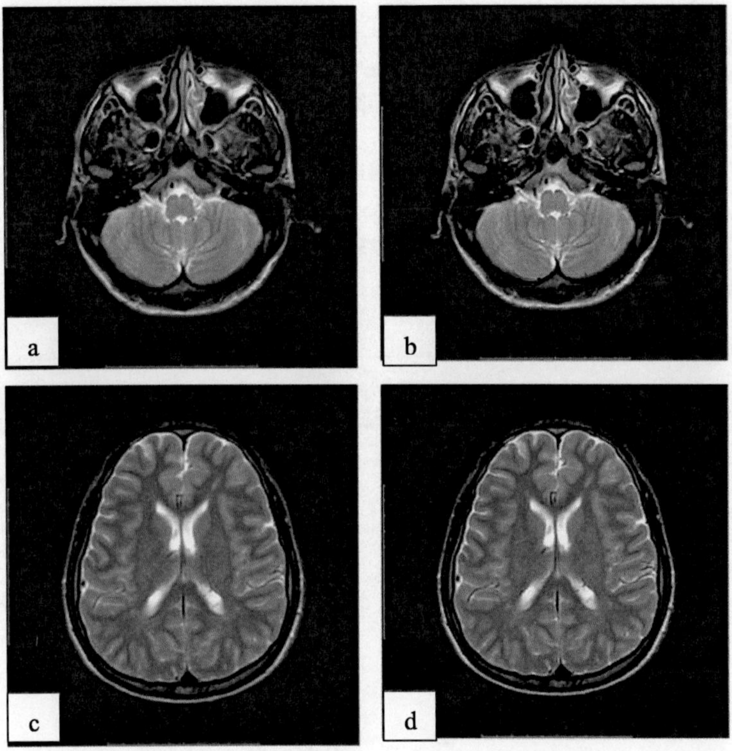


**Fig. 1** The results of MR brain T2 TSE sequence axial sections in non-cooperative patients, **a** and **c** before the application of WBFCT denoising showed ar-tack and noise in the anatomy; **b** and **d** after the application of de-noising WBFCT, it appears that there is reduced noise in the anatomy with a clearer and clearer appearance of boundaries and image structures

will be very susceptible to the emergence of movement artifacts and the possibility of unexpected noise.

## 4.2 *Quantitative Analysis*

Evaluation of the performance of the WBFCT denoising image processing is done by looking at the MSE and PSNR values to see the error sensitivity or the size of the image quality assessment. MSE is calculated by averaging the squared intensity of the original image (input) and the resulting image pixels (output). The lower the MSE value, the better the resulting image. While PSNR is calculated based on the comparison between the maximum value of the measured signal and the amount of noise that affects the signal, in other words, the higher the PSNR value, the better the image reconstruction [11]. A PSNR value falling below 30 dB indicates a relatively low image quality, where distortion due to embedding is evident. However, the image quality is said to be high when the PSNR is at a value of >40 dB [18].

Image assessment is done using MSE and PSNR calculations. The following calculation results have been obtained as in the Table 4.

**Table 4** Calculation results of MSE and PSNR images of MR brain T2 TSE sequence axial slices in non-cooperative patients between images before and after the WBFCT denoising technique

| Patients | MSE | PSNR (dB) |
|---|---|---|
| 1 | 435,605 | 69,9387 |
| 2 | 396,507 | 70,3471 |
| 3 | 455,836 | 69,7415 |
| 4 | 363,491 | 70,7247 |
| 5 | 359,161 | 70,7767 |
| 6 | 216,176 | 72,9815 |
| 7 | 247,056 | 72,4016 |
| 8 | 370,551 | 70,6411 |
| 9 | 377,035 | 70,5658 |
| 10 | 355,174 | 70,8252 |
| 11 | 490,192 | 69,4259 |
| 12 | 451,425 | 69,7837 |
| 13 | 347,199 | 70,9238 |
| 14 | 417,162 | 70,1265 |
| 15 | 496,282 | 69,3723 |
| 16 | 429,069 | 70,0043 |
| Average | 387,995 | 70,5369 |

## 5 Discussion

Noise on MRI in general can arise as a result of the image acquisition (acquisition) process and transmission errors [23]. The obtained MRI image is susceptible to the emergence of Gaussian noise which has a significant effect on image quality, so that the quality of the existing image tends to decrease and causes a reduction in contrast, detail and image information. The process of acquiring T2 TSE sequenced MR brain images in non-cooperative patients is closely related to the MRI hardware instrument used, the RF coil. The coil on the MR brain examination with a 16 channel volume phased array coil type, having a small coil arrangement placed close to the anatomy will produce a low SNR compared to the surface coil and a non-uniform reception sensitivity. The reception sensitivity of the coil system to the MRI signal has a direct impact on the SNR of the image. The volume sensitivity of the coil also plays an important role in the reception sensitivity. The ideal placement for the body part of interest is on the isocenter scanner where the best place is in terms of magnetic field homogeneity and gradient uniformity [24].

The use of the volume coil is a challenge in conducting an MR brain examination. Placement of the patient's head on the isocenter requires a supine position with a distance between the RF coil and the head. This position allows the anatomy to be far from the isocenter and prone to producing low-quality images. The research of Mohan et al. [25] stated that the MRI image obtained by using a coil with a parallel channel system (multiple coil channels) causes very inhomogeneous noise, where the signal obtained in K-space is damaged by the presence of complex additive Gaussian noise. Meanwhile, the use of MRI instruments on the surface coil causes noise to decrease, but the coil volume causes noise to increase in the anatomical area, where the smaller the number of coil channels, the smaller the SNR value. This certainly greatly affects the image quality of the MR brain which uses a volume type RF coil.

In addition, the role of parallel imaging in the examination parameters is also important and has an effect on the appearance of noise in the image. Parallel imaging utilizes spatial information in the phased array RF coil to reduce acquisition time in MRI. The main potential clinical applications include reducing acquisition time, increasing spatial resolution, or a combination of both. Improvements in image quality can be achieved by reducing the ETL of the TSE sequence. However, this technique has limitations, namely SNR reduction and artifact reconstruction. Parallel imaging in an emergency is used as a technique to overcome many obstacles, especially in non-cooperative patients. Using a faster and stronger gradient to increase the acquisition time, the spatial sensitivity of the phased array coil is used to provide spatial information on the image. Parallel imaging causes a reduction in the encoding phase line while still producing good quality and spatial resolution. The role of ETL is also important in determining whether or not an MR image is optimal. TSE sequences cause time durations that can be sped up with ETL settings. Using too long an ETL will cause a blurring of the image with loss of contrast.

From Table 3 it can also be seen that the mean rank value of the MR brain image after the application of WBFCT denoising tends to be higher on all existing anatomical criteria, compared to the MR brain image before the application of WBFCT denoising. This is because the difference in image information in the MR brain after the application of WBFCT denoising undergoes image reconstruction processing using the WBFCT denoising technique, causing reduced noise in the image. In addition, the results of the T2 TSE sequence MR brain image after the application of the WBFCT denoising technique appeared to reduce noise in both overall and individual anatomy with a clearer and clearer appearance of the boundaries and image structure.

Based on Table 4, the calculation results between MSE and PSNR obtained from MR brain images in non-cooperative patients between before and after the WBFCT denoising technique showed an average MSE value of 387.995 and an average PSNR value of 70.5369 dB. MSE calculation results show a low error value or close to zero in the range of 200 and a high PSNR value in the range of 72 dB or more than 40 dB. The results of the MSE and PSNR calculations in this study are more optimal than in previous studies where applying Gaussian denoising to the T2 TSE brain sequence MRI image with the same bit ($512 \times 512$), the results obtained an average MSE value of 2100 while the PSNR value with the results in the range of 38 dB, and also more optimal than in other previous studies with the application of WBFCT denoising on grayscale images, that the image after reconstruction of WBFCT denoising produces an average PSNR value of 30 dB [9]. This means that the MSE and PSNR values on the image reconstruction with WBFCT denoising MR brain sequence T2 TSE axial slices in non-cooperative patients that have been carried out, produce images with high quality and are more optimal than the image before the WBFCT denoising technique was carried out both physically and mentally. overall as well as per anatomical criteria (see Fig. 1).

The difference in quantitative assessment of image information between before and after WBFCT in MR brain images of non-cooperative axial sections of patients, is due to the WBFCT denoising reconstruction process which can reduce overall noise. The WBFCT denoising technique has the advantage of combining a weighted bilateral filter (WBF) and a curvelet transform. WBF decomposes the input noise region into low (mostly image information) and high frequency (edge and texture details) portions, aiming to filter out noise and preserve image detail at high frequencies. Curvelet transform (hard shrinkage) processes in the high frequency region to maintain the geometric (edge/texture) and detail of the image. Then the combination of high and low frequencies is carried out, so that WBFCT can emphasize textures and artifacts from the image by eliminating noise efficiently and thoroughly and with more detailed geomteric (edges/textures).

The denoising technique is an important part in the image processing process in imaging modalities as one of the improvement efforts, especially in reducing the effect of noise in the image. From this study, it was found that the denoising image processing method applied to MR brain images of T2 TSE sequences of non-cooperative patients was the WBFCT denoising technique. This technique can efficiently maintain texture, suppress artifacts and remove noise in the image. The use of this technique can improve image quality and can be used generally in other MRI scan sequences and organs. In addition, this WBFCT denoising image processing technique can be used and implemented in other special medical imaging fields such as Ultrasonography (USG) and CT Scan images by running a program that has been created and then duplicated into the imaging modality computer.

This research certainly has potential limitations. The limitation in this study is that the object used is only the part of the body that is examined, namely only the brain, the study also uses only one brain MRI image sequence and one type of coil. Researchers only focused on non-cooperative patients with MR brain examination with T2 TSE sequences, so that the denoising technique that was tried to be applied could not fully conclude that the results were the same on other body parts, other radiofrequency coils and other sequences on MR examination.

## 6 Conclusion

This research was conducted to determine the differences in information on MRI brain images of T2 TSE se-quences in non-cooperative patients between before and after the application of denoising WBFCT. The application of the WBFCT denoising technique to the MR image of the T2 TSE brain sequence of non-cooperative patient axial sections causes differences in image information and produces more optimal image information compared to MR images without applying WBFCT. Image processing techniques by applying WBFCT denoising can efficiently maintain texture, suppress artifacts and eliminate noise in the image so that it will greatly assist doctors in establishing diagnoses, especially for non-cooperative patients.

In future studies, it is necessary to apply WBFCT denoising to MRI images for other body parts using different types of radiofrequency coils and sequences. It is important to see the effect of applying the WBFCT denoising technique on MR images in general so that it can be used as an image processing technique that can be recommended in regular patient care.

## References

1. Zhou T, Canu S, Vera P, Ruan S (2021) A dual supervision guided attentional network for multimodal mr brain tumor segmentation. In: International conference on medical imaging and computer-aided diagnosis 2021. Lecture Notes in Electrical Engineering, vol 784. Springer, pp 3–11
2. Aboubakr N, Popova M, Crowley JL (2021) Color-based fusion of MRI modalities for brain tumor segmentation. In: International conference on medical imaging and computer-aided diagnosis 2021, Lecture Notes in Electrical Engineering, vol 784. Springer, pp 89–97
3. Li P, Wang M (2021) Sparse representation label fusion method combining pixel grayscale weight for brain MR segmentation. In: International conference on medical imaging and computer-aided diagnosis 2021, Lecture Notes in Electrical Engineering, vol 784. Springer, pp 7–16
4. Sjahriar R (2011) Radiologi Diagnostik, Edisi Kedua, Balai Penerbit FKUI: Jakarta

5. Westbrook C, Carolyne, Roth K, Talbot J (2011) MRI in practice, 4th edn. Blackwell Science Ltd., United Kingdom
6. Westbrook C (2014) Handbook of MRI technique, 4th edn. Blackwell Science Ltd., United Kingdom
7. Bitar R, General Leung, Perng R, Tadros S, Moody AR, Sarrazin J, McGregor C, Christakis M, Symons S, Nelson A, Roberts TP (2006) MR pulse sequences: what every radiologist wants to know but is afraid to ask. RSNA 26(2)
8. Yang J, Fan J, Ai D, Zhou S, Tang S, Wang Y (2015) Brain MR image denoising for Rician noise using pre-smooth non-local means filter. Biomed Eng Online 14(1):1–20
9. Kalaiselvi T, Kalaichelvi N (2018) Investigation on image denoising techniques of magnetic resonance images. Int J Comput Sci Eng 6(4):104–111
10. Tamilselvan KS (2013) A histogram based hybrid approach for medical image denoising using wavelet and curvelet transforms. Int J Comput Appl 74(21):6–11
11. Isa IS, Sulaiman SN, Mustapha M, Darus S (2015) Evaluating denoising performances of fundamental filters for T2-weighted MRI images. Proc Comput Sci 60:760–768
12. Youssif AAA, Darwish AA (2010) Adaptive algorithm for image denoising based on curvelet threshold. Int J Comput Sci Netw Secur 10(1):322–328
13. Kim DW, Kim C, Kim DH, Lim DH (2011) Rician nonlocal means denoising for MR images using nonparametric principal component analysis. EURASIP J Image Video Process 1(15):1–8
14. Balamurugan R, Saranya S (2014) Enhanced nonlocal mean filter for MRI denoising with rician noise. Int J Emerg Technol Adv Eng 4(5):256–261
15. Routray S, Kumar A, Mishra C (2018) Optik Image denoising by preserving geometric components based on weighted bilateral filter and curvelet transform. Opt Int J Light Electron Opt 159:333–343
16. Javaid Q, Arif M, Shah MALI, Nadeem M (2018) A hybrid technique for de-noising multi-modality medical images by employing cuckoo's search with curvelet transform. Mehran Univ Res J Eng Technol 37(1):29–48
17. Youssif AAA, Darwish AA (2010) Adaptive algorithm for image denoising based on curvelet threshold. Int J Comput Sci Netw Secu 10(1):322–328
18. Mamta A, Dalal T (2018) Novel method for denoising medical image using 2 level discrete wavelet transform and bilinear filter. Int J Recent Innov Trends Comput Comun 6(6):110–115
19. Cheddad A, Condell J, Curran K, Kevitt PM (2010) Digital image steganography: survey and analysis of current methods. Signal Process 90(3):727–752
20. Indrati R, Juliantara IPE et al (2017) Comparing SPIR and SPAIR fat suppression techniques in magnetic resonance imaging (MRI) of wrist joint. J Med Sci Clin Res 05(06):23180–23185
21. Homsi R, Gieseke J, Luetkens JA et al (2016) Three-dimensional isotropic fat-suppressed proton density-weighted MRI at 3 Tesla using a T/R-coil can replace multiple plane two-dimensional sequences in knee imaging Drei-dimensionale isotrope Protonen-gewichtete fettunterdrückte. Fortsch Rontgenstr 188:949–956
22. Oh E, Yoon YC, Park MJ (2017) Diagnostic performance of wrist magnetic resonance (MR) arthrography: comparison of three-dimensional isotropic T1 weighted fast spin-echo MR arthrography and two-dimensional MR arthrography. Br J Radiol 90:1071
23. Abdullah RH, Khattab RT, Ahmed AR (2017) Role of magnetic resonance imaging in evaluation of anterior cruciate ligament injuries. Egypt J Hosp Me 69(7):2897–2905
24. Mohan J, Krishnaveni V, Guo Y (2014) Biomedical signal processing and control a survey on the magnetic resonance image denoising methods. Biomed Signal Process Control 9:56–69
25. Tamilselvan KS, Murugesan G, Vinothsaravanan M (2013) A histogram based hybrid approach for medical image denoising using wavelet and curvelet transforms. Int J Comput Appl 74(21):1–11
26. Homsi R, Gieseke J, Luetkens JA et al (2016) Three-dimensional isotropic fat-suppressed proton density-weighted MRI at 3 Tesla using a T/R-coil can replace multiple plane two-dimensional sequences in knee imaging. Fortschr Rontgenstr 188:949–956

# Skin Cancer Classification Systems Using Convolutional Neural Network with Alexnet Architecture

**Dian Ayu Nurlitasari, R. Yunendah Nur Fuadah, and Rita Magdalena**

**Abstract** Skin cancer is one of three malignant cancers that are often found in Indonesia and can cause death, apart from cervical cancer and breast cancer. Skin cancer diagnosis done manually by a dermatologist through a biopsy and microscopic process. However, this process takes a long time and has a risk of accidents in the biopsy process. Whereas early diagnosis shows that more than 90% can be cured, while delay in diagnosis shows less than 50% can be cured. For this reason, this research was conducted to design and implement a system that can classify skin cancer in order to facilitate the skin detection process to be faster. This study applied the Convolutional Neural Network (CNN) method using the Alexnet architecture to classify skin cancers into four categories, namely dermatofibromas, melanoma, nevus pigmentosus, and squamous cell carcinoma. Experiments were carried out using a dataset obtained from the International Skin Imaging Collaboration (ISIC) dataset of 4000 images of skin cancer conditions of dermatofibroma, melanoma, nevus pigmentosus, and squamous cell carcinoma, consisting of 1000 images in each class. The amount of training data used is 2700 skin cancer images. While the number of validation data used is 900 images. Then the remaining 400 images were used as test data. The experimental results using training data and validation data show that the best optimizer is Adam and the use of a learning rate of 0.001 produces an accuracy value of 99% and a loss value of 0.0596 on the applied Alexnet architecture. From the Alexnet model, the test data were successfully detected according to their respective classes with the test data accuracy value of 97.5%, loss value of 0.1272 and the precision, recall and f1-score value around 0.96–0.99. Based on the results of the system performance, it shows that the applied model promises to be an early detection tool for skin cancer by dermatologists so that it can reduce the dangerous effect due to the delay in diagnosing skin cancer.

**Keywords** Skin cancer · Convolutional neural network · Alexnet

D. A. Nurlitasari · R. Y. N. Fuadah (✉) · R. Magdalena
School of Electrical Engineering, Telkom University, Bandung, Indonesia
e-mail: yunendah@telkomuniversity.ac.id

 
T. Triwiyanto et al. (eds.), *Proceedings of the 2nd International Conference on Electronics, Biomedical Engineering, and Health Informatics*, Lecture Notes in Electrical Engineering 898, https://doi.org/10.1007/978-981-19-1804-9_18

# 1 Introduction

Skin cancer is one of a triad of malignant cancers that are often found in Indonesia that can cause death, in addition to cervical cancer and breast cancer. In the United States, more than 5.4 million cases of skin cancer are found each year and make skin cancer the most common type of cancer in the country [1]. One of the main causes of skin cancer is the intensity of frequent exposure to ultraviolet radiation from the sun. The heat and radiation from the sun directly hits the earth which should be absorbed by the ozone layer as much as 93–99%. However, due to the depleting capacity of ozone, the Ultra Violet (UV) rays that reach the earth are getting bigger and can cause various problems for humans, one of which is skin cancer [2].

Generally, the diagnosis of skin cancer is done by a doctor with a biopsy and microscopic process. The biopsy process is done by taking small pieces of cancer cells to be examined and tested in detail by a doctor or dermatologist. Using this testing technique will take a long time for a dermatologist and have the risk of an accident during the biopsy process [1]. From the research that has been done, early diagnosis of skin cancer shows more than 90% can be cured, while delay in diagnosis shows less than 50% can be cured [3]. Therefore, if the diagnosis process can be carried out early, it will help reduce the risk of late diagnosis of skin cancer. Several studies have been developed for skin cancer detection. Previous study mentioned that melanoma skin cancer was detected using Linear Discriminant Analysis-Fuzzy k-Nearest Neighbor Lp-Norm. The result of this research showed an accuracy of 72% using 200 various dermoscopy images for melanoma and non-melanoma types [4].

In 2018 a study was carried out by Munthe et al. [1] with the title Skin Cancer Image Classification Based on the Level of Cancer Malignancy in Melanocytes using the Deep Convolutional Neural Network. They achieved 84% for the accuracy by using 1500 images consisting of nevus, melanoma in situ and malignant melanoma. Hosny et al. [5] did classification of skin cancer using Deep Learning and Transfer Learning. Deep Convolutional Neural Network method was applied to classify images of skin cancer. By applying the AlexNet classification and replacing the last layer with softmax to classify melanoma, common nevus, and atypical nevus they achieved 98.61% for the accuracy. Previous study has also classified skin cancer using the CNN method with a proposed architectural model for several types of skin cancer, namely dermatofibroma, nevus pigmentosus, melanoma, and squamous cell carcinoma with 95% validation accuracy [6]. In this study, the authors carried out a performance analysis of skin cancer classification system using CNN method and Alexnet architecture to classify four classes of skin cancer, namely dermatofibroma, melanoma, nevus pigmentosus, and squamous cell carcinoma. Alexnet was able to reduce the error rate of the other top 5 winners from 26 to 15.3% with fewer layers. In addition to the small number of layers, the use of relu in the alexnet architecture can make the training process faster than the usual CNN model. Therefore, the Alexnet architecture is used in this research [7]. The system performanced are tested by using test data.

# 2 Material and Methods

## 2.1 Dataset

The dataset used in this research is the International Skin Imaging Collaboration (ISIC) dataset. The number of training data used is 3600 and 400 images are used for test data. Then the data is processed using the CNN method. There are four skin cancer classes used in this study, namely dermatofibroma, melanoma, nevus pigmentosus and squamous cell carcinoma.

**Dermatofibroma**. Dermatofibromas are benign fibrous nodules commonly found on the lower skin. Dermatofibromas are also called cutaneous fibrous histiocytoma. Some minor trauma such as insects, or stab wounds such as rose thorns is the appearance of dermatofibroes [8]. The characteristics of dermatofibromas are about 2–3 mm in size, purplish brown in color, have a hard structure, and are painful when pressed [9].

**Melanoma**. Melanoma is the deadliest type of skin cancer. About 75% of skin cancer cases are Melanoma type. This type of cancer grows in skin melanocytes, the cells that produce melanin, and the dark pigment responsible for giving hair and skin its color. The main cause of melanoma type cancer is sun exposure. In addition, genetic factors, melacynotic nevi or moles, gender, and family history of having had melanoma are also causes of melanoma [1].

**Nevus Pigmentosus**. The most common benign melanocytic lesion affecting all ages is Nevus Pigmentosus. The features of Nevus Pigmentosus are like birthmarks or moles [10]. If the number of nevus is more than 100, it can have 8–10 times the risk compared to the number of nevus more than 50. This makes Nevus Pigmentosus, although benign, can potentially become melanoma, which is a very deadly skin cancer. The number of nevus will increase to a peak at the age of from 25 to 26 years which will then gradually shrink and disappear over time and it has been reported that by the age of 80 the nevus will disappear [11]. Side effects of the disease for patients affected by complications will experience neurological disorders such as seizures, fainting and vomiting [10].

**Squamous Cell Carcinoma**. About 20% of skin cancer cases are squamous cell carcinoma. Squamous Cell Carcinoma is also called epidermoid carcinoma, squamous cell epithelioma, planocellular carcinoma, prickle cell carcinoma, spinalioma.

## 2.2 Convolutional Neural Network

This study designed a detection system to classify four classes of skin cancer, namely dermatofibroma, melanoma, nevus pigmentosus, and squamous cell carcinoma. The system used Convolutional Neural Network (CNN) model with Alexnet architecture.

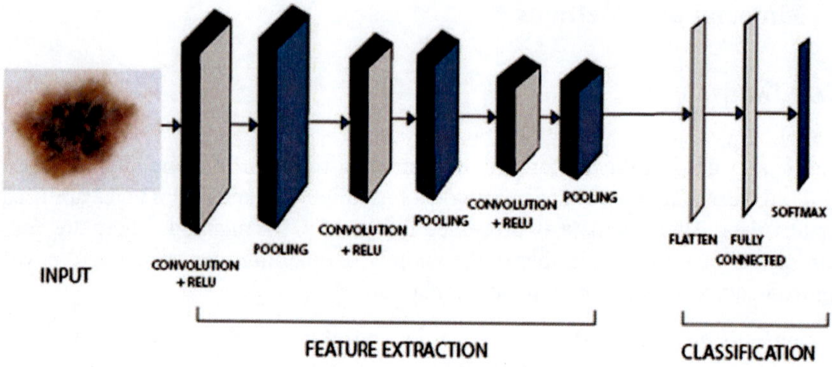


**Fig. 1** Convolutional neural network model

The development of Multilayer Perceptron (MLP) which is designed to process two-dimensional data is called Convolutional Neural Network [12]. Convolutional Neural Networks usually consist of a set of layers that can be grouped according to their function. CNN is used to analyze visual images, detect and recognize objects and images, which are high-dimensional vectors that will involve many parameters to characterize the network. CNN networks are of the feed-forward or non-repeating type, and it is proposed to reduce the number of parameters and adapt the network architecture specifically for the visual task [1]. Convolutional Neural Network consists of two major parts, namely Feature Extraction Layer and Fully-Connected Layer (Multilayer Perceptron) [6]. In general, the architecture of the Convolutional Neural Network is shown in Fig. 1.

The Feature Extraction Layer consists of Convolutional Layer with ReLU activation, and the Pooling layer. In the Feature Extraction Layer, an input in the form of image will be encoded into a feature in the form of numbers that represent the image. Convolutional layer consists of neurons arranged to form a two-dimensional filter with length and height (pixels). The convolutional layers use convolutional filters to produce a feature map [1]. ReLU is an activation layer that is used to increase the training stage of an artificial neural network which has the advantage of minimizing errors [13]. Pooling Layer is used to reduce data using Max Pooling or Average or Mean Pooling. Max Pooling will select the maximum value in the filter area when shifting, while Mean Pooling will be selected from the average value on the filter [14] as shown in the Fig. 2.

## *2.3 System Design*

This study developed a detection system to classify skin cancer based on image processing. The system used the CNN model with Alexnet architecture. The Alexnet architecture has eight layers which are divided into five convolutional layers and

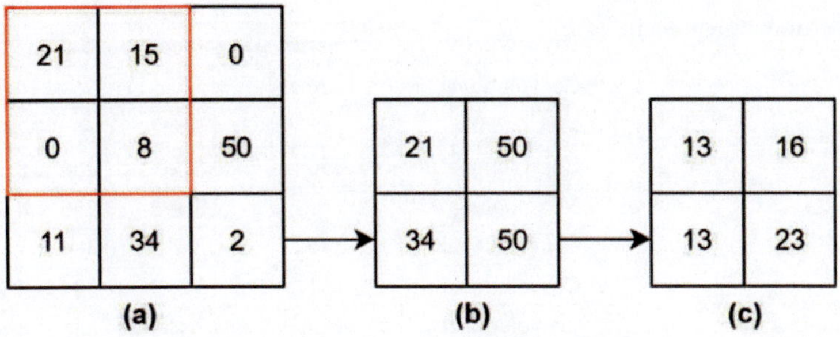


**Fig. 2** The illustration of pooling layer. **a** The 4 × 4 pixel input image; **b** max pooling; **c** mean pooling

three fully connected layers. Alexnet system model that used in this study is shown in Fig. 3.

The input image used is an image with a size of 64 × 64 × 3. Table 1 shows a summary of the kernel sizes and filters used at each layer on Alexnet architecture used in this study.

The skin cancer images are then convoluted with filters that have a specific size on each layer. Then in each hidden layer, RelU activation is used. This RelU activation will change the negative value of the feature map to zero. Then Max Pooling is

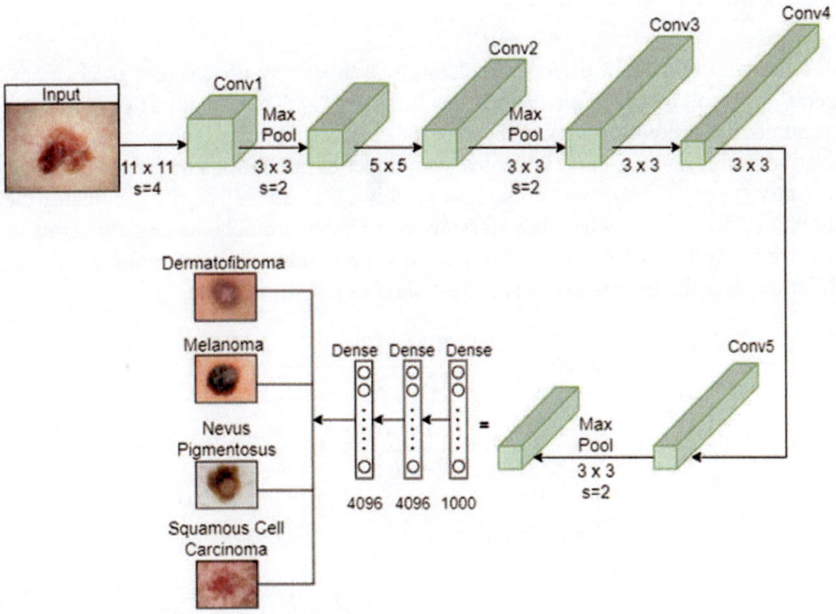


**Fig. 3** Alexnet system model used in this study

**Table 1** Alexnet architecture

| Layer type | Kernel size | Filter | Output |
|---|---|---|---|
| Convolutional | 96 | 11 × 11 | 96 × 16 × 16 |
| Max pooling | | 3 × 3 | 96 × 8 × 8 |
| Convolutional | 256 | 5 × 5 | 256 × 8 × 8 |
| Max pooling | | 3 × 3 | 256 × 4 × 4 |
| Convolutional | 384 | 3 × 3 | 384 × 4 × 4 |
| Convolutional | 384 | 3 × 3 | 384 × 4 × 4 |
| Convolutional | 256 | 3 × 3 | 256 × 4 × 4 |
| Max pooling | | 3 × 3 | 256 × 2 × 2 |
| Fully connected | | | 4096 × 1 × 1 |
| Fully connected | | | 4096 × 1 × 1 |
| Fully connected with softmax | | | 1000 × 1 × 1 |

used on the first, second and fifth layers of the Alexnet architecture to reduce image dimensions. And in the last layer, there is a softmax to classify the four classes of skin cancer.

## 2.4 System Performance

Measurement of system performance results in this study used scores of accuracy, precision, recall and f1. Calculations are shown in (1). True Positive (TP) indicates the number of predictions where the classifier correctly predicts the positive class as positive, True Negative (TN) indicates the number of predictions where the classifier correctly predicts the negative class as negative, False Positive (FP) indicates the number of predictions where the classifier incorrectly predicts the negative class as positive while False Negative (FN) indicates the number of predictions where the classifier incorrectly predicts the positive class as negative.

$$Accuracy = \frac{TP + TN}{TP + TN + FN + FP} \times 100\% \tag{1}$$

$$Recall = \frac{TP}{TP + FN} \times 100\% \tag{2}$$

$$Precission = \frac{TP}{TP + FP} \times 100\% \tag{3}$$

$$F1score = 2 \times \frac{PrecisionxRecall}{Precision + Recall} \times 100\% \tag{4}$$

## 3 Result

The skin cancer image dataset used in this study consisted of 4000 skin cancer images for dermatofibroma, melanoma, nevus pigmentosus, and squamous cell carcinoma conditions, consisting of 1000 images in each class. The amount of training data used is 2700 skin cancer images. While the number of validation data used is 900 images. Then the remaining 400 images were used as test data. Skin cancer images were trained using a CNN model with Alexnet architecture. First, the train and validation data of 3600 skin cancer images were trained with 50 epochs and learning rate of 0.001 to find the best optimizer. Some of the optimizers used are Adam, Nadam, SGD and RMSprop. Figure 4 shows a comparison of the results from using several optimizers.

From Fig. 4 it can be seen that Adam optimizer gets the best results with an accuracy value of 99% and a loss value of 0.0596. While Nadam optimizer gets accuracy value of 88.33% and loss value of 0.5628, RMSprop optimizer gets accuracy value of 97.78% and loss value of 0.1793, SGD optimizer gets accuracy value of 98.06% and loss value of 0.0633. So, the best parameter to use in Alexnet model for skin cancer classification is to use Adam optimizer and a learning rate of 0.001.

## 4 Discussion

By using the Alexnet model with the best parameter, the system is tested using 400 test data and produces an accuracy value of 97.5% and a loss value of 0.1272. Figure 5 shows the confusion matrix of the test data.

Based on Fig. 5 shows that of the 400 test data used, 391 data were correctly classified according to their class, while the remaining data were classified incorrectly. The errors occurred in two images of nevus pigmentosus detected as squamous cell carcinoma, two images of melanoma detected as dermatofibroma, four images of dermatofibroma detected as melanoma, and one image of squamous cell carcinoma detected as nevus pigmentosus. The five parameters used to measure system performance, using values from 0 to 1, the closer the value to 1 means the less error there is. Detailed scores for the five parameters from each class are shown in Table 2.

Previous study has also classified skin cancer using the CNN method with a proposed architectural model for several types of skin cancer, namely dermatofibroma, nevus pigmentosus, melanoma, and squamous cell carcinoma with 95% validation accuracy [6]. It can be seen that using the Alexnet model can increase accuracy up to 99% compared to the previous studies.

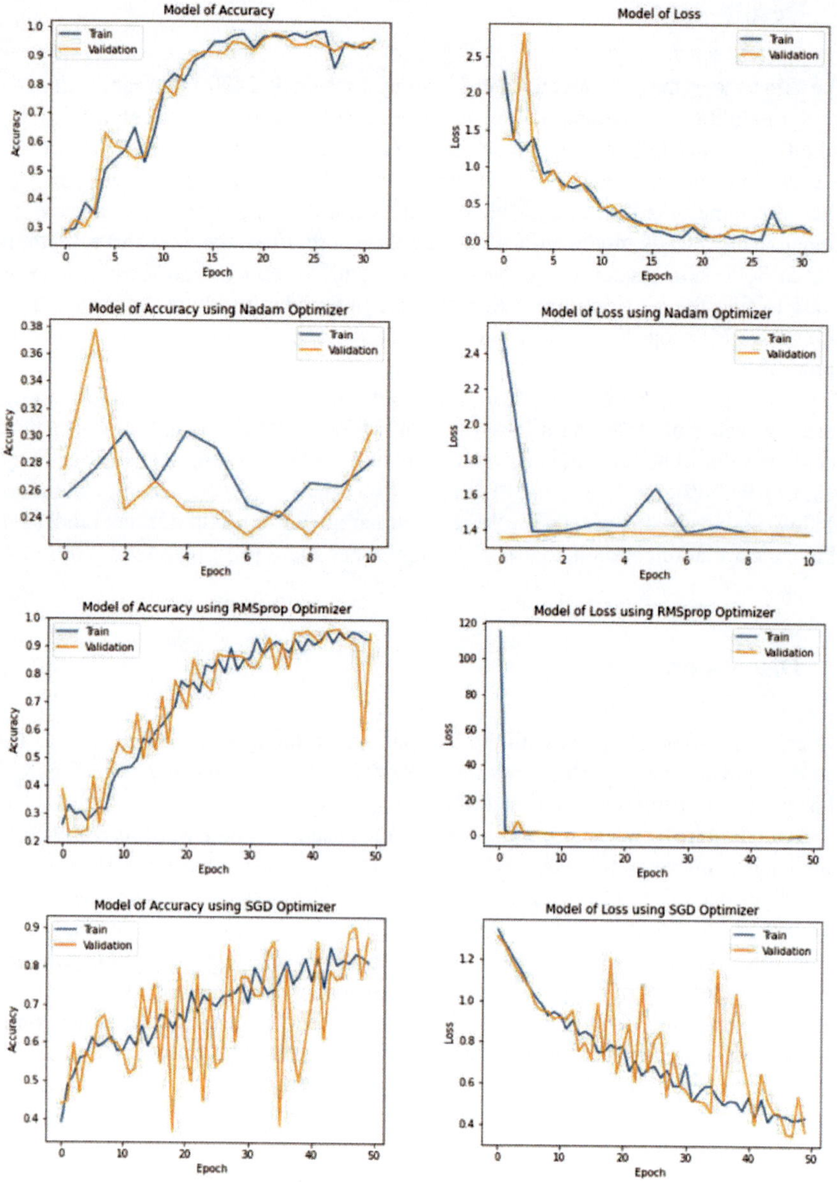


**Fig. 4** System performance result comparison

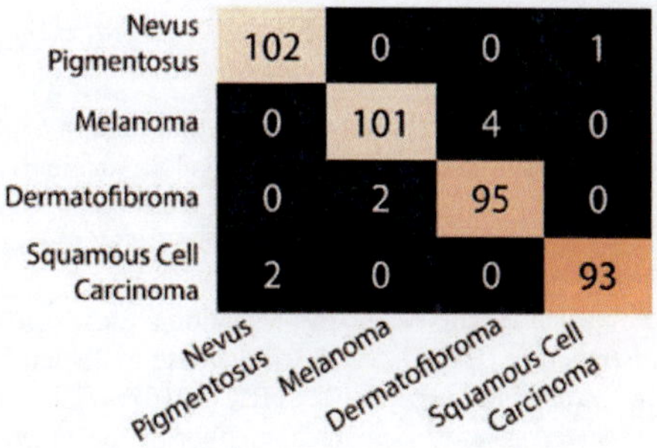


**Fig. 5** Confussion matrix of the test data

**Table 2** The performance of the system

| Class | Precision (%) | Recall (%) | F1-score (%) | No of images |
|---|---|---|---|---|
| Nevus pigmentosus | 98 | 99 | 99 | 103 |
| Melanoma | 98 | 96 | 97 | 105 |
| Dermatofibroma | 96 | 98 | 97 | 97 |
| Squamous cell carcinoma | 96 | 98 | 98 | 95 |
| Total | 97 | 98 | 98 | 400 |

## 5 Conclusion

In this study, an automatic skin cancer classification system has been designed to facilitate the skin detection process to be faster using the CNN method with the Alexnet architecture which consists of 5 hidden layers and 3 fully connected layers. Optimization was carried out on the applied model using the Adam, Nadam, RMSprop and SGD optimizers. The experimental results using training data and validation data show that the best optimizer is Adam and the use of a learning rate of 0.001 produces an accuracy value of 99% and a loss value of 0.0596 on the proposed Alexnet architecture. From the Alexnet model, the test data were successfully detected according to their respective classes, namely dermatofibroma, nevus pigmentosis, melanoma and squamous cell carcinoma with the test data accuracy value of 97.5%, loss value of 0.1272 and the precision, recall and f1-score value around 0.96–0.99. Based on the results of the performance of the system, it shows that the proposed model promises to be a tool for early skin cancer detection by dermatologists. In further research, a system can be developed to classify skin cancer with more types and number of classes.

## References


1. Munthe TLD (2018) Classification of skin cancer images based on cancer malignancy levels in melanocytes using deep convolutional neural network. University of North Sumatra, pp 74
2. Foeady AZ (2019) Skin cancer classification system based on dermoscopic image data using deep extreme learning machine method. Sunan Ampel State Islamic University Surabaya, pp 1
3. Wahaninggar K (2016) Melanoma skin cancer image classification using support vector machine (SVM). Surabaya Institute of Technology, pp 73
4. Mentari M, Sari YA, Dewi RK (2016) Melanoma skin cancer detection with linear discriminant analysis-fuzzy k-nearest neighbor LP-norm. Brawijaya University, pp 6
5. Hosny KM, Kaseem MA, Foaud MM (2018) Skin cancer classification using deep learning and transfer learning. IEEE, pp 4
6. Fu'adah YN et al (2020) Convolutional neural network (CNN) for automatic skin cancer classification. In: IOP conference series: materials science and engineering
7. Alom M Z et al (2018) The history began from alexnet: a comprehensive. Cornell University
8. Amanda O (2016) Dermatofibroma
9. Bandyopadhyay MR (2016) Dermatofibroma: a typical presentations. Indian J Dermatol
10. Tsaniyah, Delila RA, Aspitriana A, Fatmawati F (2015) The prevalence and histopathological features of nevus pigmentosus in the anatomical pathology section of Dr. Mohammad Hoesin Palembang. Sriwijaya University
11. Nisa Islamiati E, Nia Irasanti S, Kusmiati M, Hikmawati D, Nur MI (2019) Characteristics of nevus pigmentosus based on histopathological features. J Health Sci Integr 1
12. Phill K (2017) MATLAB deep learning: with machine learning, neural networks and artificial intelligence. Apress, Berkeley, CA
13. Agarap AF (2018) Deep learning using rectified linear units (ReLU). pp 2–8
14. Karpathy (2018) Introduction to convolutional neural networks. Cornell University

# Deep Learning Approach to Detect the Covid-19 Infection Using Chest X-ray Image: A Review

**Triwiyanto Triwiyanto, Lusiana, Levana Forra Wakidi, and Farid Amrinsani**

**Abstract** The COVID 2019 outbreak has been designated by WHO as a pandemic since 2020. Various methods of diagnosis of COVID 19 have been developed by several researchers to cope with COVID 19. A proper and accurate diagnosis is crucial for the next treatment step. Deep learning has been widely applied in the image classification process with high accuracy. However, the selection of the right deep learning model for the detection of lung disorders caused by COVID-19 based on x-ray images of the chest has not been widely reviewed by several reference sources. Therefore, the purpose of this study is to do a paper review that reviews a deep learning approach to detect COVID 19 through chest X-ray images. The reference sources used in the preparation of this review paper are from various databases such as PubMed, IEEE-explore, and ScienceDirect in the period of 2020–2021. The results of the review and discussion show that deep learning with the convolution neural network (CNN) algorithm is more widely applied in the process of recognizing patterns of lung abnormalities caused by COVID 19. However, deep learning with transfer learning has the potential for better accuracy because it applies the architecture that has been used to solve the same previous problem. The conclusion that can be drawn from this study is that CNN is still the right method for diagnosing lung disorders caused by COVID 10 compared to conventional machine learning.

**Keywords** COVID 19 · Chest X-ray · Deep learning · CNN

## 1 Introduction

In 2020, WHO has determined that the corona virus disease 19 (COVID 19) outbreak is a pandemic disease [1]. At the time this article was written, the COVID-19 outbreak had caused 200,518,280 people to be infected and 4,250,000 people died worldwide. The COVID-19 virus is a new variant of SARS that attacks the respiratory tract, especially the lungs. The pre-diagnosis of someone being infected with the COVID-19

T. Triwiyanto (✉) · Lusiana · L. F. Wakidi · F. Amrinsani
Poltekkes Kemenkes Surabaya, Jl. Pucang Jajar Tengah No. 56, Surabaya 60282, Indonesia
e-mail: triwi@poltekkesdepkes-sby.ac.id

 
T. Triwiyanto et al. (eds.), *Proceedings of the 2nd International Conference on Electronics, Biomedical Engineering, and Health Informatics*, Lecture Notes in Electrical Engineering 898, https://doi.org/10.1007/978-981-19-1804-9_19

virus is having a high fever, decreased sense of taste and sense of smell, experiencing a prolonged dry cough, and experiencing shortness of breath. Currently, the diagnostic process to detect whether a person is positively infected by the COVID-19 virus is carried out in three ways, using viral, blood, and chest X-ray image methods [2, 3]. Meanwhile, the examination of COVID 19 using the blood method or known as the Antigen method, is through a reagent reaction with a sample of the blood of a patient suspected of being infected with COVID 19. Actually, the examination of COVID 19 using the blood method is to detect COVID 19 indirectly, namely by seeing whether there is the formation of antibodies through the patient's blood sample. This is due to the human body; when it is infected with a virus, can naturally produce antibodies, causing the examination using the blood method to be less accurate. The diagnosis of COVID 19 using the viral method is taking samples from the nose or throat. This method is also known as a rapid test through the examination of antigens. Another alternative, viral examination of specimens, is to use polymerase chain reaction (PCR) [4]. However, to get accurate results, the examination using PCR must be carried out repeatedly within 14 days for patients who have indications with COVID 19 symptoms by using X-ray images which can be done for diagnostic purposes. Examination of chest X-rays must be done by an expert to determine lung disorders or abnormalities. Manual chest X-ray examination requires a high level of time and expertise, so as an alternative to the development of the COVID-19 identification process in the lungs, it can be done using machine learning.

Machine learning is an algorithm that is embedded in a computer machine in such a way that the machine is able to learn and make decisions like humans [5]. In general, machine learning is built using three basic components, namely, pre-processing, processing, and post-processing [6]. Pre-processing is the most important part of machine learning, including processing, thresholding, scaling, and feature extraction. Several conventional machine learnings have been used to help diagnose COVID 19 through chest X-ray images, including artificial neural network, support vector machines, and linear discriminant analysis. In conventional machine learning, it requires a feature extraction process before processing so that the accuracy of the system depends on the choice of the feature extraction model used [6]. Feature extraction models that are often used are time, frequency, and team-frequency domain features. Furthermore, in the last decade, machine learning has experienced very significant developments, especially in the pre-processing and architecture sections, namely deep learning. Several researchers have developed deep learning using the convolution neural network (CNN) algorithm [2, 7, 8], which has advantages in terms of pre-processing, namely, it has learning features through the convolution process [9] so that the deep learning model that uses the CNN algorithm does not require pre-processing in the form of feature extraction.

Several researchers have applied deep learning for the purposes of X-ray image classification to detect abnormalities in an object, such as cancer in organs, diabetes mellitus through the retina of the eye, disorders of the lungs and other medical illnesses [10–14]. During the COVID-19 pandemic, deep learning has been developed by several previous researchers to assist doctors in the diagnosis process, especially through chest X-ray images. COVID 19 attacks the respiratory tract, especially the lungs, which can be clearly seen by the symptoms of the patient experiencing shortness of breath. Shortness of breath is due to bronchial cells in the lungs have been infected by the virus and inhibit the lungs in producing oxygen for the blood. In the X-ray photo, it will be seen visually the part of the lung infected with COVID 19 with the result in the form of clouding in the image section. Deep learning methods have enormous potential to be applied to various applications, especially helping doctors in diagnosing COVID 19 in patients. Therefore, this article aims to clearly and completely review the Deep learning approach in helping the process of diagnosing patients experiencing symptoms caused by COVID 19 through chest X-ray images.

This article is expected to be able to contribute to researchers who are developing COVID-19 detection using chest X-ray images, namely architectural models and appropriate hyper parameters, in the application of deep learning. Furthermore, in this article, readers can find reliable sources of datasets so that they can be used for development purposes. Overall, the rest of the discussion of this article consists of a background section that discusses related to deep learning, and the Review Section reveals previous studies related to the diagnosis of COVID 19 based on chest X-ray images. The results and discussion section discusses the results of the review, and finally, the conclusion section concludes the results of the article review.

## 2 Deep Learning Method

The artificial neural network was first introduced in 1943 by Warren McCulloch, which is a network that imitates the working system of human brain cells that have the ability to learn new things. Basically, a neural network is composed of three main layers, namely, the input layer, the hidden layer, and the output layer. Each layer is composed of several neurons that will be active. Activation of each neuron can use sigmoid activation or other activation. In the development of artificial neural network research, the architecture of the artificial network has developed from one hidden layer to multilayer, hereinafter known as deep learning. Figure 2 shows examples of deep learning architectures used to recognize patterns in an image. The architecture shows six hidden layers, one input layer and one output layer. In order to prevent over fitting during the training process, the number of nodes in the hidden layer can be reduced by using the dropout function (5–90% of the total nodes in one layer). The number of hidden layers can be determined based on the complexity of the patterns that will be recognized by the network.

In general, the process of recognizing an image is shown in Fig. 2, which consists of pre-processing, segmentation, feature extraction, and machine learning. At the pre-processing stage, it can be in the form of stages, among others, thresholding, scaling, filtering, and morphological opening. The feature extraction stage can be carried out using time, frequency, and time–frequency domains, and this depends on the needs and complexity of the image patterns to be recognized. Feature extraction in the time domain, for example, mean, standard deviation, kurtosis, etc., is often used because it has a very fast calculation process compared to other feature domains.

The deep learning architecture shown in Fig. 2 is the development of an artificial neural network architecture model with more than one hidden layer; in this case, there are six hidden layers. In the deep learning model, as illustrated in Fig. 1, the model still requires pre-processing, segmentation, and feature extraction stages. However, the weakness of the deep learning model with the architecture, as shown in Fig. 1, is that the model still uses feature engineering to extract the learned input patterns. Feature engineering must be selected, combined, and tested, which results in the highest machine learning accuracy, so this requires more time and effort. In order to improve the model, the next deep learning development is an artificial neural network model that has feature learning so that the model can perform the feature extraction process without using feature engineering (for example, time, frequency, and time–frequency domain). In this case, the feature learning process is carried out using a convolution process between the images to be recognized by a filter or commonly referred to as the kernel.

The basic concept of feature learning is to find the dominant features in the image by utilizing the convolution process between the image and the filter (kernel). Kernel weight at the beginning is randomly generated. Kernel dimensions are generally chosen based on experimentation with the indicators that yield the highest accuracy. An example of a two-dimensional (2D) convolution process between a $7 \times 7$ image and a $3 \times 3$ two-dimensional kernel is shown in Fig. 3. The $3 \times 3$ kernel will be convoluted with a $7 \times 7$ image successively from column 1 to column 5. Each convolution image and kernel return one value. The convolution process between image (I) and kernel (K) runs sequentially from the 1st column to the 5th column with 1 column overlap from left to right. Thus, the final result of the convolution produces a new matrix with a size of $5 \times 5$ (I*K). The result of this convolution process is referred to as a feature map.

In addition to the convolution process, to reduce noise in a feature map, a max-pooling process can be applied. The max-pooling process, as shown in Fig. 4, will select the maximum values in the feature map in the matrix so as to produce a feature map with the new matrix dimensions. This process is similar to the convolution

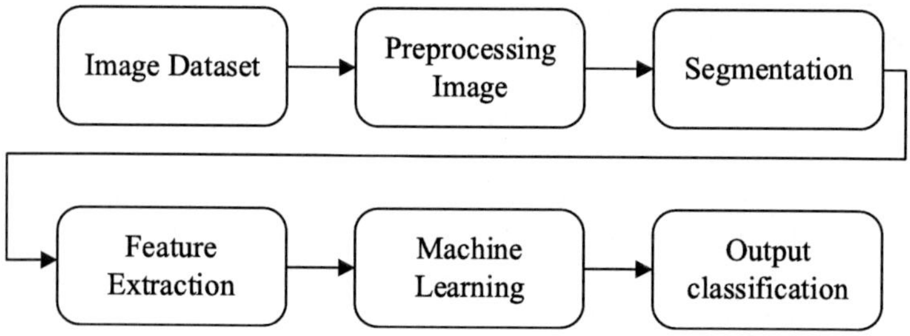


**Fig. 1** Standard image processing using machine learning

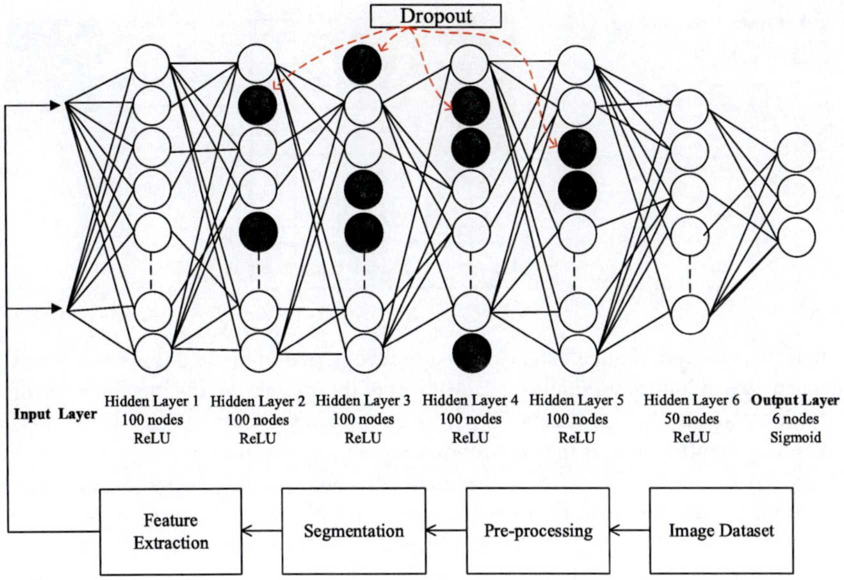


**Fig. 2** Introduction of image pattern using deep learning

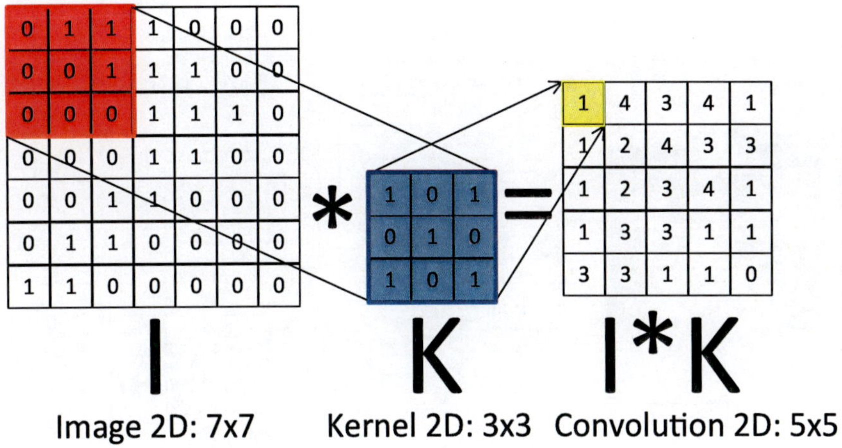


**Fig. 3** Convolution image and kernel

process, but there is no overlap between cells, and there is no multiplication and matrix addition process between the kernel and image.

Deep learning with feature learning using a convolution algorithm, hereinafter referred to as a convolution neural network (CNN). Deep learning using the CNN algorithm has been applied in various kinds of research, especially image and signal

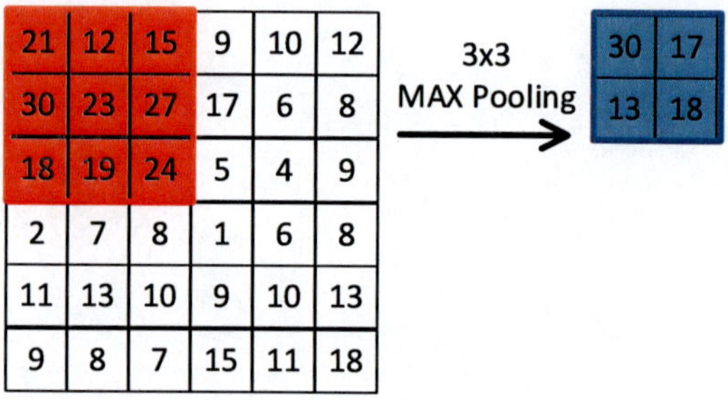


**Fig. 4** Proses max-pooling feature map 6 × 6

pattern recognition. Figure 5 shows an example of a pattern recognition chest X-ray image to detect lung abnormalities. The object of this research is the images from the chest X-ray photo. In Fig. 3, the CNN deep learning model is composed of 10 layers which is a combination of the convolution model and the standard neural network model. At the front of the CNN, the model is composed of 2 convolutions, two max-pooling, and flattened layers which are then followed by five fully connected layers (4 hidden layers and one output layer). In the convolution process, layer 1, a 32 × 32 two-dimensional image, is convoluted with a 4 × 4 kernel to produce a two-dimensional feature map with a feature map size of 28 × 28. In the 2nd layer,

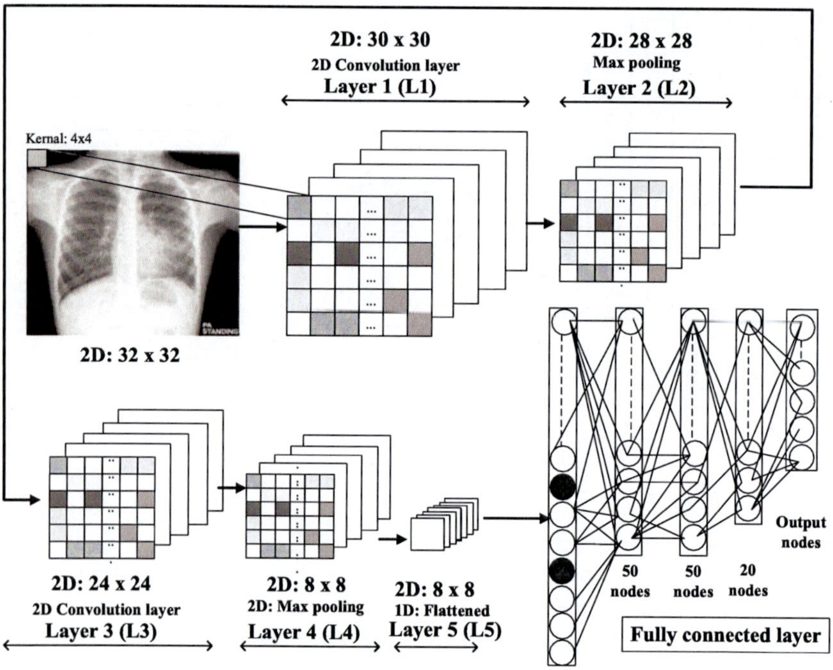


**Fig. 5** Recognition of abnormal image patterns in the lungs using CNN-based deep learning

the result of the 1st layer feature map will go through the max-pooling layer. The max-pooling process will reduce the number of previous feature maps.

The final stage of a feature learning process (Fig. 4) is the flattened layer process, which is the process of changing a 2-dimensional matrix into an N $\times$ 1 one-dimensional matrix, which then forms a hidden layer. In the next stage, the deep learning model with CNN consists of a conventional artificial neural network structure, which consists of several hidden layers and an output layer. The selection of the number of output layer nodes is determined by the number of classes in the developed model. In the next section, we review the studies that have been carried out by previous researchers in applying machine learning in more detail for the purposes of diagnosing COVID 19 based on X-rays.

## 3 Materials and Method

The research materials were taken from various reference sources such as PubMed, IEEE-explore, and ScienceDirect databases. The focus materials taken as material for making this review paper are those related to the diagnosis of COVID-19 based on x-ray images using a deep learning approach. The references we used to compile review papers are articles published from 2020 until now (July 2021). The keywords for searching in the database are deep learning, covid-19, and x-ray images. To perform keyword bibliographic analysis, we used the VosViewer application with clustering results, as shown in Fig. 6.

The analysis results showed that the proposed keywords based on the reference source database were grouped into four major groups, namely COVID-19/Deep learning, tomography, human and male clusters. The results of the VOSviewer (Fig. 5) show that each cluster contains the x-ray keyword. In more detail, the keywords for each cluster are shown in Table 1, which consists of four clusters, namely clusters 1, 2, 3, and 4, each of which is shown in red, blue, green, and yellow.

## 4 Review

In this study, we reviewed 41 articles that focused on deep learning methods to detect Covid-19 using chest X-rays images. The reference for this research is articles from 2020 to 2021, using a deep learning classifier with several algorithms, including CNN, DNN, Transfer Learning, and several other algorithms. Generally, in order to classify the image, the deep learning classifier follows several steps, including pre-processing, segmentation, feature learning, classification, and prediction. The feature learning was done by performing the convolution process between the image and kernel. The convolution process was done in two dimensional.

Table 2 shows the summary of several studies that have studied the classification of the COVID-19 images based on deep learning with the CNN algorithm. In

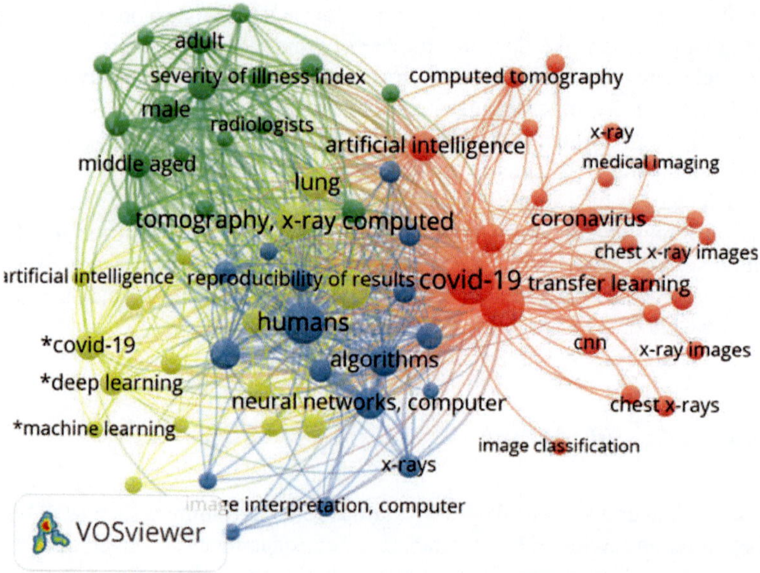


**Fig. 6** Bibliographic analysis of deep learning approach for COVID 19 detection using chest X-ray images

**Table 1** Clustering bibliographic based on deep learning, covid-19, and x-ray image keywords

| Cluster | Keywords | Colors |
|---|---|---|
| 1 | Artificial intelligence, chest CT, chest x-ray, classification CNN, computed tomography, computer-aided diagnosis, coronavirus, covid-19, covid-19 detection, deep learning, feature extraction, image classification, machine learning, medical imaging, pandemic, radiology, segmentation, transfer learning, x-ray, x-ray images | Red |
| 2 | Adolescent, adult, aged, aged 80 and over, area under curve disease prognosis, female, Italy, male, middle aged, prognosis, radiography, radiologist, retrospective studies, severity of illness index, thorax, young adult | Blue |
| 3 | Chest x-ray, algorithm, chine, computer simulation, covid-19 testing, databases, factual, human, image interpretation, image Processing, neural network, pneumonia, radiography, thoracic, reproducibility of result, roc curve sensitivity and specificity, x-rays | Green |
| 4 | Artificial intelligence, covid-19, deep learning, machine learning, transfer learning, datasets as topic, diagnosis, differential early diagnosis, lung, pandemics, pneumonia, viral, the predictive value of tests, radiographic image, sarscov-2, tomography, x-ray | Yellow |

**Table 2** Deep learning using CNN algorithm for classification of abnormalities on image x-ray caused by COVID-19

| Authors | DL algorithm | Results |
|---|---|---|
| [2] Pelaez, Enrique, Loayza, Francis et al. (2020) | CNN | Accuracy: 98.2% |
| [15] Saddam Bekhet et al. (2020) | CNN | Accuracy: 96% |
| [16] Julian D. Arias-Londono et al. (2020) | CNN | Accuracy: 91.5% |
| [17] T. Padma et al. (2020) | CNN | Accuracy: 99% |
| [9] Asma Channa et al. (2020) | CNN | Accuracy: 91.67% |
| [18] Joaquim De Moura et al. (2020) | CNN | Accuracy: 90.27% |
| [19] Rachna Sethi et al. (2020) | CNN | Accuracy: 99% |
| [20] Malaya Kumar et al. (2020) | CNN | Accuracy: 99.68% |
| [7] Areej et al. (2021) | CNN | Accuracy: 91.67% |
| [21] Sohaib Asif et al. (2021) | CNN | Accuracy: >98% |
| [22] Abhishek Panwar et al. (2021) | CNN | Accuracy: 98% |
| [23] Zehra Karhan et al. (2021) | CNN | Accuracy: 99.5% |
| [24] Shivani Sharma et al. (2021) | CNN | Accuracy: 94% |
| [25] Raghav Kandhari et al. (2021) | CNN | Accuracy: 98.9% |
| [26] Emrah Irmak. (2021) | CNN | Accuracy: 99.20% |
| [27] Nayeeb Rashid et al. (2021) | CNN | Accuracy: 96:33% |
| [28] Samira Lafraxo et al. (2021) | CNN | Accuracy<br>Binary Classification: 94%<br>Multi-class classification: 5.77% |
| [1] Mohammed Seghir et al. (2021) | CNN | Precision: 98.9% |
| [29] Ahmed Mabrouk et al. (2021) | CNN-XGB | Normal, pneumonia, and COVID-19 |
| [30] Hanan S. Alghamdi et al. (2021) | CNN | Diagnosis of COVID-19 via CXR images |
| [31] Sabrina Nefoussi et al. (2021) | CNN | Normal, pneumonia, and COVID-19 |
| [4] Mehmet Sevi et al. (2021) | CNN | COVID-19, viral pneumonia, and healthy patients |
| [32] Naveen Paluru et al. (2021) | CNN | Abnormal and normal regions |

summary, the number of classes used in this study range between two and four classes. In the two classes classification, deep learning classified the lung x-ray images in normal condition or infected by COVID-19. Furthermore, in the four classes classification, the authors classified the x-ray image into normal, pneumonia/COVID-19, pneumonia/viral, and pneumonia/bacterial infection. Moreover, the accuracy value of the CNN was obtained in the range of 92–99%, as well as the classification of CT images for normal, pneumonia, and COVID-19 [19, 19, 19]. CNN also performed a segmentation stage in which the classes were categorized as normal/abnormal images of covid-19 [23, 23].

Table 3 describes some of the deep learning methods which used algorithms other than CNN, including DTL (deep transfer learning), TL (transfer learning), DNN (deep neural network), K-EfficientNet, EfficientNet, EDL (ensemble deep learning), Mask RCNN (recurrent CNN), NN (neural network), GAN (generative adversarial network), and CovAI-Net by using CXR (Chest radiograph).

Several algorithms such as DTL [26], CovAI-Net [28], DNN [32], TL [37], Mask RCNN (recurrent CNN) [42] performed a classification from CT images which classified the image into covid-19, normal, pneumonia. Furthermore, the pneumonia locations could be located with accuracy values ranging from 90 to 99%.

## 5 Discussion

We have analyzed the keyword bibliographic using VOSviewer. We found that all of the related keywords were clustered into four clusters. The most dominant keyword was shown in cluster 1, which is indicated with the red color. In this cluster, it was shown that COVID-19 and deep learning intersect each other. Another related keyword that supports this cluster was tomography, medical imaging, x-ray, CNN, and transfer learning. The second cluster which is indicated with blue color, is more concerned with discussing the relationship among humans, neural networks, and algorithms. The third cluster (green color) discussed the relationship between tomography, radiologist, and human. The last cluster (yellow color) is related to lung, COVID-19, x-ray tomography, and deep learning keyword. In this bibliographic analysis, mostly all of the clusters were interconnected with each other, especially for clusters one and four. Based on 44 articles that have been reviewed, it can be concluded that CNN is a deep learning algorithm that performs many classification methods on CT images through a segmentation process [23, 23]. The DTL (deep transfer learning) algorithm has successfully detected COVID-19 using CT images [26]. Some deep learning algorithms such as K-EfficientNet [39], EfficientNet [40], EDL-COVID [41], and Mask RCNN [42] in detecting covid-19 produce up to 97% accuracy. Transfer learning is one of the best deep learning algorithms in performing classification methods because it has a very high accuracy of up to 99.87% [36].

In the present study, the CNN and transfer learning algorithm mostly resulted in high accuracy values. Several studies developed a deep learning classifier with a CNN algorithm to classify a number of classes. Furthermore, the authors preferred to select the CNN algorithm because this deep learning CNN architecture can be customized according to the complexity of the model. Other studies favor using deep learning using transfer learning algorithms. The benefit of using a transfer learning algorithm is that the knowledge from previous learning could be transfer for the next task. Generally, the authors used the CNN architecture from InceptionnetV3, ResNet18, ResNet50, SqueezeNet, and DenseNet-121 as the transfer learning for image classification. Basically, the architecture was developed based on a convolution neural network.

**Table 3** Deep learning based on transfer learning and other algorithms for classification of abnormalities on image x-ray caused by COVID-19

| Author | DL algorithm | Results |
|---|---|---|
| [33] Taki Hasan Rafi et al. (2020) | DTL | Accuracy: 98.43% |
| [34] O. F. Layode et al. (2020) | DTL | Covid-19 and other abnormal pulmonary and cardiothoracic conditions in CXRs |
| [35] Sanhita Basu et al. (2020) | DETL | Accuracy: 90.13% $\pm$ 0.14 |
| [36] Mohit Mishra et al. (2020) | CovAI-Net | Non-Pneumonic and Pneumonic, Covid-19 Positive and Covid-19 Negative |
| [37] Khosro Rezaee et al. (2021) | DTL | level for infectious diseases similar to bacterial and viral pneumonia |
| [38] Mohammad Mahmudur Rahman Khan et al. (2021) | DNN | Accuracy: 96.91% |
| [39] Yifan Peng et al. (2021) | DNN | COVID-19 CXR and COVID-19 CT |
| [40] Fian Yulio Santoso et al. (2021) | DNN | Normal, pneumonia and pneumonia caused by COVID-19 |
| [41] Yash Chaudhar et al. (2021) | DNN | Accuracy: 95% |
| [42] D. Haritha et al. (2020) | TL | Accuracy: 99.49% |
| [43] Stephany Octaviani et al. (2021) | TL | Accuracy: 99.35% |
| [44] Naufal Hilmizen et al. (2021) | TL | Accuracy: 99.87% |
| [45] Nikhil Bhatia et al. (2021) | TL | Healthy, pneumonia, and COVID-19 |
| [46] Amina Baseer et al. (2021) | TL | Accuracy: 97.36% |
| [47] Papa Abdou Karim et al. (2021) | K-EfficientNet | Accuracy: 97.3% |
| [48] Talha Anwar et al. (2021) | EfficientNet | Accuracy: 0.897 |
| [49] Shanjiang Tang et al. (2021) | EDL-COVID | Accuracy: 95% |
| [50] Junfeng Li et al. (2021) | NN | Accuracy: 94.1% |
| [6] Zhaohui Liang et al. (2021) | generative adversarial network (GAN) | Accuracy: 97.8% |

Based on chest X-ray images, abnormalities in the lungs can be detected based on differences in color or contrast in the images. Pneumonia, apart from being caused by COVID-19, can also be caused by another virus known as viral pneumonia. In addition, pneumonia can be caused by bacterial pathogens or referred to as bacterial pneumonia. To improve the accuracy of the deep learning classifier, some researchers only classified images into two classes, namely normal and COVID-19. Furthermore, some researchers distinguish chest X-ray images into four classes, namely, normal, COVID-19 pneumonia, viral pneumonia, and bacterial pneumonia.

## 6 Conclusion

This present study was proposed to review some paper which concern to study the implementation of the deep learning to detect the infection of the COVID-19 to the lung using chest x-ray images. A bibliographic analysis using VOSviewer was applied to obtain the keyword clustering and relationship, among others. From the analysis, it has been shown that the keyword of deep learning, COVID-19 and x-ray image was clustered into four groups. From the data collection, we confirmed that the deep learning based on convolution neural network and transfer learning algorithm resulted in high accuracy among others in the images classification. Deep learning with transfer learning (TL) algorithm was the approach that is often used among others. Generally, authors developed a deep learning approach to classify the images between 2 and 4 classes. Finally, further review paper could be proposed to classify the x-ray image chest, which comes from with and without symptoms.

## References

1. Guellil MS et al (2020) WEB predictor COVIDz: deep learning for COVID-19 disease detection from chest X-rays. In: 2020 international conference on decision aid sciences application DASA 2020, pp 601–606
2. Pelaez E, Loayza F (2020) A deep learning model to screen for Corona Virus Disease (COVID-19) from X-ray chest images, 2020. Ieee Andescon
3. Kirana AP, Bhawiyuga A (2021) Novel Coronavirus pandemic in Indonesia : cases overview and daily data time series using naïve forecast method. Indones J Electron Electromed Eng Med Inform 3(1):1–8
4. Sevi M, Aydin I (2020) COVID-19 detection using deep learning methods. In: 2020 international conference on data analytics for business industry way towards a sustainable economy ICDABI
5. Ben-David S, Shalev-Shwartz S (2014) Understanding machine learning: from theory to algorithms
6. Liang Z, Huang JX, Li J, Chan S (2020) Enhancing automated COVID-19 Chest X-ray diagnosis by image-to-image GAN translation. In: Proceeding of 2020 IEEE international conference on bioinformatics and biomedicine BIBM 2020, pp 1068–1071

7. Musleh AAWA, Maghari AY (2020) COVID-19 Detection in X-ray images using CNN algorithm. In: Proceeding of 2020 international conference on promising electronic technology ICPET, pp 5–9
8. Fangoh AM, Sahar S (2020) Using CNN-XG boost deep networks for COVID-19 detection in chest X-ray images. In: 2020 15th international conference on computer engineering and systems (ICCES)
9. Channa A, Popescu N, Malik R (2020) Robust technique to detect COVID-19 using Chest X-ray images. In: 2020 International conference on e-health and bioengineering (EHB)
10. Serener A, Sertan S (2021) Deep learning to distinguish COVID-19 from other lung infections, pleural diseases, and lung tumors. In: 2020 medical technologies congress (TIPTEKNO)
11. Mishra S (2021) Malaria parasite detection using efficient neural ensembles. J Electron Electromed Eng Med Inform 3(3):119–133
12. Mekha P (2019) Deep learning algorithms for predicting breast cancer based on tumor cells. In: 2019 joint international conference on digital arts, media technology with ECTI Northern section conference on electrical, electronics computer and telecommuncation engineering (ECTI DAMT-NCON), pp 343–346
13. Hussein S, Kandel P, Bolan CW, Wallace MB, Bagci U, Member S (2019) Lung and pancreatic tumor characterization in the deep learning era : novel supervised and unsupervised learning approaches. IEEE Trans Med Imaging 1
14. Ismail NS, Engineering E, Iskandar BS, Sovuthy C, Engineering E, Iskandar BS (2019) Breast cancer detection based on deep learning technique. In: 2019 international UNIMAS STEM 12th engineering conference (EnCon), pp 89–92
15. Bekhet S, Hassaballah M, Kenk MA, Hameed MA (2020) An artificial intelligence based technique for COVID-19 diagnosis from chest X-ray, 2nd Nov. Intell Lead Emerg Sci Conf NILES 2020:191–195
16. Arias-Londono JD, Gomez-Garcia JA, Moro-Velazquez L, Godino-Llorente JI (2020) Artificial intelligence applied to chest X-ray images for the automatic detection of COVID-19. A thoughtful evaluation approach. IEEE Access 8:226811–226827
17. Padma T, Kumari CU (2020) Deep learning based chest x-ray image as a diagnostic tool for covid-19. In: Proceedings of the international conference on smart electronics and communication (ICOSEC 2020) 2020(Icosec), pp 1–4
18. Moura JDE et al (2020) Deep convolutional approaches for the analysis of covid-19 using chest x-ray images from portable devices. IEEE Acces 8
19. Sethi R, Mehrotra M (2020) Deep learning based diagnosis recommendation for covid-19 using chest x-rays images. In: Proceedings of the second international conference on inventive research in computing applications (ICIRCA-2020), pp 3–6
20. Nath MK, Kanhe A, Mishra M (2020) A novel deep learning approach for classification of COVID-19 images. In: 2020 IEEE 5th international conference on computing communication and automation ICCCA 2020, pp 752–757
21. Asif S, Wenhui Y, Jin H, Jinhai S (2020) Classification of covid-19 from chest x-ray images using deep convolutional neural network. In: 2020 IEEE 6th international conference computer and communications ICCC 2020 (March 2020), pp 426–433
22. Panwar A, Dagar A, Pal V, Kumar V (2021) COVID 19, pneumonia and other disease classification using chest x-ray images. In: 2021 2nd international conference for emerging technology (INCET), pp 1–4
23. Karhan Z, Akal F, (2020) Covid-19 classification using deep learning in chest x-ray images. TIPTEKNO 2020—Tip Teknol Kongresi—2020 Med Technol Congr TIPTEKNO 2020, pp 3–6
24. Sharma S, Tiwari S (2021) COVID-19 diagnosis using x-ray images and deep learning. In: Proceeding of international conference artificial intelligence and smart system ICAIS 2021, pp 344–349
25. Kandhari R, Negi M, Bhatnagar P, Mangipudi P (2021) Use of deep learning models to detect covid-19 from chest x-rays. In: 2021 international conference on computer communication and informatics (ICCCI -2021), 2021

26. E. Irmak (2021) A novel deep convolutional neural network model for COVID-19 disease detection, 2021, June 2020, pp 94–97
27. Rashid N, Faisal Hossain MA, Ali M, Sukanya MI, Mahmud T, Fattah SA (2020) Transfer learning based method for COVID-19 detection from chest X-ray images. In: IEEE Proceedings of the Regional 10 Annual International Conference on TENCON, November 2020, pp 585–590
28. Lafraxo S, El Ansari M (2020) CoviNet: automated COVID-19 detection from X-rays using deep learning techniques. Colloq Inf Sci Technol Cist 489–494
29. Fangoh AM, Selim S (2020) Using CNN-XGBoost deep networks for COVID-19 detection in chest X-ray images. In: Proceedings of the 15th international conference of the computing engineering system on ICCES 2020
30. Alghamdi HS, Amoudi G, Elhag S, Saeedi K, Nasser J (2021) Deep learning approaches for detecting COVID-19 from chest X-ray images : a survey. IEEE Eng Med Biol Soc Sect 9
31. Nefoussi S, Amamra J, Amarouche IA (2021) A comparative study of deep learning networks for COVID-19 recognition in chest X-ray images. In: 2020 2nd international workshop on human-centric smart environments for health and well-being (IHSH), 2021, pp 237–241
32. Paluru N et al (2021) Anam-Net : anamorphic depth embedding-based lightweight CNN for segmentation of anomalies in COVID-19 chest CT images. IEEE Trans Neural Networks Learn Syst 32(3):932–946
33. Rafi TH (2020) An ensemble deep transfer-learning approach to identify COVID-19 cases from chest X-ray images. In: 2020 IEEE conference on computational intelligence in bioinformatics and computational biology (CIBCB)
34. Layode OF, Rahman M (2020) A chest X-ray image retrieval system for COVID-19 detection using deep transfer learning and denoising auto encoder. In: 2020 international conference on computational science and computational intelligence (CSCI) 2020, 2021, pp 1635–1640
35. Basu S, Mitra S, Saha N (2020) Deep learning for screening COVID-19 using chest X-ray images. SIEEE Symp Ser Comput Intell SSCI 2020:2521–2527
36. Mishra M, Parashar V, Shimpi R (2020) Development and evaluation of an AI system for early detection of Covid-19 pneumonia using X-ray (Student Consortium). In: Proceedings of the IEEE 6th international conference on multimedia big data, BigMM 2020, pp 292–296
37. Rezaee K, Badiei A, Meshgini S (2020) A hybrid deep transfer learning based approach for COVID-19 classification in chest X-ray images. In: 2020 27th international and 5th international iranian conference on biomedical engineering (ICBME 2020), 2021, November 2020, pp 234–241
38. Khan MMR et al (2020) Automatic detection of COVID-19 disease in chest X-ray Images using deep neural networks. In: IEEE regional 10 humanitarian technology conference on R10-HTC, December 2020, pp 7–12
39. Peng Y, Tang Y, Lee S, Zhu Y, Summers RM, Lu Z (2021) COVID-19-CT-CXR: a freely accessible and weakly labeled chest X-ray and CT image collection on COVID-19 from biomedical literature. IEEE Trans Big Data 7(1):3–12
40. Santoso FY, Purnomo HD (2020) A modified deep convolutional network for COVID-19 detection based on chest X-ray images. In: 2020 3rd international seminar research information technology intelligence systems, ISRITI 2020, pp 700–704
41. Chaudary Y (2021) Efficient-CovidNet : deep learning based COVID-19 detection from chest X-ray images. Yash. Multimed Tools Appl
42. Haritha D, Pranathi MK, Covid prediction from X-ray images. In: 2020 5th international conference on computing, communication and security (ICCCS)
43. Ngesthi SO, Setyawan I (2021) Optimized deep transfer learning for Covid-19 screening using chest X-ray image. In: 2020 3rd international conference on information and communications technology (ICOIACT), pp 342–347
44. Hilmizen N, Bustamam A, Sarwinda D (2020) The multimodal deep learning for diagnosing COVID-19 pneumonia from chest CT-scan and X-ray images. In: 2020 3rd international seminar on research of information technology and intelligent systems (ISRITI), 2020, pp 26–31

45. Bhatia N, Bhola G (2021) Transfer learning for detection of COVID-19 infection using chest X-ray images. In: Proceedings of the 5th international conference on computing methodology communication on ICCMC 2021, Iccmc, pp 1602–1609
46. Baseer A, Bhatti N (2020) Deep networks based classification of COVID-19 chest X-ray images. In: 2020 Proceedings of the 14th international conference open source system technology ICOSST 2020
47. Diallo PAKK, Ju Y (2020) Accurate detection of COVID-19 using K-EfficientNet deep learning image classifier and K-COVID chest X-ray images dataset. In: 2020 IEEE 6th international conference on computing communication ICCC 2020, pp 1527–1531
48. Anwar T, Zakir S (2020) Deep learning based diagnosis of COVID-19 using chest CT-scan images. In: 2020 IEEE 23rd international multitopic conference (INMIC)
49. Tang S et al (2021) EDL-COVID: ensemble deep learning for COVID-19 case detection from chest X-ray images. IEEE Trans Ind Inform 17(9):6539–6549
50. Li J, Zhang D, Liu Q, Bu R, Wei Q (2020) COVID-GATNet: a deep learning framework for screening of COVID-19 from chest X-ray images. In: 2020 IEEE 6th international conference on computing communication ICCC 2020, pp 1897–1902

# Parkinson's Disease Detection Based on Gait Analysis of Vertical Ground Reaction Force Using Signal Processing with Machine Learning

**Yunendah Nur Fuadah, Fauzi Frahma Taliningsih, Inung Wijayanto, Nor Kumalasari Caecar Pratiwi, and Syamsul Rizal**

**Abstract** Parkinson's Disease (PD) is a type of brain disorder caused by dopaminergic neuron loss. People with Parkinson's disease have symptoms such as tremors and stiffness which caused the affected people difficulty to control their movement. The diagnosis of PD is usually based on measures neurologist analyses of medical history, review of the symptoms, neurological and physical examination. Therefore, it requires along procedure to identify Parkinson's disease and considerable risk of misdiagnosis. This study proposes automatic detection of Parkinson's disease formed on gait analysis of Vertical Ground Reaction Force (VGRF) signals. The raw data of VGRF signals obtained from the Physionet database is filtered using a Butterworth high-pass filter with a cut-off frequency of 0.8 Hz. Afterward, the features were used based on the maximum amplitude value, the minimum amplitude value, and the maximum power value of VGRF signals after filtering. K-Nearest Neighbor was performed as a classifier to classify PD and healthy subjects. The total data used are 165 data that consists of 93 PD and 72 healthy subjects. The proposed model was evaluated using 42 test datasets and obtained a 77% AUC score by using the most optimal parameter of K-NN with K = 7 and Chebyshev as a distance matrix. The performance of accuracy and AUC score obtained in classification was acceptable even though only used 3 features as input for the KNN classifier model. In addition, the proposed method simplifies the previous algorithm in detecting Parkinson's disease. Early detection of Parkinson's disease is very important; hence it can provide the proper treatments that can delay the disease progression.

**Keywords** Parkinson detection · K-Nearest neighbor · Machine learning · And Signal processing

Y. N. Fuadah (✉) · F. F. Taliningsih · I. Wijayanto · N. K. C. Pratiwi · S. Rizal
School of Electrical Engineering, Telkom University, Bandung, Indonesia
e-mail: yunendah@telkomuniversity.ac.id


T. Triwiyanto et al. (eds.), *Proceedings of the 2nd International Conference on Electronics, Biomedical Engineering, and Health Informatics*, Lecture Notes in Electrical Engineering 898, https://doi.org/10.1007/978-981-19-1804-9_20

# 1 Introduction

Parkinson's disease (PD) is a neurodegenerative disorder that primarily modify dopamine-producing (dopaminergic) neurons in the substantia nigra area of the brain [1]. According to the Parkinson's Foundation, more than 10 million people worldwide suffer from Parkinson's disease [2]. This disease affects more men than women which has different disease progression in each person. The disease may not be noticeable at first, but over time this disease will gradually be visible. Although the cause of Parkinson's disease is unknown, it is possible to reduce symptoms in the early stages [3]. In the early stages of PD people may have tremors, stiffness, and difficulties walking and coordinating. Moreover, people with PD may also have mental and behavioral changes, depressions, and fatigue.

Diagnosis of PD is often based on measures neurologist analysis of medical history, review of the signs and symptoms, and neurological and physical examination. Therefore, it takes a long time to diagnose PD and has high possibility of misdiagnosing PD. The misdiagnosis rate of Parkinson's disease is roughly 25%, with 40% of PD cases has being misdiagnosed for other neurological illnesses [4]. Early detection and accurate diagnosis of PD is very critical due to early detection of PD possible can provide better medicament and control the outcome of the symptoms. Several studies on detecting PD have been carried out by several researchers. Shyam et al. [4] used a wearable sensor and the Linear Discriminant Analysis (LDA) classifier for the extracted gait parameters. The average accuracy of classifying between PD patients and healthy control subjects is 86.9%. Gusty et al. have examined PD diagnosis through a gait analysis by combining the wavelet packet coefficients of the Vertical Ground Reaction Force (VGRF) and classified by Support Vector Machine (SVM) [5]. The results showed an accuracy of 83.45% with 141.22 s. Enas Abdulhay et al. proposed a method to diagnose PD using the gait analysis [6]. The Chebyshev II high pass filter is used to reduce sounds due to the subject's body orientation and other environmental changes during the measurement. They reported an average accuracy of 92.7%. Lazzaro di Biase et al. have researched an overview of the most accurate markers for diagnosis and symptoms monitoring for PD gait analysis [7]. This research only reported studies at least have 80% sensitivity and specificity. Zuo et al. and Mittra et al. used K-NN as classification method [3, 8]. Their study reported accuracy performance 97.47% and 93.08% respectively in classifying PD and healthy condition. A. Bourouhou et al. presented a comparison of classification methods for Parkin-son's disease identification. They used three types of classifiers, which are K-Nearest Neighbor (K-NN), Naive Bayes (NB), and Support Vector Machine (SVM). The classifier (SVM, KNN, and NB) achieved an accuracy of 80%, 70%, and 65% respectively [9]. Apart from the aforementioned studies, there are several studies that also developed a system to categorize Parkinson's disease and healthy subjects based on machine learning [10–18] and deep learning models [19–23].

Among of various studies that classify PD and healthy subjects, K-Nearest Neighbor classifier model showed the highest accuracy performance. However, the algorithm proposed in the previous studies required 22 features [3] and 133 features [8] as input of K-NN classifier model that required complex calculation in classification process. Therefore, this study narrowed this gap by reducing the number of features to 3 as the input of KNN. This study proposed the simple automated detection of PD based on gait analysis of VGRF using signal processing and K-Nearest Neighbor (K-NN) as classifier method. The VGRF signals of PD and healthy subjects will be analyzed in time domain, frequency domain and power spectral density to extract features (the maximum amplitude value, the minimum amplitude value, and the maximum power value of VGRF signals). The extensive simulation conducted to select the best parameter of K-NN that achieved the best system performance. Furthermore, the proposed model will be evaluated using test datasets to obtain the value of precision, recall, F1-score, accuracy, and AUC score.

## 2 Material and Methods

### *2.1 Vertical Ground Reaction Force (VGRF)*

This study used VGRF datasets which can be accessed in Physionet [24]. The data contain of 279 gait recordings from 93 subjects of Parkinson's Disease (PD) and 73 subjects of healthy controls. The subjects normally walked while recording the vertical ground reaction force (VGRF). The position of force sensors to generate VGRF signals are shown in Fig. 1. Eight sensors were placed in each the subject's feet, so each datum of VGRF signals contains of 16 VGRF time series. During the recording, subjects were under minimum tremor induction medication and 60 s of data were collected based on the length of each subject's tremor at a frequency of 100 Hz [6].

Everyone has a unique gait pattern. However, there are strict differences between the gait patterns of normal people and PD patients. The VGRF signal in the time

**Fig. 1** The position of force sensors [6]

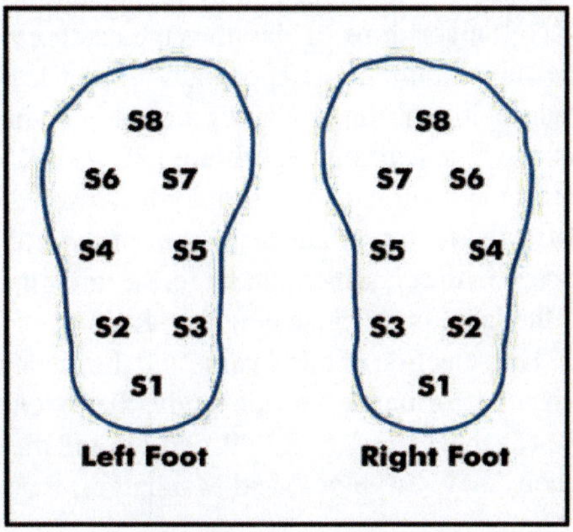

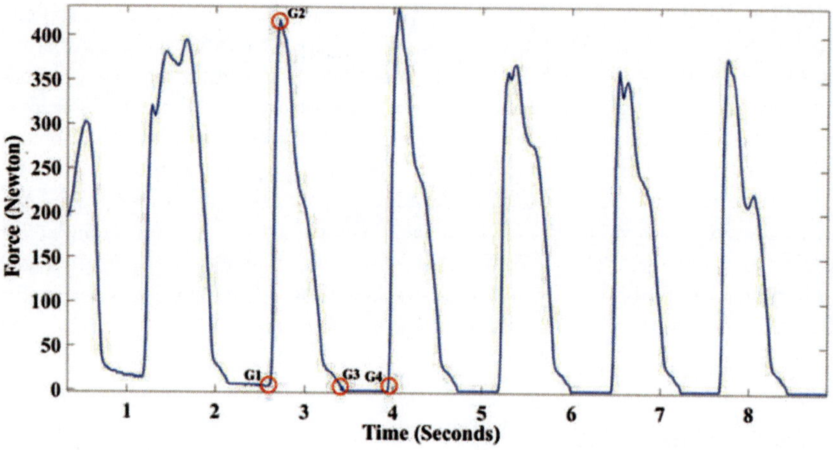


**Fig. 2** The VGRF signal in time domain

domain, as shown in Fig. 2, executes the force exerted by the foot in units of Newtons. The force generated by each person during normal walking is an important parameter that determines the gait pattern of any person. According to Fig. 2, the period from point G1 to point G4 is called the gait cycle. The duration of the gait cycle is defined as the number of steps. The time from point G1 to point G3 is called standing time or the time when the foot is in contact with the ground while walking. Finally, the period from point G3 to point G4 is defined as the swing period or time difference between the first and last point in the period [7].

## *2.2 K-Nearest Neighbor*

The one of uncomplicated machine learning algorithms is the K-Nearest Neighbor (KNN) algorithms. It classifies the category of a new instance based on determining the most common category among the k nearest neighbors. Due to its simplicity and flexibility, the K-NN algorithm is commonly used to solve many issues, based on machine learning algorithms [25–28]. KNN algorithm projected the training data into a multi-dimensional space which each dimension representing the training data's extracted features. The algorithm of the training process stores features vectors and labels. In the classification stage, the untagged test data is directly classified according to the label of its close neighbor K.

The selection of the K value and the distance metric is necessary to achieve the best KNN performance. In this study, the extensive simulation conducted to determine the K value (K = 1, 3, 5, 7, 9, and 11) and the distance metric (Euclidean, Minkowski, Chebyshev, Cityblock, and Manhattan) that achieved the best performance.

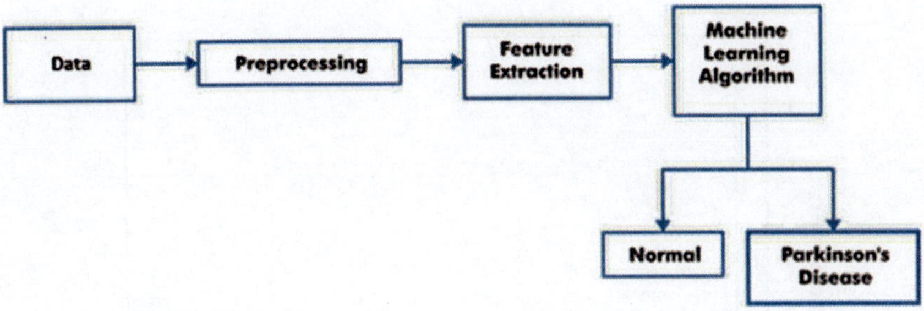


**Fig. 3** The proposed system design

### 2.3 System Design

Figure 3 shows the diagram block of the system proposed in this study. Raw data of VGRF with a total data amount of 165 data consisting of 93 subjects with Parkinson's disease and 72 data subjects in healthy condition. The VGRF recording is generated from 8 force sensors mounted on the sole of the left foot and 8 sensors mounted on the sole of the right foot. Due to the change of the body direction during the measurement process, the vertical ground reaction force values obtained using force sensors include low frequency components. The effect of time domain gait analysis can be affected by these variables. Therefore, in the preprocessing stage, a Butterworth high-pass filter with a cut-off frequency of 0.8 Hz is used to remove it.

In the feature extraction stage, the transformation from time domain to frequency domain is carried out using Fast Fourier Transform. The features used in this study consist of the maximum amplitude, minimum amplitude, and maximum power values of the VGRF after filtering stage. The results from the feature extraction stage are called features vector that will be trained using K-Nearest Neighbor to be classified into normal conditions and Parkinson's disease conditions.

## 3 Results

As shown in Figs. 4 and 5, the fast Fourier transform result of the VGRF signal after filtering, the frequency range of the signal gives a detailed description of the signal distribution. In healthy subjects, the signal amplitude in this frequency range is higher than that of Parkinson's disease subjects. In extracting some important features, this representation is crucial because the frequency domain characteristics provide a simpler approach to diagnose the disease.

As shown in Figs. 6 and 7, the power spectral density plots the amplitude of the signal power along the frequency axis. The amplitude of the power distributed over the frequency indicates the presence of Parkinson's disease. According to Fig. 6, in the initial stage of PD, the force is near the origin, while moving toward the negative

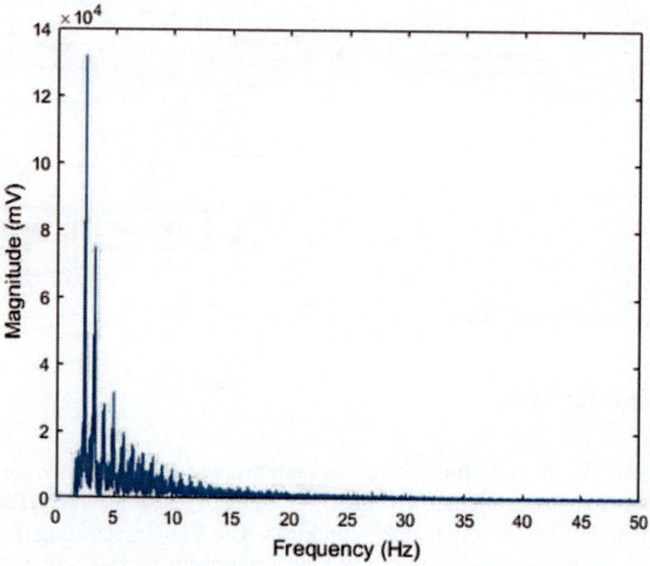


**Fig. 4** FFT of VGRF signal (healthy)

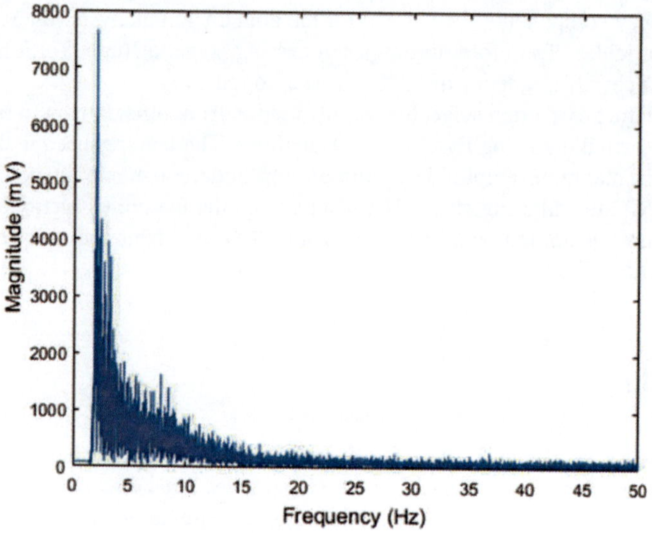


**Fig. 5** FFT of VGRF signal (Parkinson's disease)

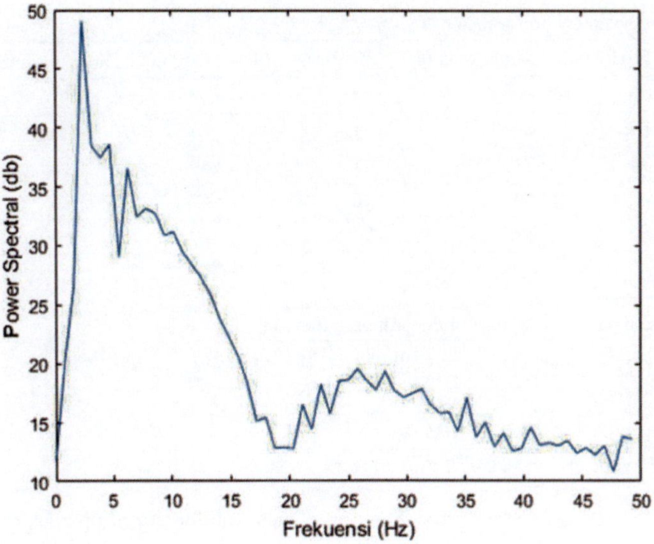


**Fig. 6** Power spectral density (healthy)

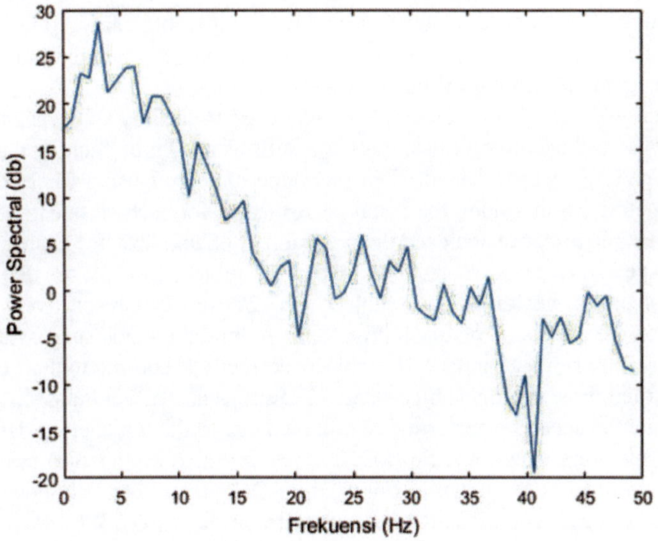


**Fig. 7** Power spectral density (Parkinson's disease)

**Table 1** The accuracy performance of K-NN

| K-value | Euclidean | Minkowski (%) | Chebyshev (%) | Cityblock (%) | Manhattan (%) |
|---|---|---|---|---|---|
| k = 1 | 60 | 60 | 74 | 55 | 55 |
| k = 3 | 67 | 67 | 71 | 64 | 64 |
| k = 5 | 74 | 74 | 71 | 69 | 69 |
| k = 7 | 69 | 69 | 76 | 67 | 67 |
| k = 9 | 62 | 62 | 74 | 60 | 60 |

**Table 2** The detail performance of the proposed method

| Condition | Precision (%) | Recall (%) | F1-score (%) | Acc (%) | Auc (%) |
|---|---|---|---|---|---|
| Healthy | 65 | 81 | 72 | 76 | 77 |
| PD | 86 | 73 | 79 | | |

force axis to increase the severity. The power spectral density of the vertical ground reaction force signal is one of the important parameters for analyzing the tester's gait pattern to assist in the diagnosis of Parkinson's disease. Based on the representations signal in the time domain, frequency domain and power spectral for healthy and PD conditions, this research used some important features that can represent healthy and PD conditions such as the maximum value of amplitude, the minimum value of amplitude, and the maximum value of power.

The total number 42 test datasets that consist of 16 healthy subjects and 26 PD subjects was used according to simulation results as shown in Table 1, the highest test accuracy 76% was obtained when the value of K = 7 using Chebyshev as a distance metric. Furthermore, the detail performance for each class can be seen in Table 2. The performance achieved the precision of 65 and 86% for healthy and PD subject respectively, recall score 81% for healthy subject and 73% for PD subject. While F1-score for healthy and PD subject was 72% and 79% respectively.

Based on the confusion matrix in Fig. 8, the proposed method successfully classified 13 healthy subjects and 19 PD subjects correctly according to their class and miss-classified three healthy subjects and 7 PD subjects. To avoid underestimate or overestimate the accuracy performance obtained due to the imbalanced dataset, the Receiver Operating Characteristic (ROC) curve was also provided to evaluate the system performance. As shown in Fig. 9, the ROC curve plots True Positive Rate (TPR) on the y-axis against False Positive Rate on the x-axis. While Area Under Curve (AUC) represents the capability of the system to distinguish between classes. The AUC score obtained in this study was 77% which means the proposed method is still affected by false detection in classifying PD and Healthy subjects.

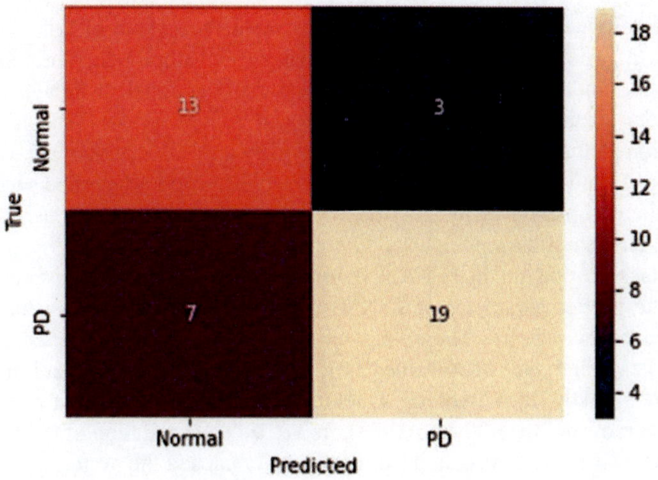


**Fig. 8** Confusion matrix of the test datasets

**Fig. 9** Receiver operating characteristic (ROC)

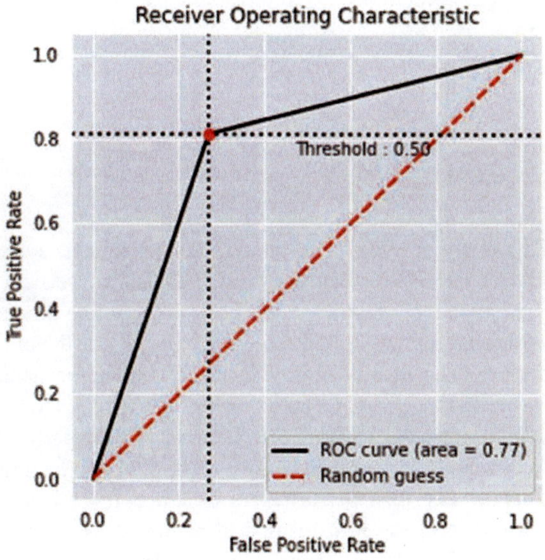


# 4 Discussion

Similar research has been shown that K-Nearest Neighbor has an excellent performance in detecting PD conditions, providing mean accuracy of 97.47% using 22 features [3] and accuracy of 93.8% using 133 features as input of K-NN [8]. The large number of features used will affect the complexity at the classification stage using

K-NN. Therefore, we reduced the number of features as input of K-NN classifier method. In this study, we used three features (maximum amplitude, minimum amplitude, and maximum power values of VGRF signals) as input of K-NN. However, based on the accuracy performance of 76% and AUC score of 77%, K-NN as a classification method provided acceptable accuracy and AUC performance results in classifying PD and healthy conditions. Moreover, the proposed method successfully reducing the complexity of the classification stage by using only three features as input of K-NN classifier model.

As a classification method, KNN required the proper features as input of K-NN and the proper parameter of K-NN such as the number of K-value and the distance equation selected. Therefore, we also conducted extensive simulation to select the best parameter of K value (1, 3, 5, 7, 9) and the best equation distance (Euqlidean, Minkowski, Cityblock, Chebyshev and Manhattan) that obtained the highest accuracy and the highest AUC score value. The limitation of the number of features and the number of data used in this study caused the system performance still to be affected by false detection as shown in Fig. 8. Therefore, this condition caused the performance accuracy and AUC score value did not reach the maximum value. However, compared with manual detection of Parkinson's disease that required complex procedures, the automatic detection based on a machine learning algorithm can be used as an assisting tool for medical experts to diagnose Parkinson's disease most simply.

## 5 Conclusion

This study develops a computer-aided diagnosis system for automatic Parkinson's disease detection formed on gait analysis of vertical ground reaction force using K-Nearest Neighbor as classifier algorithm. The proposed method can be used as an additional method in the screening process for the clinical diagnosis of Parkinson's disease. The results show that the classification accuracy had directly influenced by the K-values and distance metric used in K-NN. The convenient combination of parameters used will provide optimal system performance. The proposed method had evaluated using test datasets, containing 16 healthy subjects and 26 Parkinson's disease. The best performance obtained is 76% accuracy and 77% AUC score. Furthermore, the best result had achieved using $K = 7$ for the K-NN parameter with the Chebyshev distance metric. The proposed method used three features as input, i.e., maximum amplitude, minimum amplitude, and maximum power values. The proposed method can reduce the complexity of the classification process by using only three features. The results obtained have acceptable performance for the detection of PD, although not optimal. Finding the proper features extraction method and increasing the number of data to improve the system performance can be used for further development.

## References

1. Corona F, Pau M, Guicciardi M, Murgia M, Pili R, Casula C (2016) Quantitative assessment of gait in elderly people affected by Parkinson's Disease. In: 2016 IEEE international symposium on medical measurements and applications (MeMeA) [Internet]. IEEE, 2016. pp 1–6. Available from: http://ieeexplore.ieee.org/document/7533772/
2. Dewanjee AN, Hossain QD, Muhury A (2019) Quantitative deviation of spatial parameters of Gait in Parkinson's Disease. In: 2019 international conference on wireless communications signal processing and networking (WiSPNET) [Internet]. IEEE, 2019. pp 304–309. Available from: https://ieeexplore.ieee.org/document/9032870/
3. Zuo WL, Wang ZY, Liu T, Chen HL (2013) Effective detection of Parkinson's disease using an adaptive fuzzy k-nearest neighbor approach. Biomed Signal Process Control 8(4):364–373. Available from: https://linkinghub.elsevier.com/retrieve/pii/S1746809413000359
4. Perumal S V., Sankar R. Gait and tremor assessment for patients with Parkinson's disease using wearable sensors. ICT Express 2(4):168–174. Available from: https://doi.org/10.1016/j.icte.2016.10.005
5. Arrazaq GA, Safitri I (2018) VGRF wavelet packet decomposition for Parkinson ' s Disease. Detection 13(5):2648–2653
6. Abdulhay E, Arunkumar N, Narasimhan K, Vellaiappan E, Venkatraman V (2018) Gait and tremor investigation using machine learning techniques for the diagnosis of Parkinson disease. Futur Gener Comput Syst 83:366–373. Available from: https://linkinghub.elsevier.com/retrieve/pii/S0167739X1731631X
7. di Biase L, Di Santo A, Caminiti ML, De Liso A, Shah SA, Ricci L et al (2020) Gait analysis in Parkinson's disease: an overview of the most accurate markers for diagnosis and symptoms monitoring. Sensors 20(12):3529. Available from: https://www.mdpi.com/1424-8220/20/12/3529
8. Mittra Y, Rustagi V (2018) Classification of subjects with Parkinson's disease using Gait data analysis. In: 2018 international conference on automation and computational engineering (ICACE). IEEE, pp 84–89. Available from: https://ieeexplore.ieee.org/document/8687022/
9. Bourouhou A, Jilbab A, Nacir C, Hammouch A (2016) Comparison of classification methods to detect the Parkinson disease. In: 2016 international conference on electrical and information technologies (ICEIT). IEEE, pp 421–424. Available from: http://ieeexplore.ieee.org/document/7519634/
10. Chen X, Yao X, Tang C, Sun Y, Wang X, Wu X (2018) Detecting Parkinson's disease using Gait analysis with particle swarm optimization. In: 2018. pp 263–75. Available from https://doi.org/10.1007/978-3-319-92037-5_20
11. Alharthi AS, Casson AJ, Ozanyan KB (2021) Gait spatiotemporal signal analysis for Parkinson's disease detection and severity rating. IEEE Sens J 21(2):1838–1848
12. Javed Mehedi Shamrat FM, Asaduzzaman M, Rahman AKMS, Tusher RTH, Tasnim Z (2019) A comparative analysis of parkinson disease prediction using machine learning approaches. Int J Sci Technol Res 8(11):2576–2580
13. Manap HH, Md Tahir N, Yassin AIM (2011) Statistical analysis of Parkinson disease gait classification using artificial neural network. IEEE Int Symp Signal Process Inf Technol ISSPIT 2011:060–065
14. Andrei AG, Tautan AM, Ionescu B (2019) Parkinson's disease detection from Gait patterns. In: 2019 E-health and bioengineering conference (EHB). IEEE, pp 1–4. Available from https://ieeexplore.ieee.org/document/8969942/
15. Asmae O, Abdelhadi R, Bouchaib C, Sara S, Tajeddine K (2020) Parkinson's Disease identification using KNN and ANN algorithms based on voice disorder. In: 2020 1st international conference on innovative research in applied science, engineering and technology (IRASET). IEEE, pp 1–6. Available from: https://ieeexplore.ieee.org/document/9092228/

16. Shirvan RA, Tahami E (2011) Voice analysis for detecting Parkinson's disease using genetic algorithm and KNN classification method. In: 2011 18th Iranian conference of biomedical engineering (ICBME). IEEE, pp 278–283. Available from: http://ieeexplore.ieee.org/document/6168572/
17. Wibawa MS, Nugroho HA, Setiawan NA (2015) Performance evaluation of combined feature selection and classification methods in diagnosing Parkinson disease based on voice feature. In: 2015 international conference on science in information technology (ICSITech) [Internet]. IEEE, pp 126–31. Available from: http://ieeexplore.ieee.org/document/7407790/
18. Solana-Lavalle G, Galán-Hernández J-C, Rosas-Romero R (2020) Automatic Parkinson disease detection at early stages as a pre-diagnosis tool by using classifiers and a small set of vocal features. Biocybern Biomed Eng 40(1):505–516. Available from: https://linkinghub.elsevier.com/retrieve/pii/S0208521620300085
19. Shivangi, Johri A, Tripathi A (2019) Parkinson disease detection using deep neural networks. In: 2019 12th international conference on contemporary computing (IC3). IEEE, pp 1–4. Available from: https://ieeexplore.ieee.org/document/8844941/
20. El Maachi I, Bilodeau GA, Bouachir W (2020) Deep 1D-Convnet for accurate Parkinson disease detection and severity prediction from gait. Expert Syst Appl 143:1–27
21. Awatramani V, Gupta D (2021) Parkinson's disease detection through visual deep learning. In: 2021. pp 963–972. Available from: https://doi.org/10.1007/978-981-15-5148-2_83
22. Sivaranjini S, Sujatha CM (2020) Deep learning based diagnosis of Parkinson's disease using convolutional neural network. Multimed Tools Appl 79(21–22):15467–79. Available from: https://doi.org/10.1007/s11042-019-7469-8
23. Kaur S, Aggarwal H, Rani R (2021) Diagnosis of Parkinson's disease using deep CNN with transfer learning and data augmentation. Multimed Tools Appl 80(7):10113–39. Available from: https://doi.org/10.1007/s11042-020-10114-1
24. Goldberger AL, Amaral LAN, Glass L, Hausdorff JM, Ivanov PC, Mark RG et al (2000) PhysioBank, PhysioToolkit, and PhysioNet. Circulation 101(23). Available from: https://doi.org/10.1161/01.CIR.101.23.e215
25. Caecar Pratiwi NK, Magdalena R, Fuadah YN, Saidah S (2019) K-Nearest neighbor for colon cancer identification. J Phys Conf Ser 1367:012023. Available from: https://doi.org/10.1088/1742-6596/1367/1/012023
26. Fuadah YN, Sa'idah S, Wijayanto I, Patmasari R, Magdalena R (2020) Non invasive anemia detection in pregnant women based on digital image processing and K-nearest neighbor. In: 2020 3rd international conference on biomedical engineering (IBIOMED) [Internet]. IEEE, 60–64. Available from: https://ieeexplore.ieee.org/document/9487605/
27. Ekaputri C, Fu'adah YN, Pratiwi NKC, Rizal A, Sularso AN (2021) Drowsiness detection based on EEG signal using discrete wavelet transform (DWT) and K-Nearest neighbors (K-NN) methods. In 2021, pp 487–498. Available from: https://doi.org/10.1007/978-981-33-6926-9_42
28. Fuadah YN, Setiawan AW, Mengko TLR (2015) Performing high accuracy of the system for cataract detection using statistical texture analysis and K-Nearest neighbor. In: 2015 international seminar on intelligent technology and its applications (ISITIA) [Internet]. IEEE, pp 85–88. Available from: http://ieeexplore.ieee.org/document/7219958/

# Performance Analysis of an Automated Epilepsy Seizure Detection Using EEG Signals Based on 1D-CNN Approach

**Nor Kumalasari Caecar Pratiwi, Inung Wijayanto, and Yunendah Nur Fu'adah**

**Abstract** Epilepsy affects approximately 50 million people worldwide, is a neurological disorder associated with abnormal brain activity that result in seizures, unusual behavior, and every once in a while loss of consciousness. Seizures appear unexpectedly, posing a risk of injury and even death, particularly when they operate heavy machinery or drive a vehicle. As a result, developing a system that can predict the emergence of epileptic seizures is essential. Research on the identification of epileptic seizures using CNN can also be done by first translating EEG signals into 2D/3D images. To alleviate this challenge, we introduce a methodology that uses a 1D-CNN architecture to diagnose epileptic seizures based on raw EEG data. The 1D-CNN model consists of five convolutional layers followed by flatten and dense layers. The proposed method is tested using three scenarios, the first scenario is normal versus pre-ictal, the second is normal versus ictal, and the third is classifying EEG signal into three classes (normal vs. pre-ictal vs. ictal). The proposed 1D-CNN model delivers a great performance by providing precision, recall, and f1-score up to 0.99. The accuracy ranged between 94.9 and 96.30% for seizure detection scenario, 97.92–99.58% for seizure prediction scenario and 89.79–97.01% for three classes problem classification. This result indicates that the proposed method can be utilized as input to relevant stakeholders for additional clinical studies, and it may be employed in the medical field in the future.

**Keywords** Epilepsy seizure detection · EEG signal · 1D-CNN

## 1 First Section

Epilepsy affects approximately 50 million people worldwide. It also known as a neurological disorder associated with abnormal brain activity that result in seizures, unusual behavior, impulses, and every once in a while loss of consciousness [1]. With a prevalence of 0.75%, Indonesia has more than two million people with epilepsy,

N. K. C. Pratiwi (✉) · I. Wijayanto · Y. N. Fu'adah
School of Electrical Engineering, Telkom University, Bandung, Indonesia
e-mail: caecarnkcp@telkomuniversity.ac.id

 
T. Triwiyanto et al. (eds.), *Proceedings of the 2nd International Conference on Electronics, Biomedical Engineering, and Health Informatics*, Lecture Notes in Electrical Engineering 898, https://doi.org/10.1007/978-981-19-1804-9_21

360,000 of whom are refractory, and half of them are candidates for epilepsy surgery (ES). The ES rate continues to increase each year [2]. Epilepsy prevalence and occurrence studies are becoming more frequent, particularly in low- and middle-income countries (LMIC) [3]. Study in the context of developing a system that capable of detecting seizures based on EEG brain activity signals observation has been rampant in recent years.

Traditional machine learning algorithms, such as SVM, KNN, LDA, PLS, and random forest have been used in previous studies involving the development of wearable technology to diagnose epileptic seizures based on EEG signals [4–10], and [11]. The system's performance varies, with sensitivity ranging from 32% through 100% and accuracy starting from 69% towards 99%. As seen in studies [12] and [13] investigations into the identification of epileptic seizures were conducted using various feature extraction algorithms and SVM as the classifier. The developed system performs effectively, with accuracy reaching from 94.3% through 100%. Proven, traditional machine learning approaches have been effective and efficient in solving a variety of pattern recognition problems, including epileptic seizure detection. However substantial changes are needed to handle increasingly complex real-world applications.

Deep learning, another branch of machine learning derived from artificial neural networks, has demonstrated significant success in a variety of fields, including medicine, industry, and government [14]. Deep Learning shown a potential use for biomedical signal analysis since it simplifies raw input signals and improves classification performance [15]. Recently, the number of studies on deep learning for biomedical signal processing are beginning to rise rapidly, which demonstrated an outstanding reliability, for instance is the studies on the identification of epileptic seizures using CNN. Research on the identification of epileptic seizures using CNN can also be done by first translating EEG signals into 2D/3D images [16–20], and [21], in comparison with using raw EEG data as input model. The results of the study reveal that the system performs very well. Nevertheless, it must be compensated by adding the procedure of converting raw data into images, which requires additional memory and takes more computation time. The use of raw data to diagnose epileptic seizures is being investigated. As an input, EEG signals do not need image conversion. Furthermore, pre-processing method such as noise filtering, normalization, and signal preparation (segmentation or windowing) [22] are commonly used. The study in [23] and [24], used a dataset from the University of Bonn that included 5 classes and 500 samples in total. Non-Epileptic with Eyes Opened, Non-Epileptic with Eyes Closed, Epileptic-Interictal, Epileptic-Interictal, and Epileptic-Ictal are the five classes. In [24], the model was made up of three convolutional blocks, each contains a convolutional layer, Batch Normalization, RelU as an activation method, dropout technology to avoid over-fitting, and a max-pooling layer. The result study showed that two-class classification obtained an accuracy of 97.63–99.52%, while the three-class EEG classification obtained an accuracy of 96.73–98.06%, and 93.55% for five-class problem. Ali Emami et al. conducted a study to classify the 5 classes of EEG signal using Pyramidal one-dimensional convolutional neural network (P-1D-CNN) models [23]. Using a fixed-size overlapping window, the signal was broken down into sub-signals and augmented. Furthermore, the P-1D-CNN model was intended to interpret the sub-signals that appeared before it. The number of P-1D-CNN models was determined by the n window size (sub-signals). The model would be nP-1D-CNN if the EEG signal was separated into n windows (sub-signals). The P-1D-CNN model used in this analysis was made up of convolutional, batch normalization, ReLU, fully connected and dropout layers. The results of this study provide an accuracy value of 99.1 ± 0.9%. The other study was conduct by Mengni Zhou et al. [25], investigated the three classes (ictal, pre-ictal, and inter-ictal) from Freiburg and Children's Hospital Boston–Massachusetts Institute of Technology (CHB-MIT) EEG dataset. Three scenarios of experiment were analyzed in this study; two binary classification scenario (inter-ictal vs. pre-ictal and inter-ictal vs. ictal) and one three-class problem (inter-ictal vs. pre-ictal vs. ictal). Signals in the time or frequency domain were used as classification inputs. FFT has been used to transform time domain signals into frequency domain signals. In the year 2020, Gopal Chandra et al. published research related to 1D-CNN-Spectrogram-Based Approach for Seizure Detection from EEG Signal [26]. The Butterworth was used to filter the EEG raw data at the beginning of the process. After that, the spectrogram feature matrix generated from each segment of 2 s filtered EEG data was implemented using the 1D-CNN model for seizure detection. The proposed Spectrogram-CNN-based scheme was calculated to have a 77.57% of average accuracy. In comparison to other studies, the filtering process in [27] was carried out using a notch filter. The filtering method required to removes the 50 Hz power line noise and also DC offset. This study objective was classify the two classes: seizure (SZ) or non-seizure (NS) states during sleep, data obtained from Universitario de Coimbra-Portugal and EPILEPSIAE project.

The use of 1D-CNN in the detection of epileptic seizures resulted in a reliable system performance and was capable of minimizing computational complexity since it didn't require the conversion of raw EEG data to images, as can be seen in previous studies. In this study, we propose a 1D-CNN model to detect epileptic seizures by observing the RAW-EEG signal from Bonn University dataset. The rest of this paper is presented as follows: the second section presents the dataset used in this study, the proposed 1D-CNN model and the performance evaluation matrices. The third section presents the result of our study and discussion section. The conclusion is presented in the last section.

## 2 Material and Method

### *2.1 Dataset*

The dataset consisted of EEG records from healthy participants, patients with inter-ictal, and seizures phase. Set A, Set B, Set C, Set D, and Set E were used to categorize the data into five classes, created by Andrzejak et al. from Bonn University, Germany [28]. Surface EEG with eyes open (Set A) and closed (Set B) was recorded

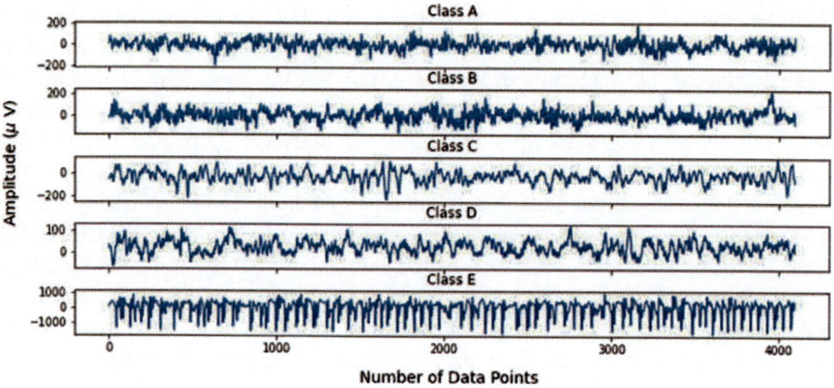


**Fig. 1** The Bonn University EEG dataset

from five healthy participants. Sets C and D, were inter-ictal (pre-ictal) intracranial EEG recordings from epilepsy patients during seizure-free periods. Electrodes in the hippocampal formation of the head were used to capture Set C, while electrodes in the epileptogenic zone were used to record Set D. Set E was documented from five patients with epilepsy who were experiencing seizure or ictal signs. The same 128-channel amplifier system has been used to archive all of the EEG signals. The data were written continuously onto the disk of a data acquisition computer system at a sampling rate of 173.61 Hz after 12 bit analog-to-digital conversion. Then, band-pass filter was configure to 0.53–40 Hz, equivalent to 12 dB/oc. Figure 1 provides several examples of EEGs. This dataset has 500 EEG recording, where each class has 100 recording. This study used all the data and using three scenarios as explained in Sect. 2.3.

## *2.2 1d-Cnn*

CNNs are built to handle data in the form of multiple arrays, organized in a sequence of stages [29]. Figure 2 illustrate the general subsystems of the 1D-CNN architecture.

CNNs are artificial neural networks with alternating convolutional and sampling layers, similar to the structure of the brain, can be utilized in any dimension scale, such as 1D-CNN for signals and time series, 2D-CNN for images and matrices, and 3D-CNN for volumetric data like medical imaging databases [30]. Figure 3 portrays a general representation of the 1D-CNN proposed method that was used in this study. We provided three scenarios, details are described in Table 1 in the next section.

The major feature of 1D-CNN over previous Artificial Neural Networks is the ability to extracts signal features by considering local information rather than the entire signal at each network layer, resulting in faster network training with a smaller

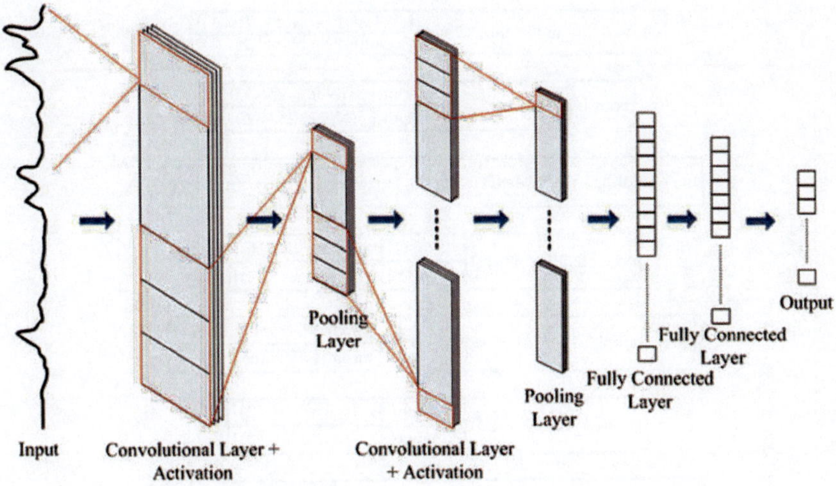


**Fig. 2** Subsystems of the 1D-CNN architecture

number of parameters to train, leading to lower cost and computing power. 1D-Convolutional layers, activation function, sub-sampling (pooling) layers, and fully connected (dense) layers are among the subsystems of the CNN architecture [13].

After each convolution operation, shift the kernel window by $s$ positions (the number of strides). Then, for stride $s$, the non-causal convolution between $x$ and $h$ is defined as in Eq. 1 [31].

$$y(n) = \begin{cases} \sum_{i=0}^{k} x(n+i)h(i), ifn = 0 \\ \sum_{i=0}^{k} x(n+i+(s-1))h(i), \quad otherwise \end{cases} \tag{1}$$

The performance of causal convolution is independent of future inputs. Let $x$ represent the input to the convolution layer of length $n$, and h represent the kernel of length $k$. After each convolution operation, shift the kernel window $s$ positions (number of strides). Then, for stride $s$, causal convolution between $x$ and $h$ is shown in Eq. 2 [31].

$$y(n) = \begin{cases} \sum_{i=0}^{k} x(n-i)h(i), \qquad ifn = k-1 \\ \sum_{i=0}^{k} x(n-i+(s-1))h(i), \quad otherwise \end{cases} \tag{2}$$

Kernel weights can be thought of as impulse responses because of their causality. The calculation is shown in Eq. 3.

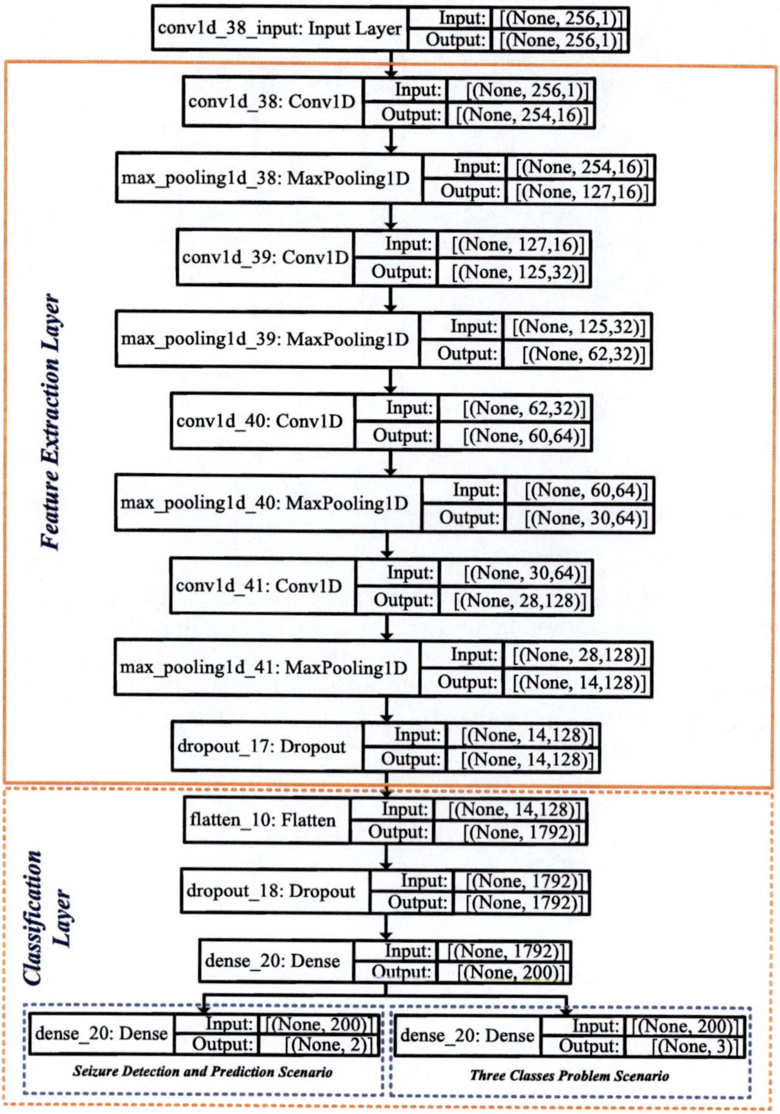


**Fig. 3** The proposed 1D-CNN model, for binary and 3 classes identification problem

$$y(n) = x(n) \circledast h(n) \tag{3}$$

When expressed in frequency domain, it is shown as in Eq. 4.

$$Y(f) = X(f)H(f) \tag{4}$$

**Table 1** Scenario and the classification issues

| Scenario | Set pairs | Classification issues |
|---|---|---|
| Seizure detection | A versus E | CI-1A |
| | B versus E | CI-1B |
| | AB versus E | CI-1C |
| Seizure prediction | A versus C | CI-2A |
| | A versus D | CI-2B |
| | B versus C | CI-2C |
| | B versus D | CI-2D |
| | AB versus C | CI-2E |
| | AB versus D | CI-2F |
| | AB versus CD | CI-2G |
| Three classes problem | A versus C versus E | CI-3A |
| | A versus D versus E | CI-3B |
| | B versus C versus E | CI-3C |
| | B versus D versus E | CI-3D |

Pooling is a technique for reducing the dimension of a mapping's convolution output while highlighting the most important features. Max pooling is the most well-known pooling procedure, which involves selecting the maximum value in a window of size $f$ and sliding this window over the input with a stride of length $s$ after each pooling operation. Dropouts are used to avoid over-fitting, which is defined as the phenomenon of memorizing inputs instead of learning general characteristics of inputs. When $P(drop) = 0.8$, each output picks a value between 0 and 1 randomly. If the number selected is less than 0.8, the output will be dropped. The depth of the output of convolution layers may be greater than one. Flatten integrates the outputs of the convolution layers into a single flat structure.

## 2.3 Evaluation Metric

The proposed system classifies the input from an EEG recording into one of two categories (for seizure detection and prediction) and classifies one of three classes' problem. To facilitate the seizure detection and prediction cycle, we create three major scenarios. Each scenario has a number of classification issues (CI). The first scenario was created to put the seizure detection mechanism with the intention of identifying between normal (healthy) and ictal states. In the second scenario, the approach to predicting the seizures was explored, with an emphasis on identifying normal versus inter-ictal conditions. The final scenario is used to classify between three conditions: normal, inter-ictal, and ictal. Table 1 shows these situations in detail.

To evaluate the system's performance, we use precision, accuracy, recall, and the f1-score, which is calculated as in Eqs. 5–8 [32] [33].

$$Accuracy = \frac{TP + TN}{TP + FP + TN + FN} \tag{5}$$

$$Sensitivity = \frac{TP}{TP + FN} \tag{6}$$

$$Specificity = \frac{TP}{TP + FP} \tag{7}$$

$$F1score = 2 \times \frac{recall \times precision}{recall + precision} \tag{8}$$

## 3 Result

Table 2 shows the comparison performance for 1D-CNN proposed model between 3 different scenarios. According to the results, the proposed method had the highest accuracy of 99.58% in predicting seizure (classify normal vs. pre-ictal condition) based on raw data of EEG. The classification between normal vs. ictal condition got the accuracy between 94.9 and 96.30% (seizure detection scenario). Meanwhile,

**Table 2** The 1D-CNN proposed model performance

| Scenario | Classification issues | Overall accuracy (%) | | Precision (%) | Recall (%) | f1-score (%) |
|---|---|---|---|---|---|---|
| | | Training | Validation | | | |
| Seizure detection | CI-1A | 99.83 | 96.04 | 95.5 | 95.5 | 95 |
| | CI-1B | 99.71 | 94.9 | 95 | 94.5 | 94.5 |
| | CI-1C | 99.73 | 96.32 | 95.5 | 96.5 | 96 |
| Seizure prediction | CI-2A | **100** | 99.17 | 98.5 | 98.5 | **99** |
| | CI-2B | 99.93 | 98.96 | 98.5 | 98.5 | **99** |
| | CI-2C | **100** | 98.65 | 98 | 98 | 98 |
| | CI-2D | **100** | **99.58** | **99** | **99** | **99** |
| | CI-2E | 99.98 | 98.26 | 97 | 98 | 97 |
| | CI-2F | 99.92 | 99.31 | 98.5 | **99** | 98.5 |
| | CI-2G | 99.75 | 97.92 | 97.5 | 97.5 | 97.5 |
| Three classes problem | CI-3A | 98.48 | 89.79 | 88.33 | 88.33 | 88 |
| | CI-3B | 99.45 | 96.53 | 95.33 | 95.33 | 95.33 |
| | CI-3C | 98.51 | 90.35 | 87.67 | 85 | 85.33 |
| | CI-3D | 99.75 | 97.01 | 96.67 | 96.33 | 96.33 |

the scenario to classify three categories (normal vs. pre-ictal vs. ictal) has slightly lower system's performance than the others, with accuracy only ranged from 89.79% towards 97.01%. The highest precision, recall and f1-score parameters were also obtained for epileptic seizure prediction scenarios (normal vs. ictal), with a value of 0.99.

## 4 Discussion

From the testing result showed in the previous section, the proposed 1D-CNN model which consists of five convolutional layers with a number of filters 16, 32, 64, 128, and 256 respectively are performed an effective, robust, and accurate automatic seizure diagnosis and prediction system based on raw-EEG data. The use of 1D-CNN in the detection of epileptic seizures resulted a reliable system performance that capable of minimizing computational complexity since it didn't require the conversion of raw EEG data into 2D-images.

Many studies have been performed on automatic epileptic seizure detection through prediction based on EEG signal (including images or raw-data) as listed in Table 3. Previous studies used traditional method that mainly required preprocessing, feature extraction and classification process. However, the proposed method in this research used 1D-CNN that can process raw data of EEG signals directly. Traditional machine learning algorithms, such as SVM, KNN, LDA, PLS, and random forest result varies performance, with accuracy ranging from 69% towards 99%. The studies [12] and [13] were investigated the identification of epileptic seizures using various feature extraction algorithms and SVM as the classifier, deliver an effective system performance, with accuracy reaching from 94.3% through 100%. It seems to be clear that traditional machine learning approaches have been effective and efficient in solving epileptic seizure detection, but substantial changes are needed to handle increasingly complex real-world applications.

Research on the identification of epileptic seizures using CNN can also be done by first translating EEG signals into 2D images [18, 21], and [17] in comparison with using raw EEG data as input model. The results of the study reveal that the system performs very well, nevertheless, it must be compensated by adding the procedure of converting raw data into images, which requires additional memory and takes a bit longer computation time. The study in [24] classify the 5 classes of Bonn University dataset, the model is made up of three convolutional blocks, each contains a convolutional layer, Batch Normalization, RelU as an activation method, dropout technology and a max-pooling layer. The result study showed that two-class classification obtained an accuracy of 97.63–99.52%, while the three-class EEG classification obtained an accuracy of 96.73–98.06%, and 93.55% for five-class problem. These results show a higher rate of performance than the model we developed, which may be due to the deeper neurons model's complexity. The proposed method can be utilized as input to relevant stakeholders for additional clinical studies, and it may be employed in the medical field in the future. This

**Table 3** The performance comparison with other research

| References | No. of classes | Classifier | Accuracy (%) |
|---|---|---|---|
| [4] | Normal versus seizure EEG | KNN<br>RBSVM<br>LDA | 98.6<br>99<br>95.7 |
| [17] | Two classes (healthy vs. epileptic subjects) | 2D-CNN | 99.48 |
| [5] | | SVM-Lin<br>SVM-RBF<br>KNN (k = 1)<br>KNN (k = 3)<br>KNN (k = 5)<br>Random forest<br>Tree-boost | 77<br>7471<br>72<br>73<br>73<br>69 |
| [18] | Ictal versus interictal (from CHB-MIT and EPILEPSIAE dataset) | FCN | 99.3<br>98 |
| [26] | CHB-MIT dataset | 1D-CNN | 77.57 |
| [21] | Inter-ictal, pre-ictal, and ictal stages | 2D-CNN | > 90 |
| [12] | Normal, pre-ictal, and seizure | SVM | 98.7 |
| [13] | 4 class: FNSZ, GNSZ, SPSZ, and TNSZ (Temple University dataset) | SVM | 95 |
| [24] | 5 classes of Bonn University dataset | 1D-CNN | 97.63–99.52 (2-class problem)<br>96.73–98.06 (3-class problem)<br>93.55 (5-class problem) |
| [25] | Ictal, preictal, and interictal (freiburg and CHB-MIT dataset) | 1D-CNN | 47.9–96.7 |
| Proposed model | 5 classes of Bonn University dataset | 1D-CNN | 94.9–96.3 (seizure detection)<br>97.92–99.58 (seizure prediction)<br>89.79–97.01 (3 classes problem) |

research has the potential to contribute to the academic understanding of biomedical signal processing, but more than this, it may have an impact on wider society by improving the quality of life of epilepsy patients.

## 5 Conclusion

Epileptic seizures appear unexpectedly, posing a risk of injury and even death, particularly when they operate heavy machinery or drive a vehicle. As a result, developing a system that can predict the emergence of epileptic seizures is essential. The 1D-CNN model that consists of five convolutional layers with number of filters 16, 32, 64, 128, and 256 respectively is chosen to construct an effective, robust, and accurate automatic seizure diagnosis and prediction system based on raw-EEG data. The classification layers consist of flatten process and two dense layers to classify EEG signal into two conditions which are normal versus pre-ictal and normal versus ictal, and other scenario are classify EEG signal into three classes (normal vs. pre-ictal vs. ictal). The proposed 1D-CNN model delivers a great performance by providing precision, recall, and f1-score up to 0.99 during prediction epileptic seizure. The accuracy ranged between 94.9 and 96.30% for seizure detection scenario, 97.92–99.58% for seizure prediction scenario and 89.79–97.01% for three classes problem classification. The proposed method can be used to assist neurologists in the precise diagnosis of epilepsy. Future studies may investigate the multichannel EEG signal and applying the channel selection process. A more in-depth investigation process can be carried out to combine the neural network as a features extractor and several classifier algorithms such as random forest, Naive Bayes, logistic regression, decision tree, KNN, and SVM.

## References


1. WHO (2019) EPILEPSY. A Public Health Imperative. Geneva
2. Muttaqin Z et al (2019) Desperately needed in Indonesia: basic epilepsy surgery centers with simple but reliable pre-surgical investigations, based on Semarang's experience. https://doi.org/10.15562/bmj.v8i2.1361
3. Fiest KM et al (2017) Prevalence and incidence of epilepsy; a systematic review and meta-analysis of international studies. Neurology 88:296–303
4. Aldana YR et al (2019) Nonconvulsive epileptic seizure detection in scalp EEG using multiway data analysis. IEEE J Biomed Health Inform 23(2):660–671. https://doi.org/10.1109/JBHI.2018.2829877
5. Van Eyndhoven S et al (2018) Single-channel EEG classification by multi-channel tensor subspace learning and regression. In: IEEE international workshop on machine learning for signal processing (MLSP), pp 1–6, Aalborg, Denmark. https://doi.org/10.1109/MLSP.2018.8516927
6. Gu Y et al (2018) Comparison between scalp EEG and behind-the-ear EEG for development of a wearable seizure detection system for patients with focal epilepsy. Sensors (Switzerland) 18(1):1–17. https://doi.org/10.3390/s18010029
7. Rizal A et al (2021) Seizure classification on epileptic EEG using IMF-entropy and support vector machine. In: Proceedings of the 1st international conference on electronics, biomedical engineering, and health informatics, pp 387–395, Springer Link
8. Rodríguez Y et al (2019) Using partial least squares for nonconvulsive epileptic seizure detection. Revista Cubana de Ciencias Informáticas 13(1):1–13

9. Tjandrasa H, Djanali S (2016) Classification of EEG signals using single channel independent component analysis, power spectrum, and linear discriminant analysis. In: 2015 international conference on machine learning and signal processing (lecture notes in electrical engineering), pp 259–268. https://doi.org/10.1007/978-3-319-32213-1
10. Vandecasteele K et al (2017) Automated epileptic seizure detection based on wearable ECG and PPG in a hospital environment. Sensors (Switzerland) 17(10):1–12. https://doi.org/10.3390/s17102338
11. Vandecasteele K et al (2020) Visual seizure annotation and automated seizure detection using behind-the-ear electroencephalographic channels. Epilepsia 61(4):766–775. https://doi.org/10.1111/epi.16470
12. Wijayanto I et al (2019) Seizure detection based on EEG signals using Katz Fractal and SVM classifiers. In: Proceeding—2019 5th international conference on science in information technology: embracing industry 4.0: towards innovation in cyber physical system, ICSITech 2019, pp 78–82. https://doi.org/10.1109/ICSITech46713.2019.8987487
13. Wijayanto I et al (2019) Seizure type detection in epileptic EEG signal using empirical mode decomposition and support vector machine. In: Proceedings—2019 international seminar on intelligent technology and its application, ISITIA 2019, pp 314–319. https://doi.org/10.1109/ISITIA.2019.8937205
14. Alaskar H (2019) Convolutional neural network application in biomedical signals. J Comp Sci Inform Technol 1100:287–297. https://doi.org/10.1007/978-981-15-0399-3_23
15. Chaabene S et al (2021) Convolutional neural network for drowsiness detection using EEG signals. Sensors 21(5):1–19. https://doi.org/10.3390/s21051734
16. Antonoudiou P, Maguire JL (2020) How deep learning solved my seizure detection problems. Epilepsy Cur 20(5):306–308. https://doi.org/10.1177/1535759720948430
17. Bouaziz B et al (2019) Epileptic seizure detection using a convolutional neural network. In: Digital health approach for predictive, preventive, personalised and participatory medicine (Advances in predictive, preventive and personalised medicine), Vol 79–86. https://doi.org/10.1007/978-3-030-11800-6_9
18. Gómez C et al (2020) Automatic seizure detection based on imaged-EEG signals through fully convolutional networks. Sci Rep 10(1):1–13. https://doi.org/10.1038/s41598-020-78784-3
19. Thanaraj KP et al (2020) Implementation of deep neural networks to classify EEG signals using Gramian Angular summation field for epilepsy diagnosis. arXiv
20. Ullah I et al (2018) An automated system for epilepsy detection using EEG brain signals based on deep learning approach. arXiv. Ml
21. Wei X et al (2018) Automatic seizure detection using three-dimensional CNN based on multi-channel EEG. BMC Med Inform Decis Mak 18(5). https://doi.org/10.1186/s12911-018-0693-8
22. Shoeibi A et al (2020) Epileptic seizure detection using deep learning techniques: a review. arXiv
23. Emami A et al (2019) Seizure detection by convolutional neural network-based analysis of scalp electroencephalography plot images. Neuro Image Clin 22:101684. https://doi.org/10.1016/j.nicl.2019.101684
24. Zhao W et al (2020) A novel deep neural network for robust detection of seizures using EEG signals. Comput Math Meth Med. https://doi.org/10.1155/2020/9689821
25. Zhou M et al (2018) Epileptic seizure detection based on EEG signals and CNN. Front Neuroinform 12(December):1–14. https://doi.org/10.3389/fninf.2018.00095
26. Jana GC et al (2020) A 1D-CNN-spectrogram based approach for seizure detection from EEG signal. Proc Comp Sci 167(2019):403–412. https://doi.org/10.1016/j.procs.2020.03.248
27. Pisano F et al (2020) Convolutional neural network for seizure detection of nocturnal frontal lobe epilepsy. Complexity. https://doi.org/10.1155/2020/4825767
28. Andrzejak RG et al (2001) Indications of nonlinear deterministic and finite-dimensional structures in time series of brain electrical activity: dependence on recording region and brain state. Phys Rev E Stat Phys Plasmas Fluids Rel Interdiscip Top 64, 6, 8. https://doi.org/10.1103/PhysRevE.64.061907

29. Lecun Y et al (2015) Deep learning. Nature 521(7553):436–444. https://doi.org/10.1038/nature14539
30. Mozaffari MH, Tay LL (2020) A review of 1d convolutional neural networks toward unknown substance identification in portable Raman spectrometer. arXiv
31. Sakrepatna Srinivasamurthy R (2018) Understanding 1D convolutional neural networks using multiclass time-varying signals. Clemson University
32. Fawcett T (2006) An introduction to ROC analysis. Pattern Recogn Lett 27(8):861–874. https://doi.org/10.1016/j.patrec.2005.10.010
33. Sasaki Y (2007) The truth of the F-measure. Teach Tutor Mater 1–5

# Comparative Analysis of Various Optimizers on Residual Network Architecture for Facial Expression Identification

**Ardityo Dimas Ramadhan, Koredianto Usman, and Nor Kumalasari Caecar Pratiwi**

**Abstract** In recent years, the interaction between humans and computers has become a popular global challenge. The emergence of social robot technology, also known as Humanoid robot technology, is one manifestation of this interaction. How to create communication with humans is one of the most essential components of social robots. Nonverbal communication, such as reading body language and recognizing facial expressions, is one approach for robots to communicate. This study will design a facial expression recognition system using CNN method, which has been proven to be superior in the field of digital image-based classification. In the future, facial expression recognition will become increasingly common in human–computer interface devices. Residual Network 34 architecture was used to classify the Cohn Kanade (CK+) data set consisting of 981 images, divided into seven classes of facial expressions; angry, disgust, fear, happy, sadness, surprise, and contempt. The investigation process is carried out by comparing three optimization algorithms: Adaptive moment (Adam), Stochastic Gradient Descent (SGD), Root Mean Square Propagation (RMSProp). Based on the results of system testing, it shows that the ResNet-34 architecture has a fairly optimal performance in the classification of facial expressions, with an average accuracy of 99.3%, precision of 99.6%, recall of 99.3% and F1-Score of 99.4%.

**Keywords** Facial expression · Convolutional neural network (CNN) · Residual network 34 · Optimizer

## 1 Introduction

Human–computer interaction has become a prominent global problem in recent years, and it is one of the most discussed research topics. Many studies have contributed to the development of social robot technology, also known as Humanoid robot technology, which is designed to assist humans in all aspects of their lives in

A. D. Ramadhan · K. Usman · N. K. C. Pratiwi (✉)
School of Electrical Engineering, Telkom University, Bandung, Indonesia
e-mail: caecarnkcp@telkomuniversity.ac.id



T. Triwiyanto et al. (eds.), *Proceedings of the 2nd International Conference on Electronics, Biomedical Engineering, and Health Informatics*, Lecture Notes in Electrical Engineering 898, https://doi.org/10.1007/978-981-19-1804-9_22

the future. Artificial emotional systems have been presented as a way to improve human–robot interaction [1]. Nonverbal communication, such as body language and facial expressions, is required for robots to develop meaningful communication with humans [2]. Various robot projects have established facial expressions as the most essential element for communicating emotional messages [2]. Intelligent robots which could interact with humans have a lot of potential applications. A social robot with advanced artificial intelligence will serve as a capable companion for users of various ages. For children, this robot serves as a babysitter who assists parents in monitoring their children; for adults, the robot will act as a personal assistant; and these robots perform as buddies for the elderly, helping them to conquer loneliness [3]. Social robot applications are extensively used in the worlds of education and entertainment, in addition to being a companion to humans. The Convolutional Neural Networks (CNNs) method has been proven to be accurate in various facial expression classification studies. CNNs are customized neural networks that employ convolution instead of matrix multiplications. CNN relies based on three fundamental concepts: parameter sharing, sparse interactions, and equivariant representations, utilized to extract features from images successfully. CNNs are also scalable to large data sets and more computationally efficient than standard Artificial Neural Networks (ANNs) [4].

A number of studies related to the topic of facial expressions have been carried out with various proposed models such as the Identity-Aware Convolutional Neural Network (IACNN) which was added by preprocessing by Zibo Meng with 7 classes data, 981 images and obtained a fairly good accuracy of 71.29% [5]. Then, the Boosted Deep Balief Network (BDBN) model has a much better accuracy than IACNN. BDBN used 8 classes with 1308 images which is have an accuracy 96.7% [6]. A Deep Temporal Appearance-Geometry Network (DTAGN) model has also been proposed with an accuracy rate of 97.25% with 7 classes and 327 image [7]. Some of the models that have been proposed are several innovations in digital image processing of facial expressions which are the development of the previous CNN model. In-kyu Choi and colleagues developed a system to classify six expression recognition by using Convolutional Neural Network (CNN) [8]. The pre-processing and data augmentation are applied to optimize the training efficiency and performance. The investigation results show good performance compared to the cross validation and the cross database, also compared to other conventional models. Z. Hammal and colleagues design a method for six classes' facial expressions classification based on the transferable belief model (TBM) framework compared with a Bayesian classifier. Both classifiers were investigated on three different databases [9]. Facial expression classification p lays crucial role in human–computer interaction. A large number of automated methods have been proposed since the past decades. Seven classes of facial expression classification with deep convolutional neural networks (CNNs) was also carried out by Thitiphong Raksarikorn and colleagues [10]. The experimental results show that the CNN model offers accuracy of 0.7169. A student's facial expressions recognition using a feed-forward learning model was built to involve teacher's behavior and student's responses in classroom [11]. The regularized extreme learning machine (RELM) classifier is employed for fast learning and algorithm. The results indicate significant performance gain on parameters such as accuracy, F1-score, and recall. A review and insights on facial emotion identification based on deep learning with various architecture of CNN and CNN-LSTM was studied by Wafa Mellouk and colleagues [12]. The recognition rate was varies in range of 65% through 99.8%.

As evidenced by the research mentioned above showed that deep learning may generate a robust Facial Expression Recognition (FER) system with a high level of recognition rate. The Residual Network (ResNet) offers numerous advantages, including the ability to speed up the training of deep networks, the reduction of the influence of the Vanishing Gradient problem, and the ability to increase the depth of the network results in fewer additional parameters. He et al. first introduced the residual network to address the performance failure in training very deep CNNs by design skip connections in the architecture, allowing information to flow to the next layer through identity mappings without additional parameters or higher computational [13]. The ResNet architecture is used in this study to create a system that can classify seven classes of facial expressions from Cohn Kanade (CK+) dataset. The seven classes are angry, disgust, fear, happy, sadness, surprise, and contempt. In the investigation process, observations were made on the effect of the ratio of training data and testing data as well as the use of three different optimizer algorithms. The training and testing data ratios are 80:20 and 75:25, and the three optimizer algorithms utilized are Adaptive moment (Adam), Stochastic Gradient Descent (SGD), Root Mean Square Propagation (RMSProp).

## 2 Material and Method

The proposed system, is divided into several main process, first is data retrieval stage, followed by the preprocessing stage, feature extraction and classification with ResNet-34 architecture, illustrated in Fig. 1.

This study obtained a dataset from Chon Kanade with PNG file formats [14], as shown in Fig. 2.

Due to the limited amount of data in the Cohn Kanade dataset, we performed data augmentation to increase the data variation. The total data used are 981 images, divided into seven classes: angry, disgust, fear, happy, sadness, surprise,

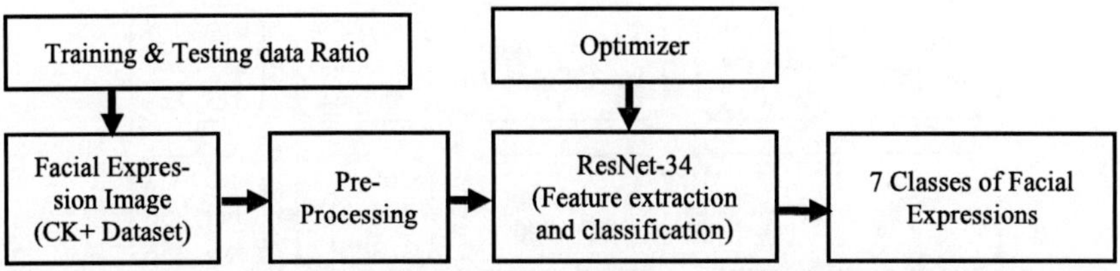


**Fig. 1** Proposed system for facial expressions classification using ResNet-34 architecture

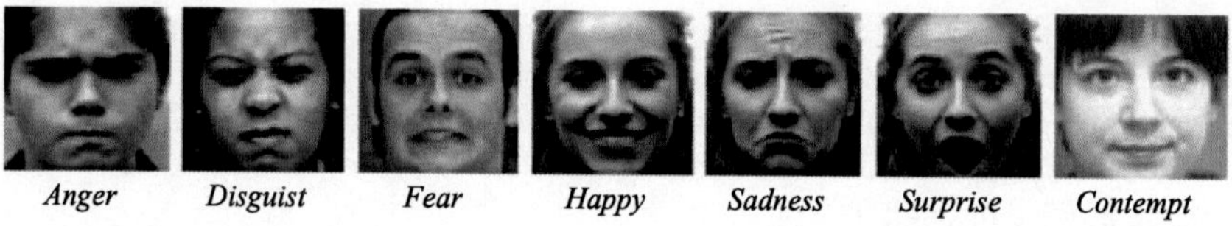


**Fig. 2** Face expression dataset

and contempt. The whole image will be divided into training data and testing data, which is one of the test scenarios, we use a ratio of 80:20 and 75:25. From these two ratios, it will be seen how they affect to the level of system accuracy.

The training process aims to instruct the ResNet-34 model in recognizing its datasets and classifying them into seven classes properly. This proposed system are using Convolutional Neural Network (CNN), with ResNet-34 architecture as feature extractor and classifier. CNN is a type of neural network that can used to detect objects in an image [13]. Figure 3 is a block diagram of the CNN model with the ResNet-34 architecture.

In the ResNet-34 architecture, the first convolution is carried out using a $7 \times 7$ filter and stride 2 so that 64 filters are obtained, then enter the pooling layer, to reduce the dimensions of the image. Max pooling used in ResNet34 has a filter size of $3 \times 3$ and stride 2. Multiple convolution processes make up the second, third, fourth, and fifth phases of the convolution. The overall multiple convolutional layer are using a filter size of $3 \times 3$ with three residual blocks. After all the convolution processes are passed, the feature map size is again reduced by using average pooling [13]. The results of each filter will pass through average pooling and enter the fully connected layer with the softmax activation function to find out the classification results. Optimizer is used to improve the learning process on the system. Every optimizer uses specific learning rate values that determine the ability of the system to learn. This study uses three types of the optimizer that are Adaptive Moment Estimation (Adam), Root Mean Square Propagation (RMSprop), and Stochastic Gradient Descent (SGD) [15].

Adam is the result of the derivation of the SGD method based on moment adaptive estimation first and second order. Optimization algorithm that calculates the learning rate adaptively for each parameter. Adam keeps the mean of the gradient of the previous process exponentially the same as RMSprop. The standard learning rate value at Adam is 0.001 [16]. Equation (1) below is used to update the neuron weights

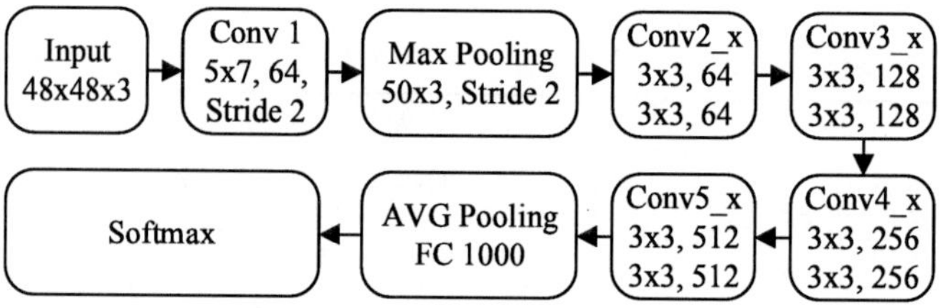


**Fig. 3** ResNet-34 architecture

in the Adam optimizer [16].

$$\theta_{t+1} = \theta t - \frac{\partial}{\sqrt{\hat{v}t} + \varepsilon} . \hat{m}_t \quad (1)$$

where $\theta_{t+1}$ is the update result parameter, $\theta_t$ is the result parameter of the previous update, $\hat{m}_t$ is the gradient of the square first order moment, $\hat{v}t$ gradient of the square of the order moment second, $\varepsilon$ and is a small scalar to prevent division by zero.

**Root Mean Square Propagation or RMSprop** is a particular version of Adagrad developed by Professor Geoffrey Hinton in his neural network class. RMSprop is similar to Adaprop, another optimizer that attempts to resolve some of the issues that Adagrad has left open. The standard learning rate value at RMSProp is 0.001 [17]. Equation (2) below is used to update the neuron weights in the RMSProp optimizer [17].

$$Mean\ Square(w, t) = \rho * Mean\ Square(w, t-1) + 0.1\left(\frac{\partial E}{\partial w}(t)\right)2 \quad (2)$$

where w is weight, t is timestamp, $\rho$ is 0.9, $\frac{\partial E}{\partial w}$ is gradient.

**SGD** is a variation of optimization gradient descent, constantly updating parameters for each data being trained. SGD does not loop when performing parameter updates, so the performance is better for large datasets. Learning value the standard rate on SGD is 0.01. Process parameter update on SGD can be defined on Eq. (3):

$$\theta_{t+1} = \theta_t - \eta d_t \quad (3)$$

where $d_t$ is gradient from objective function based on parameter $\theta$ at time step t and $\eta$ is learning rate. Loss is the comparison or difference between the predicted value and the actual value. The loss used in this study is categorical cross entropy loss [18]. The ground-truth value is expressed in $y_i$ and $\widehat{y_i}$ represents the predicted value. The formulation of loss in Eq. (4):

$$Loss = -\sum_{i=1}^{M} yi \log(p) \quad (4)$$

In order to evaluate the models, test parameters are needed as comparison values for each model. The test parameter values are the results of calculations using four performance metrics generated by the confusion matrix. The values contained in the confusion matrix are the predicted and actual results of each class. Multiclass has a predicted value and an actual value in four different combinations of values, namely Total True Positive (TTP), Total True Negative (TTN), Total False Positive (TFP), and Total False Negative (TFN) or can also be called system performance metrics [19]. Performance metrics are used to compare the quality of the predictions of the whole system. The performance parameters used in this study are accuracy, recall, precision, and F-1 score. The formulation of each metric is in the Eqs. (5) through (8) [19].

$$Accuracy = \frac{TTP_{all} + TTN_{all}}{TotalNumberOfTestingEntries} \times 100 \quad (5)$$

$$Recall = \frac{TTP_{all}}{TTP_{all} + TFN_i} \times 100 \quad (6)$$

$$Precision = \frac{TTP_{all}}{TTP_{all} + TFP_i} \times 100 \quad (7)$$

$$F1{-}Score = 2 \times \frac{(Recall \times \text{precision})}{(Recall + \text{precision})} \quad (8)$$

## 3 Result

This testing scenario is to determine the effect of the ratio between training and testing data, as well as the using of three difference optimizer algorithm. The training and testing data ratios are 80:20 and 75:25, and the three optimizer algorithms utilized are Adaptive moment (Adam), Stochastic Gradient Descent (SGD), Root Mean Square Propagation (RMSProp). All optimizers using a learning rate of 0.0001 and batch size 8. Table 1 shows the result of the ratio of training and testing data, and three different optimizer.

Based on Table 1, it can be observed that when training and testing data are compared, 80:20 performs better than 75:25. Meanwhile, Adam and RMSProp provide a very dependable system performance, surpassing 98% when examined

**Table 1** The accuracy and loss system by comparing ratio of training and testing data, as well as three different optimizers

| Ratio of training data and testing data | Optimizer | Accuracy (%) | | Loss | |
|---|---|---|---|---|---|
| | | Training | Testing | Training | Testing |
| 80:20 | Adam | 99.87 | 98.48 | 0.0123 | 0.0607 |
| | SGD | 50.89 | 49.24 | 1.4727 | 1.5045 |
| | RMSProp | 99.62 | 98.98 | 0.0173 | 0.0417 |
| 75:25 | Adam | 98.78 | 94.72 | 0.0497 | 0.1175 |
| | SGD | 46.12 | 45.12 | 1.5753 | 1.5745 |
| | RMSProp | 99.46 | 98.37 | 0.0303 | 0.0472 |

through the optimization process. Four performance parameters: accuracy, precision, recall and F1, are compared in this study. Table 2 is the confusion matrix for proposed ResNet-34 for facial expression classification system.

Of the total 198 images, 195 of them can be correctly predicted by the system according to their respective classes, and the 2 remaining were incorrectly predicted. Based on the values of the confusion matrix, the performance parameters of accuracy, precision, recall, and F-1 Score for each class can be shown as Table 3.

**Table 2** The confusion matrix for proposed ResNet-34 for facial expression classification

| | | Predicted | | | | | | |
|---|---|---|---|---|---|---|---|---|
| | | Anger | Contempt | Disgust | Fear | Happy | Sadness | Surprise |
| Actual | Anger | 20 | 0 | 0 | 0 | 0 | 0 | 0 |
| | Contempt | 0 | 12 | 0 | 0 | 0 | 0 | 0 |
| | Disgust | 0 | 0 | 33 | 0 | 0 | 0 | 0 |
| | Fear | 0 | 0 | 0 | 15 | 0 | 0 | 0 |
| | Happy | 0 | 0 | 0 | 0 | 43 | 0 | 0 |
| | Sadness | 0 | 0 | 0 | 0 | 0 | 18 | 0 |
| | Surprise | 0 | 0 | 1 | 1 | 0 | 0 | 54 |

**Table 3** Performance of prior research compared to proposed system

| Method | Dataset | Class | Performance |
|---|---|---|---|
| IACNN [3] | 981 images | Seven classes (angry, disgust, fear, happy, sadness, surprise, and contempt) | Accuracy of 71.29% |
| BDBN [4] | 1308 images | Eight classes (angry, disgust, fear, happy, sadness, surprise, contempt, and natural) | Accuracy of 96.7% |
| DTAGN [5] | 327 images | Seven classes (angry, disgust, fear, happy, sadness, surprise, and contempt) | Accuracy of 97.25% |
| Proposed method (ResNet-34) | 198 images | Seven classes (angry, disgust, fear, happy, sadness, surprise, and contempt) | Accuracy of 99.87% and Loss of 0.0123 |

# 4 Discussion

Based on Table 1 the ratio of training and testing data of 80:20 shows the best performance, suggests that the more data sent into the system for training, the better the system will be in recognizing objects. While from Table 2, shows that the surprise class fall on a prediction error, where the data are predicted to be in the Disgust and Fear classes. In the future, this deficiency can be minimized, one of which is by adding the amount of data and variations of expression in each class. For optimization algorithm, showed in Table 1 and Fig. 4, RMSprop got the best accuracy and the lowest loss rate, shows that RMSprop has the advantage of calculating individual adaptive learning rates for different parameters of the first and second moment estimates of the gradient. For each class, this section compare system performance. ResNet-34 architecture has a fairly optimal performance in the classification of facial expressions. The average accuracy of 99.3%, precision of 99.6%, recall of 99.3% and F1-Score of 99.4%. Table 3 compares the proposed system's performance with those of prior research' systems.

Several previous studies have performed automatic facial expression detection using face expression images but used eight classification classes. The method proposed in this study uses ResNet-34 to classify expression using seven face expression classes. Based on Table 3, this study shows a good level of performance by using a more significant number of classes.

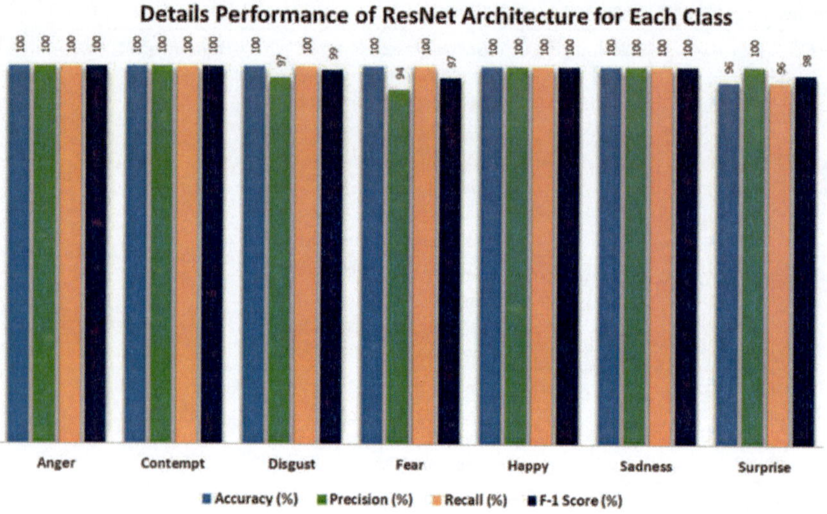


**Fig. 4** Details performance model for each class

# 5 Conclusion

The CNN model with the ResNet-34 architecture is good enough to classify face expression into seven classes: anger, sadness, happy, fear, disgust, surprise and contempt. The system can identify face expression into 7 classes with an accuracy of 98,98% for testing and 99,62% for training. The loss obtained is 0.0417 for testing and 0.0173 for training. From test results, without preprocessing on image and using RMSProp optimizer can improve the performance of the face expression classification system. In further research, it is attempted to build a real-time video-based system that can be directly implemented on human–computer interaction machines, using a more varied database and Indonesian facial expressions.

# References


1. Reyes ME, Meza IV, Pineda LA (2019) Robotics facial expression of anger in collaborative human–robot interaction. Int J Adv Rob Syst 16(1):1–13
2. Doroftei I, Adascalitei F, Lefeber D, Vanderborght B, Doroftei IA (2016) Facial expressions recognition with an emotion expressive robotic head. IOP Conf Ser Mater Sci Eng 147(1):0–11
3. Duncan B, Lorenz T (2008) Facial expression imitation for human robot interaction, National University of Singapore
4. Wang R et al (2021) Deep residual network framework for structural health monitoring. Struct Health Monit 20(4):1443–1461
5. Meng Z, Liu P, Cai J, Han S, Tong Y (2017) Identity-aware convolutional neural network for facial expression recognition. In: Proceedings—12th IEEE international conference on automatic face and gesture recognition, FG 2017—1st international workshop on adaptive shot learning for gesture understanding and production, ASL4GUP 2017, biometrics in the wild, Bwild 2017, Heteroge, pp 558–565
6. Liu P, Han S, Meng Z, Tong Y (2014) Facial expression recognition via a boosted deep belief network. In: 2014 IEEE conference on computer vision and pattern recognition, 2014, pp 1805–1812
7. Jung H, Lee S, Yim J, Park S, Kim J (2015) Joint fine-tuning in deep neural networks for facial expression recognition. In: Proceedings of the IEEE international conference on computer vision, Vol 2015 Inter, pp 2983–2991
8. Choi IK, Ahn HE, Yoo J (2018) Facial expression classification using deep convolutional neural network. J Electr Eng Technol 13(1):485–492
9. Hammal Z, Couvreur L, Caplier A, Rombaut M (2007) Facial expression classification: an approach based on the fusion of facial deformations using the transferable belief model. Int J Approxi Reason 46(3):542–567
10. Raksarikorn T, Kangkachit T (2018) Facial expression classification using deep extreme inception networks. In: 2018 15th international joint conference on computer science and software engineering (JCSSE), pp 1–5
11. Bhatti YK, Jamil A, Nida N, Yousaf MH, Viriri S, Velastin SA (2021) Facial expression recognition of instructor using deep features and extreme learning machine. Comput Intell Neurosci 2021
12. Mellouk W, Handouzi W (2020) Facial emotion recognition using deep learning: review and insights. Proc Comp Sci 175:689–694
13. He K, Zhang X, Ren S, Sun J (2016) Deep residual learning for image recognition. In: Proceedings of the IEEE computer society conference on computer vision and pattern recognition, pp 770–778

14. Miao Y, Dong H, Al Jaam JM, El Saddik A (2019) A deep learning system for recognizing facial expression in real-time. ACM Trans Multimed Comput Commun Appl 15(2)
15. Bera S, Shrivastava VK (2020) Analysis of various optimizers on deep convolutional neural network model in the application of hyperspectral remote sensing image classification. Int J Remote Sens 41(7):2664–2683
16. Kingma DP, Ba JL, ADAM (2015) A method for stochastic optimization. In: 3rd international conference on learning representations, pp 1–15
17. Ghafoor M et al (2021) Fingerprint Identification with shallow multifeature view classifier. IEEE Trans Cybernet 51(9):4515–4527
18. Andono PN, TSM (2021) Pengolahan citra digital. ANDI
19. Pratiwi NKC, Fu'adah YN, Edwar E (2021) Early detection of deforestation through satellite land geospatial images based on CNN architecture. J Infotel 13(2):54–62

# Automatic Glaucoma Classification Using Residual Network Architecture

**Fira Mutia Ramaida, Koredianto Usman, and Nor Kumalasari Caecar Pratiwi**

**Abstract** Glaucoma is an eye disease with special characteristics such as neuropathy optic nerve damage and visual field abnormalities. An increased intraocular pressure is a significant risk factor for glaucoma. Glaucoma is the second largest cause of blindness worldwide, behind cataracts, based on the current World Health Organization (WHO). Ophthalmologists usually detect glaucoma using the Cup to Disc Ratio (CDR) parameter, and manual CDR calculations should be performed by trained doctors and use expensive and relatively limited devices. This research was made to overcome this problem by creating a system that can classify glaucoma through fundus images using the Convolutional Neural Network (CNN) with Residual Network-34. A total of 2156 fundus images were used in the research, the data divided into five types of glaucoma: early, moderate, deep, OHT, and normal. The ratio between training against testing data, as well as the effect of utilizing three different optimizers: Adam, SGD, and RMS are investigated in the system testing scenario. According to the study results, the suggested approach is capable to correctly classifying Glaucoma based on fundus images, with 94% accuracy rate.

**Keywords** Convolutional neural network · Glaucoma · ResNet-34 · Optimizer

## 1 Introduction

Glaucoma is one of the diseases that cause abnormalities in the eye with unique characteristics such as optic nerve damage, neuropathy, and visual field abnormalities. Elevated intraocular pressure is a significant risk factor for glaucoma. Early diagnosis and treatment can prevent vision loss from the disease [1]. Glaucoma is the second largest cause of blindness worldwide, behind cataracts, based on the current World Health Organization (WHO) [2]. Primary Open Angle Glaucoma (POAG) is projected to afflict 57.5 million people worldwide, with a global incidence of 2.2%. Glaucoma is more common as people become older, as are age-related illnesses

F. M. Ramaida (✉) · K. Usman · N. K. C. Pratiwi
School of Electrical Engineering, Telkom University, Bandung, Indonesia
e-mail: firamutiar@student.telkomuniversity.ac.id

 
T. Triwiyanto et al. (eds.), *Proceedings of the 2nd International Conference on Electronics, Biomedical Engineering, and Health Informatics*, Lecture Notes in Electrical Engineering 898, https://doi.org/10.1007/978-981-19-1804-9_23

including retinal degeneration, vascular disease, and sleep apnea [3]. Ophthalmologists usually detect glaucoma using the Cup to Disc Ratio (CDR) parameter. However, determining the Cup to Disc Ratio (CDR) is quite tricky because of the low contrast between the cup and the environmental area. In addition, manual CDR calculations must be performed by trained doctors and expensive devices such as the relatively limited Heidelberg Retinal Tomography (HRT) [4]. Accurate Glaucoma Detection is one of the essential requirements for reducing the risk of blindness and control its development [2].

A huge number of clinical data are produced per day in the era of digital medicine, and there is a large market need intelligent adjuvant diagnosis equipment to assist health professionals [5]. Machine learning has lately witnessed some significant advancements, one of which has been fueled by discoveries in artificial neural networks, a package of techniques and algorithms that enables computers to identify complex patterns in massive data sets [6]. Convolutional neural networks are quickly gaining traction as a viable alternative to medical image analysis, and they are commonly regarded as one of the most extensively used deep learning techniques in image analysis. Convolutional neural networks have the advantage of a wide application range, fast analysis speed, and high accuracy [7]. Convolutional layers can extract deep features from medical images. By extracting features, convolutional neural networks can perform set of medical image analysis tasks including detection, classification, and detection [5]. In the context of computer-aided detection (CAD) systems and screening programs for eye disorders, CNN has been effectively applied to color fundus images, reaching advanced performance or surpassing earlier implementations [8].

One of the first automatic glaucoma diagnosis systems employed a 6-layer CNN architecture to distinguish between non-glaucoma and glaucoma patients [9]. The model was constructed from the ground up using a collection of input images and a region of interest around the optic disc taken from two publicly available datasets. In both dataset, the area under the curve (AUC) of the receiver operating characteristic curve in glaucoma detection is 0.831 and 0.887. A set of 295 fundus videos and 1810 fundus images from 206 and 489 participants attending Vision Research Clinic (UTS) and the Center for Eye Health (University of New South Wales, Sydney, Australia), were utilized in the study which employed a mixed CNN and repetitive neural network (RNN) [10]. The combined CNN/RNN model achieved a mean F size of 96.2% in separating healthy eyes and glaucoma. The basic CNN model achieves an average F-measure of 79.2%. Convolutional neural networks have shown to be effective in automatically detecting subtle characteristics of images. The ResNet-50 model was used to examine the study for early detection of glaucoma utilizing residual network, which produced an accuracy of 96.95% using a dataset from RETINA [11]. To classify glaucoma and normal, researchers used five different CNN architectures: standard CNN, DENet, GoogLeNet, VGG19, and ResNet50 with two different public datasets DRASHTI-GS and RIM-ONE, one private dataset from Hospital de la Esperanza-Barcelona (Spanish). The highest result was achieved applying a transfer learning strategy, with VGG19 reaching an AUC of 0.94 for glaucoma diagnosis in color fundus pictures using Convolutional Neural Networks

(CNN) approaches [12]. The results of the studies, which used three distinct data sets totaling 2313 images, show that this approach might be a great option for developing a computer aid system for glaucoma detection in sizable screening tests. Pinto and colleagues [13] used five alternative CNN-trained models for automated glaucoma evaluation utilizing fundus pictures; VGG16, VGG19, InceptionV3, ResNet50, and XCeption. Using the XCeption architecture, the testing procedure was tested using five public datasets (1707 images), yielded an average AUC of 0.9605 with a 95% confidence range of 95.92–97.07%, an average specificity of 0.8580, and an average sensitivity of 0.9346. Based on data from Heidelberg retina tomography (HRT), a deep neural network model for glaucoma diagnosis has been created [14]. The suggested model achieved a 94.0% AUC, the sensitivities were 91.2 and 78.3% for the two HRT imaging modalities, respectively, with specificities of 0.85 and 0.95. Elangovan and Nath compared and analyzed three different optimizers; stochastic gradient descent with momentum (SGDM), adaptive moment estimation (Adam), and root mean square propagation (RMSProp) for detecting glaucoma from fundus images using three different CNN architectures (AlexNet, VGG-19, and ResNet-101) [15]. The Adam optimizer outperforms the other optimizers in most databases, VGG-19 had the greatest classification accuracy of 91.71, 87.8, and 97.12% for DRISHTI-GS1, RIM-ONE, and LAG databases respectively.

In this study, we proposed a system for glaucoma classification using five classification classes: early, moderate, deep, OHT, and normal. The input is a fundus image obtained from the RIM-ONE r1 dataset [16] using the Convolutional Neural Network (CNN) method and using one of CNN's neural network models, residual neural network (ResNet). ResNet was used in this study because it solved the vanishing gradient problem on CNN models with many deep layers.

## 2 Materials and Method

This study is divided into four stages, the data input stage, the preprocessing stage. The next step is classification using CNN with ResNet-34 architecture. Then the testing stage. This study uses two testing scenarios, the first scenario is the optimizer test, and the second scenario is the epoch value test.

This study obtained a dataset from RIM-ONE r1 in color retinal fundus images with different dimension and .bmp file formats, consist of five classes; deep, early, moderate, OHT and Normal. Due to the limited amount of data in the RIM-ONE r1 dataset, we used data augmentation to enhance the dataset's variation and solved imbalance issues. Random rotation, shearing, zooming, and horizontal flipping were used to enhance the images. Thus, the total image used is 2.156 images. Due to the different sizes of the input images to the network, we resize the images to $50 \times 50$. The purpose of resizing is to make the computing process faster.

CNN is one of the deep learning approaches that has been drawn to this idea in recent years and has grown in prominence [17]. A convolution layer, pooling layer, and fully connected layer compose up a complete CNN architecture. The convolution layer has two main elements: filters (or kernels) and bias. The filters are designed to extract particular characteristics from an image. By lowering the resolution of the activation maps, the Pooling layer offers translation invariance. To create a classification map, the fully connected layer combines the knowledge from all activation maps from the preceding layer [18]. The model we used in this study to train our images is residual network model (ResNet-34). The training process aims to train the ResNet-34 model in recognizing its datasets and classifying them into five classes. As shows in Fig. 3, the model's input comprises of fundus images with a dimension of 50 × 50 × 3 pixels. The model's first layer is a convolutional layer with a 7 × 7 kernel size and 64 filter, then enter the pooling layer, to decrease the image's size. Max pooling used in ResNet34 has a filter size of 3 × 3 and stride 2. The second, third, fourth and fifth phase of the convolution is made up of multiple convolution operations. The first is a convolution with a filter size of 3 × 3, and then three residual modules are stacked on top of each layer. The second layer is convolution with a filter size of 3 × 3, and there are four residual blocks. After the entire convolution process is complete, the size of the feature map is again reduced by using average pooling. The results of each filter will pass through average pooling and enter the fully connected layer with the softmax activation function, which classified into five classes glaucoma.

By comparing the actual label of the input (training dataset) to the predicted label, the model trains the dataset and minimizes the loss value. If the loss value is 0, the model has learned the dataset correctly, theoretically. To achieve the minimum loss value, an optimization algorithm is required. Optimizer is used to improve the learning process on the system. Every optimizer uses specific learning rate values that determine the ability of the system to learn [19]. This study uses three types

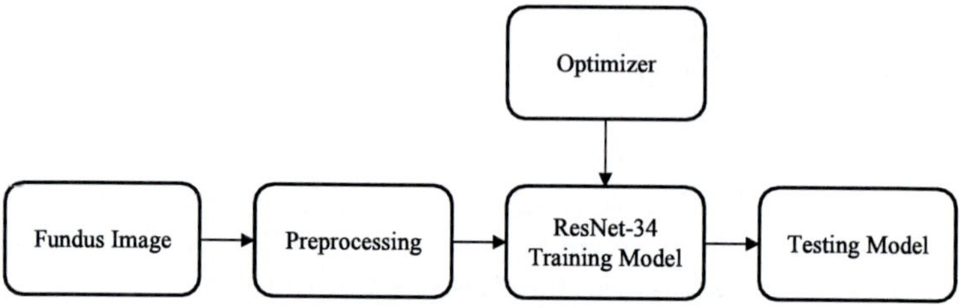


**Fig. 1** Proposed system for Glaucoma classification based on fundus images

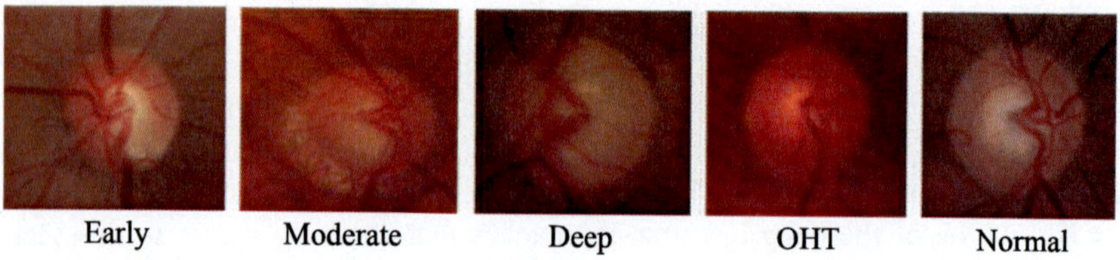


**Fig. 2** Examples five classes of color fundus images from RIM-ONE R1 dataset

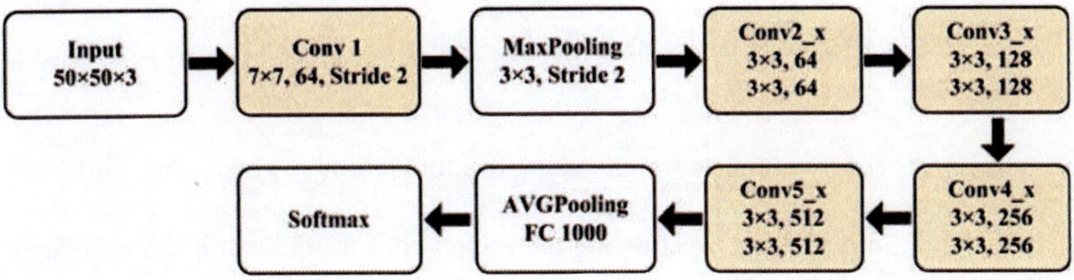


**Fig. 3** ResNet-34 architecture

of the optimizer that are Adaptive Moment Estimation (Adam), Stochastic Gradient Descent (SGD) and Root Mean Square Propagation (RMSprop).

Adam optimizer is a combination of adaptive and momentum methods. Adam is a derivation of the SGD method which is based on first and second time adaptive estimates. The mean value of the previous process gradient will be stored by the Adam optimizer exponentially the same as RMSprop [20].

$$\theta_{t+1} = \theta_t - \frac{\partial}{\sqrt{\hat{v}t + \varepsilon}} .\hat{m}t \tag{1}$$

where $\theta_{t+1}$ is the update result parameter, $\theta_t$ is the result parameter of the previous update, $\hat{m}t$ is the gradient of the square first order moment, $\hat{v}t$ gradient of the square of the order moment second, $\varepsilon$ and is a small scalar to prevent division by zero.

SGD is a variation of optimization gradient descent, constantly updating parameters for each data being trained. The SGD optimizer is a basic optimizer that maintains the learning rate to remember the weights so the learning rate will not change during the training process [20]. The SGD optimizer will calculate each parameter on each data sample that will be randomly sampled. Process parameter update on SGD can be defined on the equation:

$$\theta_{t+1} = \theta_t - \eta * (\theta; (i); (i)) \tag{3}$$

where $\theta_{t+1}$ is the parameter of the update result, $\eta$ is the learning rate hyper parameter, $(i)$ and $(i)$ is the data trained.

Root Mean Square Propagation (RMSprop) is a particular version of Adagrad that performs better on non-convex settings by converting the accumulated gradient to an exponentially weighted moving average [21]. RMSprop was established to address the problem of AdaGrad's learning speed dropping monotonically. Because each successive term is positive, AdaGrad has a flaw in its learning pace, which reduces monotonically. After a certain number of epochs, the learning speed is so slow that the weights are no longer updated [22]. The following equations demonstrate how the RMSprop gradients are calculated:

$$MeanSqu(w, t) = \rho * MeanSquare(w, t-1) + 0.1\left(\frac{\partial \mathrm{E}}{\partial \mathrm{w}}(t)\right) \quad (2)$$

where $w$ is weight, $t$ is timestamp, the value of momentum ($\rho$) is usually set to 0.9, $\frac{\partial \mathrm{E}}{\partial \mathrm{w}}$ is gradient.

Loss function is the key to adjusting neural network training weights to create a better model [23]. Deep neural network training models commonly use cross-entropy loss in (multi-class) classification problems. Loss applied to probability estimates leading to the minimization of the probability from misclassification to the fullest maximization correct labeling [24]. The following equations is standard categorical cross-entropy:

$$l_{CCE} = -\frac{1}{M}\sum_{M=1}^{M}\sum_{k=1}^{k} y_m^k log(h_\theta(x_m, k)) \quad (3)$$

where M is the example number of training, K is the number of classes, $y_m^k$ is the target label for training example, $x$ input training, and $h_\theta$ is model with neural network weights $\theta$.

Confusion matrix is an output matrix from the system's prediction results that describes the system's performance in classifying the input data. From the confusion matrix, various system performance parameters can be calculated to see how well the system model designed is performing the classification task [25]. Multiclass confusion matrix is used for classifying three or more classes. There are four terms as a representation of the results of the classification process in a multiclass confusion matrix as following:

TP (True Positive) is the number of data in the actual positive class and the positive prediction class.
FP (False Positive) is the amount of data in the actual class with the actual negative value and the positive prediction class.
FN (False Negative) is the number of data in the actual class with the actual positive value and the negative class prediction.
TN (True Negative) is the number of data in the actual class with the actual negative value and the negative prediction class.

The following are the performance metrics on a multiclass confusion matrix. From the confusion matrix, accuracy, precision, recall, and f1-score can be calculated to evaluate the system's performance.

$$Accuracy = \frac{TTP_{all} + TTN_{all}}{totalnumberoftestingentries} \quad (4)$$

$$Precision = \frac{TTP_{all}}{TTP_{all} + TTF_i} \quad (5)$$

$$Recall = \frac{TTP_{all}}{TTP_{all} + TFN_i} \quad (6)$$

$$F1 - Score = 2 \times \frac{(Precission \times Sensitivity)}{Precission + Sensitivity} \quad (7)$$

## 3 Result

In this study, the data were trained using a CNN model with ResNet-34 architecture to find the best optimizer, either Adam, SGD, or RMSprop. In addition to evaluating the effects of utilizing different optimizers, the study also investigated the impact of the testing-to-training data ratio. The hyper-parameters utilized in this scenario are learning rate 0.001, batch size 32, and epoch 25. Figures 4 and 5 shows test results of comparison of training and testing data on the different optimizer.

This test shows that Adam has training accuracy 94%, testing accuracy 89%, training loss 0.05, and testing loss 0.13. SGD has training accuracy of 41%, test accuracy 43%, training loss 0.43, and test loss 0.43.

Meanwhile, the results of RMSprop are not too different because Adam is a combination of RMSprop and Momentum. RMSprop has 91% for training accuracy, accuracy testing 80%, training loss 0.12, and testing loss 0.23. Figures 6 and 7 shows test results of the epoch value.

This test shows that the number of epochs experienced a saturation point when the epochs were valued at 75 and 100.

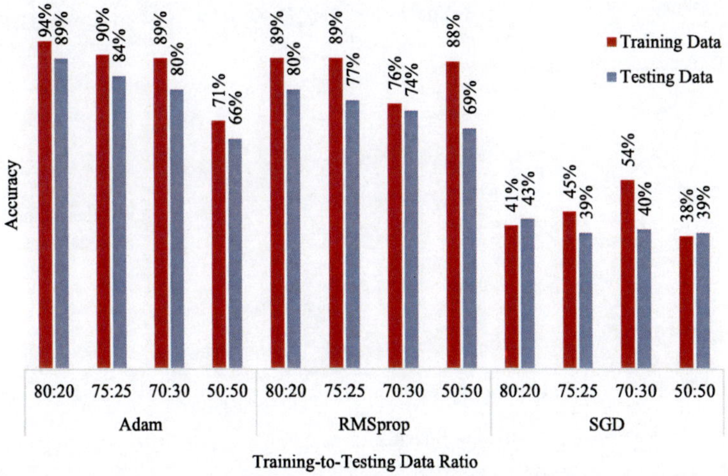


**Fig. 4** The accuracy over comparison of training and testing data on different optimizer

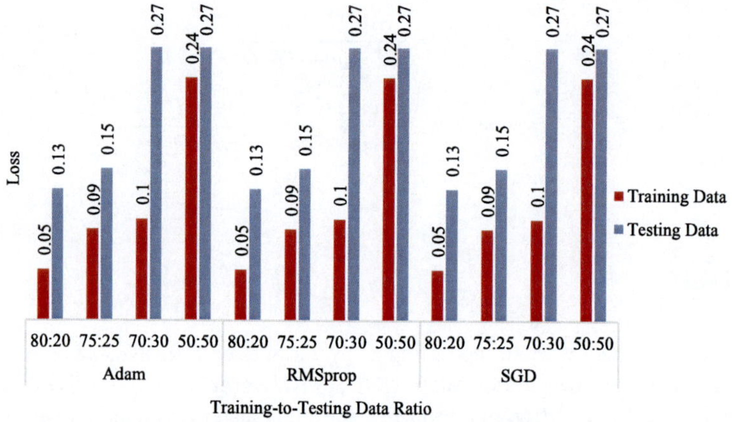


**Fig. 5** The loss over comparison of training and testing data on different optimizer

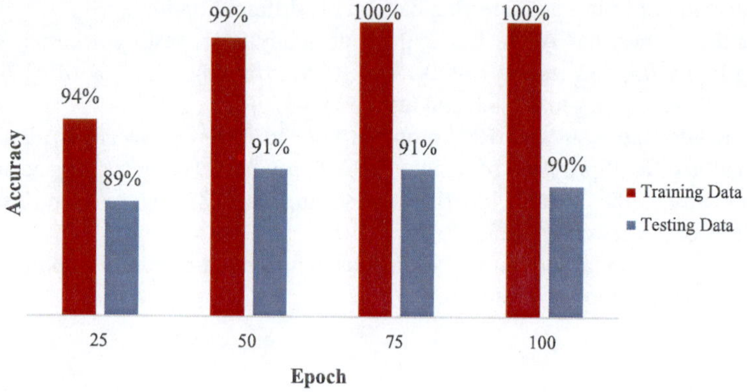


**Fig. 6** The accuracy over epoch

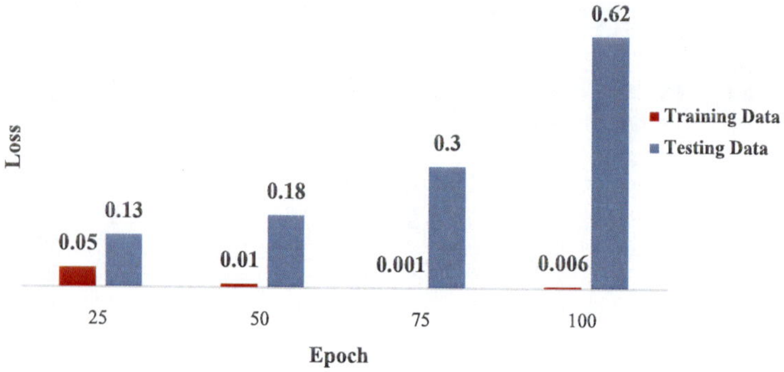


**Fig. 7** The loss over epoch

## 4 Discussion

According to the results shown in Figs. 4 and 5, it can be seen that Adam gets the best accuracy and the lowest loss value with a comparison ratio of 80% training data and 20% test data from the total data. Adam is considered as the best optimizer for classifying glaucoma using the CNN model with the ResNet-34 architecture. From Figs. 6 and 7, the epoch value of 50 was chosen as the most optimal test result, which has a good accuracy rate of 99% for training accuracy and 91% for testing and has the lowest loss value of 0.001 for training 0.18 for testing. This test shows that the number of epochs experienced a saturation point when the epochs were valued at 75 and 100. This indicates that the addition of more epoch will not significantly affect system performance. Table 1, shows the confusion matrix for the system model with the Adam optimizer. It can be seen that of the 431 validation images used, 391 were classified correctly according to class, and 40 were classified incorrectly according to their class.

Table 2 shows the detail performance of model using Adam optimizer with learning rate of 0.001 and epoch 50.

Based on the data shown in Table 2, the system performance parameter values obtained in this study are good because the results are close to 100%, so it can be concluded that the model proposed in this study, namely CNN with ResNet-34 architecture, can classify glaucoma into five classes: early, medium. OHT, and normal with high accuracy and minimum loss value.

Several previous studies have performed automatic glaucoma detection using fundus images with different methods but only used two classification classes. The

**Table 1** The confusion matrix for proposed ResNet-34 Glaucoma classification

| | | Predicted | | | | |
|---|---|---|---|---|---|---|
| | | Deep | Early | Moderate | OHT | Normal |
| Actual | Deep | 79 | 8 | 3 | 1 | 3 |
| | Early | 0 | 66 | 2 | 0 | 4 |
| | Moderate | 5 | 6 | 77 | 0 | 0 |
| | OHT | 1 | 0 | 0 | 93 | 6 |
| | Normal | 0 | 1 | 0 | 0 | 76 |

**Table 2** Details performance of ResNet-34 model

| Class | Accuracy (%) | Precision (%) | Recall (%) | F-1 score (%) |
|---|---|---|---|---|
| Deep | 84 | 93 | 83 | 88 |
| Early | 92 | 81 | 92 | 86 |
| Moderate | 86 | 93 | 88 | 90 |
| OHT | 93 | 85 | 99 | 92 |
| Normal | 99 | 99 | 93 | 96 |

**Table 3** Performance of prior research compared to proposed system

| Method | Dataset | Class | Performance |
|---|---|---|---|
| Combined CNN and RNN [8] | 1810 Fundus images and 295 fundus video | Two classes (Glaucoma vs. healthy) | Mean-F 92.6% |
| Residual network-50 [9] | 78 Fundus images | Two classes (Glaucoma vs. normal) | Accuracy of 96.95% |
| Standard CNN, VGG19, ResNet50, DENet, and GoogLeNet [10] | 2313 Fundus images | Two classes (Glaucoma vs. normal) | 0.94 AUC, 87.01% Sensitivity and 89.01% specificity |
| Proposed method (residual network-34) | 2156 Fundus images | Five classes (deep, early, moderate. OHT, and normal | Accuracy of 99% and loss of 0.01 |

method proposed in this study uses ResNet-34 to classify glaucoma using five glaucoma classes. Based on Table 3, this study shows a good level of performance by using a more significant number of classes. This study has limitations in that the current system only uses fully connected as a classifier and has not tried to analyze different classifiers (e.g., KNN, SVM, Naive Bayes, Decision Tree, etc.).

The research implies that the proposed system has a good performance. It takes endurance of clinical trials to eventually become one of the problem solvers to facilitate caregiver performance in diagnosing glaucoma.

## 5 Conclusion

Glaucoma is a chronic eye disorder that can cause blindness, if not detected early. For this reason, automatic glaucoma detection is needed. CNN model with ResNet-34 architecture was chosen to build a system that can classify glaucoma into five classes. The CNN model with the ResNet-34 architecture proposed in this study is quite good in classifying glaucoma into five classes, namely deep, early, moderate, OHT, and normal. The system can classify glaucoma into five classes with 91% accuracy for testing and 99% for training. The loss obtained is 0.013 for testing and 0.18 for training. These results are obtained by using the Adam optimizer with a ratio of training-to-testing data 80:20. In further research, a system can be developed to classify glaucoma with more data and types of class. The system is expected to be clinically tested in a real environment.

## References


1. Weinreb RN, Aung T, Medeiros FA (2014) The pathophysiology and treatment of glaucoma: a review. JAMA311(18):1901–1911
2. Benzebouchi NE, Azizi N, Bouzine SE (2018) Glaucoma diagnosis using cooperative convolutional. Int J Adv Electron Comp Sci 5(1):38
3. Allison K, Patel D, Alabi O (2020) Epidemiology of Glaucoma: the past, present, and predictions for the future. Cureus12(11):e11686
4. Nikam SM, Patil CY (2017) Glaucoma detection from fundus images using MATLAB GUI. In: 2017 3rd international conference on advances in computing, communication and automation (ICACCA) (fall), 2017, pp 1–4
5. Yang R, Yu Y (2021) Artificial convolutional neural network in object detection and semantic segmentation for medical imaging analysis. Front Oncol 11:638182
6. Lundervold AS, Lundervold A (2019) An overview of deep learning in medical imaging focusing on MRI. Z Med Phys 29(2):102–127
7. Wang J, Zhu H, Wang SH, Zhang YD (2021) A review of deep learning on medical image analysis. Mob Netw Appl 26
8. Fu H, Xu Y, Wong DWK, Liu J (2016) Retinal vessel segmentation via deep learning network and fully-connected conditional random fields. In: 2016 IEEE 13th international symposium on biomedical imaging (ISBI), pp 698–701
9. Chen X, Xu Y, Wong DWK, Wong TY, Liu J (2015) Glaucoma detection based on deep convolutional neural network. In: 37th annual international conference of the IEEE engineering in medicine and biology society (EMBC)
10. Gheisari S, Shariflou S, Phu J, Kennedy P, Agar A, Kalloniatis M, Golzan SM (2021) A combined convolutional and recurrent neural network for enhanced glaucoma detection. Sci Rep
11. Ovreiu S, Cristescu I, Balta F, Sultana A, Ovreiu E (2020) Early detection of Glaucoma using residual networks. In: 2020 13th international conference on communications (COMM), pp 161–164
12. Gómez-Valverde JJ et al (2019) Automatic glaucoma classification using color fundus images based on convolutional neural networks and transfer learning. Biomed Opt Expr 10(2):892
13. Diaz-Pinto A, Morales S, Naranjo V, Köhler T, Mossi JM, Navea A (2019) CNNs for automatic Glaucoma assessment using fundus images: an extensive validation. Biomed Eng Online 18(1):1–19
14. Wang H, Hu J, Zhang J (2021) SCRD-Net: a deep convolutional neural network model for Glaucoma detection in retina tomography, complexity
15. Elangovan P, Nath MK (2021) Performance analysis of optimizers for Glaucoma diagnosis from fundus images using transfer learning. In: Gopi ES (eds) Machine learning, deep learning and computational intelligence for wireless communication. Lecture notes in electrical engineering, Vol 749, pp 507–518
16. Fumero F, Alayon S, Sanchez JL, Sigut J, Hernandez MG (2011) RIM-ONE: an open retinal image database for optic nerve evalution. In: International symposium on computer-based medical systems (CBMS), Briston
17. Bera S, Shrivastava VK (2020) Analysis of various optimizers on deep convolutional neural network model in the application of hyperspectral remote sensing image classification. Int J Rem Sens 41(7):2664–2683
18. Rawat W, Wang Z (2017) Deep convolutional neural networks for image classification: a comprehensive review. Neural Comput 29(9):2352–2449
19. Kandel I, Castelli M, Popovič A (2020) Comparative study of first order optimizers for image classification using convolutional neural networks on histopathology images. J Imaging 6(9):92
20. Ruder S (2016) An overview of gradient descent optimization algorithms. arXiv:1609.04747
21. Sharma N, Sharma K, Bhatnagar S, Sharma D, Vij D (2019) Digit classification using convolutional neural network. Int J Eng Res Technol (IJERT) 08(11)

22. Jangid M, Srivastava S (2019) Deep convnet with different stochastic optimizations for handwritten devanagari character. Proc IC4S 1
23. Ho Y, Wookey S (2019) The real-world-weight cross-entropy loss function: modeling the costs of mislabeling. IEEE Access, pp 1–1
24. Rodriguez EG, Ganem GL, Pleiss G, Cunningham JP (2020) Uses and abuses of the cross-entropy loss: case studies in modern deep learning
25. Manliguez C (2016) Generalized confusion matrix for multiple classes

# State-of-the-Art Method Denoising Electrocardiogram Signal: A Review

**Anita Miftahul Maghfiroh, Syevana Dita Musvika, Levana Forra Wakidi, Dyah Titisari, Singgih Yudha Setiawan, Farid Amrinsani, and Dandi Hafidh Azhari**

**Abstract** Electrocardiography is a device used to record the electrical performance of the heart. ECG signals have a very important role in diagnosing various heart diseases. Signal disturbances are often a significant concern in denoising ECG signals that affect diagnostic readings of heart disease. From this explanation, an appropriate denoising method is needed to get a real signal visualization. The purpose of this paper is to provide a specific description of the ECG signal denoising method to make it easier for other researchers to develop the denoising method. The denoising method discussed in this article focuses more on deep learning methods and the decomposition process, data collection, and analysis of each method are collected from several references from several articles on ECG signal denoising. The results showed that the deep learning method used for denoising the MSE value was 0.167 and the cross-correlation was 0.476. While the average value of the SNR with the decomposition method is 7.75. The benefit for further researchers is that they can process ECG signals accurately without signal denoising, so that signal analysis for the diagnosis of heart disease can be read accurately.

**Keywords** ECG signal · Denoising · Review

## 1 Introduction

Electrocardiography is a tool that is used to record the electrical performance of the heart [1, 2]. ECG signal is a non-stationary biomedical signal, the ECG signal has a frequency that changes with time according to the physiological events of the heart. Information about the work of the heart can be obtained through the principle of electricity in the heart. Electrocardiography (ECG) has an important role in the process of monitoring and preventing heart attacks [3]. ECG signals have a very important role in diagnosing various heart diseases [4]. The frequency of the ECG

A. M. Maghfiroh (✉) · S. D. Musvika · L. F. Wakidi · D. Titisari · S. Y. Setiawan · F. Amrinsani · D. H. Azhari
Poltekkes Kemenkes Surabaya, Jl. Pucang Jajar Tengah No. 56, Surabaya 60283, Indonesia
e-mail: anitamiftah@poltekkesdepkes-sby.ac.id



T. Triwiyanto et al. (eds.), *Proceedings of the 2nd International Conference on Electronics, Biomedical Engineering, and Health Informatics*, Lecture Notes in Electrical Engineering 898, https://doi.org/10.1007/978-981-19-1804-9_24

signal has a bandwidth in the range of 0.05–100 Hz, to get the right ECG signal reading, an appropriate method is needed for signal analysis, one of which is the detection of R peaks [5], and an appropriate denoising method is needed to get a real signal visualization. Denoising is a method for estimating an unknown true signal from a signal that has been corrupted by noise [6]. The purpose of denoising is to reduce noise in the original image to minimize loss of original features and improve signal-to-noise ratio (SNR) [7]. Many factors affect the quality of the ECG signal, including noise interference and movement artifacts that can affect the P and Q signals from the original signal [8] so the denoising method is very important to overcome these problems to get a real signal visualization. Several methods have been used by several researchers to remove noise interference in the ECG signal. To obtain an ECG signal in lead I, lead II, and lead III electrodes are positioned according to the Eintovhen triangle rule [1]. Carlos Lastre et al., method of shifting unbiased finite impulse response filter (UFIR) was used for feature extraction of ECG signal denoising [4]. This algorithm is quite good in reducing noise to be smooth with a $p$-value $< 0$. However, the computations used are quite heavy. The decomposition method is also still being developed by researchers to reduce noise in the ECG signal [9–13]. The decomposition algorithm is considered efficient for reducing noise in the ECG signal. Broadly speaking, the Ensemble Empirical Mode Decomposition (EEMD) method system consists of (1) Target data added with noise (2) then the data is decomposed into IMFs (3) then steps 1 and 2 are repeated continuously by adding each time the white series different noise (4) The next step means of ensemble IMFs with appropriate decomposition values is used as the final result [13]. Deep learning methods were also developed for signal processing [14], several deep learning methods including Convolutional Neural Network (CNN) and a Long Short-Term Memory (LSTM) model were used for denoising ECG signals with the average RMS error = 0.0299.

The conventional denoising process is also carried out with an analog filter design [15] to eliminate the noise frequency by Rodbing Lundberg [16]. The experiment is to eliminate noise interference on the sound wave by estimating the frequency disturbance and then given an adaptive notch filter to be able to reduce noise interference. From the several studies mentioned, it proves that there have been many researchers discussing the ECG signal denoising process algorithm with their respective advantages and disadvantages. Therefore, a special study is needed to discuss these methods further. To make it easier for other authors to develop an ECG signal denoising method to produce an accurate ECG signal.

## 2 State-of-the-Art

In this section the author will discuss several methods in more detail, the methods discussed are Deep learning and decomposition methods. Figure 1 is an example of a signal before and after the denoising process.

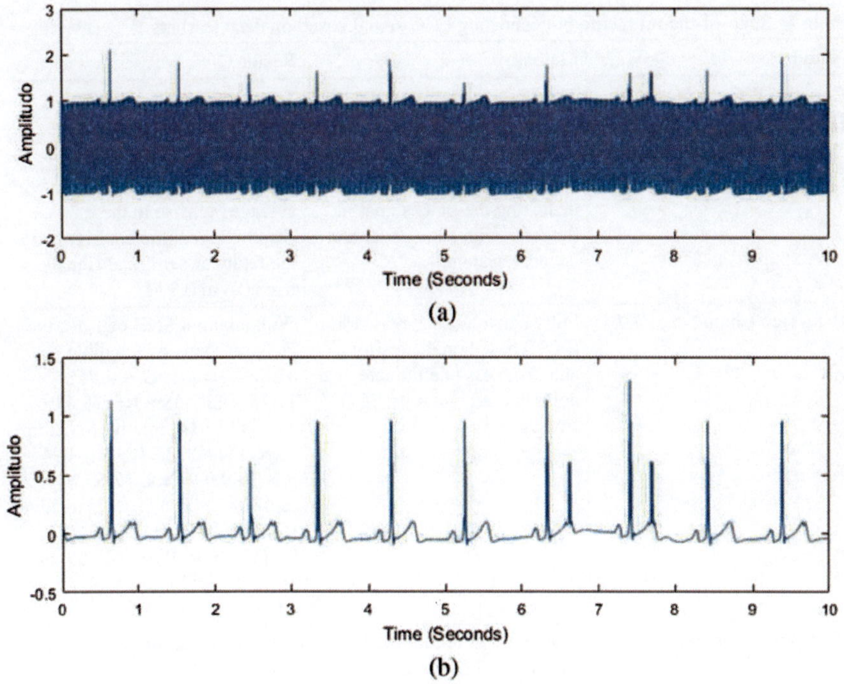


**Fig. 1** **a** ECG signal due to 50 **Hz** frequency interference **b** ECG signal denosing with digital filter

In figure it is explained that the ECG before the denosing process contained 50 Hz frequency interference from the power lines, then the denoising process was carried out using a digital IIR filter [17].

## *2.1 Denoising Based Deep Learning*

Convolutional Neural Networks (CNNs) models are used by several researchers to eliminate denoising with deep learning methods. Table 1 describes the state-of-the-art method for denoising ECG signals based on deep learning.

CNNs model used by Corneliu T. C. Arsene et al. for denoising the ECG signal [18] the denoising process used six convolution and two-dimensional layers, each layer has 36 filters with a kernel size of 19 × 1 per filter.

The data set used consists of 3 datasets, namely: consisting of 2 synthetic data generated by soft [25], while the third data was obtained from the real data set. Each data set is divided into two, namely test data (1/4) and (3/4) are datasets for practice. The first synthetic dataset has 6888 clean ECG signal with time duration of 10 s

**Table 1** State-of-the-art method to denoising ECG signal based on deep learning

| Author | Method | Result |
|---|---|---|
| Corneliu T. C. Arsene et al. [18] | The CNN model is used with six convolution and two-dimensional layers | The test results using 200 epochs resulted in an average RMS = 0.0299 |
| Eleni Fotiadou et al. [19] | Deep convolutional is used for denoising the ECG signal in the fetus with an encoder and decoder system | The test results produce an average increase in the correlation coefficient between the faulty and original signals from 0.6 to 0.8 M |
| Hsin-Tien Chiang et al. [20] | Fully convolutional network (FCN) based on denoising autoencoders to eliminate noise caused by faulty ECG signals | With an input SNR of 1 dB, the FCN reached an incredible 31.83% [= (15.49 – 1.75) / 11.75] and 9.55% [= (15.49 – 14.14) / 14.14] relative SNRimp increase and 32.98% [=(0.094 – 0.063)/ 0.094] and 12.50% [= (0.072 – 0.063) / 0.072] relative RMSE reduction and 36.29% [= (30.89 – 19.68) / 30.89] and 14.77% [= (23.09–1968) / 23.09] |
| Zhongyao Zhao et al. [21] | Combination of modified frequency slice wavelet transform (MFSWT) and convolutional neural network (CNN) for signal denoising | The level of accuracy obtained is 86.3% |
| Tanvir Mahmud et al. [22] | DeepArrNet (CNN) is used for automatic detection of arrhythmia classification of denoised ECG signals | The level of accuracy obtained is 99.28% |
| Wei Zhao et al. [23] | Deep learning method is used to classify arrhythmia ECG signals | The overall accuracy was 98.6% and sensitivity of N, S, V, F were 99.4%, 85.4%, 96.6%, 90.6% respectively |
| Pratik Singh et al. [24] | GAN-based CNN is used to denoise the ECG signal | Average RMSE value 0.17 |

with 30,000 samples per ECG signal. The sampling frequency is 3000 Hz, with time variations from 57 to 67 heart beats per minute as test case scenario.

An LSTM model with two layers and 140 hidden nodes is also used [18]. Of the two models, CNN is superior to LSTM with an average value of RMS = 0.0299. The structure of the CNNs model is described in Fig. 2. The CNN model used is the Adam optimizer with a training batch size of 300 with an average Root Mean Squared (RMS) error of 0.0346 with 40 training epochs and to get RMS = 0.0299 iterations are carried out up to 200 epochs with a duration of 58 min.

The explanation of the CNN system is described in the diagram block in Fig. 3.

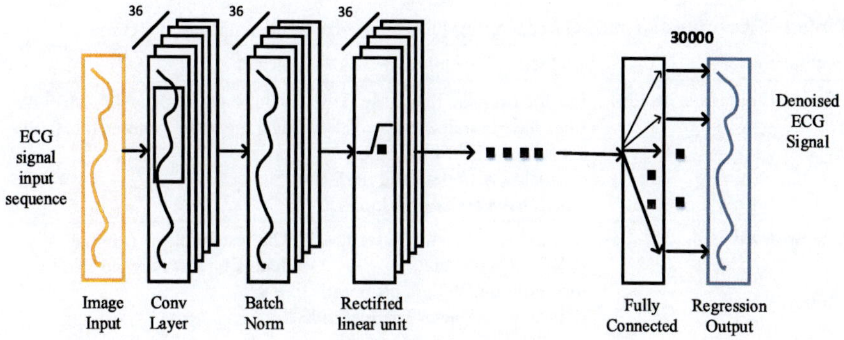


**Fig. 2** CNN's deep learning model structure [18]

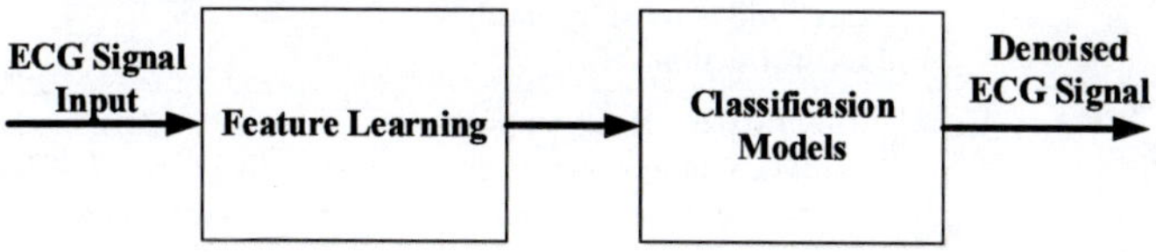


**Fig. 3** Diagram block CNN system

Figure 3 describes the ECG signal input through feature learning, feature learning or also known as feature extraction. In this section, the encoding process is carried out from an image to features in the form of numbers that represent the image (ECG signal) as described in Fig. 2. The feature extraction layer consists of two parts. Convolutional Layer and Pooling Layer. In the discussion of this article only use the Convolutional Layer. After the learning process, the next process is classification and then the output is a real ECG signal.

## *2.2 Denoising Based Decomposition Method*

The method of discrete wavelet transform (DWT) decomposition is used by researchers to remove denoising [26–29]. The approximation process to level-2 is then used for signal denoising using soft thresholding. This process resulted in a fairly good approach with an average MSE value = 0.002 [26]. Table 2 describes the state-of-the-art method for denoising the ECG signal based on the decomposition method.

DWT analyzes signals in different frequency bands with different resolutions by breaking down the signal into rough approximations and detailed information. DWT uses two sets of functions, called scale functions and wavelet functions, which are related to low pass and high pass filters [37]. In the decomposition of the signal in the frequency band, there are high pass and low pass filters which are signals based

**Table 2** State-of-the-art method to denoising ECG signal-based decomposition method

| Author | Method | Result |
|---|---|---|
| Yaprak Eminaga et al. [30] | Infinite Impulse Response (IIR) filter based on discrete wavelet transform (DWT) for ECG denoising with ilet3 and ilet5 which have better performance | With input SNR = 4db MSE the average value generated is 0.004 |
| Xiaowen Xu et al. [31] | Empirical wavelet transform (EWT) and wavelet thresholding (WT) is proposed to remove artifacts. The method consists of five steps, namely spectrum preprocessing, spectrum segmentation, EWT decomposition, wavelet threshold denoising, and EWT reconstruction | The results of the average denoising test resulted in SNR = 9.74 |
| Dengyong Zhang et al. [32] | Empirical mode decomposition (EMD), sample entropy, and increasing threshold function were used to approach denoising the ECG signal | The results of the input SNR dB 10 with a data set of 100 obtained the value of Proposed = 7.75, NLM = 6.85 and CEEMDAN = 6.04 |
| P. Karthikeyan et al. [33] | Discrete wavelet transform (DWT) is used for denoising with mother wavelets (db4, coif5 and sym7) | Mother wavelet coif 5 is said to have the best performance compared to db4 and sym7 |
| Young In Jang et all [34] | Selection of the right mother wavelet for the decomposition method to eliminate signal denoising. It is proven that the db9 and sym9 type mother wavelets have better performance than other types of mother wavelets | SNR performance result db9 = 35,726 level 7 |
| Reeta Devi et al. [35] | Comparison of three methods used for LMS, RLS and DWT. denoising techniques | Better filter performance with 2db SNR value |
| Udit Satija et al. [36] | The denosing of the ECG signal is decomposed using the method consists of the modified ensemble empirical mode decomposition (CEEMD) then feature extraction and classification to produce a real ECG signal | Average sensitivity 99.12%, specificity 98.56%, and overall accuracy by 98.90% |

on the time domain. The original x[n] signal is first passed through a half-band high pass filter denoted g[n] and a lowpass filter h[n]. After filtering, half of the sample can be omitted, since the signal has the highest frequency of π / 2 radians instead of π [38]. Therefore, the signal can be added to a new sample by removing every other sample. This process is one level of decomposition and can be mathematically expressed in Eq. 1

$$\mathrm{yhigh}[k] = \sum_{n} x[n].g[2k - n]$$
$$\mathrm{ylow}[k] = \sum_{n} x[n].h[2k - n] \tag{1}$$

In Fig. 4 it is explained about the wavelet decomposition process by breaking the signal into approximation coefficients ($y_{low}$) and detailed information ($y_{high}$).

The dataset used for the ECG signal denoising process using the DWT method is the MIT-BIH database in MATLAB, simulation experiments and comparisons are carried out by selecting different thresholds of wavelet coefficients at different scales [39]. Schematic discrete wavelet transforms (DWT) to remove noise there are three stages to overcome the denoising of the ECG signal which is described in Fig. 5.

In the first stage, the wavelet decomposition is chosen to eliminate de-noising by selecting the wavelet coefficient, then the second stage of the wavelet threshold process is carried out to obtain the wavelet coefficient. The third stage is a signal reconstruction after the threshold denoising process which results in denoising the y(n) signal.

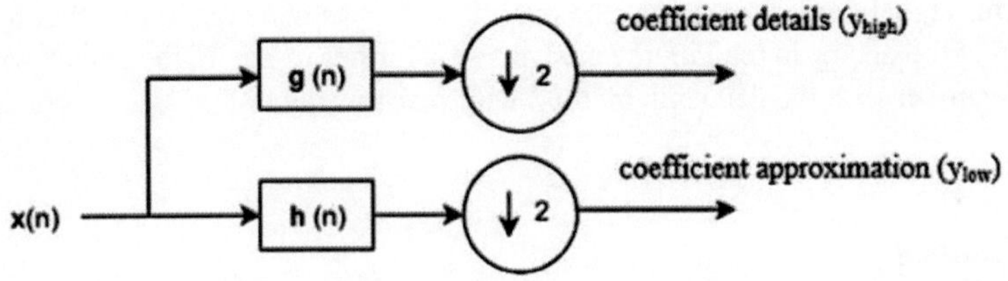


**Fig. 4** Block diagram of the decomposition process

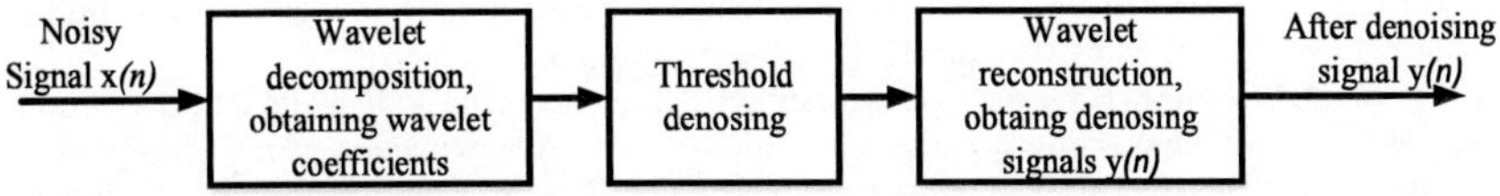


**Fig. 5** DWT schematic for denoising process

## 3 Discussion

In some of the methods discussed by the author in the previous chapter, it was found that the CNN Deep learning model method takes 58 min and 200 epochs to achieve better results on the test dataset by producing an average RMS value = 0.0299 [18]. Meanwhile, in the wavelet decomposition method, it is explained that the simulation results show that the improved threshold algorithm is effective in eliminating noise and produces better and more efficient visual effects [39]. Of the two methods, each has its own advantages and disadvantages, the deep learning method has high accuracy but has a long learning time, whereas the decomposition method has a fairly good performance for denoising EK signals with time efficiency.

## 4 Conclusion

This article aims to review the development of the ECG signal denoising algorithm from several researchers with its advantages and disadvantages. As in the deep learning method used for the denoising process, the MSE value is 0.167 and the cross-correlation is 0.476. The deep learning method is considered capable of signal denoising with a high level of accuracy, but the data training process takes a long time. Meanwhile, for the decomposition method, the average value of SNR is 7.75. This method is also considered capable of denoising signals with good SNR levels, but the computation of this decomposition method is quite heavy. However, several things can be improved by further researchers, namely the selection of the right algorithm for signal denoising so that the output signal has good quality so that it does not affect the doctor in reading the analysis. For further research, the author will try to experiment with the denosing method with real-time work.

## References


1. Wilkins LW (2011) ECG interpretation made incredibly easy! (5th edn). Pdf, pp 1–174
2. Diah Zuhroini R, Titisari D, Hamzah T, Kho TK (2021) A two channels wireless electrocardiograph system using bluetooth communication. J Electron Electromed Eng Med Inform 3(3):134–140. doi: https://doi.org/10.35882/jeeemi.v3i3.3
3. Labate D, La Foresta F, Occhiuto G, Morabito FC, Lay-Ekuakille A, Vergallo P (2013) Empirical mode decomposition vs. wavelet decomposition for the extraction of respiratory signal from single-channel ECG: a comparison. IEEE Sens J 13(7):2666–2674. doi: https://doi.org/10.1109/JSEN.2013.2257742
4. Lastre-Domínguez C, Shmaliy YS, Ibarra-Manzano O, Munoz-Minjares J, Morales-Mendoza LJ (2019) ECG signal denoising and features extraction using unbiased FIR smoothing. Biomed Res Int. doi: https://doi.org/10.1155/2019/2608547
5. Maghfiroh AM et al (2021) State-of-the-art method to detect r-peak on electrocardiogram signal: a review 10:321–329. https://doi.org/10.1007/978-981-33-6926-9_27

6. Taswell C (2000) The what how, and why of wavelet shrinkage denoising. Comput Sci Eng 2(3):12–19. doi: https://doi.org/10.1109/5992.841791
7. Fan L, Zhang F, Fan H, Zhang C (2019) Brief review of image denoising techniques. Pdf 7
8. Aiboud Y, El Mhamdi J, Jilbab A, Sbaa H (2016) Review of ECG signal de-noising techniques. In: Proceedings of the 2015 IEEE world conference on complex system. WCCS 2015. doi: https://doi.org/10.1109/ICoCS.2015.7483313
9. Singh P, Shahnawazuddin S, Pradhan G (2017) Significance of modified empirical mode decomposition for ECG denoising. In: Proceedings of the annual international conference on IEEE engineering medical biological society EMBS, pp 2956–2959. doi: https://doi.org/10.1109/EMBC.2017.8037477
10. Mohguen W, Bekka RE (2019) Comparative study of ECG signal denoising by empirical mode decomposition and thresholding functions. In: Proceedings of the 6th international conference on electrical and electronics engineering ICEEE 2019, pp 126–130. doi: https://doi.org/10.1109/ICEEE2019.2019.00032
11. Karagiannis A, Constantinou P (2011) Noise-assisted data processing with empirical mode decomposition in biomedical signals. IEEE Trans Inf Technol Biomed 15(1):11–18. doi: https://doi.org/10.1109/TITB.2010.2091648
12. Jain S, Bajaj V, Kumar A, Liouvelle R (2018) Fractional integral based empirical mode decomposition for ECG Denoising. IEEE J Biomed Heal Inform 22(4):1133–1139. doi: https://doi.org/10.1109/JBHI.2017.2753321
13. Gandham S, Anuradha B (2016) An iterative method of ensemble empirical mode decomposition for enhanced ECG signal denoising. In: Proceedings of the International Conference on Wireless Communication, Signal Process, Networking, WiSPNET 2016, IEEE, pp 1477–1480. doi: https://doi.org/10.1109/WiSPNET.2016.7566382
14. Kido K et al (2019) A novel CNN-based framework for classification of signal quality and sleep position from a capacitive ECG measurement. Sensors (Switzerland) 19(7). doi: https://doi.org/10.3390/s19071731
15. Chen B, Li Y, Cao X, Sun W, He W (2019) Removal of power line interference from ECG signals using adaptive notch filters of sharp resolution. IEEE Access 7:150667–150676. doi: https://doi.org/10.1109/ACCESS.2019.2944027
16. Lundberg R (2017) Notch filters for removing common noise frequencies
17. Rachman RA, Wisana IDGH, Nugraha PC (2021) Development of a low-cost and effisient ECG devices with IIR digital filter design. Indones J Electron Electromed Eng Med Inform 3(1):21–28. https://doi.org/10.35882/ijeeemi.v3i1.4
18. Arsene CTC, Hankins R, Yin H (2019) Deep learning models for denoising ECG signals. Eur Signal Process Conf 220:1–5. doi: https://doi.org/10.23919/EUSIPCO.2019.8902833
19. Fotiadou E, Konopczyński T, Hesser J, Vullings R (2019) Deep convolutional encoder-decoder framework for fetal ECG signal denoising. Comput Cardiol Conf 45:1–4. doi: https://doi.org/10.22489/cinc.2019.015
20. Chiang HT, Hsieh YY, Fu SW, Hung KH, Tsao Y, Chien SY (2019) Noise reduction in ECG signals using fully convolutional denoising autoencoders. IEEE Access 7:60806–60813. doi: https://doi.org/10.1109/ACCESS.2019.2912036
21. Zhao Z et al (2019) Noise rejection for wearable ECGs using modified frequency slice wavelet transform and convolutional neural networks. IEEE Access 7:34060–34067. https://doi.org/10.1109/ACCESS.2019.2900719
22. Mahmud T, Fattah SA, Saquib M (2020) DeepArrNet: an efficient deep CNN architecture for automatic arrhythmia detection and classification from denoised ECG beats. IEEE Access 8:104788–104800. doi: https://doi.org/10.1109/ACCESS.2020.2998788
23. Zhao W et al (2019) Deep learning based patient-specific classification of arrhythmia on ECG signal. Proc Annu Int Conf IEEE Eng Med Biol Soc EMBS, 1500–1503. doi: https://doi.org/10.1109/EMBC.2019.8856650
24. Singh P, Pradhan G (2021) A new ECG denoising framework using generative adversarial network. IEEE/ACM Trans Comput Biol Bioinform 18(2):759–764. doi: https://doi.org/10.1109/TCBB.2020.2976981

25. Kumar GA, Tech M, Vegi S, Year BTF (2015) Analyzing of an ECG signal mathematically by generating ii:39–44
26. Singh P, Pradhan G (2018) Significance of non-local means estimation in DWT based ECG signal denoising. In: 2018 5th international conference on signal processing integra networks, SPIN 2018, pp 18–22. doi: https://doi.org/10.1109/SPIN.2018.8474133
27. Ranjeet K, Farida (2011) Retained signal energy based optimal wavelet selection for denoising of ECG signal using modifide thresholding. In: International conference on multimedia, signal processing and communication technology IMPACT 2011, no 1, pp 196–199. doi: https://doi.org/10.1109/MSPCT.2011.6150473
28. Castillo E, Morales DP, García A, Martínez-Martí F, Parrilla L, Palma AJ (2013) Noise suppression in ECG signals through efficient one-step wavelet processing techniques. J Appl Math. doi: https://doi.org/10.1155/2013/763903
29. Mure T, Wavelet transform based ECG signal filtering, pp 90–93
30. Eminaga Y, Coskun A, Kale I (2018) IIR wavelet filter banks for ECG signal denoising. Sign Proc Algor Archit Arrange Appl Conf Proceed SPA 5:130–133. doi: https://doi.org/10.23919/SPA.2018.8563418
31. Xu X, Liang Y, Yang J, He P (2019) Adaptive motion artifact reduction based on empirical wavelet transform and wavelet thresholding for the non-contact ECG monitoring systems
32. Zhang D et al (2020) An efficient ECG denoising method based on empirical mode decomposition, sample entropy, and improved threshold function. Wirel Commun Mob Comput 2020. doi: https://doi.org/10.1155/2020/8811962
33. Karthikeyan P, Murugappan M, Yaacob S (2012) ECG signal denoising using wavelet thresholding techniques in human stress assessment. Int J Electr Eng Inform 4(2):306–319. doi: https://doi.org/10.15676/ijeei.2012.4.2.9
34. Jang YI, Sim JY, Yang JR, Kwon NK (2021) The optimal selection of mother wavelet function and decomposition level for denoising of DCG signal. Sensors 21(5):1–17. doi: https://doi.org/10.3390/s21051851
35. Devi R, Tyagi HK, Kumar D (2019) Performance comparison and applications of sparsity based techniques for denoising of ECG signal. In: 2019 6th international conference on signal process. Integra Networks, SPIN 2019, pp 346–351. doi: https://doi.org/10.1109/SPIN.2019.8711632
36. Satija U, Ramkumar B, Manikandan MS (2018) Automated ECG noise detection and classification system for unsupervised healthcare monitoring. IEEE J Biomed Heal Inform 22(3):722–732. doi: https://doi.org/10.1109/JBHI.2017.2686436
37. Polikar R (1994) The wavelet tutorial. Internet Resour. httpengineering rowan edu polikarWAVELETSWTtutorial html, pp 1–67. doi: https://doi.org/10.1088/1751-8113/44/8/085201
38. Maghfiroh AM, Arifin A, Sardjono TA (2019) Wavelet-based respiratory rate estimation using electrocardiogram. In: Proceedings of the international seminar on intelligent technology its application ISITIA 2019, pp 354–359. doi: https://doi.org/10.1109/ISITIA.2019.8937201
39. Zhang J, Lin JL, Li XL, Wang WQ (2017) ECG signals denoising method based on improved wavelet threshold algorithm. In: Proceedings of the advanced information management, communication, electronic, automatics control conference on IMCEC 2016, IEEE, pp 1779–1784. doi: https://doi.org/10.1109/IMCEC.2016.7867525

# Development of Monitoring System for Room Temperature, pH and Water Level Hydroponic Cultivation Using IoT Method

Rismayani, S. Y. Hasyrif, Asma Nurhidayani, and Nirwana

**Abstract** The problem in this research is how to redesign the monitoring system for room temperature, pH and water level on hydroponic plants using the android platform and analyze the performance test of the monitoring system. This research aims to develop a system design for monitoring room temperature, pH, and water level on hydroponic plants that are run on the android platform using Internet of Things (IoT) based technology. The materials used in this research are data related to room temperature, ideal water level, and water pH from hydroponic plants. The method or technology used in IoT (Internet of Things) is run on the Android platform; IoT is a concept where different or the same information can exchange internet connectivity with objects around which are controlled using a Smartphone. The monitoring system created is used by farmers who cultivate the hydroponic plant industry. The results of this study are the construction of a hydroponic cultivation monitoring management system using the android platform with IoT-based technology; the system is connected to a prototype device consisting of sensors that detect temperature, water level and water pH, a system with an android platform built to help aquaculture farmers in remote control, anytime and anywhere. Based on black-box testing to determine system functionality, valid results are obtained and based on system service level; there are 83.4% very satisfied.

**Keywords** Monitoring · IoT (internet of things) · Android · Hydroponic

Rismayani (✉) · S. Y. Hasyrif · Nirwana
Dipa Makassar University, Makassar 90000, South Sulawesi, Indonesia
e-mail: rismayani@dipanegara.ac.id; rismayani@undipa.ac.id

A. Nurhidayani
Puangrimaggalatung University, Sengkang, South Sulawesi, Indonesia

 
T. Triwiyanto et al. (eds.), *Proceedings of the 2nd International Conference on Electronics, Biomedical Engineering, and Health Informatics*, Lecture Notes in Electrical Engineering 898, https://doi.org/10.1007/978-981-19-1804-9_25

# 1 Introduction

Hydroponics is the cultivation of plants using water as a growing medium, hydroponic plant cultivation in Indonesia has existed for a long time, namely in 1980. Currently, many hydroponic industries cultivate this plant which is spread throughout Indonesia. The increasing number of Korean and Japanese-style restaurants opening in Indonesia has made hydroponic plants the target of restaurant entrepreneurs. Many hydroponic industries have developed and produced hydroponic products. As for the research that the author previously carried out in 2020 with the title Design of Web-Based Hydroponic Plants Room Temperature and Water Nutrition Monitoring System [1]. This study creates a web-based system that uses WIFI and Microcontroller technology; a prototype has been built in this study to Room temperature and water nutrition hydroponic, but in previous research, even though the system is already running on a web platform, the system is still stand-alone and cannot be used anywhere. As for the problems in previous studies, the system built is standalone and can only be used on computer devices and can be monitored while in the hydroponic garden, but with a system that runs on the android platform, monitoring can be done anytime and anywhere as long as it is connected to the internet network. Therefore, in this study, the authors developed an android-based system for monitoring hydroponic plant cultivation, which consists of monitoring room temperature, water pH, and water level that affect water nutrients in hydroponic plants. In compiling and completing this research, there are several other supporting theories as follows.

Hydroponics is a technique of planting using water media instead of soil; hydroponic plants also do not require a lot of water; therefore, setting the water level of hydroponic plants greatly affects plant growth [2]. Hydroponics is a technique of planting using water media instead of soil; hydroponic plants also do not require a lot of water; therefore, setting the water level of hydroponic plants greatly affects plant growth. Then hydroponic water culture using a solution of macro and micronutrients and hydroponic nutrient film technique is a technique of planting in narrow and long trenches.

Furthermore, the system is built using an android-based platform; android is a mobile-based operating system and is the most popular today, especially on Smartphone [3]. The advantages of Android are open source, various prices, many applications and easy to modify.

The technology used is the Internet of Things (IoT), a concept where objects can transfer data over a network that does not have to have human-to-human or human-to-computer interaction [4]. The way Internet of Things works is by utilizing arguments and algorithms from the programming that has been compiled. The arguments are formed to result in interactions that help hardware or machines perform functions or work. The most important factor lies in the internet network, which is the liaison between the system and hardware, which is the main task of humans, namely supervisors, to monitor every action and behavior of machines while working. The elements of Internet of Things are sensors, connections, data processing, and user interfaces.

As for some work related to the monitoring implementing Internet of Things that previous authors, namely research that develops an Internet of Things-based intelligent hydroponic system using Deep Neural Networks and a prototype made for tomato plant growth as a case study was developed [5]. Research that designs and develops a hydroponic plant growth automation control and monitoring system evaluates the effect of using a prototype on a system capable of controlling significant environmental factors that affect plant growth, including temperature, humidity, and water in the solution mixing process [6, 7]. Research on Internet of Things Internet of Things based hydroponic plant control called ANDES, ANDES is configured with the connection of various sensors and microcontrollers via Smartphone that effectively lowers or increases the pH concentration in the range of values from 5.5 to 6.5 [8]. Build an Internet of Things system to monitor and control all hydroponic system parameters such as water level, pH, humidity, and temperature through a mobile application using a pump-controlled ESP32 microcontroller and draw water from a reservoir connected to a regular water line [9]. Discussion of intelligent innovations that optimize remote electronic control systems that collaborate agriculture and fisheries into one system [10]. Discussion on detecting and monitoring lettuce internal changes in real-time [11]. Discussion about Plant Talk, which can flexibly configure the connection of various sensors and actuators of hydroponic plants via Smartphone [12]. Research that tested the sensors used and accurate response to the output to control the motor as a refill water pump, plant watering pump and nutrient pump [13]. Research that develops a water quality management system for catfish ponds by utilizing aquaponics technology and Internet of Things technology with a water quality control system using fuzzy logic to control temperature and ammonia levels is important in maintaining water quality [14]. This study focuses on the nutrients preserved in lettuce and the automation of parameters that affect plant growth in an NFT type hydroponic system, such as temperature, water acidity (pH), water level and light intensity [15]. Research that designs and builds automatic vertical hydroponic systems indoors and does not depend on outdoor climate [16]. Research developing a smart greenhouse for hydroponic agriculture based on the Internet of Things, which measures the chlorophyll content of mustard leaves grown hydroponically in a greenhouse system, determines mustard plants' nitrogen status [17, 18]. Research that makes a water pH control system, filling water reservoirs, giving Arduino-based nutritional liquids automatically, which can help expedite the cultivation process with hydroponic media using the Fuzzy method [19]. Research that conducts data acquisition on an Internet of Things-based hydroponic plant automation system using ESP8266 [20]. Discusses the manufacture of devices that use Internet of Things to maintain water conditions to increase lobsters' viability in ponds [21]. Discussion on building real-time agricultural applications with low-cost Internet of Things devices and detecting malicious packet drop attacks on Internet of Things platforms [22].

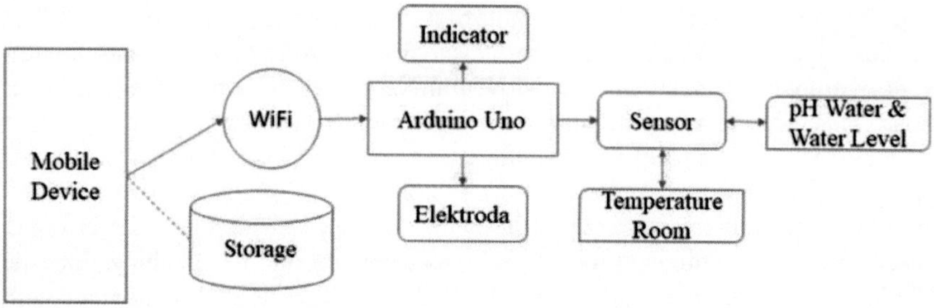


**Fig. 1** System architecture

# 2 Method

## *2.1 Architecture System*

Figure 1 is a system architecture where mobile devices with the android platform are connected to the Internet of Things technology by controlling using indicators; the indicators used are Arduino microcontrollers interconnected with electrodes, prototypes, and sensors made in previous research in 2020 [1].

## *2.2 Materials*

The materials used is normal room temperature data for hydroponic plants, water pH data is required for hydroponic plants and water level data is required for hydroponic plants. The method and technology used is android-based technology. Monitoring data for room temperature, water pH and water level for hydroponic cultivation will be sent and displayed on mobile phones with the android platform starting from the current state, history, and graph.

## *2.3 Hardware and Software*

The hardware used is PC Device, Mouse Logitech K150, Android Smartphone, Arduino Mega, LDR sensor, LED, Electrodes, Cooling/Space Heating, Water Pump and software used is windows 10, Microsoft Word 2016, Android Studio 2017, Visual Studio 2016, SQL Lite, UML Star, Google Chrome and OS Android Oreo. The data processing used is statistical data processing using ANOVA.

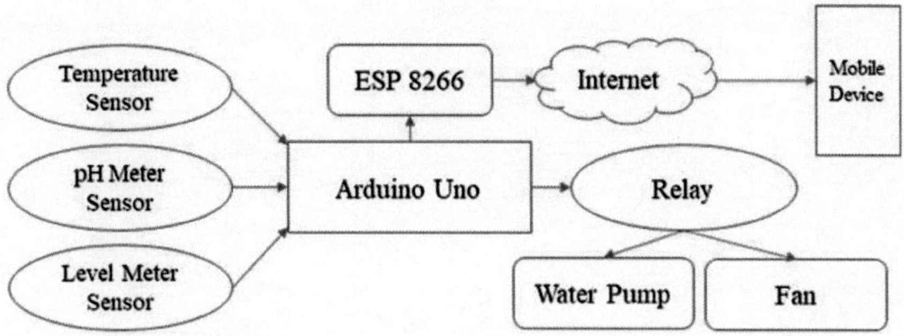


**Fig. 2** Analysis prototype

### *2.4 Data Collection*

The data collection process is carried out is observation, the author makes observations of the research site and discusses the development of the monitoring system design that was built. Interview, the author conducted interviews with several hydroponic plant cultivators to determine what parts had to be done or what was lacking from the monitoring system in previous studies. Document, author collects image data and explanations of other related information from the internet, books and journals related to the research carried out.

Figure 2 explains that the system is made mobile using a standalone application, and the device used is a mobile, namely Smartphone. In making a monitoring system for room temperature, water pH and water level for hydroponic plants, there are 3 sensors used, namely temperature sensors, proximity sensors and pH sensors that are connected to Arduino, and there are tools used in the form of water pumps and fans for monitoring used by the internet. To send data to mobile devices to control room temperature, water pH, and water level of hydroponic plants.

Figure 3 is a system use case diagram design which is an overview of the system; there is one actor, namely hydroponic farmers, where hydroponic farmers can carry out activities in the form of logging into the system and then view the latest data from Water PH, Room Temperature and Water Height. The actor's next activity is looking at graphs, graphs that are seen about the movement of water, temperature movements, and water level movements.

## 3 Result

This research was previously conducted in 2020 by building a prototype and a web-based system [1]; Then, in this study, the author developed the system to the android platform and synchronized it with the prototype that had been made previously.

The system displays produced in this study are:

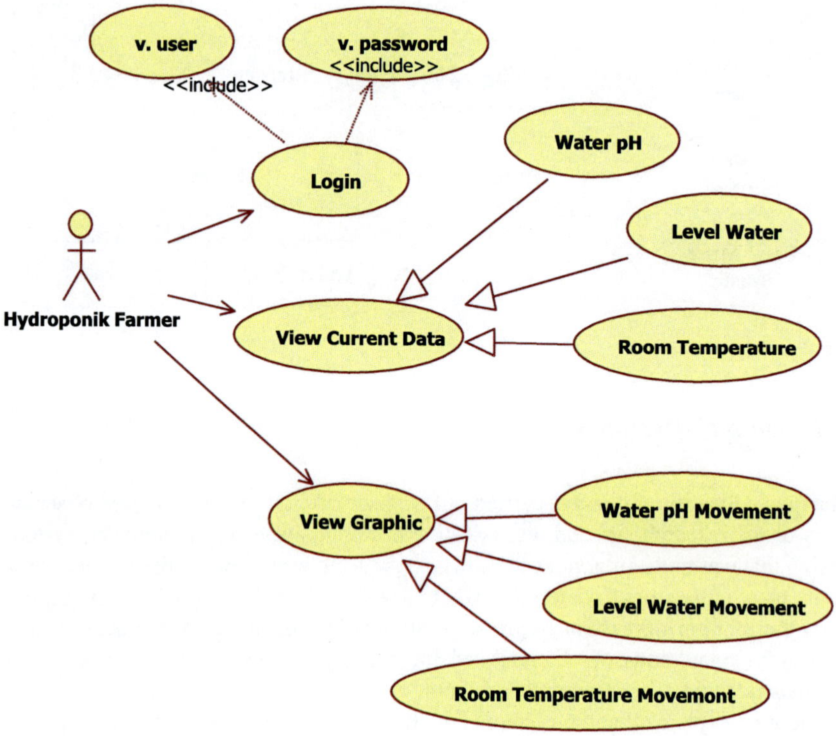


**Fig. 3** System overview

Figure 4 shows a display system, where there are two inputs, namely username, input in the form of an email address and input in a password, main menu display which contains several menus, namely profiles, temperature graph displays, pH and water level graphs, and then monitoring the latest data from the hydroponic system. The latest monitoring data at room temperature, water pH and water level from hydroponic plants.

Figures 5, 6 and 7 are graphic displays of movement of room temperature, water pH and water level for hydroponic plants. Figure 5 is a graphical display of trials regarding monitoring of hydroponic plant systems that observe the room temperature of hydroponic plants periodically for 7 days whose tests are carried out in addition to the rainy season. Where the average room temperature observed is at a temperature of 30 degrees. Figure 6 shows a graphic depiction of monitoring water levels in hydroponic plant storage containers, this is monitored so that the system can inform every time farmers in the hydroponic industry can add water.

Figure 7 is a graph that shows the results of monitoring the pH of water from hydroponic plants, the system can be seen so that the monitoring of water pH remains normal, because basically water pH and water level are one of the factors that play an important role in the growth of hydroponic plants.

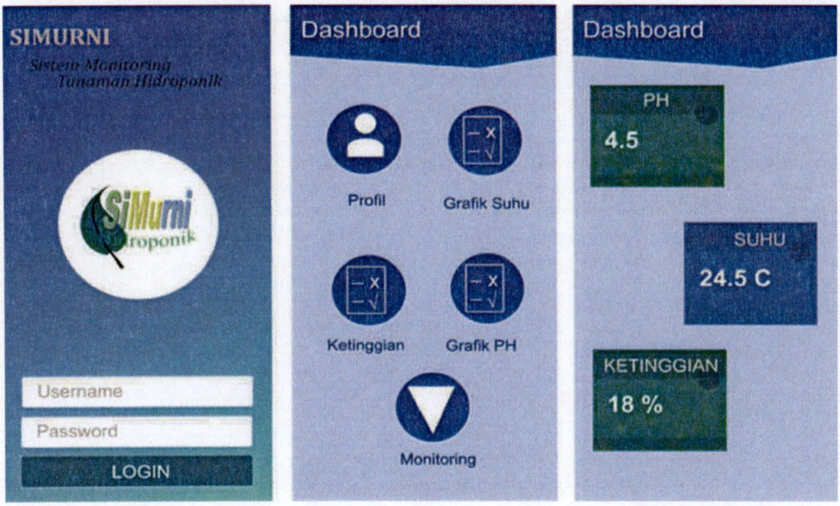


**Fig. 4** Display system

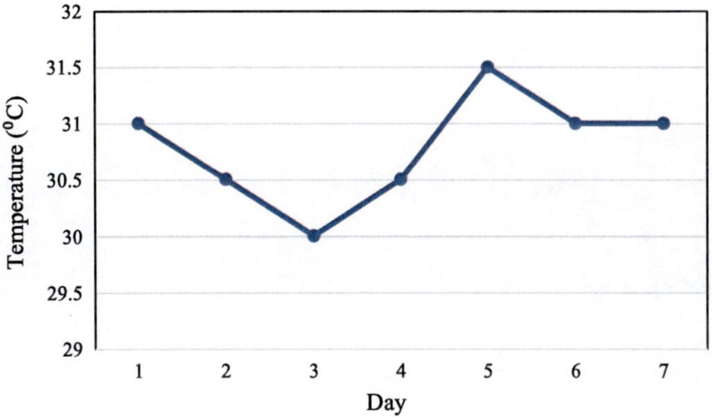


**Fig. 5** Room temperature graphic

Table 1 is a dataset parameter table that is managed based on the results of the monitoring system performance. Tables 2 and 3 are the results of statistical analysis using Two-factor without Replication ANOVA analysis with alpha data of 0.05. Based on the Black Box testing that has been carried out in general, it can be concluded that the application test results are as follows Table 4.

Further testing was carried out to determine the level of satisfaction with the system service; a questionnaire was collected from 50 respondents consisting of hydroponic plant cultivators with the following results:

Figure 8 is a diagram of the results of the questionnaire presentation obtained from 50 respondents based on the level of service of the hydroponic plant motoring

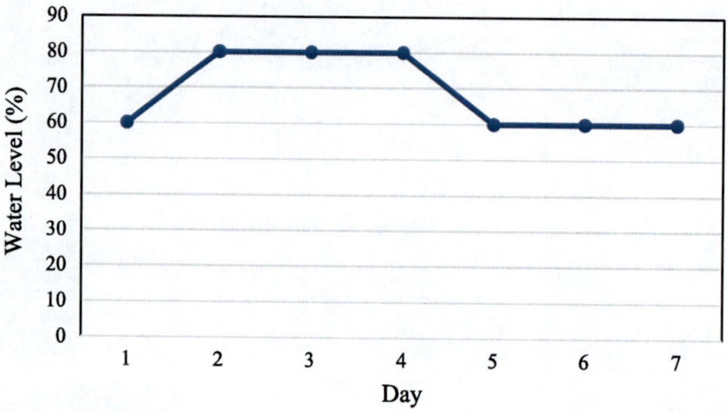


**Fig. 6** Level water graphic

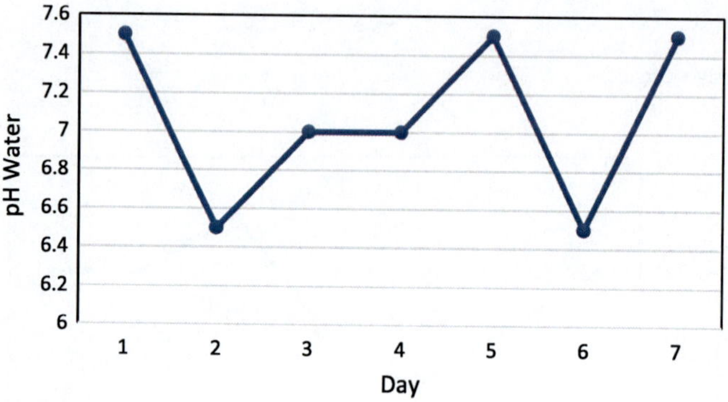


**Fig. 7** pH water graphic

**Table 1** Parameters

| No. | Testing | Day | | | | | | |
|---|---|---|---|---|---|---|---|---|
| | | 1 | 2 | 3 | 4 | 5 | 6 | 7 |
| 1 | Room temperature (°C) | 31 | 30.5 | 30 | 30.5 | 31.5 | 31 | 31 |
| 2 | Water level (%) | 60 | 80 | 80 | 80 | 60 | 60 | 60 |
| 3 | pH water | 7.5 | 6.5 | 7.0 | 7.0 | 7.5 | 6.5 | 7.5 |

management system, namely 83.4% very satisfactory, 14.2% satisfactory, 2.4% sufficient and 0% unsatisfactory.

**Table 2** Two-factor without replication

| Summary | Count | Sum | Average | Variance |
|---|---|---|---|---|
| Water level (%) | 7 | 480 | 68.57143 | 114.2857 |
| pH water | 7 | 49.5 | 7.071429 | 0.202381 |
| Room temperature (°C) | 7 | 215.5 | 30.78571 | 0.238095 |
| Day 1 | 3 | 98.5 | 32.83333 | 691.5833 |
| Day 2 | 3 | 117 | 39 | 1404.75 |
| Day 3 | 3 | 117 | 39 | 1393 |
| Day 4 | 3 | 117.5 | 39.16667 | 1388.583 |
| Day 5 | 3 | 99 | 33 | 690.75 |
| Day 6 | 3 | 97.5 | 32.5 | 717.25 |
| Day 7 | 3 | 68.5 | 32.83333 | 691.5833 |

**Table 3** Statistical analysis using Anova

| Source of variation | SS | df | MS | F | P-value | F crit |
|---|---|---|---|---|---|---|
| Rows | 13,468.88 | 2 | 6734.44 | 166.2418 | 1.79E-09 | 3.885294 |
| Columns | 202.2381 | 6 | 33.70635 | 0.832052 | 0.567554 | 2.99612 |
| Error | 486.119 | 12 | 40.50992 | | | |
| Total | 14,157.24 | 20 | | | | |

**Table 4** Black box system testing

| No. | Testing scenario | Result | Conclusion |
|---|---|---|---|
| 1 | Login | Login view successfully | Valid |
| 2 | View current data | View current data successfully | Valid |
| 3 | View temperature room graph | View temperature room graph successfully | Valid |
| 4 | View pH water graph | View pH water graph successfully | Valid |
| 5 | View water level graph | View water level graph successfully | Valid |

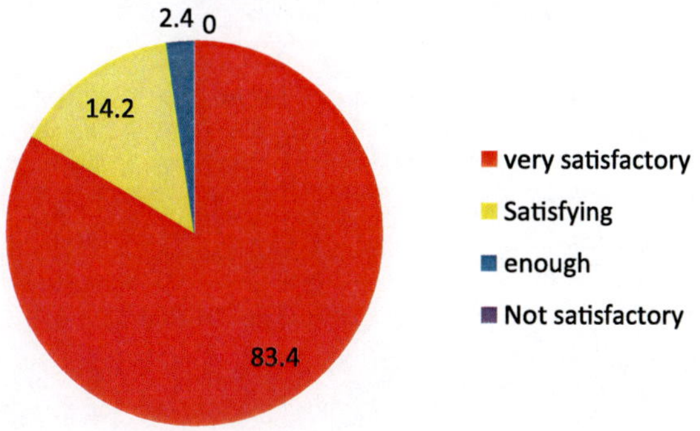


**Fig. 8** Percentage questionnaire result

## 4 Discussion

The research conducted resulted in an android-based monitoring system using the IoT method for monitoring room temperature, pH and water content of hydroponic plants. Some of the same studies that make monitoring systems are research that discusses monitoring fuel trucks [23]. Research also examines making monitoring systems to control body temperature and measure heart rate using the IoT method [24]. Then research discusses IoT monitoring in electric power consumption in rural areas, which can be monitored through the android application [25]. Furthermore, research that discusses the development of water quality management in catfish kola that applies IoT technology [14]. This research is the development and change of the system platform from previous research. In earlier research, a prototype and a series of tools and sensors were made to measure room temperature, pH and water level [1]. This research produces a monitoring system that can be run on mobile devices that use the Android platform, then the results of this study are used by farmers in the hydroponic industry.

## 5 Conclusion

This study concludes that building a monitoring system that can monitor room temperature, water pH, and water level based on android can help farmers cultivate hydroponic plants. Development of a hydroponic cultivation monitoring management system using the android platform with the Internet of Things-based technology; the system is connected to a prototype device consisting of sensors that detect temperature, water level and water pH, a system with an android platform built to help aquaculture farmers in remote control, anytime and anywhere. Based on black-box testing to determine the system's functionality, valid results were obtained and based on the results of the questionnaire to determine the service level of the system, the results were 83.4% very satisfactory. Suggestions for the development of this research are that research in the storage process can use the cloud, apply relevant algorithms, and measure room temperature, pH, and water level monitoring system services from hydroponic plants.

**Acknowledgements** This research is fully supported by SIMLITABMAS RISTEK-BRIN DIKTI grant, 395/M/KPT.KP/2018 and 4672/LL9/PG/2020. The authors fully acknowledged RISTEK-BRIN Indonesia and Dipa Makassar University for the approved fund which makes this important research viable and effective.

## References

1. Rismayani R, Sy H (2020) Design of web-based hydroponic plant's room temperature and water nutrition monitoring system. J Pekommas 5(1), 1. doi: https://doi.org/10.30818/jpkm.2020.2050105
2. Resh HM (2016) Hydroponic food production: a definitive guidebook for the advanced home gardener and the commercial hydroponic grower (7th edn). CRC Press
3. Mednieks Z, Meike GB, Dornin L, Pan Z (2013) Enterprise android: programming android database applications for the enterprise. John Wiley & Sons
4. Ismail Y (2019) Internet of things (IoT) for automated and smart applications. BoD—Books on Demand
5. Mehra M, Saxena S, Sankaranarayanan S, Tom RJ, Veeramanikandan M (2018) IoT based hydroponics system using deep neural networks. Comp Electron Agric 155:473–486. doi: https://doi.org/10.1016/j.compag.2018.10.015
6. Kularbphettong K, Ampant U, Kongrodj N (2019) An automated hydroponics: system based on mobile application. IJIET 9(8):548–552. doi: https://doi.org/10.18178/ijiet.2019.9.8.1264
7. Rico AL (2019) Automated pH monitoring and controlling system for hydroponics under greenhouse condition. J Eng Appl Sci 15:523–528. doi: https://doi.org/10.36478/jeasci.2020.523.528
8. Sihombing P, Zarlis M, Herriyance (2019) Automatic nutrition detection system (ANDES) for hydroponic monitoring by using micro controller and smartphone android. In: 2019 fourth international conference on informatics and computing (ICIC), pp 1–6. doi: https://doi.org/10.1109/ICIC47613.2019.8985851
9. Ullah A, Aktar S, Sutar N, Kabir R, Hossain A (2019) Cost effective smart hydroponic monitoring and controlling system using IoT. Intell Contr Autom 10(04), 04. doi: https://doi.org/10.4236/ica.2019.104010
10. Hartono RWT, Suwanda FH, Angraeni SP, Pratiwi E, Adi GS, Taufiqurrohman D (2019) E-aquaponics: aquaculture and hydroponic integration using electronical control and monitoring. In: 2019 international conference on electrical engineering and informatics (ICEEI), pp 315–319. doi: https://doi.org/10.1109/ICEEI47359.2019.8988855
11. Puengsungwan S, Jirasereeamornkul K (2019) Internet of things (IoTs) based hydroponic lettuce farming with solar panels. In: 2019 international conference on power, energy and innovations (ICPEI), Oct 2019, pp 86–89. doi: https://doi.org/10.1109/ICPEI47862.2019.8944986
12. Van LD et al (2019) PlantTalk.: a smartphone-based intelligent hydroponic plant box. Sensors 19(8, 8). doi: https://doi.org/10.3390/s19081763
13. Muharnis KS, Lianda J (2019) Smart green house's hydroponic with arduino uno. In: Proceeding of the 2nd international conference on applied science and technology (iCAST), Oct 2019. Accessed 3 Dec 2020
14. Rozie F, Syarif I, Rasyid MUHA (2020) Design and implementation of intelligent aquaponics monitoring system based on IoT. In: 2020 international electronics symposium (IES), Sep 2020, pp 534–540. doi: https://doi.org/10.1109/IES50839.2020.9231928
15. Saputro JS, Latifa U, Ramelan A (2020) Design of nutrition automation on lactuca sativa NFT hydroponic systems. J Electr Electron Inform Commun Technol 2(1, 1). doi: https://doi.org/10.20961/jeeict.2.1.41353
16. Chowdhury MEH et al (2020) Design, construction and testing of IoT based automated indoor vertical hydroponics farming test-bed in Qatar. Sensors 20(19, 19). doi: https://doi.org/10.3390/s20195637
17. Andrianto H, Suhardi, Faizal A (2020) Development of smart greenhouse system for hydroponic agriculture. In: 2020 international conference on information technology systems and innovation (ICITSI), pp 335–340. doi: https://doi.org/10.1109/ICITSI50517.2020.9264917
18. Lukito RB, Lukito C (2019) Development of IoT at hydroponic system using raspberry Pi—ProQuest. TELKOMNIKA 17(2):897–906. doi: https://doi.org/10.12928/TELKOMNIKA.v17i2.9265

19. Mauliddya GN, Fauziah, Hayati N (2020) Prototype automatic maintenance system on hydroponic plants using fuzzy and Arduino Uno methods. Mantik 4(3, 3). doi: https://doi.org/10.35335/mantik.Vol4.2020.1028.pp1849-1854
20. Hariono T, Putra MC (2021) Data acquisition for monitoring IoT-based hydroponic automation system using ESP8266. NEWTON Netw Inform Technol 1(1, 1)
21. Abdurrasyid A, Indrianto I, Susanti MNI, Purwanto YS (2021) Detection of water quality in crayfish ponds with IoT. Bull Electr Eng Inform 10(2, 2). doi: https://doi.org/10.11591/eei.v10i2.1968
22. Terence JS, Purushothaman G (2021) Low-cost real-time implementation of malicious packet dropping detection in agricultural IoT platform. In: Advances in distributed computing and machine learning, Singapore, pp 87–97. doi: https://doi.org/10.1007/978-981-15-4218-3_9
23. Tulloh R, Ramadan DN, Hadiyoso S, Rohmattullah, Rahmana Z, Fuel (2021) Truck tracking for real-time monitoring system using GPS and Raspberry-Pi. In: Proceedings of the 1st international conference on electronics, biomedical engineering, and health informatics, Singapore, pp 29–41. doi: https://doi.org/10.1007/978-981-33-6926-9_3
24. Raja Aris RSNA, Mohd Azhari A, Syafie LS, Azimi FH, Ridzuan Aw S (2021) Graphical user interface for heartbeat and body temperature monitoring system using internet of things (IOT). In: Proceedings of the 1st international conference on electronics, biomedical engineering, and health informatics, Singapore, pp 667–679. doi: https://doi.org/10.1007/978-981-33-6926-9_59
25. Pazikadin AR, Ali K, Rifai D, Awang NA, Ghoni R, Mamat NH (2021) IoT-based solar photovoltaic (PV) real time monitoring system for power consumption on Maahad Tahfiz School. In: Proceedings of the 1st international conference on electronics, biomedical engineering, and health informatics, Singapore, pp 281–294. doi: https://doi.org/10.1007/978-981-33-6926-9_24

# Implementation of One-Dimensional Convolutional Neural Network for Individual Identification Based on ECG Signal

**Ana Rahma Yuniarti and Syamsul Rizal**

**Abstract** Electrocardiogram (ECG) signal has been widely studied for biometric recognition (or subject identification) applications over the past decade. Many techniques have been offered as well, from traditional computing to machine learning techniques. However, most studies evaluate their proposed models by independently separating the datasets between healthy (normal) and unhealthy (abnormal/arrhythmia) heart conditions. Some studies even used the ECG signal datasets from subjects only under healthy heart conditions. We believe that developing an ECG-based biometric system that includes the heart, both under healthy and unhealthy conditions, is highly needed since the users might be in both conditions. To the best of our knowledge, this is the first study in the literature, which considers the combination of the dataset of ECG signals from subjects under the healthy heart and unhealthy (arrhythmia) conditions in training, validation, and even testing processes. We combined the datasets from MIT-BIH Normal Sinus Rhythm, MIT-BIH Arrhythmia, and St Petersburg INCART 12-lead Arrhythmia databases obtained from Physionet. From the combination of those databases, we obtained a total of 32,628 datasets from 89 subjects which were later modeled using a machine learning technique, i.e., one-dimensional convolutional neural network (CONV1D). This study aims to build a light-weight yet reliable ECG-based biometric system by implementing only two layers of the convolutional neural network into those joined datasets. We evaluated the model's performance with k-fold cross-validation (k = 5) and yielded the accuracy and F1-scores of 99.8% And 99.8% respectively. We also proved that our model is a good fitting (not under/over-fitting) by providing the visualization plot of accuracy and loss. These findings show that our model is robust enough for ECG-based subject identification, which can be implemented for healthy and unhealthy heart conditions.

**Keywords** Subject identification · Convolution neural network · Biometrics · ECG

A. R. Yuniarti
Department of Computer Engineering, Universitas Pendidikan Indonesia, Bandung, Indonesia

S. Rizal (✉)
School of Electrical Engineering, Telkom University, Bandung, Indonesia
e-mail: syamsul@telkomuniversity.ac.id

 
T. Triwiyanto et al. (eds.), *Proceedings of the 2nd International Conference on Electronics, Biomedical Engineering, and Health Informatics*, Lecture Notes in Electrical Engineering 898, https://doi.org/10.1007/978-981-19-1804-9_26

# 1 Introduction

Biometrics are biological characteristics that can identify a person digitally to grant access to systems, devices, or data [1]. Biometric applications are becoming increasingly popular and essential since the security issues arising correspond to the increasing number of data produced per day by each person in this Big Data and IoT era. Based on the Verizon Data breach investigation report [2], more than 70% of employees reuse passwords at work, and 81% of hacking-related breaches utilize either stolen or weak passwords.

To date, there are many Biometric (subject identification) methods such as signature, fingerprint, face, retinal structure or iris, voice, and even vein recognition [3–7]. Those methods were believed could replace the burden of remembering long passwords in traditional methods. However, security vulnerabilities are arising following the growth of advanced forgery techniques. For example, fingerprints and facial recognition systems can be counterfeited by 3D models. In voice recognition, the voice can be easily manipulated by using recording tools. In iris recognition, the scanners can be easily fooled by the high quality of iris images (photography).

On the other hand, ECG has also been investigated over the past decades as a novel tool in Biometric application [8], which can solve the issues arising in the previous methods. There are some reasons that ECG has a strong potential for Biometrics application. First, the ECG signal is unique. There are no two identical ECGs in the world. The ECG shape differs from one person to another depending on the anatomical and morphological features of the heart and body of each person (i.e., heart position, chest geometry, ion mechanism, and other pathological conditions) [9]. Second, ECG is invisible (can not be seen with eyes directly), making it extremely hard to forge. Finally, it exists in all living humans, making it continuously available, even in the case of physically disabled subjects [10].

However, ECG-based biometric systems are usually less accurate than traditional technologies due to some challenges such as noise and artifacts (i.e., electrode materials, sensor placement, baseline-drift, motion artifacts, etc.), signal abnormalities (i.e., physical exercise, heart rate variability, arrhythmia, etc.), or thorax geometry and tissue characteristics [11]. To increase the performance, some studies in the literature have implemented machine learning techniques for ECG-based biometrics systems [12, 13].

Hammad et al. [13] proposed Residual Network (ResNet) for ECG classification. ResNet is the model which has a deep layer and requires a two-dimensional dataset for training the model. Thus, they need to convert the ECG signal, which is one-dimensional (1D) data, into image (2D). The training process consumes more time because of the utility of many layers in this model, and it cannot be used for real-time identification. The study from the literature [12] developed an ECG-based personal authentication system using a long short-term memory (LSTM) model. The authors used two different public datasets: MIT-BIH Normal Sinus Rhythm (NSRDB), and MIT-BIH Arrhythmia database. The system obtained the accuracy (F1-score) of 100% for NSRDB and 99% for the MIT-BIH Arrhythmia database. However, they did not provide any graph regarding the training and validation accuracy, so we cannot decide whether the LSTM model is overfitting or not. Furthermore, they extracted the ECG signal with 288 samples (2.25 s), which is too much for the LSTM model. The LSTM requires more computation time than a normal one-dimensional convolutional (CONV1D) model.

The recent study from Bajare and Vaishali [14] implemented a more light-weight model using CONV1D with only two convolutional layers. They used NSRDB and ECG-ID datasets for the experiment. For NSRDB, they obtained 96,93% of accuracy, which is lesser than [12]. Whereas for the ECG-ID database, they achieved 100% of accuracy. The drawback of this study is that they only considered the ECG signals under healthy conditions. Moreover, they did not provide the training and validation accuracy graph, so we cannot see if their model is good-fitting. Furthermore, just as other previous studies in literature, for evaluating their model, they split the datasets independently, e.g., train the NSRDB and ECG-ID dataset using their model separately.

The light-weight system for ECG-based biometrics is urgently needed nowadays to minimize the computing cost so that we can implement it for more massive data. Moreover, an ECG-based biometric system needs to reckon both healthy (normal) and unhealthy (arrhythmia) heart conditions since arrhythmia exists in a large portion of the world population [15]. Besides, as we mentioned before, we cannot decide whether the biometric's users (or the tested subjects) have a normal heart or not in a real-world application. Thus, in this study, we proposed a novel light-weight system for ECG-based individual identification using two convolutional layers of CONV1D inspired by the work of Bajare and Vaishali [14], but with a different scheme. Unlike them [14], which only considered the heart under healthy conditions, we combined the dataset under healthy (normal) and unhealthy (arrhythmia) heart conditions automatically in the system. So, we did not divide the template between subjects under normal and arrhythmia conditions from training and validation to testing work. To the best of our knowledge, this is the first study in the literature which considers such conditions. Besides that, a biometric system needs to be robust to ensure security. Hence, in this study, we also aim to achieve high accuracy (i.e., as close as possible to 100% accuracy).

## 2 Research Method

The system diagram of the proposed work is shown in Fig. 1, which consists of seven steps: data collection, pre-processing (filter application), R-peak detection, segmentation (PQRST selection), DWT application, CONV1D modeling, and identification.

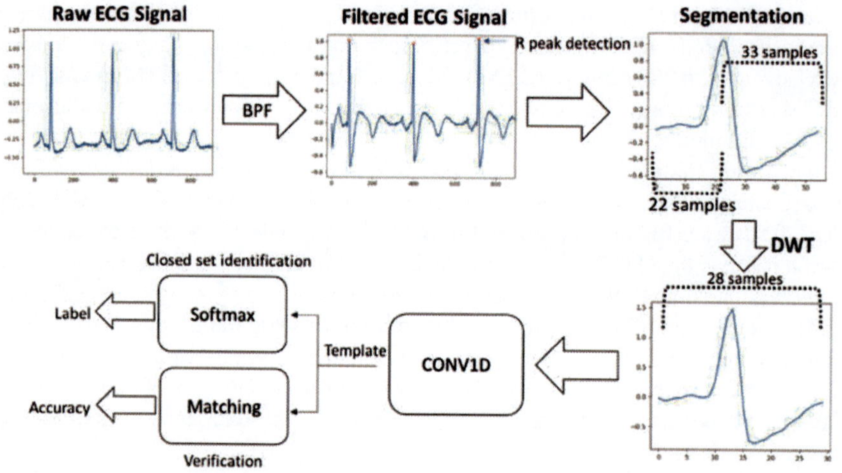


**Fig. 1** The system diagram of the proposed work

## 2.1 Data Collection

The ECG signal represents the propagation of electrical impulses generated by the heart. Figure 2 portrays one cycle of an electrical impulse generated by the human heart on normal condition along with the corresponded ECG waveforms.

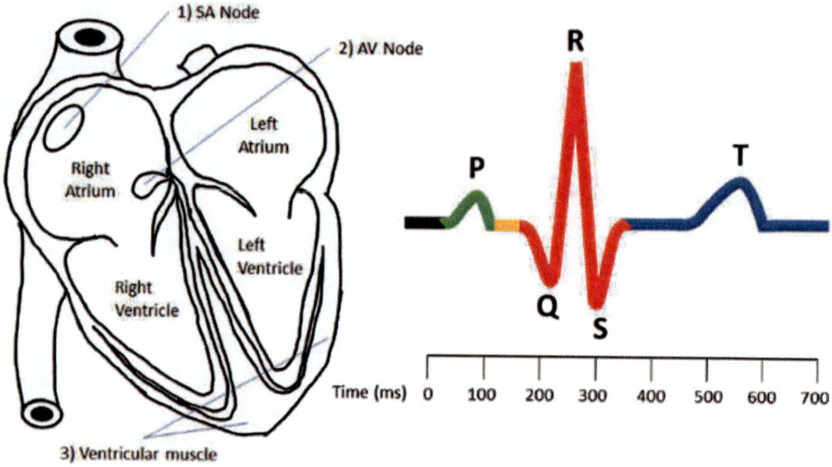


**Fig. 2** An illustration of electrical impulse (action potential) generated by the specialized cells in the heart, and their contribution to the ECG waveforms

**Table 1** The summary of the database used

| Dataset | No. of subjects | Heart condition | Sampling frequency (Hz) |
|---|---|---|---|
| MIT-BIH NSRDB | 18 | Normal | 128 |
| MIT-BIH Arrhythmia | 39 | Arrhythmia | 360 |
| INCART | 32 | Arrhythmia | 257 |
| TOTAL | 89 | | |

The P wave indicates the activation of the atria (atrial depolarization), and its duration ranges from 60 to 120 ms under normal conditions. The PQ segment indicates the elapsed time between the atrial activation to the beginning of ventricular activation and its duration ranges between 12 and 20 ms. The QRS complex (i.e., the joint of Q, R, and S waves) is associated with the activation of the ventricle (ventricular depolarization), and its duration ranges from 60 to 90 ms. The alteration of this complex gives information on the possibility of the occurrence of heart diseases such as arrhythmia, fibrillation, and a heart attack. The ST segment indicates the relaxation after the ventricle depolarization and its normal duration ranges from 230 to 460 ms. The T wave represents the ventricular repolarization in preparation for the next cycle and its standard length ranges between 100 and 250 ms [11].

Arrhythmia, an abnormal condition of heart activity, exists in a large portion of the population in the world [15]. Under arrhythmia, the duration of each segment in ECG signal may be altered. For example, prolonged QRS complex may be associated with ventricular tachycardia; flat, decline or depressed ST segments may indicate coronary ischemia [16, 17]. Hence, the ECG-based biometric system should consider not only the healthy heart condition but also the arrhythmia condition.

For this study, we combined the datasets from MIT-BIH NSRDB, MIT-BIH Arrhythmia, and St Petersburg INCART 12-lead Arrhythmia databases obtained from Physionet. The summary of these three databases is provided in Table 1. The ECG signal from those databases contains some noises, as we can see in Fig. 3. Those noises can be caused by the electrode materials, sensor placement, baseline-drift, motion artifacts, etc., during the recording or measurement process.

## 2.2 *Pre-processing*

Since the collected datasets contain some noises, we conducted pre-processing here. ECG pre-processing usually includes a low-pass filter to remove high-frequency noises due to muscle activity and a high-pass filter to remove low-frequency noise due to baseline drift (breath, etc.) [10]. In this case, we applied a 1-order Butterworth

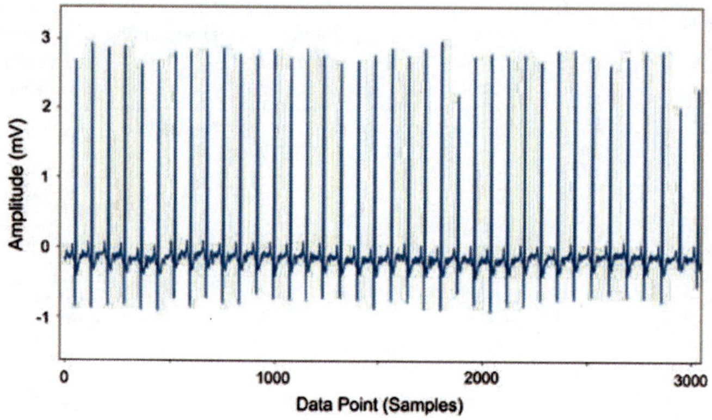


**Fig. 3** The example of RAW ECG signal

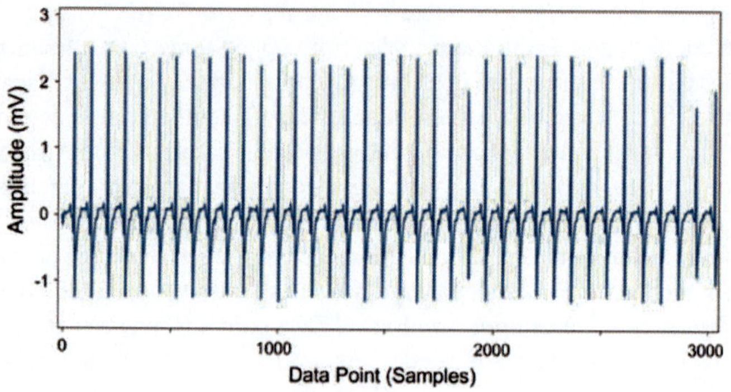


**Fig. 4** The example of ECG signal after filter application

band-pass filter (2–40 Hz) with a sampling frequency of 250 Hz to each RAW ECG signal. The example of the filtered signal can be seen in Fig. 4.

## 2.3 R-peak Detection

A previous study from Xiang et al. [18] stated that analyzing the QRS-complex wave is enough for ECG-based health evaluation. This is because QRS-complex is the most notable feature compared to other segments (i.e., P-wave or T-wave) and can be used to retrieve additional clinical information such as RR-interval and QT-interval PR-interval, and so on. However, the inclusion of P-wave has shown a significant improvement in the identification results, while T-wave inclusion resulted in a smaller improvement. Due to this reason, we decided to use the whole PQRST segment for this study.

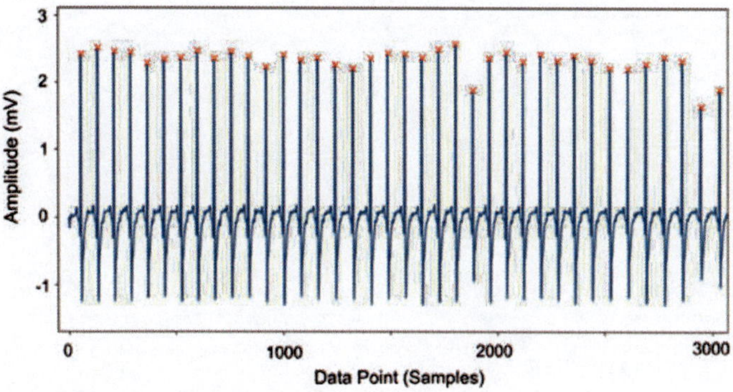


**Fig. 5** The example of the detected R-peak

To obtain the PQRST segment in this study, we first need to detect the R-peak from each ECG signal [19]. To perform R-peak detection, we used an existing library in Python, i.e., "engzee_detector" from the "ecgdetectors" package [20]. Figure 5 shows the detected R-peak on the consecutive filtered ECG signal.

## 2.4 *Segmentation*

After R-peak was detected, we performed ECG segmentation by evaluating each PQRST segment and clipping the ECG signal in interval 88 ms (or equal to 22 data-points) to the left of R-peak and 132 ms (or equal to 33 data-points) to the right. These values are based on the typical duration of the P-Q and S-T complexes [21]. So, totally, we fixed the length of the PQRST segments at 224 ms (or equal to 56 data points) of each ECG signal in the datasets. Figure 6 illustrates the procedure.

## 2.5 *DWT Application*

To enrich the signal characteristics, each PQRST segment was transformed into a wavelet domain to obtain a time–frequency representation of the signal. Compared to fast Fourier transform (FFT), Discrete Wavelet Transform (DWT) presents a more powerful technique to expose the spectral characteristics of complex and non-stationary signals such as the ECG signal [14, 22]. DWT uses scaling functions and wavelets to decompose functions. DWT divides the signal dimension into two parts: high and low frequency, or so-called decomposition. The output from the high-pass filter and low-pass filter will generate the DWT coefficient. By using this coefficient, the decomposition signal can be reconstructed back to the original, called Inverse-DWT. This research applied a 1-order of DWT to the segmented ECG signal to get

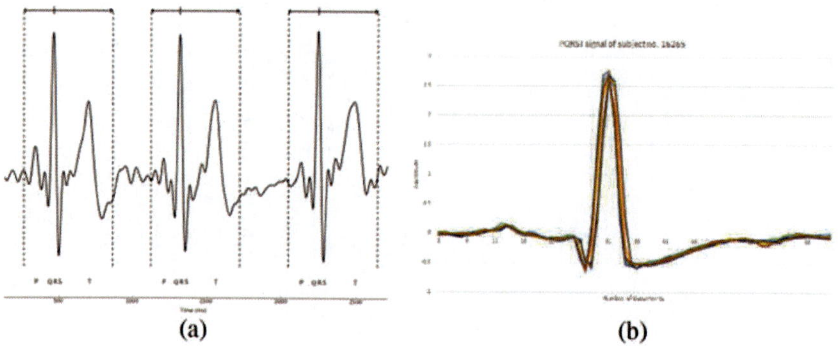

Fig. 6 The example of ECG segmentation process: **a** PQRST-segment selection procedure (the arrows and dashed lines indicate the length and limits of each segment); **b** the example of 10 cycles of PQRST-segment from one subject

**Table 2** The configuration of the CSV file of PQRST features from all subjects

| 1st columns | 2nd–28th columns | 29th columns |
|---|---|---|
| Dataset index-1 | PQRST features/cyles-1 | Subject label-1 |
| … | … | … |
| … | … | … |
| Dataset index-n | PQRST features/cyles-n | Subject label-89 |

the high-frequency signal. As a result, we obtained 28 data points for each frame, including P, QRS-complex, and T wave as the output of this process.

The features of PQRST waveforms after DWT application from all datasets (i.e., a total of 89 subjects from a combined dataset) were then stored into one CSV file. The configuration of the CSV file is shown in Table 2. The first column of the CSV file is for dataset indexing. The 2nd to 28th columns are for PQRST features. We also added one more column (column 29th) to put the label (e.g., subject-1, subject-2, … subject-89) for each PQRST feature to mark which signal belongs to whom. This file would later be used as the input in the CONV1D model (training, validation, and testing simulation).

## 2.6 CONV1D Modelling

In this study, two 1-D convolutional layers were used with the number of channels are 16 and 32 for the first and second 1-D convolutional layers. The kernel size for both layers is $5 \times 1$, and the activation function that we used is ReLU. Two Max Pooling layers were used after a 1-D convolutional layer with kernel size $2 \times 1$. The function of the Max Pooling layer is to generalize the signal and see it in the big picture without making any significant data changes. It leads to a faster convergence

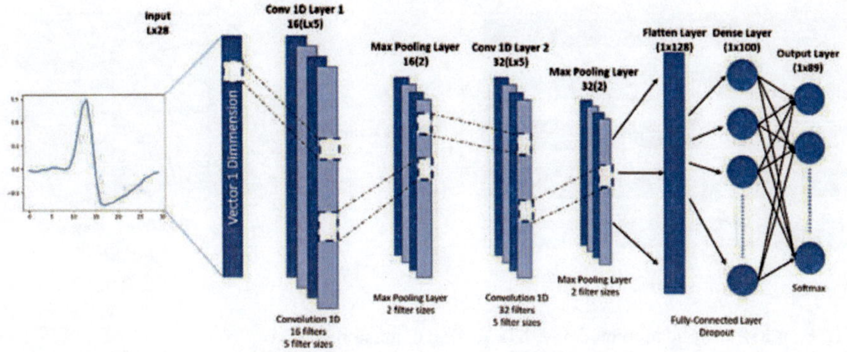


**Fig. 7** The architecture of CNN model

**Table 3** Parameters setting for convolutional neural network model

| Parameter | Value |
|---|---|
| Total epoch | 200 |
| Optimizer | Adam |
| Learning rate | 0.001 |
| Loss | Categorical cross-entropy |
| Regulation/validations | Early stopping and model validation |
| Momentum | $1 \times 10^{-6}$ |

rate [23, 24]. After getting the feature map, we do Flatten to feed forward into the classification layer, which has one Dense layer with 100 neurons and an output layer with 89 neurons. The activation function we used in the output layer was Softmax [25], as shown in Fig. 7.

The overall simulation was carried out using Keras 2.4.3 and Python 3.7.4 on the desktop computer with the specification of Ubuntu 20.04 (64 bit), 16 GB RAM, 512 GB SSD, AMD Ryzen 3 3300x, and GPU Nvidia GTX 1050 Ti 4 GB. The hyperparameter that this paper used can be seen in Table 3.

## 2.7 *Performance Evaluation*

The performance of our model was evaluated based on the accuracy, F1-score, and the loss graph. First, we randomly split the data into train-set and validation-set with the ratio of 80:20, respectively. Then, we applied k-fold cross-validation procedures to ensure that every obeservation data in the dataset has a chance to appear in train-validation sets. We used k = 5 to get a total of five accuracy scores from the train set. Using this method, we can get the average accuracy to know that our model has good accuracy even though the dataset is imbalanced. The k-fold cross-validation model

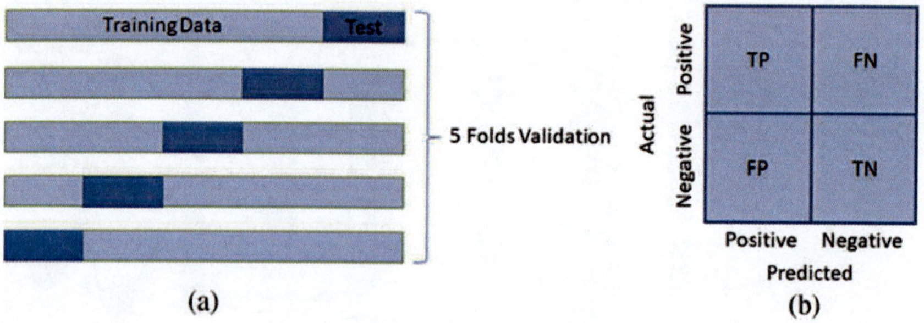


**Fig. 8** **a** K-fold validation model with (k = 5), **b** confusion matrice

can be seen in Fig. 8a. Next, we generated the confusion matrix which portrays the relation between the predicted and the actual labels in two-axis. The matrix yields four parameters: True Positive (TP), True Negative (TN), False Positive (FP), and False Negative (FN), as illustrated in Fig. 8b. TP is the total number the model predicted positive, then it is positive. FP is the total number the model predicted positive, but it is negative. FN is the total number the model predicted negative, but it is positive. TN is the total number the model predicted negative, then it is negative. Based on those parameters, we calculated the accuracy and F1-score, following equations below:

$$Accuracy = (TP + TN)/(TP + TN + FP + FN) \tag{1}$$

$$F1\text{ - }score = 2 * (Recall * Precision)/(Recall + Precision) \tag{2}$$

where recall and precission themselves are calculated as follow:

$$Recall = TP/(TP + FN) \tag{3}$$

$$Precission = TP/(TP + FP) \tag{4}$$

## 3 Results

As a result of this study, a recognition system was developed to give an alternative tool in Biometrics identification using ECG on a sufficiently large set of input data. To see the performance of our proposed model, we calculate two evaluation metrics: accuracy and F1-score.

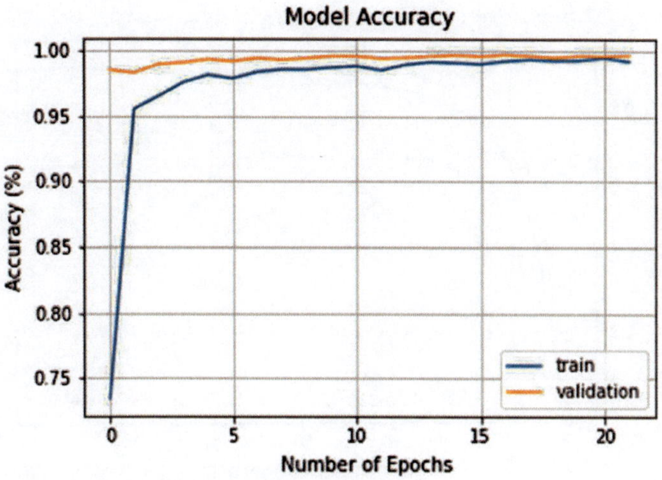


**Fig. 9** Training and testing accuracy of the proposed model

## *3.1 Model Accuracy*

Accuracy measures all the correctly identified cases (both positive and negative). As shown in Fig. 9, approximately 99.8% of accuracy was achieved in this study after 15 epochs which are high enough for the model to be considered accurate. Furthermore, as we can see in the figure, the line plot of train and validation accuracy managed to coincide, which indicates the model is a good fitting.

## *3.2 F1-Score*

F1-score measures the ratio of weighted precision and recall. Precision itself is a ratio of correctly identified positive cases from all the predicted positive cases. In contrast, recall (or so-called sensitivity) is the ratio of the correctly identified positive cases from all the actual positive cases.

F1-score is mostly used as an evaluation model if an imbalanced class distribution exists, just like in our cases, where the variation of features from subject to subject is high. There is a subject with only 400 samples, and on the other hand, another subject has up to 600 features.

Figure 10 shows the F1-score of the proposed model in training and testing simulation. Same with accuracy, the F1-score in this study was best achieved about 99.6% after 118 epochs. The high value of the F1-score indicates that the model is good enough to correctly identify actual threats and not be disturbed by the false alarm.

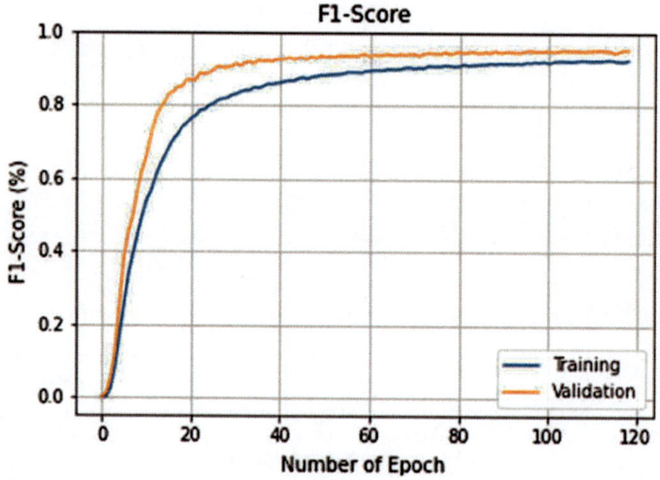


**Fig. 10** Training and testing F1-score of the proposed model

Figure 11 shows the loss graph of the proposed model. We can see from the figure that our model is not overfitting, yet the loss is close to 0.01. It means that our model is reliable in identifying the subject.

Although we previously set the epoch value 200 on the parameter setting, the simulation stopped at about 118 epochs and 140 epochs for F1-score and loss, respectively. This is because the early stopping and model checkpoint were applied as a regularization procedure to avoid overfitting the model. This is also shown by training and testing graphs (both in accuracy and F1-score) which are close to each other.

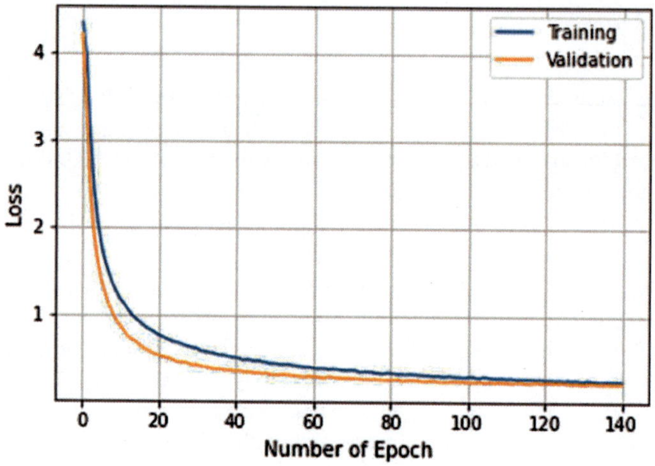


**Fig. 11** Training and testing loss of the proposed model

### 3.3 *Confusion Matrix*

Figure 12 shows the confusion matrix for each class. The confusion matrix is needed to show the number of correct predictions by the proposed model for each class. We can see that the proposed model can predict well for each class. The x-axis represents the predicted label in the confusion matrix, while the y-axis is the actual label. For example, "subject 16,273" has 166 corrected predictions and one wrong prediction as "subject 16,420".

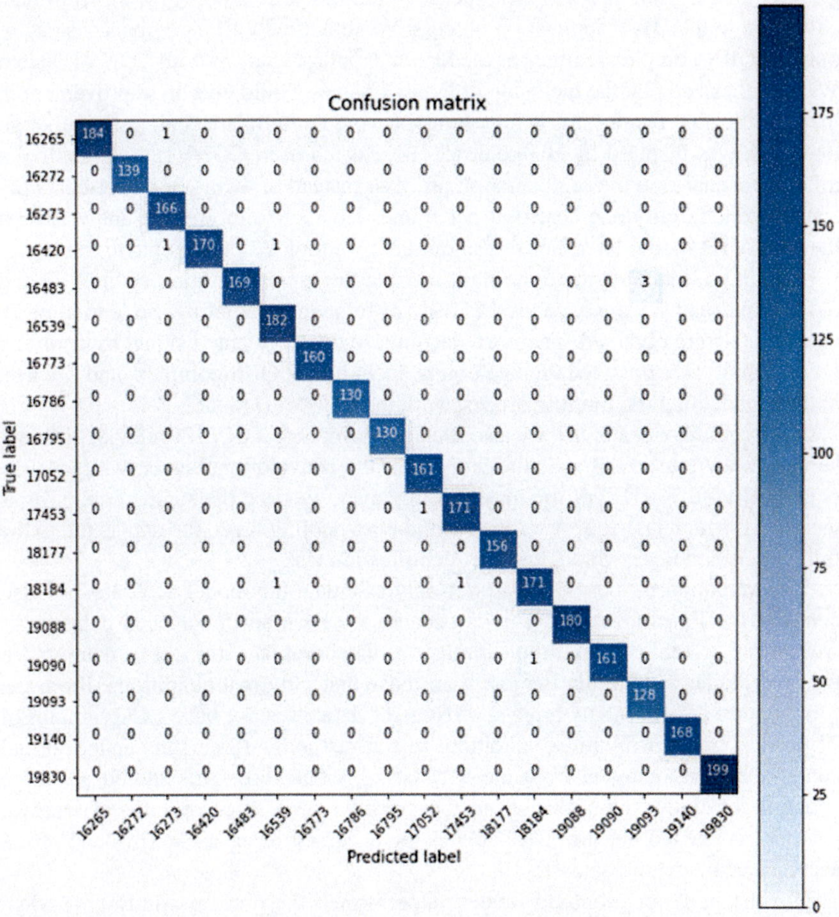


**Fig. 12** Confusion matrix of the proposed model using testing data

## 4 Discussions

Our proposed method opened an exciting new avenue of study focused on ECG-based individual identification systems by considering a mixed dataset of heart conditions (i.e., under normal and arrhythmia). For the first attempt of study, we combined three different datasets from publicly available databases: MIT-BIH NSRDB, MIT-BIH Arrhythmia, and 12-lead INCART databases. These datasets have different frequency sampling, as we summarize in Table 1. We then converted the frequency sampling for all datasets into a constant value which is 250 Hz. After that, each dataset would go through the same process as depicted in the block diagram (Fig. 1), from data collection to the DWT application process. We took the PQRST segment instead of only the QRS-complex segment as the feature input for analysis with CONV1D later. We hypothesized that the inclusion of P and T waves would give an improvement in the identification result. This is following the work from Bajare et al. [14]. Although this work was inspired by Bajare et al. [14], which used CONV1D, we applied a different scenario in the segmentation process. Instead of taking 3–4 heartbeats per frame, we took only one heartbeat per frame. This is to simplify the analysis with the CONV1D model later. For this one frame, we took 22 data points to the left of R-peak and 33 data points to the right to meet the typical duration of the P-Q and S-T complexes [17] since we used 250 Hz of frequency sampling. So, a total of 56 data points were obtained. Then, we decompose this segmented signal by applying DWT. Finally, we obtained 28 data points, including P, QRS-complex, and T wave, before conducting the training process with the CONV1D model.

Just like Bajare et al. [14], we also used two layers of CONV1D but with different kernel size. We used a $3 \times 1$ filter kernel for the convolutional layer, while Bajare et al. [14] used $7 \times 1$. For the max-pooling layer, we used the same kernel size as them [14], which is $2 \times 1$. After the second max-pooling layer, the data is fed to the fully connected layer which does the identification task.

For evaluation purposes, we do not only calculate the model accuracy but also consider the F1-score value. This is because we have an imbalanced dataset. As we can see in Table 1 about the summary of databases, the number of datasets for the heart under arrhythmia is more than those under normal conditions. From the combination of MIT-Arrhythmia and INCART databases, we have ECG samples of 71 persons under arrhythmia condition. In contrast, only 18 persons under normal conditions were obtained from the MIT-NSRDB database. This should get more attention for future studies that we need to consider the balanced number of datasets. F1 score is needed because it calculates the accuracy of each class instead of the accuracy of the whole dataset.

For instance, our proposed model outperformed the previous study [14] when using the MIT-BIH NSRDB database, but not with their experiment using the ECG-ID database. Our proposed model achieved a validation accuracy of 99.8% (see Fig. 10) and an F1-score of 99.8% (see Fig. 11) with the combined datasets. In comparison, Bajare et al. [14] achieved the highest accuracy of 96.93% using the MIT-BIH NSRDB database (see Table 4). Although when using the ECG-ID database

**Table 4** The summary of previous study on ECG-based biometric system

| Articles | Model | Database | Accuracy (%) |
|---|---|---|---|
| Hammad et al. [13] | ResNet | • PTB | 98.85 |
| | | • CYBHi | 99.27 |
| Kim et al. [15] | LSTM | • MIT-BIH NSRDB | 100 |
| | | • MIT-BIH Arrhythmia | 99 |
| Bajare et al. [17] | CONV1D | • MIT-BIH NSRDB | 96.93 |
| | | • ECG-ID | 100 |
| Proposed model | CONV1D | • MIT-BIH NSRDB<br>• MIT-BIH Arrhythmia<br>• INCART | 99.8 |

they [17] managed to achieve 100% of accuracy, they did not show whether their model is a good fit. Meanwhile, with only a 0.02% different, we can prove that our model is a good fitting based on the plot of accuracy and loss. A good fit model is essential to achieve in order the model can predict more accurately when we feed the system with new data (which is not in the dataset yet). For comparison, Table 4 shows the summary of the previous studies, and we can see that our proposed model can compete with other models, while our model can do predict more subjects.

Finally, the implication of our study will be elaborated on in this section. Investigating a light-weight yet robust system of ECG-based biometric systems could benefit for real world application. We have shown that a robust system can be developed by using only two-layer convolution instead of implementing a more complex structure. This can be a benefit regarding low computing cost, which becomes a major concern in many hardware usages. Furthermore, conducting a study with the basic consideration that we have no prior information about the heart's condition of the users (or tested individuals) will also benefit in a real-world application. Biometric systems in real-world applications such as digital transaction, entertainment industry, or other else generally do not require the information about the heart's condition of their user before hand (i.e., whether they have a normal or abnormal heart). Thus, inspecting an ECG-based biometric system with the mixture datasets (i.e., ECG data under normal and abnormal conditions) will resemble actual application. So that errors (misidentification) in the actual application can be minimized. Our findings give a new insight that a reliable system using mixture datasets is possible to build.

## 5 Conclusions

This study gives a new insight into ECG-based individual identification systems by considering combined datasets of the heart under normal and arrhythmia conditions. For forming a combined dataset, we utilized three publicly available databases on Physionet, which are: MIT-BIH Normal Sinus Rhythm Database, MIT-BIH Arrhythmia Database, and INCART 12-lead Database. A total of 32,628 datasets in the form of PQRST features from 89 persons were obtained. We implemented only two layers of a convolutional neural network to build a light-weight system that can maintain reliable performance. The results show that our proposed model is robust enough for ECG-based individual identification by providing a good accuracy of 99.8% in the form of an F1-score. We also proved that our model is a good fit (not under/over-fitting) based on the visualization plot of accuracy and loss. However, this work requires further investigation in some points, such as: utilizing a balanced dataset, implementing different kernel sizes, or using a greater combination of datasets to confirm the feasibility of our proposed approach.

## References


1. Korolov M (2019) What is biometrics? 10 physical and behavioral identifiers that can be used for authentication, 12 Feb 2019. [Online]. Available: https://www.csoonline.com/article/3339565/what-is-biometrics-and-why-collecting-biometric-data-is-risky.html. There is NO VOL, NO PP
2. NN: 81 of company data breaches due to poor passwords, 14 Aug 2018. [Online]. Available: https://www.tracesecurity.com/blog/articles/81-of-company-data-breaches-due-to-poor-passwords. There is NO VOL, NO PP
3. Marasco E, Ross A (2014) A survey on anti spoofing schemes for fingerprint recognition systems. ACM Comput Surv 47(2):1–36
4. Schroff F, Kalenichenko D, Philbin J (2015) FaceNet: a unified embedding for face recognition and clustering. In: The IEEE conference on computer vision and pattern recognition (CVPR), pp 815–823. IEEE, Boston
5. Asnawi R, Said M (2018) Testing of other languages usage in addition to the default languages for the easy voice recognition module. In: International conference on electronics technology, pp 321–324. IEEE, Chengdu
6. Karimian N, Guo Z, Tehranipoor M, Forte D (2017) Highly reliable key generation from electrocardiogram (ECG). IEEE Trans Biomed Eng 64(6):1400–1411
7. Aloudat A, Michael K, Abbas R (2016) The Implications of Iris-recognition technologies: will our eyes be our keys. IEEE Cons Electron Mag 5(3):95–102
8. Liu F, Lin G, Shen C (2015) CRF learning with CNN features for image segmentation. Pattern Recogn 48(10):2983–2992
9. Singh YN, Singh SK, Ray AK (2012) Bioelectrical signals as emerging biometrics: issues and challenges. Int Schol Res Notices 2012:1–13
10. Gargiulo F, Fratini A, Sansone M, Sansone C (2015) Subject identification via ECG fiducial-based systems: influence of the type of qt interval correction. Comput Methods Programs Biomed 121(3):127–136
11. Merone M, Soda P, Sansone M, Sansone C (2017) ECG databases for biometric systems: a systematic review. Expert Syst Appl 67:189–202

12. Kim B-H, Pyun J-Y (2020) ECG identification For personal authentication using LSTM-based deep recurrent neural networks. Sensors 20(11):1–17
13. Hammad M, Plawiak P, Wang K, Acharya UR (2020) ResNet-attention model for human authentication using ECG signals. Expert Syst 2:1–17
14. Bajare S, Vaishali I (2019) ECG based biometric for human identification using convolutional neural network. In: 10th international conference on computing, communication and networking technologies (ICCCNT), pp1–6. IEEE, Kanpur
15. Virani SS, Alonso A, Aparicio HJ, Benjamin EJ, Bittencourt MS, Callaway CW, Carson AP, Chamberlain AM, Cheng S et al (2021) Heart disease and stroke statistics-2021 update L A report from the American Heart Association. Circulation 143(8)
16. Elgendi M, Mohamed A, Ward R (2017) Efficient ECG compression and QRS detection for E-health applications. Sci Rep 7:1–16
17. Maršánová L, Němcová A, Smíšek R et al (2019) Advanced P wave detection in Ecg signals during pathology: evaluation in different arrhythmia contexts. Sci Rep 9:1–11
18. Xiang Y, Lin Z, Meng J (2018) Automatic QRS complex detection using two-level convolutional neural network. Biomed Eng Online 13(17):1–17
19. Maghfiroh AM, Musvika SD, Wakidi LF, Lamidi, Sumber, Mak'ruf MR, Pudji A, Titisari D (2021) State-of-the-art method to detect R-peak on electrocardiogram signal: a review. In: Proceedings of the 1st international conference on electronics, biomedical engineering, and health informatics, pp 321–329. Springer
20. Porr B, Howell L (2019) R-peak detector stress test with a new noisy ECG database reveals significant performance differences amongst popular detectors. bioRxiv, pp 1–27. Cold Spring Harbor Laboratory, Singapore (2019)
21. Klabunde RE (2020) Cardiovascular physiology concept. [Online]. Available: https://www.cvphysiology.com/Arrhythmias/A009. Accessed 14 Jan 2020. There is NO VOL, NO PP
22. Malleswari PN, Hima Bindu C, Satya Prasad K (2021) An improved denoising of electrocardiogram signals based on wavelet thresholding. J Biomimet Biomat Biomed Eng 51(1):11–129
23. Huang JJ, Putra W (2020) RunPool: a dynamic pooling layer for convolution neural network. Int J Comput Intell Syst 13(1):66–76
24. Yamashita R, Nishio M, Do RKG et al (2018) Convolutional neural networks: an overview and application in radiology. Insights Imaging 9:611–629
25. Cardarilli GC, Di Nunzio L, Fazzolari R et al (2021) A pseudo-softmax function for hardware-based high speed image classification. Sci Rep 11:1–10

# A Cost-Effective Multi-lead ECG Ambulatory Monitoring System Built Around ESP-32D Using ADS1293

**Harikrishna Parikh, Bhavesh Pithadiya, Jatin Savaliya, Ankitkumar Sidapara, Kamaldip Gosai, Urmi Joshi, and H. N. Pandya**

**Abstract** Cardiovascular diseases have been a major reason causing human mortality in the last half-century. It is evident that with careful monitoring and tracing precursors, the threat can be curbed to an appreciable level. Ambulatory monitoring devices with diverse features are available for the same purpose and they vary largely in the price range. Most of them are very expensive to be affordable to common people. This paper, proposes a cost-effective solution. We have devised a pocket-sized, multi-lead ECG ambulatory monitoring system prototype, capable of recording bipolar and unipolar ECG leads at 200 samples per second for a time duration, up to a week in the onboard microSD card. The system is built around SOC ESP-32D, ADS1293 front end and RTC DS1302z. ADS1293 provides 24-bit digital data for each sample from 3 channels (reading LA, RA, and LL signals with respect to RL). These samples are converted to 8-bit resolution for further processing. From the standard arithmetic established for the Einthoven's Lead System (Leads I, II and III) and the Goldberger's Lead System (Leads aVR, aVL and aVF) the actual 3 channels are converted to 6 leads and the same is stored periodically on the attached microSD card along with the timestamp. The trials carried out on human subjects are successful and ECG plots obtained from stored data are good enough not only for monitoring but also for diagnosis purposes. With some necessary upgradation, the system can be deployed for cardiac patient monitoring at the community level in a very cost-effective way. The system has been realized and tested on a couple of volunteers from the research group. During the test period recording of ECG was quite satisfying and the system generated all alerts during forced alerts. The plots of ECG derived from recorded data were found to be acceptable for monitoring as well as diagnosis. Successful implementation of such low-cost systems at the community level will help monitor cardiac patients and save many human lives, which otherwise would have been constrained due to affordability.

H. Parikh (✉) · B. Pithadiya · J. Savaliya · A. Sidapara · K. Gosai · H. N. Pandya
Department of Electronics, Saurashtra University, Rajkot, India
e-mail: harikrishna.parikh@gmail.com

U. Joshi
Government Polytechnic, Jamnagar, India



T. Triwiyanto et al. (eds.), *Proceedings of the 2nd International Conference on Electronics, Biomedical Engineering, and Health Informatics*, Lecture Notes in Electrical Engineering 898, https://doi.org/10.1007/978-981-19-1804-9_27

**Keywords** Ambulatory monitor · Multi-lead ECG · ADS1293 · ESP-32D

## 1 Introduction

Cardiovascular disease is the leading cause of death due to non-conjugative diseases across the world [1] as well as in India where the death toll has crossed the double mark from 2000 to 2015 [2]. 17.9 million people are estimated to have lost their lives due to CVDs across the world in 2015, representing 31% of all global deaths by non-conjugative diseases [3, 4]. In contrast to a general belief that CVDs are prevalent in urban areas, 40% and 56% rise in CVD cases among rural men and women respectively is recorded [2]. The majority of CVDs including, heart attacks and strokes can be prevented by the treatment of precursors such as high blood pressure, lipid profile, and diabetics, and practicing healthy living [5]. An individual's health status can be revealed by studying various physiological parameters. Tools/instruments to perform this monitoring has improved a lot in the last half-century and have proven to be very useful to reveal the onset of health issues before it exaggerates [6]. Frequent monitoring and use of smart devices can help figure out the patient and treat him/her accordingly to avoid any hostile consequences [7].

ECG is a quasi-periodical, rhythmically repeating signal, acts as an indicator of bioelectric events and in turn health of the heart. ECG is considered the most important tool in defining the health of a heart, as careful study of it can aid detection of CVD far before it actually knocks [8].

Many researchers have already contributed a lot in this field since the development of the first such monitor known as 'the cardiotachoscope' in 1952 [9]. In recent years, matured information technology and electronics industry, lead the development further in the direction of miniaturization, wearability, implantability, digital wireless operation. Now, the signals are recorded on digital media such as a flash memory or a microSD card instead of tape recorders, in such ambulatory systems [10]. With the evolution of digital signal processing, now it is possible to analyze the signal in real time with recording and each of the QRS complexes can be categorized and labeled accordingly (Romero et al. 2009). Kapse, Parikh, and Shah have earlier reported a single lead ECG recorder using Arduino UNO and AD8232 AFE, capable of recording ECG on a microSD card [11]. Junjiang Chen et al. have also reported similar heart activity monitor based on microcontroller Atmega128L [12]. Kohno, Abe, and Benditt have also reported a similar system capable of sampling ECG signal with a predefined sampling rate and converting the same to its digital equivalent, and storing it with timestamp on digital media [13]. Similar ECG ambulatory monitor is reported from Teixeira and Ferreira [14]. M. Neyja et al. have devised an IoT-Based E-Health Monitoring System Using ECG Signal. with Hidden Markov Model (HMM) to improve the timely treatment of hospitalized patients [15]. M. A. Yusof and Y. Wen Hau have reported a home-based vital sign monitor with an android mobile application facilitating the monitoring of ECG along with body temperature and blood oxygen [16]. Oresko et al. have embedded real-time data processing on a monitor, making it capable of feature extraction and beat classification [17]. The most basic ECG monitoring systems include the primary processes like signal acquisition, signal processing, feature extraction [18]. Henian Xia, Irfan Asif, and Xiaopeng Zhao have reported an IoT-based monitoring system with a primary data acquisition feature [19]. Feature extraction techniques have been divided into 3 categories by Tejedor et al. as time-based, frequency-based, and combined time and frequency [20]. Tripathi et al. have devised a wearable real-time ECG monitoring system based on smartphone [21].

Modern ECG monitors equipped with signal processing, feature extraction, beat labeling and pattern detection algorithms are smart enough to identify deviation in ECG morphology attributed to cardiac disorder very efficiently [22–24]. But such units are very expensive and not affordable in our country, where a large population and smaller budget for health is a big obstacle. Hence, we framed the objective of designing an ultra-low-cost ECG monitor. Looking into a large number of human victims and their increasing number in developing countries like India, the objective is justified. The objective of the study is to devise a multi-lead ECG ambulatory monitor, that can record Einthoven's and Goldberger's leads at 200 samples/second on the memory card attached with a resolution of 8-bits.

# 2 Materials and Methods

## *2.1 Conceptualizing the System*

Bioelectric signals generated from heart muscular activities have to be analyzed to help in diagnosis. Such signals are picked up from the surface of the body using ECG electrodes converting ionic conduction at the tissue level to electronic signals on the surface level. Here, are employed Silver-Silver Chloride pre-gelled disposable electrodes to pick up signals from the body. Such signals are extremely small in magnitude and overridden with ambient noise, motion artefacts, and bio-signals from other body parts, mandating careful signal conditioning to provide a reliable representation of heart physiology. We started designing such multi-lead ECG system with the specifications enlisted as follows.

The system is expected to offer six-lead ECG recording with 8/10-bit resolution at sampling rate of 200 Hz. The system must be able to store the sampled signals on attached microSD card with timestamping. The proposed system must generate alerts against lead-off, battery drain, microSD card error as well as real-time-clock issues.

## 2.2 Prototype Design

Several options, including discrete, op-amp based, or instrumentation amplifier-based circuits as well as analog or digital front-end single IC solutions were available. Looking forward to the higher level of integration resulting in a compact system, we searched for single IC solutions. We decided to go ahead with a multi-lead, multi-channel ECG front end with onboard ADC, lead selector, compensator, lead-off detector, right leg drive (RLD), and a common mode detector. Popular options for this category of devices include ADS1292 (2-channel) [25], ADS1293 (3-channel) [26], HM301D (3 differential, 1 impedance channels) [27], ADAS1000 (5-channel) [28], MT2511 (1-ECG, 1-PPG channel each), R1025 (1-ECG, 1-PPG channel each) [29], etc. After careful study of specifications, we have selected ADS1293 (manufactured by Texas Instrument) for the multi-lead ECG monitoring system. Some important features of ADS1293 include low power operation, low noise, 24-bit resolution 3-parallel ECG channels with Pace output, RLD, Wilson and Goldberg terminal, AC and DC lead-off detection, in-built oscillator, and reference [26].

We preferred to design a 6-lead ECG system using a single ADS1293 IC with 4 limb electrodes connected, rather than going for a complete 12-lead ECG system. Configuration of ADS1293 allows us to derive bipolar leads (Einthoven's leads) i.e. lead I, lead II and lead III, and unipolar leads (Goldberger's leads) i.e. aVR, aVL and aVF. A typical connection for deriving 5-lead ECG is adopted from the ADS1293 datasheet [26] with some modifications to fetch signals from RA, LA, and LL with RLD. Arithmetic operations (Table 1) over RA, LA, and LL signal sample values yield all bipolar/Einthoven's leads (I, II, and III) and unipolar/Goldberger's leads (aVR, aVL and aVF).

A simple, but self-explanatory block diagram shown in Fig. 1, describes the system. The block diagram depicts, signal acquisition from the limbs (right and left arm near shoulders and abdomen near both legs) using silver-silver chloride electrodes. The signals are fed to ADS1293 digital front-end configured to receive signals from RA, LA, and LL and amplify them with RLD (right leg drive). SOC ESP-32D reads from the front end and calculates the leads as shown in Table 1. The lead values (samples) are stored on a microSD card attached along with a security string and timestamp.

**Table 1** Calculation of the leads from channel values [30]

| Lead | Arithmetic operation |
|---|---|
| Lead I | Ch2–Ch1 (LA–RA) |
| Lead II | Ch3–Ch1 (LL–RA) |
| Lead III | Ch3–Ch2 (LL–LA) |
| aVR | − (Lead I + Lead II)/2 |
| aVL | (Lead I − Lead III)/2 |
| aVF | (Lead II + Lead III)/2 |

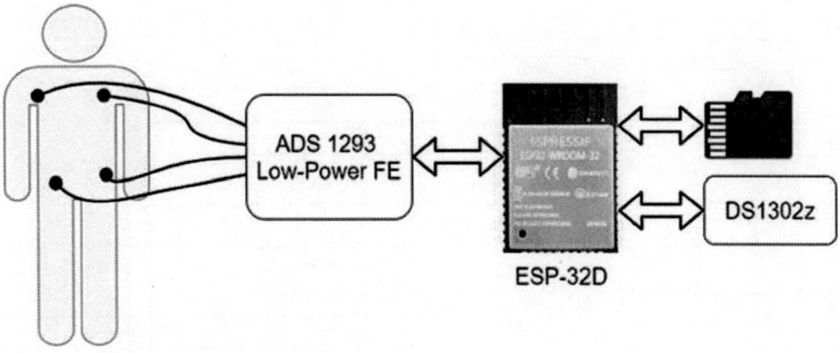


**Fig. 1** Block diagram of the multi-lead ECG ambulatory monitor

This prototype is designed with ESP-32D SOC as the brain. This 32-bit SOC from Espressif running at 160-240 MHz clock and 3.3 V battery, offers loads of features. The circuit diagram of the system is depicted in Fig. 2. The system comprises of an ECG front-end ADS1293, SOC ESP-32D, a Real-Time Clock (DS1302z), and a microSD memory card (16 GB).

ADS1293 has series of control/status registers (00-2F) and data registers (30–50) onboard accessible via serial peripheral interface (SPI) protocol (a generic 4-wire synchronous interface) [26]. The front-end is configured using control registers for desired channel switching, pace channel selection, Wilson central selection, sampling rate, filter setting, feedback, right-leg drive, and single-chip configuration. Lead-off detector registers and Error status registers are useful for the detection of poorly connected electrodes and errors due to various other reasons.

The system is designed to perform first of all configuration of ADS1293 for 3-channel ECG recording and supporting peripherals and then read digital output from each channel in accordance with the configuration and store them on a memory card. At the same time, the system is designed to generate appropriate alarms in case of lead-off condition or generation of any type of error. The ECG data is stored in binary files, each file storing data for an hour. The filename is AYYMDDHH.ECG, where, DD, M, YY, and HH are the date, the month, the year, and the hour of monitoring. This makes the identification/selection of one of several files for review/diagnosis easier. These files are comparatively smaller in size and provide better data handling capability. For uninterrupted and flawless monitoring of one hour, with 8-bit resolution at 200 Hz sampling rate, the size of the file will be $(200 \times 3 + 18 + 7) \times 3600 = 2{,}250{,}000$ bytes or 2.25 MB, aggregating to a daily data collection of $24 \times 2.25$ MB $= 54$ MB. ADS1293 and the microSD card are connected with SOC ESP-32D using SPI interface, while RTC DS1302z is connected using 3-wire interface.

After testing the system at the module level next was to design a working prototype. We designed a compact circuit board (PCB) (Fig. 3) using DipTrace. The circuit is realized using SMD components to the most, for reducing size and weight,

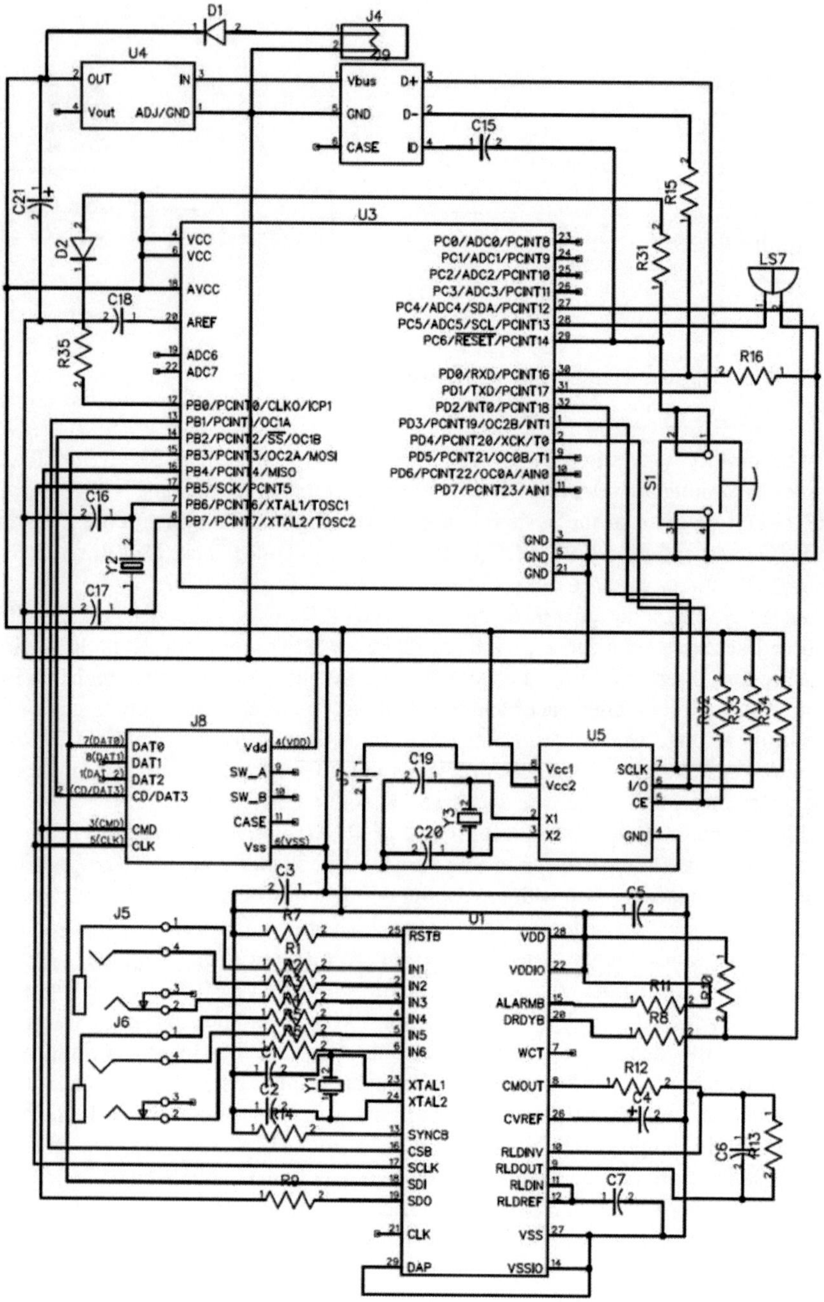


**Fig. 2** Schematic of the proposed multi-lead ECG ambulatory monitoring system

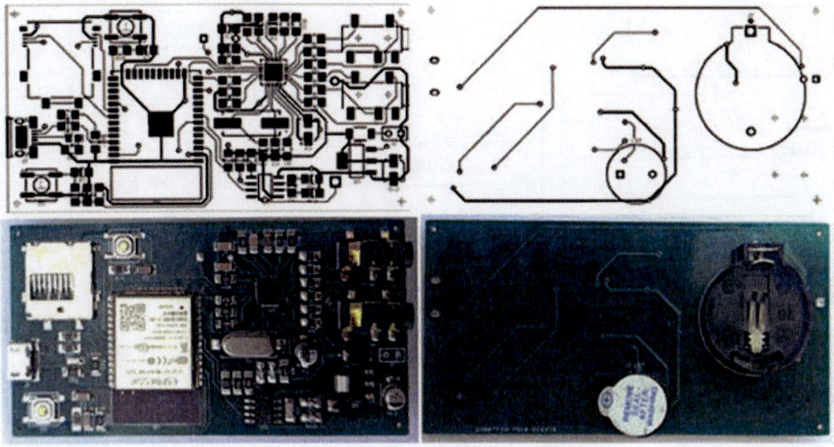

**Fig. 3** PCB layout and actual systems after assembly of components

making it comfortable to wear on the body for a long duration without significant inconvenience.

## 2.3 *Embedded Software*

The system is built around SOC ESP-32D, a 32-bit microcontroller, hence, embedded software plays an important role in defining the functionality of the system [31]. The front end provides a resolution of 24-bits for each channel, which is much higher than required for diagnosis purpose. Hence, the data is scaled down to 8-bit for monitoring purpose, making 3-bytes (1 for each channel) per sample. From, this data is calculated all 6-leads using relation mentioned in Table 1. Such data along with the system ID (1 byte), the System type (1 byte), the Security string (5 bytes), and timestamp (18 bytes) is stored on the microSD card. In the previous study, we have recorded ECG data in CSV file format [11], demanding much more data space due to text representation of data and separating character ‘,’. We switched to binary file format resulting in file size as small as up to one-fourth of the CSV file for 8-bit samples. The configuration of ECG front end ADS1293, RTC, memory card, error detection, alarm generation, deriving signal values for channels at 200 Hz, scaling and storing the same on microSD card; all these functions are governed by firmware written. For being open-source and due to ease of libraries availability and great community support, we chose Arduino as the coding platform. A flowchart, broadly defining data acquisition and warning/alert generation is shown in Fig. 4. The data is temporarily stored in file ‘heart.ecg’ and the same file is renamed when the hour changes to a name ‘AYYMDDHH.ECG’ as discussed above.

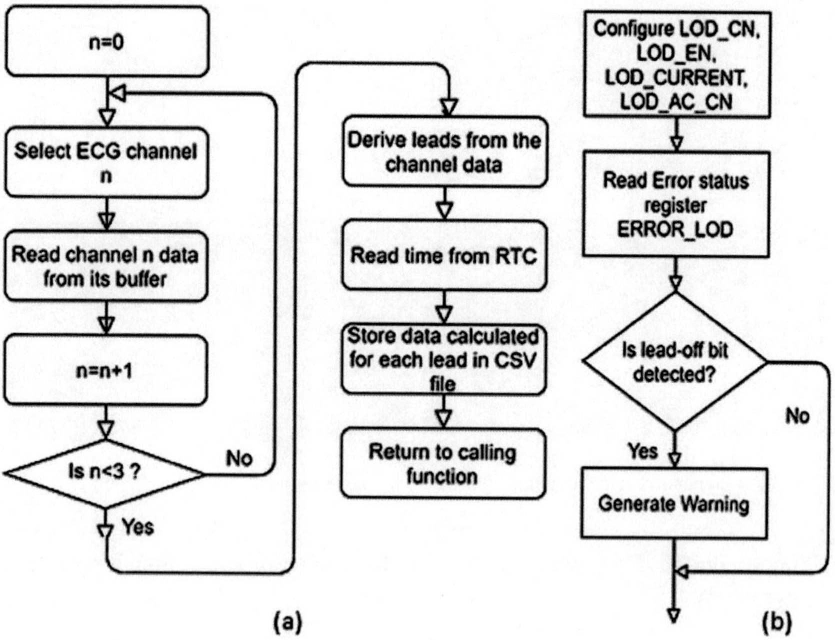


**Fig. 4** Flowchart describing **a** data acquisition and **b** alert generation

## 3 Result

Multi-lead ECG recorder is to be carried on the patient's body and ECG electrodes are to be placed on the body (on the chest near both shoulders and the abdomen near both legs). Trials of the system were carried out on a couple of subjects and the ECG data were sampled at 200 Hz. The experiment was stretched to a duration of 1 week (05–11 July 2021). We forced different types of errors on the system, namely no memory card, poorly connected or disconnected electrode, low voltage from power-bank, RTC out of time, etc. to test the reliability of the system. The system was powered by a 5000 mAh mobile power bank.

The system worked quite well and did not cause any significant discomfort (except the electrodes and cables making subject uneasy for some time) to the subject during the period of operation. We provided 5000 mAh power bank as power supply, which ran for 62 h, before draining totally. This compelled replacement of the drained power bank with another charged one twice during this tenure, causing a break in recording for not more than 2 min.

The ECG data were recorded successfully on the microSD card attached in binary data form, one file every hour. A screenshot of a typical data file is shown here in Fig. 5. The stream of characters in the file represents values for three channels (RA,

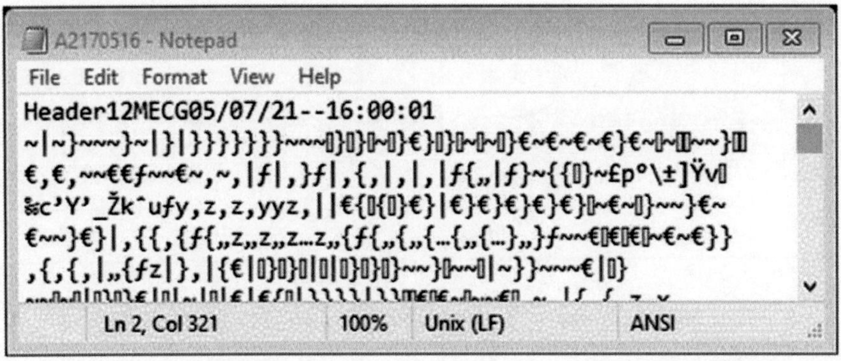


**Fig. 5** Screenshot of A2170516.ECG (3-channel data from sys#1 on 05/07/21 at 16:00:01 h)

LA, and LL) mandates the retrieval of binary data from it. After these characters are converted to binary numbers, leads, they are converted to millivolt equivalent using Eq. (1). The leads I, II, III, aVR, aVL, and aVF are calculated from RA, LA, and LL values using relations in Table 1. After extracting number values from the binary file and calculating amplitude for each lead, the ECG data appears as follows (Table 2). Here are presented only 5 samples for each lead. The sampling rate of 200 samples/second would otherwise have populated the table extensively. One sample ECG plot with the corresponding data is shown here (Table 2; Fig. 6).

Table 2 is representing simple numeric values corresponding to each lead calculated from three channel inputs corresponding to RA, LA, and LL with RLD. Being digital information, it has no unit. But, one can convert the digital information to amplitude easily using Eq. (1).

$$Amplitude = \frac{Reference\ Voltage}{(2^8 - 1) \times 1000} \times \left[sample\ value - (2^7 - 1)\right] \quad (1)$$

Prior to starting a week-long experiment, the system prototypes were tested for error detection and the alert generation. Each of the two system prototypes were

**Table 2** Multi-lead ECG signals (sample data only, actual data for a 5-s plot comprises of 1000 rows)

| S. No. | Amplitude of ECG leads (mV) | | | | | |
|---|---|---|---|---|---|---|
| | I | II | III | aVR | aVL | aVF |
| 1 | – 0.142 | – 0.103 | 0.039 | 0.122 | – 0.090 | – 0.032 |
| 2 | – 0.142 | – 0.116 | 0.026 | 0.129 | – 0.084 | – 0.045 |
| 3 | – 0.155 | – 0.129 | 0.026 | 0.142 | – 0.090 | – 0.052 |
| 4 | – 0.168 | – 0.116 | 0.052 | 0.142 | – 0.110 | – 0.032 |
| 5 | – 0.116 | – 0.103 | 0.013 | 0.110 | – 0.064 | – 0.045 |

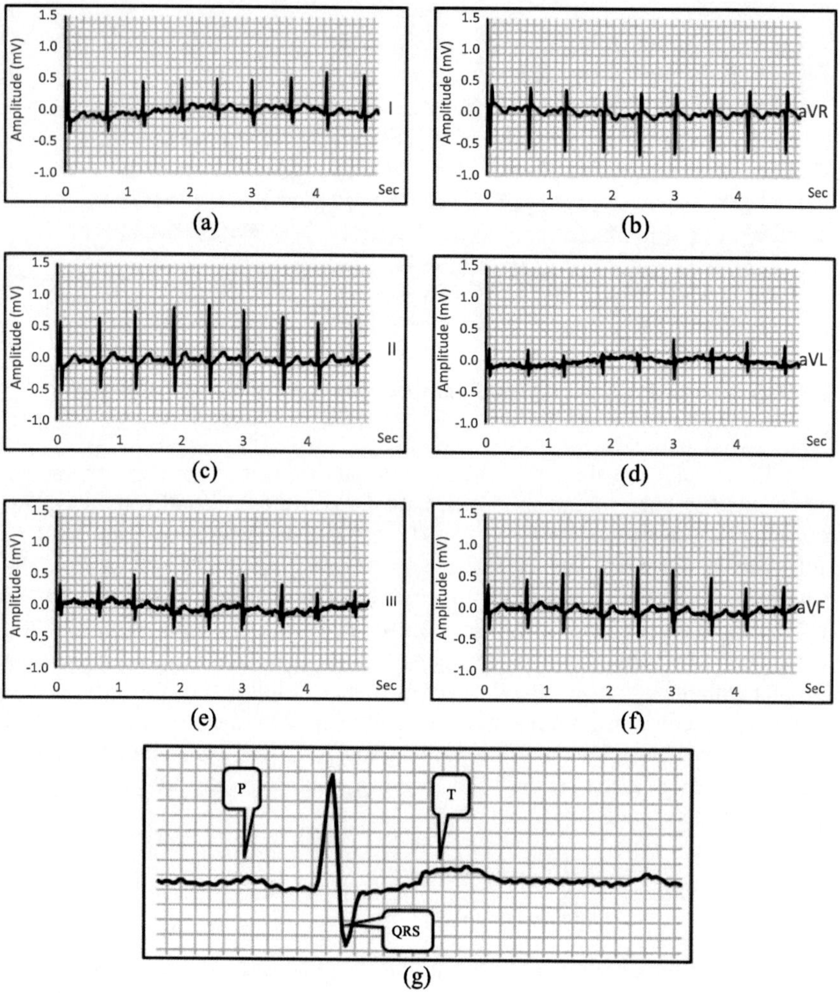


**Fig. 6** **a–f** ECG plots derived from ambulatory monitor for leads I, II, III, aVR, aVL and aVF, **g** magnified view of lead II

forced with errors 20 times in laboratory condition. The process was carried out twice aggregating to 40 tests for each type of error. The response in terms of alert generation was recorded. The outcome of the same is tabulated in Table 3.

**Table 3** Error-alert response

| S. No. | Name of the forced error | Faithful alerts (%) |
|---|---|---|
| 1 | Memory card (including bad memory, broken/rusted contact, invalid size and no card) | 100 |
| 2 | Electrode (including poorly connected or disconnected electrode and old/expired electrode offering very poor signals) | 92.5 |
| 3 | Low voltage from power bank (< 4.0 V) | 97.5 |
| 4 | RTC out of time (including no RTC, bad IC, and loss of time) | 97.5 |

## 4 Discussion

The interpretation of a result can be carried out in qualitative as well as quantitative manner. The system is designed for ambulatory ECG monitoring and the purpose is well served. ECG signals acquired by the system contain a considerably lower amount of noise. The lead signals calculated from the recorded data, when plotted, were found to be quite acceptable for diagnosis. The system has recognized errors across four categories mentioned in Table 3 with a success rate of more than 92%.

The system exhibited uninterrupted functioning for minimum of 62 h, on a fully charged 5000 mAh power bank. It can be concluded that the system offers a single charge operation of 2½ days.

The system acquired signals from ADS1293 with 24-bit resolution which is much higher than required (8-bit). Signals are scaled down to 8-bit before the calculation of limb leads (Einthoven's leads and Goldberger's leads) is carried out. The leads (I, II, III, aVR, aVL and aVF) are recorded with adequate reliability and contain adequate information for monitoring as well as diagnosis purpose.

Ngoc Thang Bui et al. has reported a similar portable ECG monitoring system using the same front-end IC [32]. But their system exhibits a considerable amount of noise, mandating the application of filters. Alessandro Zompanti et al. has devised a portable ECG device using capacitive dry electrodes and ESP32D as core microcontroller, offering BLE connectivity [33]. The system devised by them exhibits noise even after the application of filters. Compared to the abovementioned studies the signals acquired by our system has considerably lower noise.

Due to the limited number of research references on ESP32D as microcontroller and ADS1293 as a front-end, which we have used in our work, it is difficult to carry out more comparative studies.

Being our first effort to realize a multi-lead ECG ambulatory monitor, and has some limitations to be overcome. The limitations of the system are discussed here. The system has neither onboard battery nor charging facility, making it mandatory to carry a power bank along with the system. The addition of a battery operation would add value to the system. The recorded signals in binary file require decoding of embedded information, hence, cannot be processed directly with Microsoft Excel or other spreadsheet applications to generate plots readily. A dedicated supporting application is required to be developed to facilitate reading, decoding, and plotting of

ECG signals on the console. Due to infrastructure constraints, we could not compare the recorded signals with ECG phantom or other emulated signals.

The system prototype, though primitive, is working to the level of satisfaction and serves the purpose for which it is designed. Lower noise and highly reliable alerts make it more useful. The system is prepared at a very nominal cost. Such a cost-effective system can be of great help to large-scale applications.

## 5 Conclusion

Most ambulatory ECG monitors available in the market are very expensive and hence, was felt a need to devise a cost-effective multi-lead ECG ambulatory monitor. The objective of the study is to devise a multi-lead ECG ambulatory monitor, that can record Einthoven's and Goldberger's leads at 200 samples/second on the memory card attached with a resolution of 8-bits. The mentioned research has resulted in an ambulatory ECG monitoring system, which is fully functional, compact, wearable, and providing a pretty good length of operation on a single charge. In test conditions, all alerts are generated faithfully ensuring flawless operation. Even the magnified plot of ECG clearly shows the P-wave, QRS-complex and T-wave, sufficient for diagnosis purpose. The system is devised at a cost of 4000 rupees, which can be reduced substantially, if manufactured in large quantity. Such a cost-effective system with satisfactory performance will surely help to monitor the health of the community at large.

Summarizing, the system is ready for community trials. Further, an automatic ECG beat labeling software is under development, that will ease the process of diagnosis by identifying types of beats based on the morphology of the QRS complex.

**Acknowledgements** The authors wholeheartedly acknowledge the support from the Department of Electronics and Saurashtra University, in carrying out this research.

## References

1. Kevin MN, Hamzah A, John KJ (2019) Cardiovascular disease as a leading cause of death: how are pharmacists getting involved. Integr Pharm Res Practice 8:1–11
2. Calvin K, Gupta R, Xavier D, Prabhakaran D, Mathur P, Kalkonde Y, Kolpak P, Suraweera W, Jha P (2018) Divergent trends in ischaemic heart disease and stroke mortality in India from 2000 to 2015: a nationally representative mortality study. Lancet Glob Health 6(8):914–923
3. Wang H, Naghavi M, Allen C, Barber RM, Bhutta ZA, Carter A, et al (GBD 2015 Mortality and Causes of Death Collaborators) (2015) Global, regional, and national life expectancy, all-cause mortality, and cause-specific mortality for 249 causes of death, 1980–2015: a systematic analysis for the global burden of disease study 2015. Lancet 388(10053):1459–1544
4. World Health Organization (2020) Cardiovascular-diseases-(cvds). https://www.who.int/news-room/fact-sheets/detail/cardiovascular-diseases-(cvds). Last accessed 2020/05/06

5. McGill HC, McMahan CA, Gidding SS (2008) Preventing heart disease in the 21st century: implications of the pathobiological determinants of atherosclerosis in youth (PDAY) study. Circulation 117:1216–1227
6. Elliott M, Coventry A (2012) Critical care: the eight vital signs of patient monitoring. Br J Nurs 21(10):621–625
7. Mohammed M, Hayton R, Clements G, Smith G, Prytherch D (2009) Improving accuracy and efficiency of early warning scores in acute care. Br J Nurs 18(1):18–24
8. Salehi F, Kazemi T, Hajihosseini M (2017) The importance of electrocardiography parameters in healthy Iranian children. ARYA Atherosclerosis 13(3):159–160
9. Himmelstein A, Scheiner M (1952) The cardiotachoscope. Anesthesiology 13(1):62–64
10. Mark RG, Ripley KL (1987) Ambulatory ECG monitoring: real-time analysis versus tape scanning systems. In: Images, signals and devices. M. D. computing: benchmark papers. Springer, New York, pp 55–67
11. Kapse HN, Parikh HN, Shah RB (2015) Development of Arduino based low cost system for monitoring vital biomedical parameters. PRAJNA J Pure Appl Sci 22, 23:64–67
12. Chen J, Zhang Y, Cao M (2012) The study of heart monitor based atmega128L. In: Qian Z, Cao L, Su W, Wang T, Yang H (eds) Recent advances in computer science and information engineering, lecture notes in electrical engineering, vol 127. Springer, Berlin, Heidelberg, pp 15–19
13. Kohno R, Abe H, Benditt DG (2017) Ambulatory electrocardiogram monitoring devices for evaluating transient loss of consciousness or other related symptoms. J Arrhythmia 33(6):583–589
14. Teixeira JP, Ferreira A (2015) Ambulatory electrocardiogram prototype. Proc Comput Sci 64:800–807
15. Neyja M, Mumtaz S, Huq KMS, Busari SA, Rodriguez J, Zhou Z (2017) An IoT-based e-health monitoring system using ECG signal. In: GLOBECOM 2017—2017 IEEE global communications conference, pp 1–6
16. Yusof MA, Hau YW (2018) Mini home-based vital sign monitor with android mobile application (myVitalGear). In: 2018 IEEE-EMBS conference on biomedical engineering and sciences (IECBES), pp 150–155
17. Oresko JJ, Zhanpeng J, Cheng J, Huang S, Sun Y, Duschl H, Cheng AC (2010) A wearable smartphone-based platform for real-time cardiovascular disease detection via electrocardiogram processing. IEEE Trans Inf Technol Biomed 14(3):734–740
18. Banaee H, Ahmed MU, Loutfi A (2013) Data mining for wearable sensors in health monitoring systems: a review of recent trends and challenges. Sensors 13(12):17472–17500
19. Xia H, Asif I, Zhao X (2013) Cloud-ECG for real time ECG monitoring and analysis. Comput Methods Progr Biomed 10(3):253–259
20. Tejedor J, García CA, Márquez DG, Raya R, Otero A (2019) Multiple physiological signals fusion techniques for improving heartbeat detection: a review. Sensors (Basel) 19(21):4708
21. Tripathi RP, Tiwari A, Mishra GR, Bhatia D (2019) Design and implementation of a wearable real-time ECG monitoring system based on smartphone. In: Ray K, Sharan SN, Rawat S, Jain SK, Srivastava S, Bandyopadhyay A (eds) Engineering vibration, communication and information, lecture notes in electrical engineering, vol 478. Springer, Singapore, pp 495–503
22. Alarsan FI, Younes M (2019) Analysis and classification of heart diseases using heartbeat features and machine learning algorithms. J Big Data 6(81):1–15
23. Teplitzky BA, McRoberts M, Ghanbari H (2020) Deep learning for comprehensive ECG annotation. Heart Rhythm 17(5):881–888
24. Kiranyaz S, Ince T, Gabbouj M (2016) Real-time patient-specific ECG classification by 1-D convolutional neural networks. IEEE Trans Biomed Eng 63(3):664–675
25. Texas Instruments (2021) ADS1292 datasheet. https://www.ti.com/document-viewer/ADS1292/datasheet. Last accessed 2021/06/20
26. Texas Instruments (2020)ADS1293 datasheet. https://www.ti.com/document-viewer/ADS1293/datasheet. Last accessed 2020/10/09

27. STMicroelectronics (2021) HM301D datasheet. https://www.st.com/en/data-converters/hm301d.html. Last accessed 2021/06/20
28. Analog Devices Inc. (2021) Data sheet ADAS1000/ADAS1000-1/ADAS1000-2. https://www.analog.com/media/en/technical-documentation/data-sheets/ADAS1000_1000-1_1000-2.pdf. Last accessed 2021/06/20
29. RichTek Inc. (2021) R1025 datasheet. https://www.richtek.com/assets/product_file/RT1025/DS1025-00.pdf. Last accessed 2021/06/20
30. Prabhakaran D, Kumar RK, Naik N, Kaul U (2019) Tandon's textbook of cardiology, vol 1. Wolters Kluwer, pp 298–300
31. Yu C (2014) Research and application of embedded system development based on petri nets. In: Jeong H, Obaidat MS, Yen N, Park J (eds) Advances in computer science and its applications. Lecture notes in electrical engineering, vol 279, pp 1017–1021
32. Bui NT, Vo TH, Kim BG, Oh J (2019) Design of a solar-powered portable ECG device with optimal power consumption and high accuracy measurement. Appl Sci 9(10):1–19
33. Zompanti A, Sabatini A, Grasso S, Pennazza G, Ferri G, Barile G, Chello M, Lusini M, Santonico M (2021) Development and test of a portable ECG device with dry capacitive electrodes and driven right leg circuit. Sensors 21(8):1–15

# 3D Printer Movement Modelling Through Denavit–Hartenberg Theory and RoboAnalyzer

**Jatin Savaliya, Kamaldip G. Gosai, Ankitkumar Sidapara, Harikrishna Parikh, Bhavesh Pithadiya, and Haresh Pandya**

**Abstract** Despite elaborate searching, hardly we have come across the publication explaining the movement of Cartesian Fused Deposition Modelling type 3D printers. This finding inspired us to develop a mechanism which will suffice to understand the movement. Our aim is to build in the laboratory unidirectional and bidirectional movement models and corelate the theoretical aspects with proper working of these models. Pursuing the same, single and dual axis movement mechanisms are prepared to demonstrate the working of 3D printer movement. The movement analysis is carried out using D-H (Denavit-Hartenberg) theory and RoboAnalyzer. The carriage motion, the movement bounds and accuracy are discussed. We designed and developed necessary fixtures using NX-10. Movement control of stepper motor is realized using codes running on Arduino board. The front end is developed in Visual studio for better user interface. The working of models is tested through MATLAB calculations and RoboAnalyzer simulation. The result obtained by measuring the travelled distances for different number of steps for stepper motor, for single axis model reveals $\pm$ 0.27 to $\pm$ 0.96 standard deviation range. Similarly, dual axis model reveals $\pm$ 0.35 to $\pm$ 0.97 for X-axis and $\pm$ 0.42 to $\pm$ 0.84 for Y-axis standard deviation ranges. Our work encourages learners to make their movement mechanism based on their ideas and can verify it through the theoretical concepts. It will help the 3D printing community in understanding the movement of FDM type 3D printer with proper analytical ideas. The use of RoboAnalyzer will inculcate a confidence among the learners.

**Keywords** A slider · 3D printer · D-H theory · RoboAnalyzer

J. Savaliya (✉) · K. G. Gosai · A. Sidapara · H. Parikh · B. Pithadiya · H. Pandya
Department of Electronics, Saurashtra University, Rajkot, Gujarat, India
e-mail: jatinele@gmail.com



T. Triwiyanto et al. (eds.), *Proceedings of the 2nd International Conference on Electronics, Biomedical Engineering, and Health Informatics*, Lecture Notes in Electrical Engineering 898, https://doi.org/10.1007/978-981-19-1804-9_28

# 1 Introduction

3D printers are wonder machines of the present age. They have attracted the industry people and academicians. Many academic institutions have included the 3D printer in their regular studies world over [1–4]. A large number of users are using different types of 3D printers. Among them, the FDM cartesian type 3D printers are most popular, easily available and very cost-effective. In this category, 3D printers having three independent and mutually perpendicular movement are the first choice of the people as they are available in abundance, have enough support of learning and DIY (Do-It-Yourself) kits are available. Academic institutions are invariably having these machines. Hence, a large number of learners are interested to know the working of these printers. Many are fascinated to make their own. The first thing they need to learn is how these 3D printers move their printing heads in three dimensions. We explored the world of research literature which offers the easy-to-understand contribution in such line of work. We came across very few research articles which were near to our work to some extent. This inspired us to develop a prototype and an easy-to-understand method guiding to help understand the movement of the cartesian type 3D printer.

Dev Singh and Rahul [5] have published their work on design and development of cartesian 3D printer. They did not explain the movement mechanism. Patel et al. [6] have reported their work on design and development of FDM (Fused Deposition Modeling) machine. They did not cover the printer movement mechanism. In a similar line of work, Tasneem and Amer [7] and Suprith et al. [8] have worked on the design and fabrication of 3D printers. 3D printer motion concepts are not covered in these works. Hitesh Dommati in his dissertation of Master of Technology in Mechatronics also described design and development of fused filament 3D printer [9]. He also has not covered the movement aspects. As the cartesian 3D printer is having similarity of the cartesian robot arm and gantry robot, we searched for translatory movement work in this field. A. Emre Cetin in his thesis work mentioned about the kinematics of the three-axis cartesian robot arm [10]. He has discussed the Denavit-Hartenberg theory nicely. His main concentration was on the forces between the object and the robot arm. Mahir Abdelwahid Ibrahim Ismail and Mohammed Khalafallah Mohammed discussed gantry robot kinematics [11]. They used MATLAB for the calculation of kinematics analysis. Their main contribution is centered about the GUI for solving the kinematics of this robot. V. V. Suryawanshi et al. have discussed planar stage [12]. They developed their model using CATIA V5 and carried out analysis through ANSYS 14. The working model prepared by them is claimed to have a good match with the expected data for XY movement. They have not covered the Denavit-Hartenberg theory and RoboAnalyzer in their work. C. V. Ferreira and V. F. Romano presented a good work on gantry manipulator [13]. They discussed kinematics and dynamic analysis in order to compensate the positional error. They used Finite Elemental Analysis method with the help of ANSYS 5.4 software for structural deformation. Eiour Orn Porsson carried out to prepare large scale 3D printer linear motion analysis [14]. They studied mainly frame structures using Makerslide and OpenRail aluminum extrusions. They used LabView software for strain experiments. Nicholas et al. [15] discussed about the design and construction of 3D printer platform construction. They adopted the core XY movement method. There was no mention of kinematics analysis in both of these works. We also searched some of the patents [16, 17] based on cartesian robots. There the main focus was on the mechanical design of the structure of this robot. Fikrul Akbar Alamsyah applied the D-H theory for the kinematics solution of robot arm to make cylindrical RPP type robot arm as 3D printer [18].

After going through above previous works, we felt that there is need to develop working models which can demonstrate the motion of 3D printer for X-direction and XY planar movement in an easy-to-understand way without involving detailed mathematical treatment and in a cost-effective way. To justify the proper working of our models, we applied Denavit-Hartenberg theory [19] and RoboAnalyzer simulation software [20].

We used locally available mechanical hardware and electronic hardware components to build our models. The hardware consisted of lead screws, guiding steel rods, sturdy platform, stepper motors, limit switches, needle pointers, graph papers and petty fastening accessories. We used Arduino UNO controller and an A4988 stepper motor driver [21]. Parts for frame structures of the model are 3D printed in-house using NX 10.0 software. To provide user-friendly environment we have created the front-end using Visual Studio 2019 (community Version).

For experimentation of our models, we first worked on the translation motion of the carriage on lead screw due to the rotation of the steeper motor. This led us to finalize the formula involving the number of steps to travel required axial distance on the lead screw. Based on this formula, we programed the Arduino controller. In the front-end we provided the facility to input the number of steps to the stepper motor and to record the distance travelled by the carriage. By pressing run button in the front-end the back-end program causes the carriage to travel specific distances. For different number of steps, the distance travelled in X-direction and on XY-plane were measured with the help of graph paper and the needle indicator. To augment the observed results, MATLAB was used for kinematics analysis based on D-H theory as well as RoboAnalyzer for simulation. The measured values and calculated values were having a good match.

Our contribution to understand the movement of 3D printer will motivate the learners as it is simple to understand, easy to fabricate using components from the local market and quite cost effective.

Compared to our target work, all explored research articles have one or another type of gap. Nobody has constructed easy to fabricate and cost-effective working models which can be easily implemented by the learners. To cater such a need we aimed to design and fabricate single axis and dual axis movement models and present theoretical concepts for verification of the working these models.

## 2 Materials and Method

In order to fill the gaps in the previous work, we fabricated two working models: one for the single direction movement (X) and another for the dual direction movement (XY). The single direction model uses one stepper motor, two guiding rods, one carriage carrying a needle indicator, one lead screw, two linear bearings, one limit switch and one linear scale. Two fixtures were fabricated using 3D printer to hold the stepper motor, guide rod and lead screw. The stepper motor and limit switch are connected to the Arduino Uno board. In a similar way the dual axis model is prepared using two stepper motors for Y-movement and one stepper motor for X-movement. Each stepper motor has a set of two guiding steel rods and one lead screw. Two limit switches are used to decide the home position. Necessary fixtures were fabricated in-house using 3D printer. The detailed description of both these models are as follows.

### *2.1 Construction of Models*

Figure 1a shows the schematic of single axis movement mechanism while Fig. 1b shows the schematic of double axis movement mechanism. In Fig. 1a,b, frame fixture supports are shown as a, b and a, b, c, d, e and f respectively. The steel rods are shown as 1, 2 and 1, 2, 3, 4 in Fig. 1a, b respectively. The frame fixtures are designed in Siemens NX 10.0 software and printed using 3D printer. In Fig. 1a carriage is having three holes to have two linear bearings and one threaded rod. Linear bearings help an easy movement of the carriage while a rod helps to slide the carriage. The linear bearings are passed through two steel rods.

Three rods are fixed on two fixtures situated on the opposite ends of the model. The carriage can be driven in the linear manner by rotational movement of leadscrew driven by stepper motor precisely. A needle is placed at the bottom of the carriage to provide precise measurement visibility. The linear ruler scale with mm graduated divisions is placed to measure the linear movement of the carriage on X-axis (for the single axis model). The head of XY-slider moves along X and Y directions by rotating the X and Y leadscrews using stepper motors. A supporting steel rods passing through linear bearings provide rigidity and work as guide to head for XY-movement. Limit switches are used as movement bounds at one end of the lead screw for both models. A graph paper of 1 mm division scale is fixed on the supporting board on which XY-slider is mounted. The fine tipped pen is attached on the carriage to draw the distance travelled on graph paper. Figure 1b shows all details of XY-slider.

Figure 1c, d shows the models of single and dual axis prepared with the help of 3D printer and in-house workshop facilities respectively. In Fig. 1c, 50 mm of distance travelled accurately by carriage after applying the relevant number of steps to stepper motor is shown. Similarly, the head has travelled 50 mm in X and Y

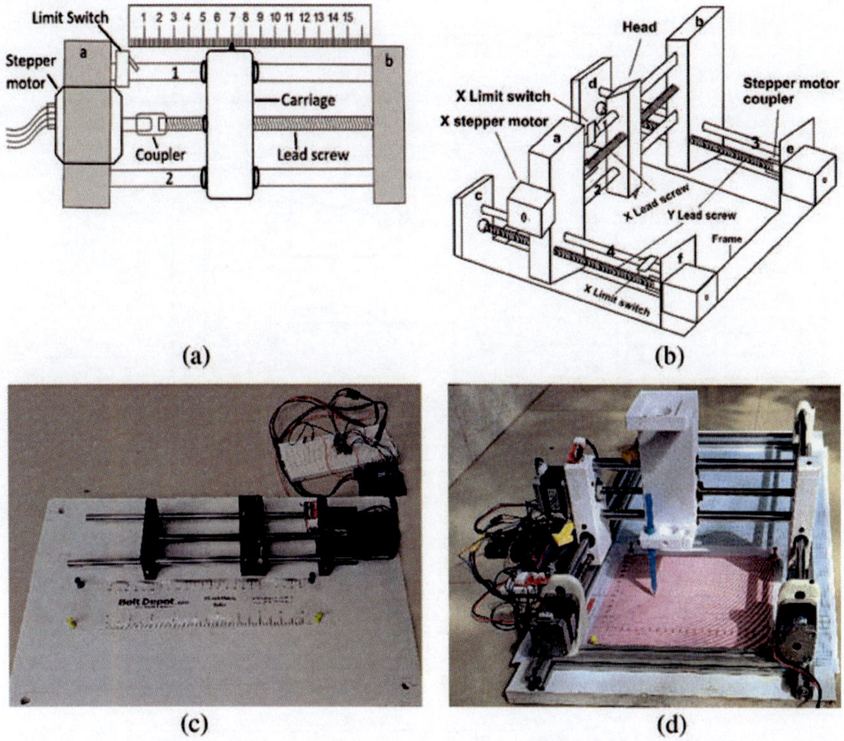


**Fig. 1** Schematic of the construction of models (**a**) and (**b**), Single (**c**) and dual (**d**) axis models prepared in laboratory

direction coordinately is shown in Fig. 1d. As we have used 1 mm scale and graph paper, the accuracy of measurement, visually, is ½ mm of X and XY models.

## 2.2 *Electronic Hardware*

Figure 2a, b shows the schematic diagrams of the electronic circuit used to energize the stepper motors and limit switches. Stepper motors are connected to Arduino UNO microcontroller board via an A4988 stepper motor driver module. Limit switches are directly connected to microcontroller. The Arduino UNO microcontroller board gives step and direction signals to an A4988 motor driver module according to the program embedded. The stepper motor shaft rotates as per given number of steps and forward or reverse direction signals from microcontroller. When any limit switch is turned ON it breaks the movement of stepper in one direction.

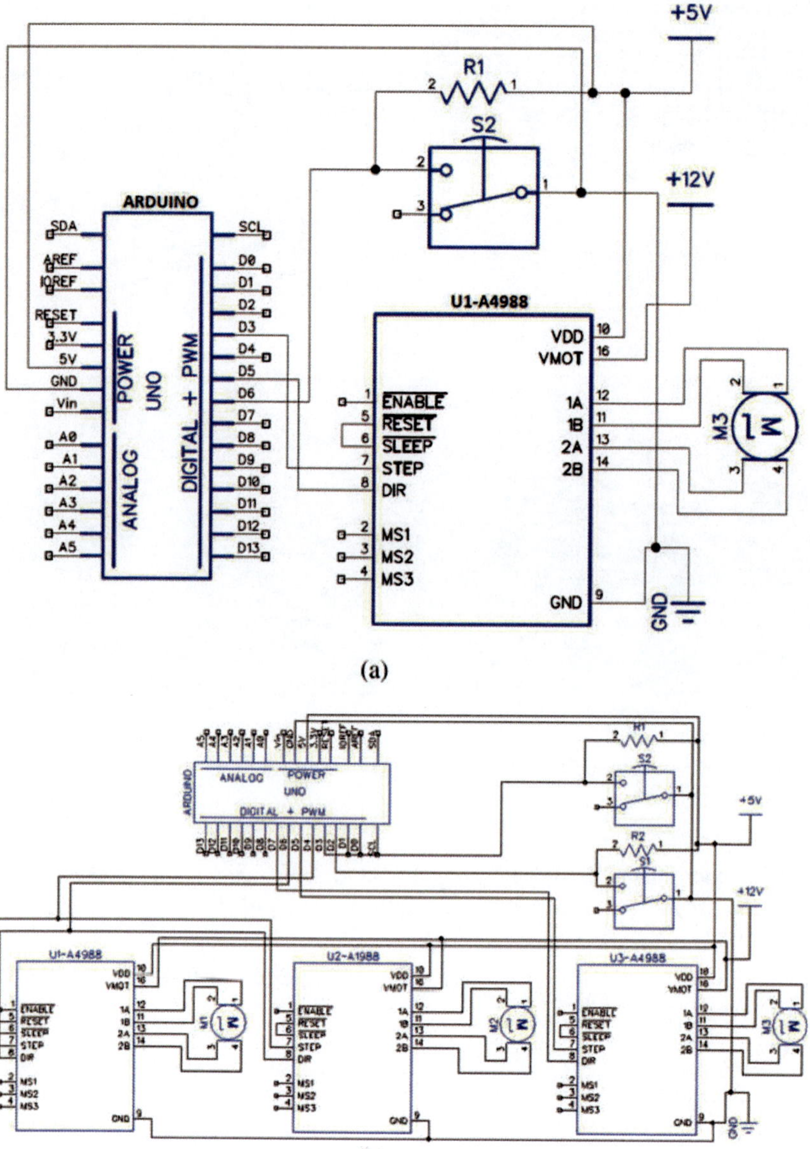


**Fig. 2** Electronics circuit schematic diagram of **a** single and **b** dual axis movement models

## 2.3 D-H Theory

3D printer is a special type of robot. The tool tip movement of the robot describes the movement of the carriage of 3D printer. The movement of tool tip is classically explained by Denavit and Hartenberg. Almost all researchers use D-H theory to explain the movement of the machine. We also have adopted D-H theory for the same reason.

Denavit and Hartenberg presented their work in 1955 describing set of rules regarding coordinate frame assignments and determination of kinematics parameters [19]. It helps to analyze the forward and inverse kinematics of the fixed arm robot. Number of books have simplified the D-H theory [22–24]. An arm robot is made of several rigid links and joints connecting these links. Basically, two types of joints are more common: revolute-joint and prismatic joint [24].

In 3D printer, X, Y and Z movements are due to translation type of motion. Such motions are attributed to the prismatic joints. We will discuss 3D printer movement by using x-axis and XY-axis movement models.

## 2.4 D-H Theory for the Single Axis Model [24]

In a single axis model, over a single rigid link carriage is performing translation motion in one direction. In order to apply D-H theory, we have to follow the set of rules to frame the basic link and frame diagram. After this, we can frame the kinematics parameter table and an arm matrix equation. Solving this equation will provide the estimated position of the carriage on the rigid link which is nothing but the distance travelled by the carriage needle over the graph.

**D-H theory Set of Rules** [24]

Draw the Single Line Drawing of the system and attach coordinate frames to every joint. Figure 3 shows the SLD diagram with coordinate frame assignment. Direction of translation motion is from left hand to right hand. So, for prismatic joint $Z^0$ of coordinate frames $L_0$, will be along the axis of movement. $X^0$ will be perpendicular

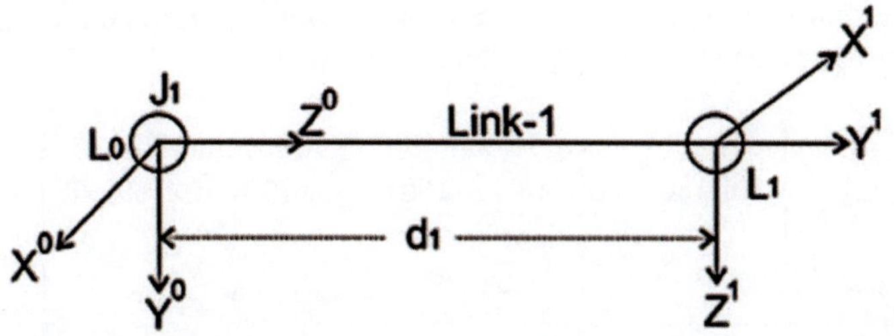


**Fig. 3** Single line diagram of the single axis model with coordinate frame assignment

**Table 1** Kinematics parameters for single axis motion

| Joint | $d_1$ (mm) | $\theta_1$ (°) | $\alpha_1$ (°) | $a_1$ (mm) |
|---|---|---|---|---|
| $J_1$ | $d_1$ | 180 | 90 | 0 |

to $Z^0$ but coming out of the page. $Y^0$ will be positioned following the right-hand rule. As the approach vector of the tool is point downwards, take $Z^1$ perpendicular to $Z^0$ and in the downward direction. $X^1$ will be going inside the page and $Y^1$ will be as per right hand rule. Refer to Fig. 3.

For determination of kinematic parameter, we have only one joint $J_1$, which is prismatic in nature. So, four KP parameter will be as follows.

$\theta_1$ is the rotation about the $Z^0$ axis to align $X^0$ with $X^1$. It is 180° in our case. $d_1$ is the translation along $Z^0$ to align/intersect $X^0$ with $X^1$. In our case, it is total distance travelled by carriage. So, $d_1 = d_1$. $a_1$ is the translation along $X^1$ to align/intersect $Z^0$ with $Z^1$. In our case, they already intersect. Hence, $a_1 = 0$. $\alpha_1$ is the rotation about $X^1$ to align $Z^0$ with $Z^1$. In our case, it is 90°.

So, kinematics parameters taken will be as shown in Table 1.

## 2.5 *An Arm Matrix Calculation for Single Axis [24]*

An arm matrix equation is derived from the kinematics parameter table and a general link coordinate transformation matrix denoted by $T_{k-1}^{k}$ and given as follows [24].

$$T_{k-1}^{k} = \begin{bmatrix} \cos\theta_1 & -\cos\alpha_1\sin\theta_1 & \sin\alpha_1\sin\theta_1 & a_1\cos\theta_1 \\ \sin\theta_1 & \cos\alpha_1\cos\theta_1 & -\sin\alpha_1\cos\theta_1 & a_1\sin\theta_1 \\ 0 & \sin\alpha_1 & \cos\alpha_1 & d_1 \\ 0 & 0 & 0 & 1 \end{bmatrix} \tag{1}$$

$T_{k-1}^{k}$ is the matrix which provides the transformation of homogeneous coordinate frame from the frame k to k − 1. As in a single axis model, we have only one prismatic joint we will have only one arm matrix giving transformation from k = 1 frame to k − 1 = 0 frame, i.e., transformation from tool tip to the base. These frames are shown as $L_1$ and $L_0$ respectively as shown in Fig. 3. Following Eq. (1) and kinematics parameter table, $T_0^1$ will be as follows [24].

$$T_0^1 = \begin{bmatrix} \cos(180) & -\cos(90)\sin(180) & \sin(90)\sin(180) & 0 \\ \sin(180) & \cos(90)\cos(180) & -\sin(90)\cos(180) & 0 \\ 0 & \sin(90) & \cos(90) & d_1 \\ 0 & 0 & 0 & 1 \end{bmatrix} \tag{2}$$

$$T_0^1 = \begin{bmatrix} -1\,0\,0\,0 \\ 0\;\,0\,1\,0 \\ 0\;\,1\,0\,d_1 \\ 0\;\,0\,0\,1 \end{bmatrix} \tag{3}$$

In Eq. (3), $d_1$ is the distance travelled in a single direction.

In our single axis model, rotation of the stepper motor and lead screw gives translation. The Lead of lead screw depends on the pitch of the lead screw and number of starts and relation is given below [25].

Lead of lead screw = pitch × No. of starts

In our case, pitch is 2 mm and start is 4.

So,

$$Lead, l = 2 \times 4 = 8\,\text{mm}$$

Also,

$$Lead, l = distance/revolution \tag{4}$$

Now, 360° makes 1 revolution, then $\theta$ degree (The amount of rotation of the spindle of stepper motor) will make, say R revolution, then

$$R = \theta/360^0 \tag{5}$$

Substituting Eq. (5) in Eq. (4),

$$l = (d \times 360^o)/\theta \tag{6}$$

In our stepper motor, 0.45° is the angle of rotation for a single step given to the stepper motor.

For any random angle $\theta$, the number of steps, say n, will be

$$\begin{aligned} n &= \theta/0.45^\circ \\ \theta &= 0.45^\circ \times n \end{aligned} \tag{7}$$

Substituting Eq. (7) in Eq. (6),

$$\begin{aligned} l &= \frac{d}{\frac{0.45}{360} \times n} \\ d &= l \times \frac{0.45}{360} \times n \end{aligned}$$

But lead l, is 8 mm, Hence,

$$d = 8 \times \frac{0.45}{360} \times n$$
$$d_1 = d = 0.01 \times n \quad (8)$$

Hence, for direct kinematics, input will be the number of steps applied to stepper motor and output will be the distance travelled by the carriage.

## 2.6 D-H Theory for the Dual Axis Model [24]

In this case, there are two types of translation motion perpendicular to each other.

SLD diagram is shown in Fig. 4. The coordinate frames $L_0$, $L_1$ and $L_2$ are assigned to prismatic joints $J_1$, $J_2$ and tool, respectively. The orientation of X, Y and Z axis of each frame is shown following D-H theory. Following the procedure done for the single axis model, the kinematic parameter table can be obtained as shown in Table 2.

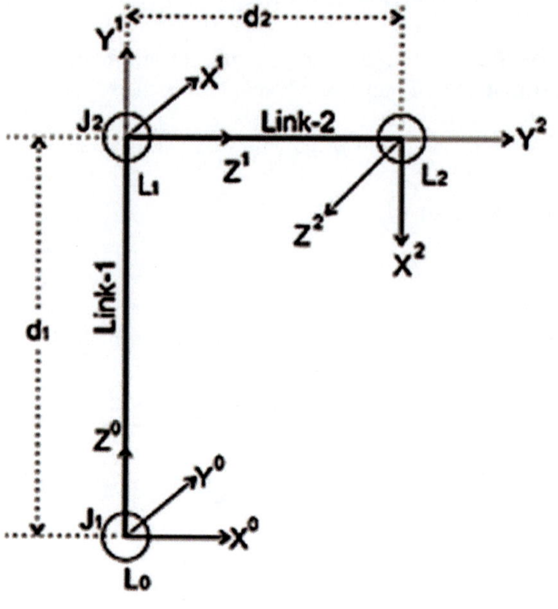


**Fig. 4** Single line diagram of the dual axis model with the coordinate frame assignment

**Table 2** Kinematic parameters for the dual axis motion

| Joint | d (mm) | $\theta$ (°) | α (°) | a (mm) |
|---|---|---|---|---|
| $J_1$ | $d_1$ | 90 | 90 | 0 |
| $J_2$ | $d_2$ | – 90 | 90 | 0 |

## 2.7 Arm Matrix Calculation for Dual Axis [24]

The General Link Coordinate Transform matrix (GLCTM) is used to determine the tool position in XY-plane. The multiplication of matrices of the both directional movements determines the XY-coordinates of position of the head. In other words [24],

$$T_0^2 = T_0^1 \times T_1^2 \tag{9}$$

$$T_0^1 = \begin{bmatrix} \cos\theta_1 & -\cos\alpha_1 \sin\theta_1 & \sin\alpha_1 \sin\theta_1 & a_1 \cos\theta_1 \\ \sin\theta_1 & \cos\alpha_1 \cos\theta_1 & -\sin\alpha_1 \cos\theta_1 & a_1 \sin\theta_1 \\ 0 & \sin\alpha_1 & \cos\alpha_1 & d_1 \\ 0 & 0 & 0 & 1 \end{bmatrix}.$$

$$= \begin{bmatrix} \cos(90) & -\cos(90)\sin(90) & \sin(90)\sin(90) & 0 \\ \sin(90) & \cos(90)\cos(90) & -\sin(90)\cos(90) & 0 \\ 0 & \sin(90) & \cos(90) & d_1 \\ 0 & 0 & 0 & 1 \end{bmatrix} \tag{10}$$

$$T_0^1 = \begin{bmatrix} 0 & 0 & 1 & 0 \\ 1 & 0 & 0 & 0 \\ 0 & 1 & 0 & d_1 \\ 0 & 0 & 0 & 1 \end{bmatrix}. \tag{11}$$

$$T_1^2 = \begin{bmatrix} \cos(-90) & -\cos(90)\sin(-90) & \sin(90)\sin(-90) & 0 \\ \sin(-90) & \cos(90)\cos(-90) & -\sin(90)\cos(-90) & 0 \\ 0 & \sin(90) & \cos(90) & d_1 \\ 0 & 0 & 0 & 1 \end{bmatrix}$$

$$T_1^2 = \begin{bmatrix} 0 & 0 & -1 & 0 \\ -1 & 0 & 0 & 0 \\ 0 & 1 & 0 & d_1 \\ 0 & 0 & 0 & 1 \end{bmatrix} \tag{12}$$

Now, the multiplication of Eqs. (11) and (12) gives $T_0^2$, which decides the tool position in XY-plane.

$$T_0^2 = \begin{bmatrix} 0 & 1 & 0 & d_2 \\ 0 & 0 & -1 & 0 \\ -1 & 0 & 0 & d_1 \\ 0 & 0 & 0 & 1 \end{bmatrix} \tag{13}$$

In Eq. (13), $d_1$ and $d_2$ are distances travelled in two different perpendicular directions for XY-motion. They are calculated just like Eq. (8).

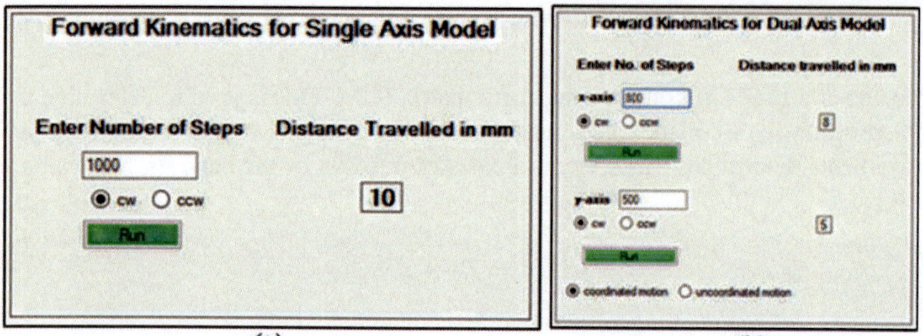


(a) (b)

**Fig. 5** Front-end user interface developed for **a** single-axis and **b** dual-axis forward kinematics

For direct kinematic, input will be the number of steps applied to stepper motors and output will be distance travelled by the carriage on XY-plane.

### *2.8 Front-End Development*

We have developed front-end to provide a convenient user interface using Visual Studio 2019. Figure 5a, b shows the front-end developed to operate stepper motor in a desired manner. Two different front-ends are developed for the forward kinematics of single and dual axis models. For both the front-ends, in forward kinematics the number of steps should be entered with the selection of clockwise or counterclockwise direction of stepper motor shaft rotation. After clicking on the Run button, distance travelled by the carriage will be displayed in mm. In Fig. 5b the coordinated and uncoordinated radio buttons are employed to achieve X-axis and Y-axis coordinated and uncoordinated movements.

## 3 Result

### *3.1 For Single Axis Model*

As discussed in the introduction section, we fabricated the single axis movement demonstrating the model as shown in Fig. 1c. While experimenting we connected the stepper motor and the limit switch with the Arduino Uno board. Thereafter the front-end was opened in the computer. We inputted the number of steps, n, of the same value in the text box five times while selecting the clockwise rotation of the stepper motor. The translatory motion was measured for each time. We obtain the mean value of translation data d1 and also calculated the standard deviation. The similar type

**Table 3** Translation, d, for the number of steps for Direct Kinematic

| S. No. | Calculated data | | | | Observed data |
|---|---|---|---|---|---|
| | As per Eq. (8) | | MATLAB | RoboAnalyzer | |
| | n input in (no. of steps) | d output in (mm) | d output in (mm) | d output in (m) | d output in (mm) |
| 1 | 2500 | 25 | 25 | 0.025 | $24.5 \pm 0.42$ |
| 2 | 5000 | 50 | 50 | 0.050 | $48 \pm 0.96$ |
| 3 | 7500 | 75 | 75 | 0.075 | $74.5 \pm 0.57$ |
| 4 | 10,000 | 100 | 100 | 0.100 | $99.5 \pm 0.35$ |
| 5 | 12,500 | 125 | 125 | 0.125 | $123.5 \pm 0.79$ |
| 6 | 15,000 | 150 | 150 | 0.150 | $150.5 \pm 0.27$ |

of process was carried out for different values of n. For all these different values of n, mean values and standard deviations were obtained. These processed data are indicated in Table 3.

To find out the proper working of the single axis model, we calculated the translation motion using Eq. (8), MATLAB and RoboAnalyzer. To simulate single axis model, we configured the single axis environment in RoboAnalyzer with proper data using kinematic parameters found from the D-H theory. When we run the simulation, we obtained the data, d, showing the translation for the relevant values of n. These data are also shown in Table 3.

## 3.2 *For Dual Axis Model*

Here also we did the proper connection of all three stepper motors and two limit switches with microcontroller. We inputted the same, n, values ($n = 5000$) to both the Y-axis stepper motors and the different value of n ($n = 2500$) for the X-axis motor. This caused all the three motors to rotate and provide the XY-motion of the needle on the graph paper. We performed the experiment for five times with the same, n, values mentioned above and measured the position of the needle on the graph paper every time. We calculated the mean value and standard deviation for X-position ($d_1$) and the Y-position ($d_2$) on the graph paper. In a similar way, we inputted different, n, values and measured $d_1$ and $d_2$. Theoretical calculations were carried out using Eq. (8), MATLAB and simulation was performed in RoboAnalyzer. Table 4 shows the calculated translation data and observed data.

**Table 4** Translation, $d_1$ and $d_2$, for the number of steps for Direct Kinematic

| S. No. | Calculated data | | | | | | | | Observed data | |
|---|---|---|---|---|---|---|---|---|---|---|
| | As per Eq. (8) | | | | MATLAB | | RoboAnalyzer | | | |
| | n (no. of steps) | | Output in (mm) | | Output in (mm) | | Output in (m) | | Output in (mm) | |
| | X-axis | Y-axis | $d_1$ | $d_2$ | $d_1$ | $d_2$ | $d_1$ | $d_2$ | $d_1$ | $d_2$ |
| 1 | 2500 | 5000 | 25 | 50 | 25 | 50 | 0.025 | 0.050 | 24.5 ± 0.57 | 49 ± 0.84 |
| 2 | 5000 | 10,000 | 50 | 100 | 50 | 100 | 0.050 | 0.100 | 50 ± 0.35 | 99.5 ± 0.61 |
| 3 | 7500 | 15,000 | 75 | 150 | 75 | 150 | 0.075 | 0.150 | 74.5 ± 0.45 | 149 ± 0.79 |
| 4 | 10,000 | 20,000 | 100 | 200 | 100 | 200 | 0.100 | 0.200 | 99 ± 0.90 | 199 ± 0.67 |
| 5 | 12,500 | 25,000 | 125 | 250 | 125 | 250 | 0.125 | 0.250 | 125 ± 0.57 | 250 ± 0.42 |
| 6 | 15,000 | 30,000 | 150 | 300 | 150 | 300 | 0.150 | 0.300 | 150 ± 0.65 | 299 ± 0.76 |

## 4 Discussion

Both the models which we fabricated in our laboratory and put into operative environment have successfully provided good results. From Tables 3 and 4, one can learn that the expected translation data calculated by theory and simulated by RoboAnalyzer have a very good match. One can also find out from the observed data that the repeatability of the movements is also fair.

For direct kinematics, we provided the number of steps to the stepper motor from 2500 to 15,000. As per theoretical calculation these inputs were supposed to provide the translation, d, from 25 to 150 mm. The same inputs when simulated in RoboAnalyzer provided the values 0.025 m to 0.150 m. When we performed the actual experiment on the models, the range of translation we obtained is 24.5 mm ± 0.42–150.5 mm ± 0.27. Thus, the calculated translation matches well with the observed data. Similarly, for dual axis model, we performed calculation for 2500–15,000 as number of steps to stepper motor as input for X-direction movement. For Y-direction movement, the number of steps started from 5000 to 30,000. The theoretical estimation from MATLAB script provided the output from 25 to 150 mm for X-direction translation while 50–300 mm for Y-direction translation. The RoboAnalyzer provided the results for X-direction as 0.025–0.150 and 0.05–0.3 m for Y-direction. The experiment performed revealed the X-direction translation to be 24.5 mm ± 0.57–150 mm ± 0.65. For Y-direction translation the experimental result ranges from 49.0 mm ± 0.84–299 mm ± 0.76. These results exhibit quite good agreement with the theoretically calculate counterpart using MATLAB and RoboAnalyzer.

Our work based on observed data on homemade models, calculation using MATLAB and RoboAnalyzer is not seen in the relevant type of works. Ismail and Mohammed [11] discussed D-H theory and measured movement data on a GUI platform on a robot CAD model of Cartesian (gantry) robot. They represented their data in the form of screenshots and not in the processed data format. Emre Cetin [10] in his thesis discusses a detail of the D-H theory, mathematics including position control, velocity and acceleration variation as well as results of the control mechanisms. He has not highlighted positioning data in tabular form. Suryawanshi et al. [12], have done good work on XY-scanning stage along with the table showing expected translation data and observed translation data for different values of the number of steps. But in their work, they have not used D-H theory and/or RoboAnalyzer. Ferreira and Romano [13] reported the similar type of work on the positioning deviation of Cartesian robot. They used D-H theory and have shown their results in the number of graphs. Their work involves extensive mathematics and elastic deformation of the components. This work lacks of simple design, simple mathematics and is not cost effective. On the other hand, in our work we have used simple models, simple calculations and open-source simulation software. All these factors make the learner comfortable in learning.

In our models, distances travelled are measured on a graph paper or a linear scale having maximum resolution of half mm. Actually, data taken are for the minimum step angle of 0.45° which can be reduced up to 0.1° with the help of an A4988 driver. We also have not included frictional forces, velocity and acceleration to make the model simple.

Our both the working modules are simple in nature and use. Any user can easily fabricate and perform the experiment to gain the knowledge of 3D printer movement. RoboAnalyzer being open-access simulation software is also an added advantage for the learners.

## 5 Conclusion

Our idea to develop the single and dual axis movements was aimed to understand the movement of the extruder as it is vital to understand the working of 3D printer. Our literature survey suggested that there was no exact work reported which can guide the learners to gain knowledge of movement of 3D printer movement in an easy-to-understand way, easy to fabricate the required hardware with cost consideration. This framed our target to build such system consisting of models prepared for single direction movement and dual direction movement that can be verified theoretically.

In the process, we fabricated the single and dual axis movement mechanism using mechanical and electronic hardware. We tested the working of these prototypes. We collected the data showing the single direction motion and planar motion. Repeated data we processed and tabulated them. We also calculated the expected data based on D-H theory. We also configured the model environment in the RoboAnalyzer simulation software and obtained the data for single axis and dual axis motion.

All these finding we compared. The results showed that the theoretical estimation matches well with the motion of the models. The mean value was calculated for every input (number of steps) while preforming experiment. From range of data obtained we also calculated standard deviation which ranges from 0.27 to 0.96 for single axis and 0.35–0.9 for X-translation and 0.42–0.84 for Y-translation in the case of dual axis model. We feel that our work will be very useful to them who want to gain the knowledge of working of 3D printer. The measurement means of the motions was based on the graph paper and a scale. This did not reveal the capability of the system.

We hope that some more improvement in our models will make them useful in the real 3D printers. For this, the understanding of the belt driven XY movement and lead screw-based Z movement will be extremely useful. Models can be augmented to facilitate to measure its minimum movement capability.

**Acknowledgements** We, all contributors who carried out this research work warmly thank to the Saurashtra University, Rajkot, Gujarat, India for valuable support. We also express our special thanks to the Department of Electronics, Rajkot for providing the laboratory facilities to complete this work.

## References

1. Pai SS, Gourish B, Moger P, Mahale P (2018) Application of 3D printing in education. Int J Comput Appl Technol Res 7(7):278–280
2. Mehta PU, Berdanier CGP (2019) A systematic review of additive manufacturing education: toward engineering education research in AM. In: 126th American society for engineering education annual conference and exposition 2019, vol 9, pp 6810–6819. American Society for Engineering Education, Tampa, Florida, USA
3. Despeisse M, Minshall T (2017) Skills and education for additive manufacturing: a review of emerging issues. In: IFIP international conference on advances in production management systems, pp 289–297
4. Alabi MO, de Beer DJ, Wichers H, Kloppers CP (2020) Framework for effective additive manufacturing education: a case study of South African universities. Rapid Prototyping J 26(5):801–826
5. Dev Singh D, Rahul G (2018) Design and development of Cartesian co-ordinate-based 3D printer. Int J Mech Prod Eng Res Dev 8(1):263–270
6. Patel N, Bhatt K, Thesiya D, Vora R, Ranjanna Srinivas A (2017) A design, development and mechanical characterization of FDM machine. In: Proceedings of 10th international conference on precision, Meso, micro and nano engineering (COPEN 10). Indian Institute of Technology, Madras, Chennai, India, pp 107–112
7. Tasneem MHB, Amer GT (2019) Design, fabrication and testing of a 3D printer. In: Proceedings of the international conference on industrial engineering and operations management, Pilsen, Czech Republic, pp 2334–2344
8. Suhas Suprith G, Dhanush B, Mustafa JMD, Sai Naveen N, Srinivas S (2020) Design and fabrication of Cartesian 3D printer at low cost. Int J Sci Eng Res 11(6):73–79
9. Dommati H (2015) A dissertation on design and development of an affordable and commercial 3D printer based on fused filament fabrication. Central Institution of tool design, Hyderabad, India
10. Emre Cetin A (2002) Handling interaction forces between an object and Cartesian robot arm in Plana motion, a thesis. In: Olgun Ceilk AS, pp 52–55

11. Ismail MAI, Mohammed MK (2015) Gantry robot kinematic analysis user interface based on visual basic and MATLAB. Int J Sci Res 4(2):482–485
12. Suryawanshi VV, Sonawane PM, Deshmukh SP (2015) Design and development of stepper motor based XY scanning stage. Int J Innov Res Sci Eng Technol 4(9):8161–8169
13. Ferreira CV, Romano VF (2002) A design methodology for the compensation of positioning deviation in gantry manipulator. J Brazilian Soc Mech Sci 24(2):83–92
14. Þórsson EÖ (2013) Analysis of linear motion systems for a large scale FDM 3D printer, final project in mechanical and energy technology. Reykjavík University, Menntavegur 1, 101 Reykjavík
15. Borowski N, Danielson P, Wray M (2017) Design and construction of a 3D printer platform, a major qualifying project. Worcester Polytechnic Institute, UK
16. Costa (1995) Tree-axis Cartesian robot, U.S. Patent 5,476,358
17. Lomerson Jr, Parnel GJ, Dye RD, Prill J (2003) Cartesian robot, U.S. Patent 6,626,630 B1
18. Alamsyah FA (2019) The kinematics analysis of robotic arm manipulators cylindrical robot RPP type for FFF 3D print using Scilab. Int Conf Mech Eng Res Appl IOP Conf Ser Mater Sci Eng 494(1):1–8
19. Denavit J, Hartenberg RS (1955) A kinematic notation for lower-pair mechanisms based on matrices. J Appl Mech 22:215–221
20. Othayoth RS, Chittawadigi RG, Joshi RP, Saha SK (2017) Robot kinematics made easy using RoboAnalyzer software. Comput Appl Eng Educ 25(5):669–680
21. Patil SK, Patil RT (2018) Controlling stepper motor using Arduino Uno. Int Res J Eng Technol (IRJET) 5(4):3540–3542
22. Robert J (2015) Schilling: fundamentals of robotics: analysis and control, 1st edn. Pearson Publications, US
23. Craig JJ (2017) Introduction to robotics: mechanics and control, 4 edn. Pearson Publications, USA
24. Manjunath TC (2013) Fundamentals of robotics, 5 edn. Nandu Printers and Publishers Pvt. Ltd., Mumbai (reprint)
25. Patil AN, Patil AB, Narkhede SS, Mane PD (2018) Design of eccentric load carrying lead screw mechanism: an application of auxiliary rolling shutter system. In: Proceeding of 2nd international conference on engineering trends in science, engineering and technology, Mahratta chamber of commerce, industries and agriculture, Pune (India), vol 8, Issue 9, pp 668–676, 29–30 Sept 2018

# An Arm Robot for Simplified Robotic Pedagogy: Fabrication Method, DH Theory and Verification Through MATLAB and RoboAnalyzer

**Kamaldip G. Gosai, Jatin Savaliya, Ankitkumar Sidapara, Harikrishna Parikh, Bhavesh Pithadiya, and Haresh Pandya**

**Abstract** Robotics has attracted learners from schools to universities being one of the fastest emerging fields in electronics and mechatronics. In most institutions, robotics teaching is carried out through the ready-made robot trainers from various manufacturers. Such teaching style lacks design, creativity and deprives learner from making and testing robots in one's own way. The present paper discusses how one can design, make and put the robot in working condition through the knowledge of basic robotic theory like coordinate frames, coordinate transformations, D-H theory, arm equation and matrix manipulations. Design procedure of enhanced two-axis planar robot, its model making process, application of D-H theory and verification of the relationship between the angular displacements and the position through MATLAB and RoboAnalyzer are presented in this paper. Two Laser sources are employed to mark position on graph paper as well as angular displacement on the circular scale respectively. It is noteworthy that programming skill is not mandatory for learning the basics of robotics. We obtained satisfactory results of the proper working of our robot by comparing the practical observations with the theory and simulation software. The model will be very helpful to the learners who are not having plush laboratory facilities.

**Keywords** D-H theory · MATLAB · RoboAnalyzer · Two-axis planar robot · Coordinate frames · Kinematics parameters

## 1 Introduction

To produce better manpower, teaching–learning methods are to be modified such that it should generate learners who can come up with working products after the completion of their education or during the education phase. To generate expert manpower in the field of robotics, educational institutions need to train learners who can digest the theoretical concepts, nourish their thinking to design one's own robot and who can

K. G. Gosai (✉) · J. Savaliya · A. Sidapara · H. Parikh · B. Pithadiya · H. Pandya
Department of Electronics, Saurashtra University, Rajkot, Gujarat, India
e-mail: kmlgosai11@gmail.com



T. Triwiyanto et al. (eds.), *Proceedings of the 2nd International Conference on Electronics, Biomedical Engineering, and Health Informatics*, Lecture Notes in Electrical Engineering 898, https://doi.org/10.1007/978-981-19-1804-9_29

fabricate well-thought robot. Exploring the ways in which institutions train the inquisitive minds, we found in most of the cases that teaching–learning of robotics involves readymade robots provided by the branded manufacturers. Though colleges and universities cover good theoretical concepts, practical or hands on training is carried out using manufacturer supplied robots or robotic kits along with given programs. We also explored research activities which help simplifying the teaching–learning robotics. We hardly found such research articles. Instead, people have contributed quite a bit in how to use robots in education.

Ghaleb and Aly [1] published the article based on Final year capstone project. They discussed the modelling design and control of 2-DOF robot arm using MATLAB/simulation software. Mustafa and Al-Saif [2], Gouasmi et al. [3], Okubanjo et al. [4], Krisbudiman et al. [5], Othayoth et al. [6] have reported similar work. Their works are around the model making by the use of some or other software and then performing simulation for verification of the theory. Actual robot making and theoretical verification of the proper working of self-made robot is not seen in these works. Amr Nasr A. E. Gaber et al. have published a good work [7]. They mentioned the word Experimentally but physical robot making is not mentioned. They used Autodesk and MATLAB SimMechanics. Rana and Roy [8] reported the design and construction of robot arm. They have not included the design aspects based on theoretical concepts. Raquel E. Patino-Escarcina et al. have prepared an educational curriculum for kids, named EDUROSC-kids to help education in robotics [9]. Child-education is focused in this work.

Some have described elaborately about assembling the robots and make them work as per given software programs. One example of such an attempt is Chap. 11 of a book [10].

Some online training courses are available for building robots using kits. Robotrix India offers coding and robo-training for kids [11]. Mechatron robotics offers similar type of robotic training [12].

In higher education institutions like colleges or universities robotic training courses are somewhat of the higher level. SRM University based at Chennai, India offers robotic training supported by robotic laboratory [13]. They use IRB 1410, IRB 360 robots manufactured by ABB, Zurich, Switzerland. They also use Lego kits. On the other hand, there are different high-tech institutions engaged in robotic education and research [14, 15]. These institutions are costly and beyond the reach of learners from developing or under developed countries.

Looking at such previous works contributing to teaching–learning robotics we feel that there is an imbalance of theory, designing and robot making through practical consideration. Through this paper we present a simplified learning method for robots which is easy to understand, can be verified with established theory presented in several books [16–19], includes guidance for fabrication and verification tools to justify the learning. Also, this learning is very cost effective.

We adopted the theoretical results for two axis planar robot for forward and inverse kinematics [20]. The forward kinematics using DH-theory provides the final transformation matrix $T_0^2$ to find out the position of tool-tip as follows.

$$T_0^2 = \begin{bmatrix} C_{12} & -S_{12} & 0 & a_1C_1 + a_2C_{12} \\ S_{12} & C_{12} & 0 & a_1C_1 + a_2S_{12} \\ 0 & 0 & 1 & 0 \\ 0 & 0 & 0 & 1 \end{bmatrix} \quad (1)$$

From Eq. (1) the position of tool-tip on X-axis and Y-axis can be obtained as

$$X = a_1C_1 + a_2C_{12} and Y = a_1C_1 + a_2S_{12} \quad (2)$$

where, $C_{12} = \cos(\theta_1 - \theta_2)$, $S_{12} = \sin(\theta_1 - \theta_2)$, $C_1 = \cos\theta_1$ and $S_1 = \sin\theta_1$.

Note that, $\theta_1$ and $\theta_2$ are the angular displacements of joint $J_1$ and $J_2$.

Similarly for inverse kinematics, we use X and Y values found with the help of Eq. (2) to calculate the angular values $\theta_1$ and $\theta_2$ from the following formulae.

$$\theta_2 = \pm\cos^{-1}\left[\frac{w_1^2 + w_2^2 - a_1^2 - a_2^2}{2a_1a_2}\right] \quad (3)$$

$$\theta_1 = \pm\tan^{-1}\left[\frac{(a_1 + a_2C_2)w_2 - (a_2C_2)w_1}{(a_1 + a_2C_2)w_1 + (a_2C_2)w_2}\right] \quad (4)$$

Thereafter we discuss materials and method to fabricate the enhanced two-axis planar robot. One can easily manipulate this robot for different orientation of both links. The circular scales are available to record the orientation. MATLAB is used for solving the direct and inverse kinematics. For further verification we also used RoboAnalyzer.

We found that the robot model works properly as theoretical calculations and simulation software supports the recorded data of the robot motion. We hope that such robot designing and fabrication will help learners to grasp the knowledge of robot-making in easy-to-simple way with cost-effectiveness.

## 2 Materials and Method

We discuss here the detailed aspects of what materials are required and the method of how to fabricate the working prototype of the two-axis planar robot. In the making of this prototype, we have included the provision to observe the movement of the robot and its final reach point for direct kinematics. The same is also made available for inverse kinematics.

### 2.1 Design and Fabrication of the Two-Axis Planar Robot Model

To make enhanced two-axis planar robot model, first take a piece of light weight wood (Link 1) as shown in Fig. 1a.

The area in which you want the robot to work determines the length of this wood-piece. Near the proximal-end of this wood piece drill the hole to prepare joint $J_1$. At the left of this hole, drill number of holes to insert counter weights (so that the robot can be placed vertically up). At the right side and near to the hole for $J_1$ joint, drill hole to accommodate the line laser which can help to read the angle $\theta_1$. At the far-end of this wood-piece drill another hole to make a joint $J_2$. Now, take another light weight wood-piece (Link 2) smaller in length to the previous one. At the proximal-end of this second wood-piece drill a hole to match the hole of joint $J_2$ of previous wood shown in Fig. 1b. At the far-end of Link 2 wood-piece, drill a hole to accommodate the laser beam torch. Laser torches and counter weights are not shown in Fig. 1.

Now, take a piece of plywood having area which can accommodate the movement of the robot. Take a graph paper having size which can cover the robot movement on plywood. Paste it on the one surface of the plywood. Now, drill a hole at the origin of the graph paper passing through the plywood. Place a circular scale on the hole you just drilled, to measure angle $\theta_1$. Insert a threaded rod through this hole. With the help of two nuts, fix the rod on the plywood as shown in Fig. 2. Now, insert the link 1 wood-piece through the threaded rod from side, where the graph paper and the circular scale is seen. Tighten this link 1 through a nut and a fly nut on the threaded

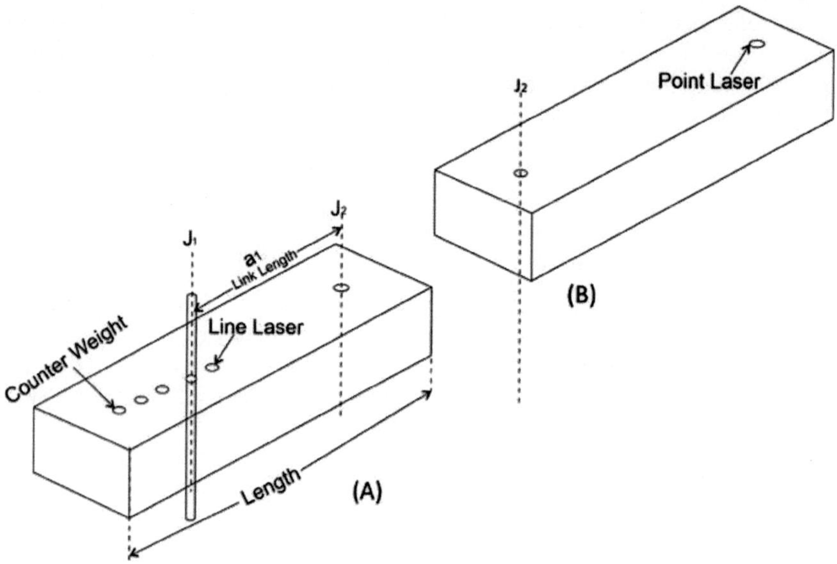


**Fig. 1** Link selections for the two-axis planar robot

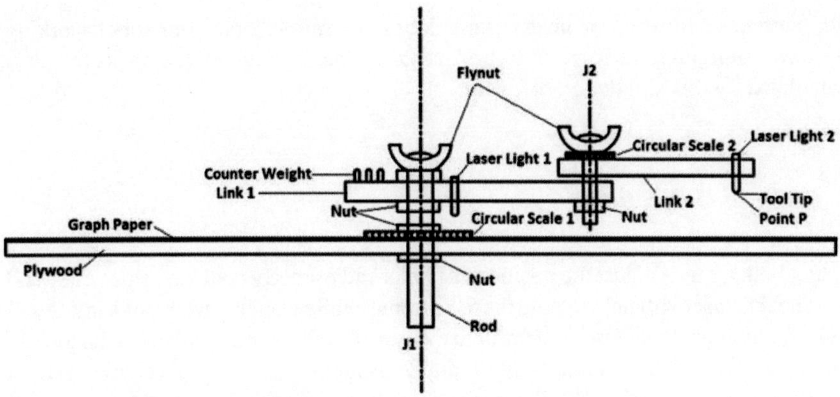


**Fig. 2** Schematic showing assembly of the two-axis planar robot

rod. Insert the line laser with its power connections at its hole on the link 1. At the hole $J_2$ pass another threaded rod through both the links. At the top surface of Link 2 insert a second circular scale through the rod to measure angle $\theta_2$. Draw a line on the middle of the top surface of Link2 where the circular scale is fixed to enable the user to measure the angle $\theta_2$. Fix Link 2 with Link 1 using a nut and a fly nut as shown in Fig. 2. At the far end of Link 2 insert the point laser which works as the tool to accurately measure the X-Y coordinates of the position of the planar robot. Now, the complete two-axis planar robot is assembled.

## 2.2 *Method to Use the Robot*

To make this robot cost-effective, we have eliminated the use of motors and other electronic gadgets. We also dropped the gripper mechanism. The concentration was given to make a working model through which one can justify the theoretical knowledge. The fly nuts are employed to manually activate the robot links. As there are two revolute joints, two fly nuts are used. By loosening and tightening these fly nuts one can change the positions of both links on the graph paper on plywood. To measure the position of the tool tip of the robot the point laser is used. From this laser point incident on XY-graph paper one can manually find out the X and Y position of the tool tip. For finding out the angular movements of the links we have implemented two circular scales, one for $\theta_1$ and second for $\theta_2$. Thus, by moving links one can note the values of $\theta_1$ and $\theta_2$. The corresponding tool tip XY position can be measured from the graph paper. One can tabulate the observations. MATLAB is used to calculate the theoretical expected values of X and Y positions. The comparison of observed values and calculated values should confirm the direct kinematics. Similarly, by manually adjusting the known XY values of the tool tip one can find out the orientation $\theta_1$ and $\theta_2$ of the links. Once again MATLAB will provide theoretical expectations. This will suffice verification of inverse kinematics. To further boost our robot working we have configured the robot in RoboAnalyzer. One can find out the respective data calculated by this simulation software.

### 2.3 Data Collection

Using both fly nuts adjust the positions of links and properly read the values of $\theta_1$ and $\theta_2$. The line laser will help to note the $\theta_1$ readings while center marking of Link-2 will help $\theta_2$ readings. Point laser is helpful to measure X values and Y values of the tool tip positions. Thus, data is collected for $\theta_1$ and $\theta_2$ as inputs and X and Y values as output for the direct kinematics. Similarly, use point laser for recording round values of X and Y positions considering them as input and record the $\theta_1$ and $\theta_2$ values as output for inverse kinematics. These observed data can be compared to the theoretical data calculated by the MATLAB. Augmented calculations of RoboAnalyzer can also be included in the data collection.

## 3 Results

Figure 3 shows the photo of the robot assembled in our laboratory. Two circular scales are visible which measure $\theta_1$ and $\theta_2$ values. The counter weights are also seen which are helpful for vertical positioning of the robot. A line laser is available to indicate $\theta_1$ values on the circular scale. The central mark on Link-2 on its top surface

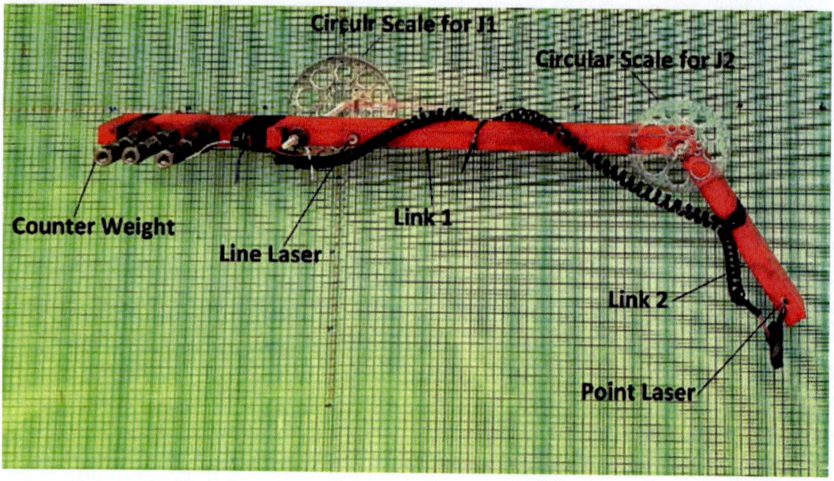


**Fig. 3** Two-axis planar robot model constructed in the laboratory

(may not be visible) helps to record $\theta_2$ values. A point laser will help to record the X and Y values of the tool tip.

The accuracy of recorded data for X and Y position of the tool-tip is 0.05 cm due to the graph we have used. As our robot is manual robot the repetitive data can be obtained by careful adjustment.

## 3.1 *Direct Kinematics*

The direct or forward kinematics is discussed in three ways: experimentally measured values from the model, theoretical calculation using MATLAB and performing simulation on RoboAnalyzer.

**Measurements from the Planar Robot Model**

For the forward kinematics, loosen the fly nuts at the joints $J_1$ and $J_2$ and manually move both the links. Now tighten nuts to measure known values of these angles $\theta_1$ and $\theta_2$. Now, measure the X-distance and Y-distance on the graph where the sharp beam of point laser falls. Do this for different values of both the angles. Record the measurement readings as shown in Table 1.

**Theoretical Calculation using MATLAB**

Run the script written using Eq. (1) for forward kinematics in MATLAB (We have not provided the script in this paper due to space constraint). Obtain the values of X and Y coordinates from it and record the same as shown in Table 1.

**Simulation from RoboAnalyzer**

For further verification RoboAnalyzer [21] is used. Configure the two-axis planar robot in RoboAnalyzer. Run the simulation and note the X and Y coordinates. Record these readings as shown in Table 1.

The results of forward kinematics by theoretical calculations using MATLAB, through the simulation software RoboAnalyzer and through the practically measured on the model robot are shown Table 1.

Figures 4 and 5 show the screen shots of MATLAB and RoboAnalyzer, respectively, for forward kinematics.

## 3.2 *Inverse Kinematics*

Inverse kinematics of the two-axis robot is inspected using three different methods: measurements using robot model, theoretical calculations using MATLAB and simulation using RoboAnalyzer.

**Table 1** Forward kinematics reading for 2-R planar robot

| Quadrant | $\Theta_1$ (°) | $\Theta_2$ (°) | Translation from the model | | Calculated through MATLAB | | Verified by RoboAnalyzer | |
|---|---|---|---|---|---|---|---|---|
| | | | X (cm) | Y (cm) | X (cm) | Y (cm) | X (cm) | Y (cm) |
| 1 | 20 | 50 | 49.02 ± 0.1789 | 34.925 ± 0.2630 | 49.17 | 35.42 | 49.16 | 35.42 |
| 1 | 50 | 70 | 17.26 ± 0.2408 | 52.82 ± 0.1483 | 17.85 | 52.71 | 17.85 | 52.70 |
| 1 | 20 | 26 | 55.58 ± 0.1923 | 31.46 ± 0.1673 | 56.75 | 30.69 | 56.75 | 52.70 |
| 2 | 80 | 70 | – 11.36 ± 0.2302 | 54 ± 0.2739 | – 10.89 | 54.57 | – 10.89 | 54.57 |
| 2 | 110 | 70 | – 37.7 ± 0.2121 | 40.45 ± 0.1291 | – 36.72 | 41.82 | – 36.71 | 41.81 |
| 2 | 120 | 60 | – 43.72 ± 0.2387 | 37.64 ± 0.1140 | – 43.75 | 38.54 | – 43.75 | 38.53 |
| 3 | 180 | 10 | – 64.44 ± 0.1816 | – 2.6 ± 0.3162 | – 65.67 | – 3.73 | – 65.67 | – 3.73 |
| 3 | 250 | – 60 | – 36.54 ± 0.3578 | – 42.68 ± 0.1924 | – 36.39 | – 45.55 | – 36.39 | – 45.54 |
| 3 | 270 | 90 | – 21.48 ± 0.3633 | – 43.5 ± 0.3536 | – 21.50 | – 44.50 | – 21.5 | – 44.5 |
| 4 | 300 | – 30 | – 22.46 ± 0.3209 | – 59.58 ± 0.3114 | – 22.25 | – 60.04 | – 22.25 | – 60.03 |
| 4 | 330 | – 70 | 31.14 ± 0.2966 | – 43.46 ± 0.3361 | 34.80 | – 43.42 | 34.80 | – 43.42 |
| 4 | 360 | – 30 | 61.18 ± 0.2775 | – 11.58 ± 0.2280 | 63.12 | – 10.75 | 63.11 | – 10.75 |

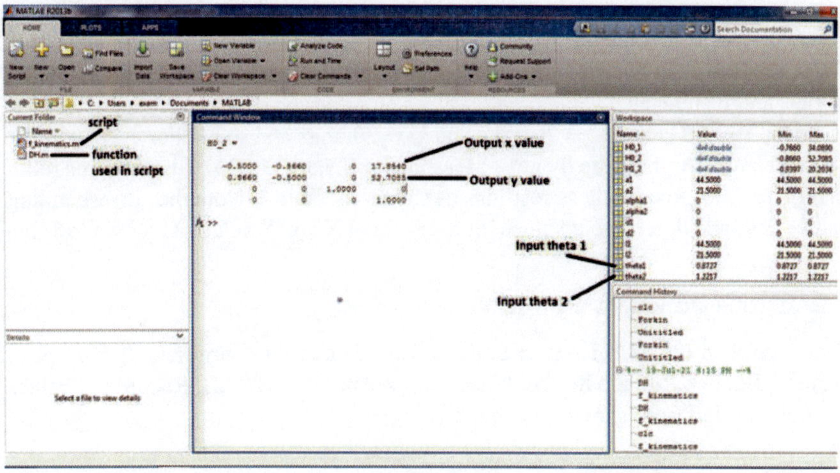


**Fig. 4** Screenshot, showing X and Y values in MatLab for direct kinematics

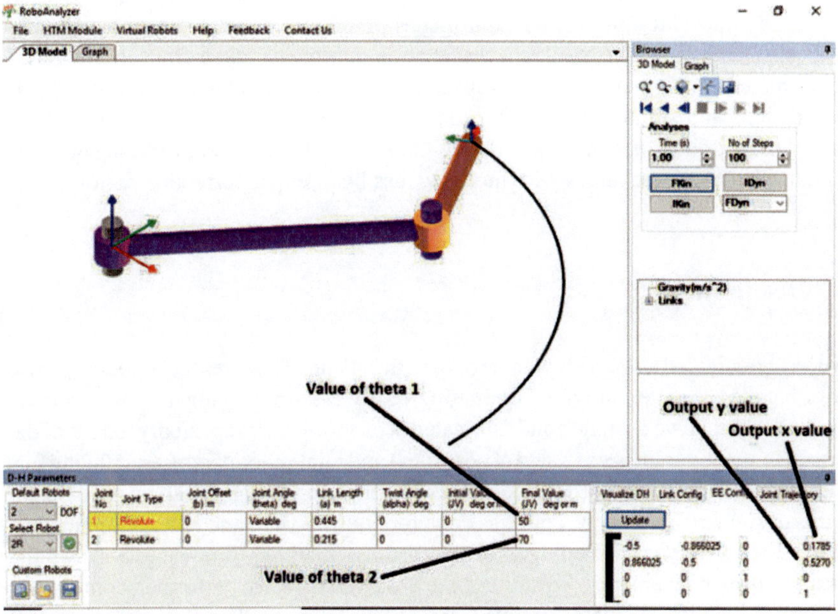


**Fig. 5** Screenshot, showing X and Y value in RoboAnalyzer for direct kinematics

**Measurements using the two-axis planar robot**

For noting the practical measurements, loosen the fly nuts. Move the links manually to measure the integer X values and Y values on the graph paper which read like X = 10 units, Y = 20 Units, X = 20 units and Y = 20 units and so on. For every setting, you will have to tighten the fly nuts. Measure the X values and Y values on this robot as input values. Record these readings as shown in Table 3. Note the corresponding values of $\theta_1$ and $\theta_2$ as output values for every set of X and Y values as shown in Table 2.

**Theoretical calculations using MATLAB**

Write script in the MATLAB to evaluate Eq. (3) and then write another script to evaluate Eq. (4). Run the inverse kinematics script in MATLAB. Record the values of angles $\theta_1$ and $\theta_2$ as shown in Table 2.

**Simulation through RoboAnalyzer**

Perform simulation for the configured two-axis robot in RoboAnalyzer. Record the values of angles $\theta_1$ and $\theta_2$ for the set of values of position of laser point on graph paper, i.e., the values of X and Y coordinates of the tool point as shown in Table 2.

From Tables 1 and 2, we learn that the measurements taken from the two-axis robot model for forward as well as inverse kinematics match well with MATLAB calculations and simulation of RoboAnalyzer. In Table 2 one may wonder that the values of $\theta_1$ do not match. This is due to the nature of the function arctangent. One can match arctangent values with model values by a proper correction factor.

## 4 Discussion

We have fabricated a two-axis planar robot with enhanced features like circular scales, laser sources, counter weights eliminating costly electronic gadgets. The two-axis planar robot that we designed and fabricated is experimented repeatedly to record the cartesian space parameters (X and Y positions) and joint space parameters ($\theta_1$ and $\theta_2$). The observed data were processed for error estimation using statistical methods in terms of standard deviation. This was done for both, forward and inverse kinematics. Table 2 shows the processed data for forward kinematics, while Table 3 shows the data for inverse kinematics. To validate the observed data, we performed comparison of these data with calculated results from MATLAB as well as RoboAnalyzer. All these three datasets are presented in Tables 2 and 3. Comparison of the datasets reveal that the errors in the designed system are acceptably small. Even value of standard deviation reveals reasonably good repeatability of the movement. Studying the calculated data and observed data, we find that, the model prepared is working as expected. We suggest that as our two-axis planar robot movement is achieved by loosening and tightening the fly nuts care has to be taken for good repeatability and accuracy. For better judgement of X and Y values on the graph paper laser source will

**Table 2** Inverse kinematics reading for 2-R planar robot

| Quadrant | Values from model (cm) | | Measurement from model (°) | | Calculated through MATLAB (°) | | Verified by RoboAnalyzer (°) | |
|---|---|---|---|---|---|---|---|---|
| | X | Y | $\theta_1$ | $\theta_2$ | $\theta_1$ | $\theta_2$ | $\theta_1$ | $\theta_2$ |
| 1 | 32 | 41 | 28 ± 0.8944 | 82.1 ± 0.6633 | 27.86 | 82.11 | 27.85 | 82.11 |
| 1 | 3 | 62 | 74.3 ± 0.6 | 41.6 ± 0.8 | 73.69 | 42.51 | 73.69 | 42.51 |
| 1 | 51 | 32 | 16.2 ± 0.7483 | 52.1 ± 1.1135 | 15.80 | 51.83 | 15.80 | 51.83 |
| 2 | − 3 | 64.5 | 83.9 ± 0.8 | 24.3 ± 1.0770 | 84.41 | 25.52 | 84.41 | 25.52 |
| 2 | − 50 | 11 | 140.4 ± 0.5830 | 84.5 ± 0.6324 | − 37.12 | 84.65 | 142.87 | 84.64 |
| 2 | − 40 | 39 | 114 ± 0.6324 | 69.7 ± 1.1661 | − 65.37 | 69.23 | 114.63 | 69.23 |
| 3 | − 54 | − 1 | 158.4 ± 0.8 | 75.6 ± 0.9695 | − 21.62 | 75.64 | − 21.62 | 75.64 |
| 3 | − 55 | − 30 | 195.4 ± 1.0198 | 39 ± 0.8944 | 16.08 | 39.22 | − 163.93 | 39.21 |
| 3 | − 46 | − 40 | 207.4 ± 0.4898 | 47.6 ± 0.9695 | 25.75 | 48.28 | − 154.25 | 48.27 |
| 4 | 28 | − 46 | 278.6 ± 1.0198 | 75.8 ± 0.7483 | − 81.48 | 76.17 | − 81.48 | 76.16 |
| 4 | 37 | − 51 | 295.8 ± 0.7483 | 36.1 ± 0.9165 | − 65.89 | 37.03 | − 65.89 | 37.03 |
| 4 | 55 | − 24 | 320.2 ± 0.9797 | 52.4 ± 0.3741 | − 40.14 | 52.74 | − 40.14 | 52.73 |

be very helpful. It will be convenient to use the model in vertical position. Hence, the counter weight is must.

Number of researchers have worked on an ARM robot [22–25]. Saulaiman et al. [22] has presented a very short review about the development of robot arm. They have used geometrical method to find out position. A very brief overview of robot arm control is considered. Fabrication and real implementation are not seen. Htun et al. [23] discussed about the 2-DOF robot manipulator. In their work they did not use D-H theory for kinematic analysis and positioning was attained by C++ program. Similar type of work, Shekhar and Jayswal [24] has reported on 2-DOF planar manipulator. They covered the kinematic analysis by geometric means. They also performed the simulation but it was for the trajectory motion and they did not indicate in-house model fabrication and have not used D-H theory. Okubanjo et al. [4] have used mathematics to derive the Lagrange-Euler formulae and used them in Simulink for PID control implementation. The real model making is not discussed. Widodo et al. [25] describe kinematic learning through MATLAB based simulation. Our simulation method is not based on MATLAB but we used RoboAnalyzer. Again, the real implementation through model fabrication is missing in their work.

After studying all such similar looking research articles, we found that our work is very different, innovative, easy to understand and fabricate, supported by theoretical analysis and very cost-effective.

This is an academic robot helpful in learning theoretical concepts and it provides confidence to make one's own robot. Note that it is not an industrial robot. Hence, accuracy is not expected like an industrial robot. It is made from the wood. Hence, with weather effect links may warp. Of course, one can use metal links for longevity. Gripper working is not included to maintain simplicity. As the span of the movement of about five by five feet, transportation of the model by the individual may be problematic.

The present work will be very helpful to the learners who have not adequate laboratory facilities to grasp concepts of robotics. Learners can verify the knowledge gained in classes. This will also boost creativity in the learners. It will be useful to students as well as teachers, because it is easy-to-fabricate and does not cost much.

## 5 Conclusion

The necessity of having the low cost, easy to fabricate robot models which can satisfy the theoretical learning in implementing one's own robot design is envisaged and achieved in this paper. In achieving our target, we discussed two-axis planar robot preliminary concepts and D-H theory with direct and inverse kinematics. Building a two-axis planar robot is explained in detail. We have described how one can use the robot to record the necessary observations of orientations and position of the tool-tip. Method to verify the observed data with theoretical calculations using MATLAB is also presented. RoboAnalyzer is used to boost the concepts of robotic learning. The results we obtained with this robot are quite satisfactory. It is concluded that though this is an academic type of robot, it will be very helpful to achieve the learning capabilities of the learners. The cost effectiveness, easy to fabricate and operate features will be suitable to the learners who have limited laboratory facilities.

The logical extension of our work can be the use of stepper motors along with simple programmes to understand the motion concepts. Further, one can develop the systematic approach of making working model which can perform the trajectory movement as planned by the user.

**Acknowledgements** Authors are thankful to Saurashtra University, RAJKOT, INDIA for providing financial help in carrying out this research work and its publication.

## References

1. Ghaleb NM, Aly AA (2018) Modeling and control of 2-DOF robot arm. Int J Emerg Eng Res Technol 6(11):24–31
2. Mustafa AM, Al-Saif A (2014) Modeling, simulation and control of 2-R robot. Glob J Res Eng H Robot Nano-Tech 14(1):49–53
3. Gouasmi M, Ouali M, Fernini B, Meghatria M (2012) Kinematic modelling and simulation of a 2-R robot using SolidWorks and verification by MATLAB/Simulink. Int J Adv Robot Syst 9:1–13
4. Okubanjo AA, Oyetola OK, Osifeko MO, Olaluwoye OO, Alao PO (2017) Modeling of 2-DOF robot arm and control. Futo J Ser (FUTOJNLS) 3(2):80–92
5. Krisbudiman A, Nugroho TH, Musthofa A (2021) Analysis industrial robot arm with Matlab and RoboAnalyzer 7(3):75–80
6. Othayoth RS, Chittawadigi RG, Joshi RP, Saha SK (2017) Robot kinematics made easy using RoboAnalyzer software 25(5):669–680
7. Gaber ANAE, Rezeka SF, El Gamal HA (2016) Design and position control of arm manipulator; experimentally and in MATLAB SimMechanics. Int J Eng Res Technol 5(8):352–359
8. Rana MT, Roy A (2017) Design and construction of robotic arm for industrial automation. Int J Eng Res Technol 6(5):919–922
9. Patino-Escarcina RE, Barrios-Aranibar D, Bernedo-Flores LS, Alsina PJ, Goncalves LMG (2021) A methodological approach to the learning of robotics with EDUROSC-kids. J Intell Robot Syst 2:1–23
10. Manoel Carlos Ramon, Intel® Galileo and Intel® Galileo Gen 2 (2014) API features and Arduino projects for Linux programmers, Chapter-11 assembling and controlling a robotic arm. Apress Open Publisher, pp 509–577
11. Home Page. www.robotix.in. Last accessed 2021/09/07
12. Home Page. www.mechatronrobotics.com. Last accessed 2021/09/07
13. Robotics Lab. www.srmist.edu.in/mech-engg,robotics-lab. Last accessed 2021/09/07
14. Course overview. www.ri.cmu.edu/education/courses/. Last accessed 2021/09/07
15. GRASP Laboratory. www.grasp.upenn.edu. Last accessed 2021/09/07
16. Denavit J, Hartenberg RS (1955) A kinematic notation for lower-pair mechanisms based on matrices. J Appl Mech 22:215–221
17. Bruno S, Oussama K (2016) Springer handbook of robotics, 2nd edn. Springer International Publishing AG
18. Schilling RJ (2015) Fundamentals of robotics: analysis and control, 1st edn. Pearson Publications
19. Craig JJ (2017) Introduction to robotics.: mechanics and control, 4th edn. Pearson Publications

20. Manjunath TC (2013) Fundamentals of robotics, 5th end. Nandu Printers and Publishers Pvt. Ltd., Mumbai (reprint)
21. RoboAnalyzer Home page. http://www.roboanalyzer.com. Last accessed 2021/07/14
22. Sulaiman I, Salam MO, Tanimu Y (2018) Development of a robot ARM: a review, The Federal Polytechnic Bida, School of Engineering Technology. In: 8th national engineering conference
23. Htun TZ, Soe AK, Phyu KW (2020) Design of 2-DOF robot manipulator. https://www.researchgate.net/publication/341070239_Design_of_2-DOF_Robot_Manipulator. Last accessed on 2021/09/19
24. Shekhar C, Jayswal SC (2016) Task time optimization of two DOF robot ARM manipulator using genetic algorithm. Int J Mech Prod Eng 4(2):75–80
25. Widodo A, Muzakki A, Baskoro F (2018) A 2-DOF robot ARM simulation for kinematics learning, advances in social science, education and humanities research. In: 2nd international conference on vocational education and training (ICOVET 2018), vol 242, pp 249–252

# Design, Fabrication and On-Site Implementation of Steel-Framed, Tractor Mountable and Electronically Controlled Pesticide Filling, Mixing and Spraying Attachment

**Ankitkumar P. Sidapara, Jatin A. Savaliya, Kamaldip G. Gosai, Harikrishna N. Parikh, H. N. Pandya, and Bhavesh Pithadiya**

**Abstract** Most farmers in India owe a small piece of land, and hence, cannot afford expensive advanced systems and technology. Farmers use traditional backpack sprayer for spraying pesticides, which is laborious and hazardous to farmer. Preparing the solution of pesticide with water and some of the pesticides need continuous stirring because of their low solubility are issues of backpack type sprayer. These problems framed our aim to make a sprayer which can be attached with the tractor with novel feature like a motor driven tank filling, electronically height adjustment of the boom, foldable ends of the boom and automatic pesticide filling. This paper represents research on the innovative design of automated sprayer attachment. This sprayer attachment is prepared as the solution to abovementioned limitations of traditional sprayer. Using micro-controller and flow sensor, the sprayer can prepare the solution in precise ratio set by the farmer eliminating human interaction. Spray height, span and periodicity of nozzles are adjustable, facilitating the farmer to use it for any crop at any growth level. Also, the spray rate can be adjusted in order to control the dosage. In-built stirrer ensures constant concentration. This attachment is realized using Arduino, DC motor, chain, lead screw, nozzle assembly, the pressure pump and supporting signal conditioning circuits. In experimental trials it covered 3 acres in an hour. The on-site testing of the device worked as per expectations giving the field efficiency 85.82%. The spray rate and span of the coverage were good enough.

**Keywords** Pesticide spraying · Filling and mixing of pesticides · Arduino · Flow sensor

A. P. Sidapara (✉) · J. A. Savaliya · K. G. Gosai · H. N. Parikh · H. N. Pandya · B. Pithadiya
Department of Electronics, Saurashtra University, Rajkot, Gujarat, India
e-mail: sidaparaankit@gmail.com



T. Triwiyanto et al. (eds.), *Proceedings of the 2nd International Conference on Electronics, Biomedical Engineering, and Health Informatics*, Lecture Notes in Electrical Engineering 898, https://doi.org/10.1007/978-981-19-1804-9_30

# 1 Introduction

Indian economy is heavily based on agriculture. A proper yield of the crop is primary condition to boost this economy. Right from seed sowing to final harvesting, farmers face many threats for good yield, like nature dependent irrigation, attacks by pests and insects, damage by animals, insufficient storage facilities and so on. Farmer use pesticides or insecticides to save crops. Many of the Indian farmers have small land and they are not financially sound to use the most sophisticated machine for application of pesticides to their crops. They use backpack sprayer. Researchers have come forward to help the farmer with newer ideas for making good pesticide sprayers. Sprayers are mainly of two types: shoulder laden or vehicle driven. Due to painful labor, harmful to health and consumption of time, shoulder laden sprayer needs to be replaced by vehicle driven sprayers. These problems aroused our interest to develop the sprayer which can be attached to the existing vehicle like tractor. This interest finally got converted to our aim. Researchers have developed varieties of vehicle driven sprayers like human-pushed carts, remote controlled robot carts and solar powered carts. Drone technology is on the horizon to come fast in use. Dhiraj Aher et al. have devised an automatic sprayer four-wheel cart which is hand driven [1]. Here, hand driven motor activates a lobe pump to transfer the pesticide with pressure to the nozzle. Akshaya C. Shirwal et al. have developed similar push type sprayer [2]. The added feature is that, the same machine can be used for fertilizer dispensing. Another variety of push type sprayer is by Singh et al. [3]. They used beam engine principle to generate pressure in the cylinder to eject fluid. V. Pranoy et al. have designed and tested a battery-operated sprayer driven by bicycle. The system has sprayer tank mounted on the cart which is driven by bicycle and the sprayer can rotate by 360° [4]. Apart from these researchers, a number of other research groups also have published their work on sprayers [5–8]. Solar energy supported sprayers are also a category where researchers have contributed their work. Patil et al. [9], Ahalya et al. [10], Chinda [11] and Kumavat Mukesh et al. [12] are some of them. The robot vehicle-based pesticide sprayers also have contributed a lot [13–18]. Siddhi Mane et al. developed a robot vehicle with camera [19].

Compared to robot vehicular sprayer, hand operated or having an attachment of sprayer with existing vehicles like, cycle, motorcycle or tractor are cost effective and easy to fabricate. Hand operated sprayer involves human labor. Many farmers are having tractors with multiple attachments. Hence it will be affordable to fabricate the sprayer as attachment to the existing tractors. Hence, we decided to design and fabricate a device which can be attached to a tractor. We also planned to add some automation like water filling in the tank, pesticide filling and mixing, height and span adjustment of the sprayer. To find out the work done similar to our plan, we explored more literature. Unfortunately, very few research articles found having a suitable match to our expectation. One of these research works is of Mr. Nageshkumar T. who reported his work through his Ph.D. thesis [20]. He has used instead of multiple nozzles only two spraying guns. The gun boom automatic height adjustment is not seen. Also, his work is mainly concentrated on sprayed droplets. Ramchandra Sutar et al. reported one more tractor mounted sprayer work [21]. He has discussed air assisted axial flow blower sprayer. Another tractor mounted boom sprayer reported by Sanchavat et al. [22] is about the field evaluation of the sprayer. This sprayer is hydraulically height adjustable. Even though, it does not satisfy our expectation.

Our thorough search on previous work resulted in need to make the working prototype of vehicle-attachable sprayer with useful features. In the present paper, we have designed, fabricated and tested one such sprayer attachment. It is having additional facilities like mixing of an automatic and precise amount of pesticide, the constant stirring of the liquid. The boom has features like height adjustment, foldability and adjustable nozzle distance. In addition to flow, spray pressure is also adjustable. The most attractive feature is its low cost.

# 2 Materials and Method

Our device comprises of different types of hardware and electronic components. A number of accessories like Brass nozzles, valves, pressure-pipes, aluminum profile, gear-chain, a reservoir tank, lead screws and so on have been utilized in the work. After the frame designing, the frame was fabricated, electronic circuits were built and housed in the frame as well as on the dashboard of the tractor. The driver only has to turn on the tractor and press few of dashboard switches to operate the device.

## *2.1 Design and Working of the Automatic Pesticide Filling and Spraying Attachment*

Figure 1 shows the schematic of automatic pesticide filling and spraying attachment. The skeleton is designed such that it can be fitted in a regular tractor or mini tractor. A pesticide bottle can be fixed on its stand. A tube connects the bottle with the motor. The output of the motor (M4), non-return valve solenoid (V1) and flow sensors are connected in the series. Before using flow sensor, passing a known amount of liquid through it, the output signal pulses are counted. This is to establish a relation between the amount of liquid passing and the number of pulses. Four selection push button switches are provided on console panel to decide amount of the pesticide to be mixed. On pushing any of these switches, the corresponding amount of pesticide will be displayed on display as set count. When the user is satisfied, he can turn the pesticide motor ON to mix pesticide in the tank. Pesticide fluid passing through the flow sensor will increase the count. When this count equals the set count, the pesticide motor is stopped. To avoid spillover of pesticide, a solenoid valve is also activated to instantly cease pesticide going to the water tank. Some pesticides due to its viscosity don't mix with the water. For these pesticides, constant stirring is obtained through motor M3. This motor lifts the heavy pesticides that accumulate

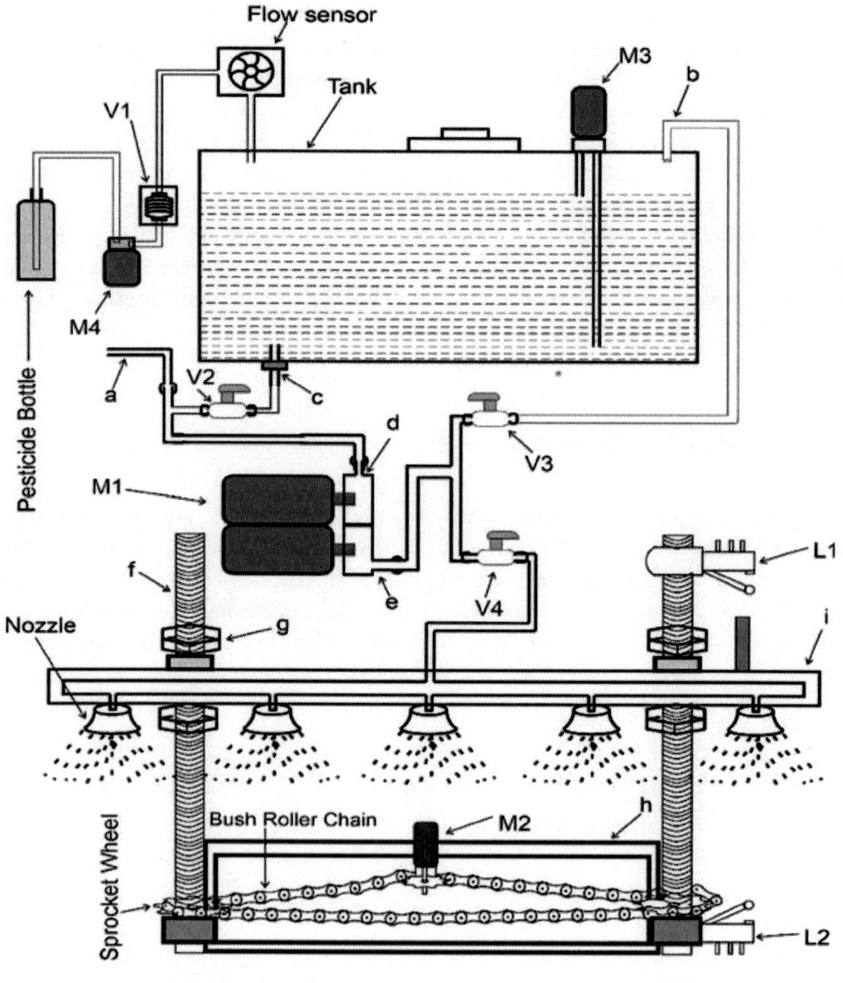


**Fig. 1** Schematic diagram of an automatic pesticide filling and sprayer attachment

on the bottom of the tank and pumps it to the top of the water surface. This brings a good mixture of water and pesticide.

In Fig. 1, 'a' and 'b' are inlet and outlet for the pesticide reservoir tank filing with water respectively. 'd' and 'e' are inlet and outlet of the double motor diaphragm water pump M1 respectively. 'h' is a base frame of structure. A double motor diaphragm water pump M1 is employed for two purposes: To fill the tank with water and to transfer pesticide mixed water to the sprayer nozzles. To fill the water in the tank, V2 and V4 are closed and valve V3 is opened manually. When M1 is turned ON in this condition, the water is pumped from the source through a tube 'a' to the top tank. When pesticide mixed water is to be sprayed, valve V2 and v4 are opened and V3 is closed. In this condition, when M1 is ON it pumps the water from the tank and sends it to the number of nozzles attached on the nozzle holding boom ‘i’.

The sprayer boom ‘i’ is fixed on the two lead screws as shown in Fig. 1 as ‘f’ through two different nuts, ‘g’. One end of each lead screw is welded to the sprocket wheel. The other ends of these lead screw are fixed with the frame. These sprocket wheels are connected with rotating motor M2 through a bush roller chain. Two console switches: up and down controlled motor M2. When UP switch is pressed, motor rotates and along with it, the lead screws also rotate to lift the nozzle bar up. When the down switch pressed, the nozzle bar moves down. This facility is to accommodate plants of different heights. At the extreme end of one lead screw, two limit witches are fixed to stop the advancement of the nozzle bar, in up and down direction.

We used the diaphragm double rotor water pump as a sprayer motor which will pump the liquid from the sprayer tank and push it to the nozzles. Another diaphragm-based water pump we used as a pesticide filling motor. For mixing viscous pesticides with the water a constant stirring heavy-duty battery sprayer motor is employed. To perform up and down motion of the sprayer boom a square gearbox DC motor is used. To achieve the desired amount of pesticide mixing with the water, the flow sensor is considered in the design. The specifications of these major components are shown in Table 1. We have not mentioned petty accessories like fasteners, a housing of the PCB boards, switches, etc. in Table 1.

The electronic part assembly and the PCB testing were carried out in the laboratory of our department. Counting the number of pulses as an output of the flow sensor for the definite amount of liquid calibrate the pesticide filling mechanism. Then from the known number of pulses required for amount of the liquid dispensing was obtained by programming the controller. We provided four switches on the control panel to preset four different pesticide amounts. By testing multiple times, the output amount of liquid measuring through the graduated cylinder we found that there was an error of $\pm$ 2 ml. Generally, farmers used a minimum of 5 ml of pesticide for 15 L of water for the specific type of pesticide. Considering the 150 L capacity of our tank, the pesticide amount required becomes 50 ml. This suggests that the accuracy of our pesticide filling device is acceptable.

## 2.2 *Operation of Filling and Spraying Attachment*

Different switches are available on the console control this attachment. The filling mechanism is explained through the flow chart shown in Fig. 2. For a given flow sensor and the known amount of fluid, the number of output pulses is noted. Based on this, four different volumes’ switches are made available on the console. These are for 1 ml or 1 L, 10 ml or 10-L, 100 ml or 100-L, 1000 ml or 1000 L. The switch named UNIT uses for the selection of ml or liter. By default, this switch is set for ml. When the user pressed any switch from 1, 10, 100, or 1000 ml, the corresponding number of counts is displayed on display. Then, if user turns ON the motor M4, the

**Table 1** Specifications of the major parts of the sprayer

| S. No. | Name of the component | Model | Specifications of the component | Source |
|---|---|---|---|---|
| 1 | Diaphragm double rotor water pump for spraying | SL-DP16 | Pressure: 140PSI (8.5BAR cut-off)<br>Open flow-rate: 7–9 LPM<br>Voltage rating: 12 V DC<br>Current rating: 4–6.5 A | Amazon online market place |
| 2 | Diaphragm based water pump for pesticide filling | R-365 | Voltage rating: 6–12 V DC<br>No load current: 0.23A<br>Maximum flow: 2–3 L/min | HNHCART, Kirtinagar, New Delhi, India |
| 3 | Diaphragm water pump for constant stirring | RO-4949 | Pressure: 130PSI (9.0BAR cut-off)<br>Open flow-rate: 6 LPM<br>Voltage rating: 12 V DC<br>Current rating: 3–4 A | Amazon online market place |
| 4 | Square gearbox DC motor for up-down mechanism | MG-555 | Operating voltage (VDC):12<br>No load speed (RPM): 100<br>Rated current (mA): $\leq 3600$<br>Rated torque (N-cm): 77.4 | Robu, Pune, Maharashtra, India |
| 5 | Flow sensor | YF-S201 | Working voltage (V): 5–18<br>Max current draw: 15 mA@ 5 V<br>Working flow rate (L/min): 1–30<br>Accuracy: $\pm$ 10%<br>Maximum water pressure: 2.0 MPa<br>Pulses per liter: 450 | [23] |

(continued)

**Table 1** (continued)

| S. No. | Name of the component | Model | Specifications of the component | Source |
|---|---|---|---|---|
| 6 | Controller board | Arduino Nano | Microcontroller: an ATmega328<br>Operating voltage:5 V<br>Flash memory:32 KB of which 2 KB used by bootloader<br>SRAM: 2 KB<br>Clock speed: 16 MHz<br>Analog IN pins: 8<br>EEPROM: 1 KB<br>DC current per I/O Pins:40 mA (I/O pins)<br>Input voltage: 7–12 V<br>Digital I/O pins: 22 (6 of which are PWM)<br>PWM output: 6<br>Power consumption: 19 mA<br>Product code: A000005 | [24] |

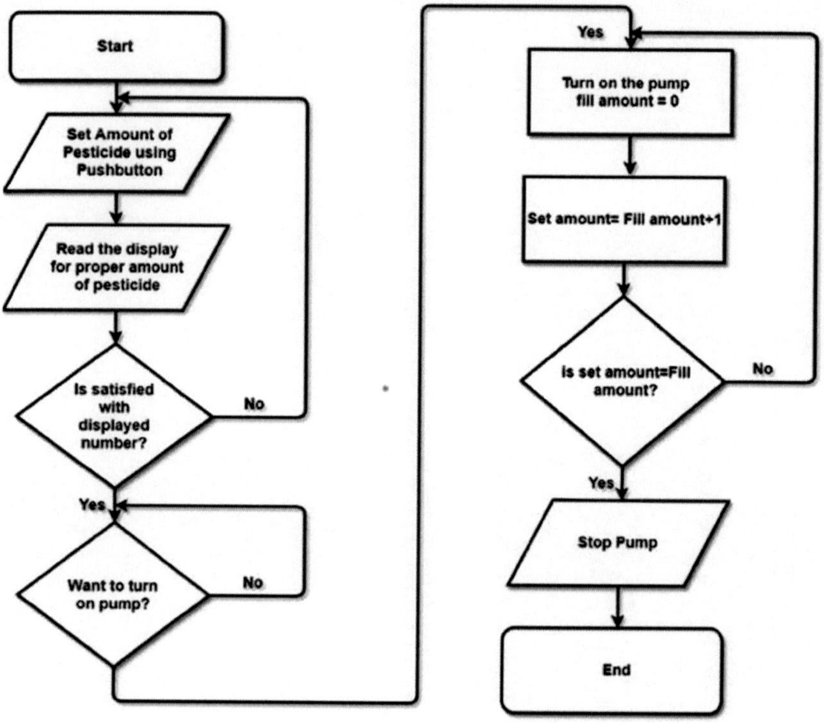


**Fig. 2** Flowchart of the pesticide filling process

pesticide flows to the tank through the flow sensor. As the fluid passes the number of counts increase. At some stage when these counts are equal to set the amount of pesticide (using the button) M4 is turned OFF and solenoid valve is activated.

For the sprayer bar up and down movement, corresponding switches are available on the console. A regular knob is available on the console to control the flow rate of the sprayer.

## 2.3 Details of Circuit Design

Various electronic circuits control the pesticide filling and spraying attachment. Figure shows five different circuits. Figure 3 shows a power supply circuit wherein the 12 V battery is taken as a source and the required output of 5 V is generated.

Figure 4 is the circuit for driving the pump for pesticide filling. It is operated through a relay which works based on the signal received from Arduino via an optocoupler.

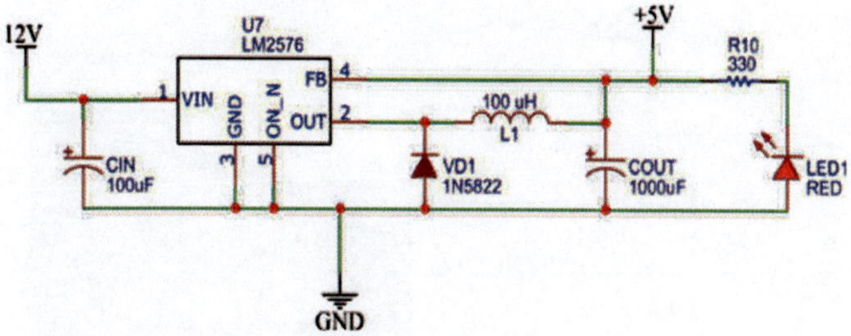


**Fig. 3** Power supply circuit of pesticide filling

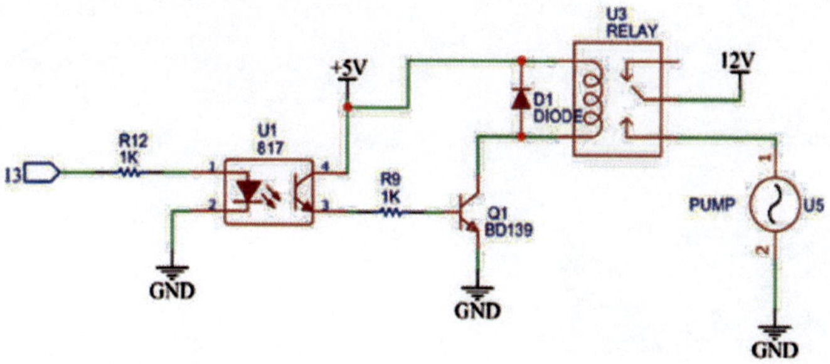


**Fig. 4** Driving circuit for pesticide filling pump

The circuit which controls the solenoid valve is shown in Fig. 5. It is similar to the circuit for the pesticide filling motor circuit. Figure 6 shows some details of flow sensor.

Figure 7 shows the Arduino Nano board circuit. The control panel switches (four switches for selection of a desire amount of pesticide volume, one START/STOP for pesticide filling motor, one for SET/RESET, the selection of the desire amount of pesticide volume, one for counter reset and another one for the ml/liter selection of pesticide fluid) feed information about their ON/OFF status on the data lines of

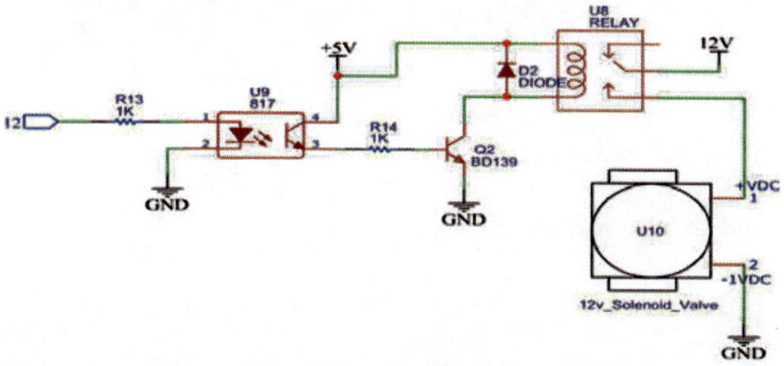


**Fig. 5** Driving circuit of solenoid valve for pesticide filling

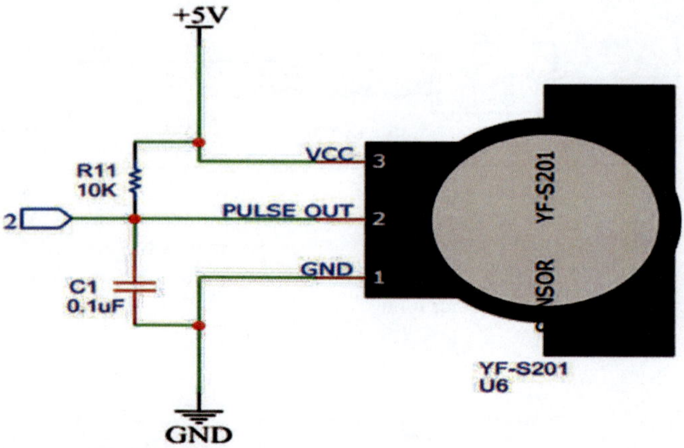


**Fig. 6** Pin out connections for flow sensor

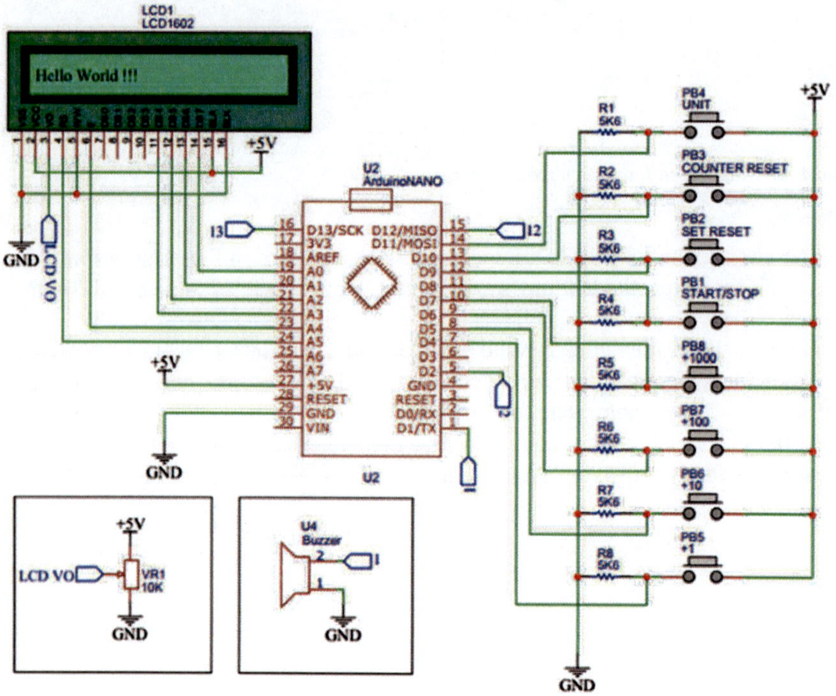


**Fig. 7** The circuit for automatic pesticide filling

the Arduino board. The address lines from the board control the display on LCD. A buzzer driven by pin1 of the board is for the audible indication of the end of the pesticide filling process. The VR1 is to adjust the brightness of LCD.

Figure 8 shows the circuit which controls the Up and Down direction of the nozzle bar. A common selection switch and the respective limit switch control Up or Down relay.

The speed of the pumping motor controls the flow rate of the sprayer. The IC LM555 based PWM concept is used for this. The variable VR1 uses for the setting of PWM pulse width for getting proper flow rate, the circuit is shown in Fig. 9.

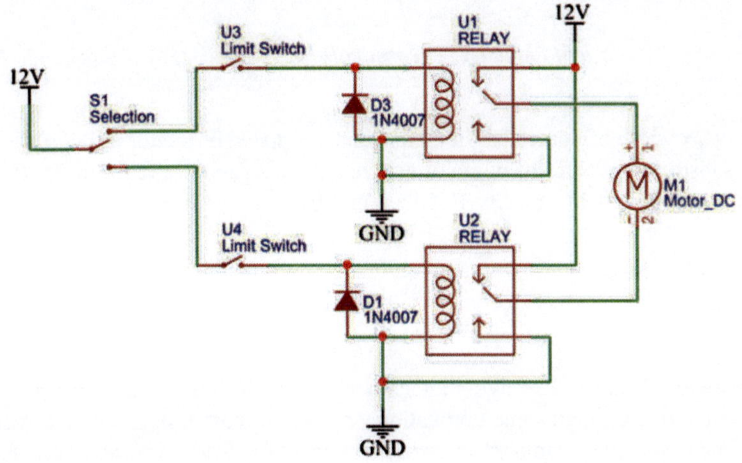


**Fig. 8** Circuit for up-down mechanism

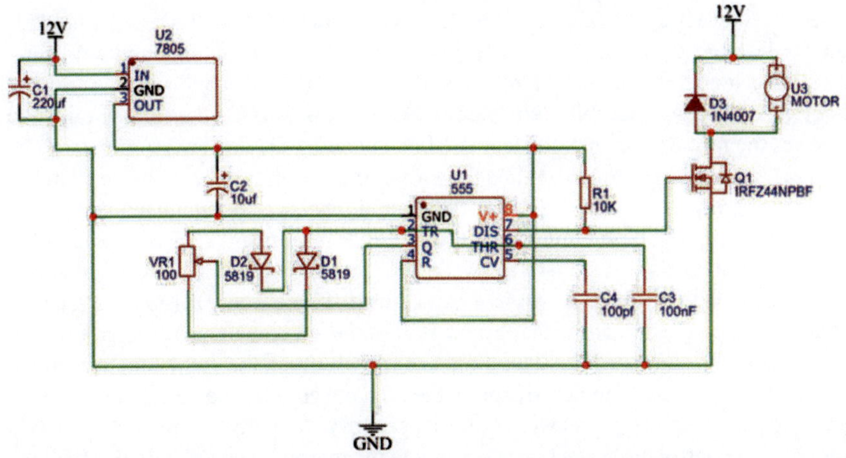


**Fig. 9** Circuit for control of the flow rate of the double motor diaphragm water pump

## 2.4 Theoretical Calculation of Field Capacity [26]

The tractor moving with the sprayer in action covers the certain area of the field which provides the field capacity. The number of nozzles and the total span of the nozzles along with the speed of the tractor's wheel play a vital role. In our case, space between two nozzles is 36 inches. Here, we have use maximum five nozzles for spraying pesticide. So, 36 (Space between two nozzles in inch) * 4 (Space between total no. of nozzles) = 144 in.

Where, 144 in. is a total length of nozzle bar 144 in. = 3.6576 m.

The theoretical average speed of the tractor is 4.5 km/h.

$$\textit{Field capacity (Theoretical)} = \frac{\mathrm{w} \times \mathrm{s}}{10} (\mathrm{ha/h}) \tag{1}$$

where, w = width of nozzle bar in meters and s = speed of tractor in km/h.

By substituting values of width of nozzle bar and speed of tractor in Eq. (1), we get the theoretical field capacity 1.65 ha/h or 4.07 Acre per hour.

# 3 Result

The pesticide filling and spraying attachment where design concepts are shown in Fig. 1 embodied through some fabrication work and circuit design and PCB making tasks. The realization of this attachment is shown in the form of photographs shown in Fig. 6, where the nozzle bar can be seen in its folded condition. In the photograph of the sprayer, parts labeled are clearly visible. The part showing the attachment with the tractor is not clearly seen in the photograph.

After completing the fabrication of the device while transporting it to the field for on-site testing, we found that only two persons can manage loading and unloading on the transport vehicle easily. It took less than a minute to attach this device with the tractor. A diaphragm double rotor water pump fills the water in the sprayer tank and relieves the farmer from manual labor. While operating the device the operator (The farmer) found it comfortable. When the farmer pressed the proper console switches the device properly reacted and mixed the desired amount of pesticide with the water. This automatic pesticide filling protects the farmer from manual handling. After the proper addition of pesticide into the water the stirrer turned on. The speed of stirrer was as per requirement. The operator can adjust the height by pressing the relevant switch on the console. Now, the farmer started the sprayer by a regulator knob on the console. We followed the tractor motion and observed the spray function on the plants. We found that the rate of spray, the area covered by the sprinkled pesticide and deposition on the plants were quite satisfactory. Actually, the regulator knob is provided to control the spray rate according to the requirement. Overall, our findings were satisfactory.

Figure 10 shows a photograph of the attachment fitted with the tractor and spraying the pesticide in the farm. In this photograph the nozzle bar is shown in its extended condition.

Figure 11 shows the photograph of actual field test of our system. If the farmer has divided his land for multiple crops, depending on the growth of those crop plants, the height adjustment facility was found very satisfactory to the farmer. Also, the distance between the rows of plants varies depending the type of crop. The nozzle span adjustment facility was realized in the actual field. In some cases, depending

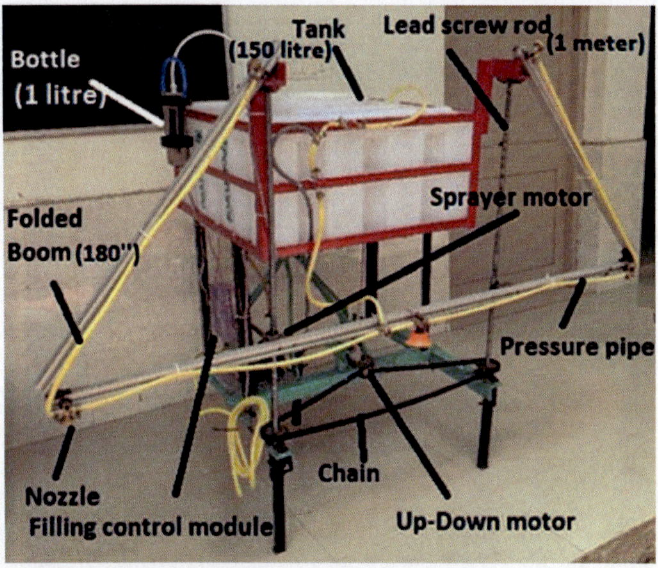


**Fig. 10** Pesticide filling and spraying attachment fabricated in-house

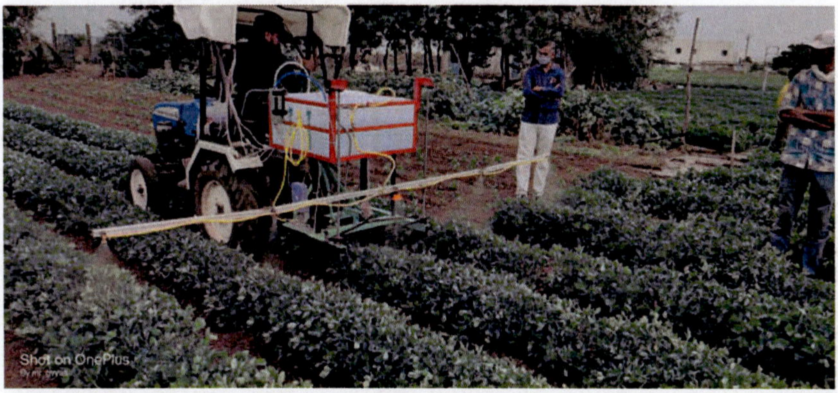


**Fig. 11** Field test of pesticide filling and spraying attachment

**Table 2** Comparison of our automatic and affordable pesticide sprayer with sprayers of branded companies

| Name of company | Automatic height adjustment (m or ft) | Automatic pesticide filling (ml) | Automatic pesticide mixing (L/min) | Pesticide reservoir tank refilling (L) | Rate in India mart in rupees |
|---|---|---|---|---|---|
| Our automatic and affordable pesticide sprayer | √ | √ | √ | √ | 15,000 |
| Shaktiman | √ | × | √ | √ | 1,176,000 |
| John Deer | × | × | √ | √ | 500,000 |
| Vasundhara Krishi Yantra | × | × | × | √ | 60,500 |
| Simple farm solution Pvt. Ltd. | × | × | × | × | 150,000 |
| Samarth services | × | × | × | × | 100,000 |
| Star agro-tech | × | × | × | × | 135,000 |
| Jagat Sukh Industries | × | × | × | √ | 75,400 |
| GTHS International Pvt. Ltd. | × | × | × | √ | 45,000 |

on the geometry of the field, the length of the nozzle bar may be a hindrance. So, manually folding the nozzle bar end segments is helpful to reduce its length.

Table 2 shows prices and some features of some of the branded manufacturers obtained from Indiamart [25]. One can learn from the table that our attachment is very cost-effective and has several features which are not available in other sprayers.

### 3.1 Performance of the Sprayer Attachment [26]

We check the performance of the sprayer attachment in terms of field efficiency by comparing the actual field area covered by the tractor along with the sprayer with the theoretical estimation. The on-site actual coverage providing field capacity was measured to be 3.5 Acre per Hour. This is the data acquisition part of our model. The efficiency is calculated as follows.

$$Field\ efficiency(\eta) = \frac{Effective\ field\ capacity(acre/h)}{Theoretical\ field\ capacity(Acre/h)} \times 100\% \quad (2)$$

By substituting the values of effective field capacity and theoretical field capacity in Eq. (2), we get the field efficiency $(\eta) = 85.82\%$ .

# 4 Discussion

The automatic pesticide filling and spraying device we have fabricated and tested on the field has produced results which are satisfying the need of small farmers. During the on-site testing, we had invited the interested farmers on the field who appraised the attempt. Most of them were concerned about the cost. When we informed about the price, they readily inquired about how to place the order.

The true interpretation of our work can be stated on the results of on-site testing. We offered the farmers to spray the pesticide by driving the tractor themselves. With a proper explanation from our side, when farmers took test run one-by-one, they expressed that every farmer should have this attachment. The farmers observed the quality of spray, how to prepare the spray liquid and the facility of folding the boom while turning the tractor at the boundaries of the farm. The height adjustment and nozzle spacing adjustment were practically explained to the farmers. We also answered the queries about maintenance cost, wear and tear and waiting time to purchase the attachment.

Our design and fabrication of automatic sprayer is not meant only for pesticide spraying. The innovative feature of our work is the automatic and required amount of pesticide filling in the tank just by pressing few switches. This feature is not available in previous works, so comparison of this feature cannot be done. We mentioned in the materials and method section that error in filling in pesticide is $\pm$ 2 ml.

We explored very hard to find out the performance of sprayer attachment on the tractor in the previous research works. We came across only one such reference. Mulatu [27] has reported the performance evaluation of the boom sprayer. His calculation reports field efficiency as 82.7%. As per our calculation, the field efficiency is 85.82%. So, the comparison turns out to be almost similar.

Our device is the first device prepared by us and tested on-site but time-testing of its wide acceptability would be justified by the users over a time-period. The pesticides which are very viscous in nature may cause a problem for the proper filling in our system. As the lead screws used are constantly exposed to the environment, a regular cleanliness and lubricating is necessary. Due to the smaller pitch of our lead screws, up and down time for boom movement is more.

Based on the live response of the farmers during on-site testing of the pesticide spraying device, we happily note that in our first attempt the sprayer device worked satisfactorily. The inquiry about the purchase of the sprayer indicates that the small farmers welcomed our effort. The reason for the device appeasements is the features like boom height adjustment, adjustable nozzle, automatic pesticide filling and mixing, liberty from the manual water filling, and the cost-effectiveness is on the top of all the other features. As the output of our research, we can state that we have design and created a device for small farmers which will satisfy the local and regional need. Our device may also be helpful to the farmers of not only India but also to the farmers of under-developed countries.

## 5 Conclusion

The automatic pesticide filling and sprayer attachment is made with a purpose to reduce the burden of a backpack, the cost and the time of farmers. The inbuilt pump replaces the manually filling of water in the tank. Also, the automatic pesticide filling mechanism replaces the manual pouring of pesticides with the water. The facility of spraying pesticide for different heighted plants is incorporated to take care of multiple crops in a single farm. Adjustable nozzle distance is useful for the variable distance between the rows of plants. A foldable nozzle arm is convenient for turns of the tractor in the field. Multiple features of our attachment with a very low price are the attractive side of our work. The field test run is very successful. The performance evaluation of the device is compared with the previous studies and the results found have a good match. Our field efficiency is 85.82%.

To mention the future works for a better modification of our design like Manual folding of the boom can be automized, for the protection of the lead screw, encapsulation can be implemented, SS-lead screw can replace the MS-lead screw, to increase the number of nozzles, a 3-rotor pressure motor is mandatory, to avoid the choking of the nozzle holes, filters can be employed before the pumps.

**Acknowledgements** The help by the department of electronics in terms of laboratory facility is noteworthy. Financial help by the Saurashtra University is highly acknowledged for publishing this work. The helping hand of Mr. Vipul and Mr. Aravind in the fabrication of the frame and other parts of attachment is also noteworthy. I also, express my thanks to Mr. Gunjan for providing valuable support to make this work live.

## References

1. Aher D, Sayyad G, Shimpi S, Sonawane D (2018) Hand driven four-wheel automatic spraying machine. Int Res J Eng Technol (IRJET) 05(04):4351–4352
2. Shirwal AC, Bharadwaj AR, Anilkumar TN, Harish T, Shanakara DR (2017) Development of mechanically operated pesticide sprayer and fertilizer dispenser. Int J Sci Res Dev 5(4):1529–1532
3. Singh RH, Akodiyawala A, Khokar J, Ingole G (2019) Mechanical agriculture sprayer vehicle (MASV). Int J Adv Res Ideas Innov Technol 5(1):476–479
4. Pranoy V, Subramanayam TDS, Mani Kumar PC, Babu R (2017) Design and fabrication of pesticide series spraying machine for multiple agricultural crops. Int J Res Appl Sci Eng Technol 5(X):1038–1042
5. Kiran CH, Sthavarmath R, Abhishek, Gowtham Raj R, Amar (2018) Fabrication of multipurpose pest sprayer. Int J Res Sci Innov V(V):12–15
6. Poratkar SH, Raut DR (2013) Development of multinozzle pesticide sprayer pump. Int J Mod Eng Res 3(2):364–368

7. Shalini DV (2016) Automatic pesticide sprayer for agriculture purpose. IJSART 2(7):150–154
8. Kumbhare DN, Singh V, Waghmare P, Ansari A, Tiwari V, Gorle RD (2016) Fabrication of automatic pesticides spraying machine. Int Res J Eng Technol 3(4):912–916
9. Patil A, Reddy H, Rajashekar K, Sagar Oburai K, Nagesh BS (2007) An innovative approach to control pesticide sprayer using solar based Bluetooth device. Int J Adv Res Electr Electron Instrument Eng 6(5):4098–4101
10. Ahalaya M, Muktha A, Veena M, Vidyashree G, Rehna VJ (2017) Solar powered semi-automatic pesticide sprayer for use in vineyard. Int J Electron Commun Eng 4(4):54–57
11. Chinda PR (2019) Solar agro sprayer. Int J Innov Technol Explor Eng 8(11):245–249
12. Kumavat Mukesh M, Wadavane D, Ankit N, Dipak V, Chandrakant G (2018) Solar operated pesticide sprayer for agriculture purpose. Int Res J Eng Technol 05(05):3365–3369
13. Kumari JS, Karim KKA, Tanaji MH, Uttamrao BY, Hussain MMAM (2018) Agriculture robotic vehicles-based pesticides sprayer. IJSRD 06(03)
14. Milan P, Jigna D, Kamlesh C, Bataviya M, Ravia K, Dhaval M (2018) Automatic pesticide spraying robot: design development and fabrication based on farming. Int J Trend Res Dev 05(02):635–637
15. Kassim AM, Termezai MFNM, Jaya AKRA, Azahar AH (2020) Design and development of autonomous pesticide sprayer robot for fertigation farm. Int J Adv Comput Sci Appl 11(02):545–551
16. Chaitanya PVR, Kotte D, Srinath A, Kalyan KB (2020) Development of smart pesticide spraying robot. Int J Recent Technol Eng 08(05):2193–2202
17. Rajesh Kanna P, Vikram R (2020) Agriculture robot—a pesticide spraying device. Int J Future Gener Commun Netw 13(01):150–160
18. Londhe SB, Sujata K (2017) Remotely operated pesticide sprayer robot in agricultural field. Int J Comput Appl 167(03):26–29
19. Mane SS, Pawar NN, Patil SA, Shirsath DO (2020) Automatic farmer friendly pesticide spraying robot with camera surveillance system. Int Res J Eng Technol 07(05):5347–5349
20. Nageshkumar T (2017) Design, development and evaluation of tractor operated automatic gun sprayer for field crops, a Ph.D. thesis submitted to Department of Farm Machinery and Power Engineering College of Agricultural Engineering, Raichur, University of Agricultural Sciences, Raichur, July
21. Sutar R, Kashid P, Patil P, Kadate G, Kalekar A, Lad A (2019) Modification on tractor mounted axial flow blower sprayer. Int J Innov Res Sci Eng Technol 8(4):3886–3892
22. Sanchavat H, Chudhary H, Bhautik G, Singh SN (2019) Field evaluation of a tractor mounted boom sprayer. Agric Eng Today 41(4):67–71
23. Karray F, Triki M, Jmal MW, Abid M, Obeid AM (2018) WiRoTip: an IoT-based wireless sensor network for water pipeline monitoring. Int J Electr Comput Eng (IJECE) 8(5):3250–3258 (2018). https://robu.in/product/yf-s201-water-flow-measurement-sensor-with-1-30liter-min-flow-rate-2/
24. Kurniawan A (2019) Arduino nano a hands-on guide for beginner, kindle edition, PE Press
25. Tractor mounted sprayers. https://dir.indiamart.com/impcat/tractor-mounted-sprayers.html. Last accessed 2021/08/11
26. Sahay J (2019) Elements of agricultural engineering: farm power, farm machinery, farm processing, farm electricity, 5th edn. Standard Publisher Distributors, New Delhi
27. Mulatu Y (2018) Fabrication and performance evaluation of ground wheel operated boom sprayer. Int J Eng Res Online 6(3):16–23

# An IoT Based Greenhouse Control System Employing Multiple Sensors, for Controlling Soil Moisture, Ambient Temperature and Humidity

**Bhavesh Pithadiya, Harikrishna Parikh, Jatin Savaliya, Ankitkumar Sidapara, Kamaldip Gosai, Dhrumil Vyas, and H. N. Pandya**

**Abstract** In order to fulfill the need of ever-growing human population, we need to increase agricultural production at a very high rate. Looking into the climatic conditions; which are beyond our control, Greenhouses are the only way out. Greenhouse offers controlled environment for optimized growth of plant. This paper proposes to apply the internet of things (IoT) technology to greenhouse, in order to monitor environmental conditions and irrigation using a web-based application and boost agricultural yield in turn. This IoT-based greenhouse monitoring system was designed for monitoring and controlling different parameters remotely. The system involves multiple-point, sensing of three vital parameters, namely soil moisture, ambient temperature and humidity (10 soil moisture sensors, 4 integrated humidity and temperature sensors), for controlling exhaust fan and water pump to maintain the desired environmental conditions inside. This system was installed in a cucumber greenhouse and found to be monitoring different parameters on a real time basis and logging them in the database. It satisfactorily controlled the parameters in accordance with predefined values. This system is low cost and easy to use for the farmer, with improvement of agriculture yield.

**Keywords** ESP-32 · Soil moisture sensor · DHT-22 (humidity and temperature) sensor · IoT · Web application

## 1 Introduction

Agriculture is India's backbone, supporting more than half of the country's population. India's population is increasing constantly, and so is the demand for food. Harvest is affected adversely by unanticipated climate changes caused by man-made

B. Pithadiya (✉) · H. Parikh · J. Savaliya · A. Sidapara · K. Gosai · H. N. Pandya
Departments of Electronics, Saurashtra University, Rajkot 360005, India
e-mail: pithadiyabh2@gmail.com

D. Vyas
Akaaish Mechatronics Ltd., Anand 388120, India

 
T. Triwiyanto et al. (eds.), *Proceedings of the 2nd International Conference on Electronics, Biomedical Engineering, and Health Informatics*, Lecture Notes in Electrical Engineering 898, https://doi.org/10.1007/978-981-19-1804-9_31

and natural factors. As a result, the greenhouse is favored to maintain optimal climatic conditions by precisely controlling the ambient temperature, relative humidity, and soil moisture required by the crops. A greenhouse can provide a more favorable shelter for plants and hence, agriculture in greenhouse is referred to as protected agriculture, protecting the crop against unfavorable environmental conditions. With help of constant monitoring the optimal climatic conditions (temperature, light intensity, soil moisture, and humidity) for crop growth may be maintained. Monitoring such system is a tedious job demanding frequent visit and care, making most farmers feel inconvenient. Although greenhouse helps increase yield, a reason for lower acceptance is that climate control failure leads to crop failure. The advancement in sensors and the internet of things has significantly altered the world, including, greenhouse monitoring and control. Wireless sensor networks can aid to effective monitoring of the same and in turn control the greenhouse [1].

Geographical area and local climate play important role in determining growth of harvest and any stress in climatic condition results in deviation of plant growth [2]. Photosynthesis, transpiration, absorption, respiration, blooming, etc. biological processes are function of ambient temperature [3]. On other hand, humidity in air influences transpiration [4]. Temperature and humidity are interrelated and collectively affect the transpiration, and harvest in turn. Optimally controlled soil moisture facilitates root growth, stretch the flowering time and resulting in increased yields [5].

Researchers have proposed and implemented diverse advancements in wireless technology over time to increase the yield. Academic researchers have proposed IoT-based greenhouse systems with real-time access in last decade. The study by M. Suresh et al. employs network based on GSM, reading signals from the associated sensors on the ground, and GUI is used for android devices and testing of its performance [6]. A Semi-automated system enabling the farmer to make a decision has been devised by K. Sreeram et al. [7]. Message Queue Telemetry Transfer (MQTT) protocol was chosen over Constrained Application Protocol and Extensible Messaging and Presence Protocol transmission, effectively providing the different quality of services to detect different parameters [8]. An enclosed micro-climate for the plant growth in which the gateway receives the sensor data and control information through a ZigBee wireless network providing real-time monitoring from the web application is also reported [9]. The photovoltaic panel powered system combined with a duplex cellular-web interface communication offering data inspection and irrigation programming from web page is reported by Joaquin et al. [10]. Raspberry Pi 3 Model B employed to automate greenhouse maintenance operations and monitors the growth conditions inside the greenhouse has been reported [11]. Irrigation and monitoring of agriculture using a cloud technique connecting an irrigation control mechanism through IoT have also been investigated [12]. Wireless Sensor Network (WSN) based embedded system; dealing with the implementation of ZigBee with different Topology used for real time monitoring based on GUI application for Greenhouse parameters has been developed on Java platform [13]. Use of Esp8266 and an AT89S52 as monitoring device for observing the framework of sensors and sending email warnings and messages to the mobiles, is already studied [14]. Greenhouse environment monitoring a system based on ZigBee was studied to control and provide real time data for agriculture [15]. WSN measurement data has been exchanged via IoT. A Smartphone application has been developed that allows users to control a series of actuator and sensors [16].

The proposed system prototype implemented at cucumber greenhouse, employs ESP-32 SOC as a web-server. Microcontroller connects to ten soil sensors and four integrated humidity and temperature sensors along with actuators. A web-based application manages it in real time. Predefined values of soil moisture, ambient temperature and humidity required for the cucumber greenhouse are set in web-application. Web-application monitors those parameters, which in turn are used to control the actuators. Also shown real time analysis is represented graphically. Thus, this system is effective to use and easy to monitor and control to improve yield.

## 2 Materials and Methods

### *2.1 Proposed System Components (Hardware)*

**ESP-32**. ESP32 is a smart, generic Wi-Fi and Bluetooth MCU SOC Microcontroller module targeting various applications from Espressif Systems [17]. The ESP32-D0WDQ6 chip is at the heart of this module designed to be scalable and adaptable [17]. Two CPU cores can be managed independently, and the CPU clock frequency is adjustable in the range of 80–240 MHz [17]. ESP32 has 30 multi-functional GPIO pins, supporting diverse peripherals, including capacitive touch sensors, Hall sensors, an SD card interface, Ethernet, high-speed SPI, UART, I2S, and I2C devices. It offers 802.11 b/g/n Wi-Fi networking at speeds of up to 150 Mbps [17]. Salient features of the ESP-32 include 18 ADC channels, 10 Capacitive I/Os, 3 UART interfaces, 3 SPI interfaces, 2 I2C interfaces, 16 PWM output channels, 2 DACs and 2 I2S interfaces [17].

**DHT-22**. DHT22, humidity and temperature sensor are extremely accurate. They are available as sensor as well as module and measure the relative humidity with a capacitive sensor element and temperature with an NTC thermistor connected to a high-performance 8-bit micro-controller [18]. It can detect relative humidity levels ranging from 0 to 100% (accuracy $\pm$ 2) and temperatures ranging from -40 to 125 degrees Celsius (accuracy $\pm$ 0.3 °C) [18]. When linked to the CPU, the DHT22 employs a single wire serial interface to communicate data via a DATA pin on the sensor, Fig. 1 shown DHT22 connect to MCU.

**Soil Moisture sensor**. The moisture of the soil is detected with resistive type soil moisture sensor module. The volumetric content of water inside the soil is measured and converted to soil moisture. It comprises two immersion gold coated probes to monitor soil moisture [19]. Such module with probe and signal conditioning circuit employing op-amp LM393 is shown in Fig. 2.

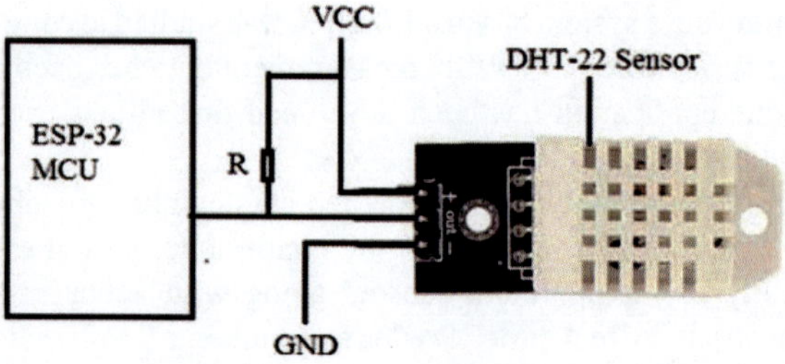


**Fig. 1** MCU connection to DHT22

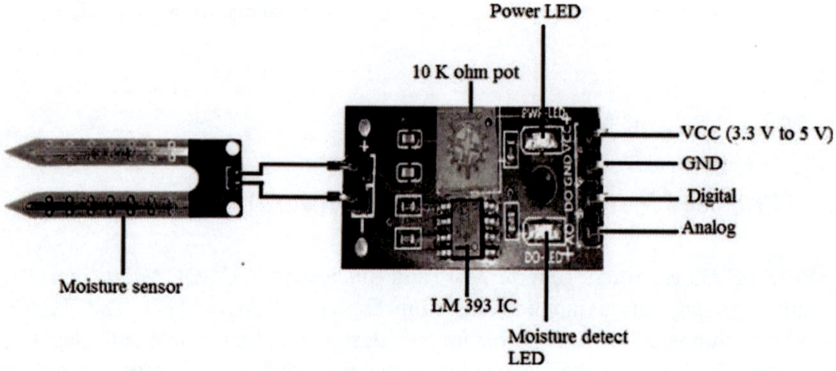


**Fig. 2** Soil moisture sensor with amplifier section

**Relay**. SLA-5VDC-SL-A 4Pin 30A Power Relay. The relay is switched with the help of a small signal from a micro-controller like an Arduino, ESP-32, and ESP8266. This relay can be used to drive 30 A devices.

## 2.2 *Web-Application*

API or Application Programming Interface [20] is used for connection between a micro-controller and PHP Server running. APIs are mainly transmitted using either of the two different methods: GET and POST. In this experiment GET method is used for inserting data, that is data of 10 soil moisture sensors and 4 pairs of temperature and humidity into a database. Data is first concatenated into one string containing domain name, location of PHP file [21] and data to be inserted. In response to this operation, a JSON response is generated containing information about relay status.

Front-end programming was carried out using HTML, CSS and JAVASCRIPT. We have used APACHE server [23] and MySQL database [24].

### 2.3 Block Diagram and Experimental Set up

Figure 3 shows, a functional block diagram of the proposed system with embedded hardware as well as wireless communication. Core part of the system is ESP-32 SOC, responsible for all data collection, processing and generating control signals. Sensors, namely: 10 resistive soil moisture sensors and 4 DHT22 (temperature and humidity sensor) are connected to the micro-controller board and logs data periodically. The logged data is sent to server for further data analysis.

The experimental setup is shown in Fig. 4. The MCP 3008 is an eight-channel, ten-bit ADC IC [25]. 8 soil moisture sensors are connected to MCP 3008 and rest 2 are connected directly to GPIO pins of ESP-32. 4 DHT22 (providing digital data packets) are directly connected to controller GPIOs using single wire serial interface. Externally powered relay module is employed to switch on/off the pump and the exhaust fan.

Once, the connection is established, controller starts acquiring data (soil moisture, temperature and humidity) from sensors. Transmitting data over the internet using HTTP protocol mandates to typecast data into string form. These strings are then concatenated in one string comprising the domain name of the web server, followed by the path of a PHP file on the server, and at last data string separated by '&'. This string then posted on to the server using the HTTP GET method. Upon successful insertion of the data to the database, a response of 200 is received, else a corresponding error code is received. Also, in response server sends time, date and status of the pumps, exhaust fan and colling system in JSON format. At the next step, the controller parses this JSON data and manipulates it to represent the status of pumps, exhaust fan and colling system on the webpage as well as to manipulate the digital output. Time information is also logged for visual representation and analysis. The same process is depicted in form of the flowchart shown in Fig. 5.

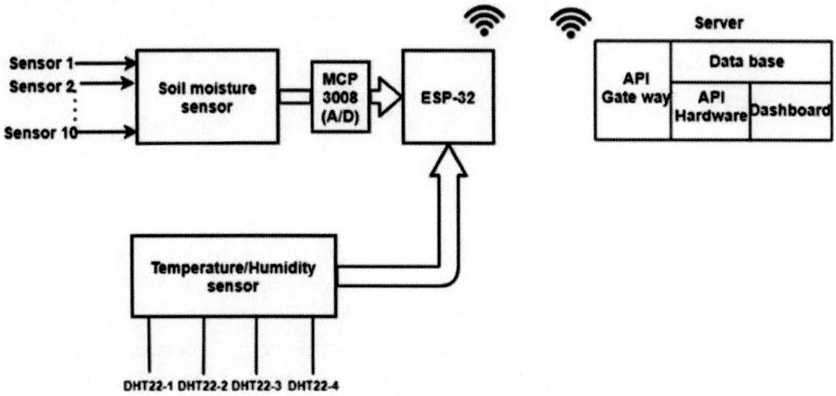


**Fig. 3** Block diagram of the proposed system

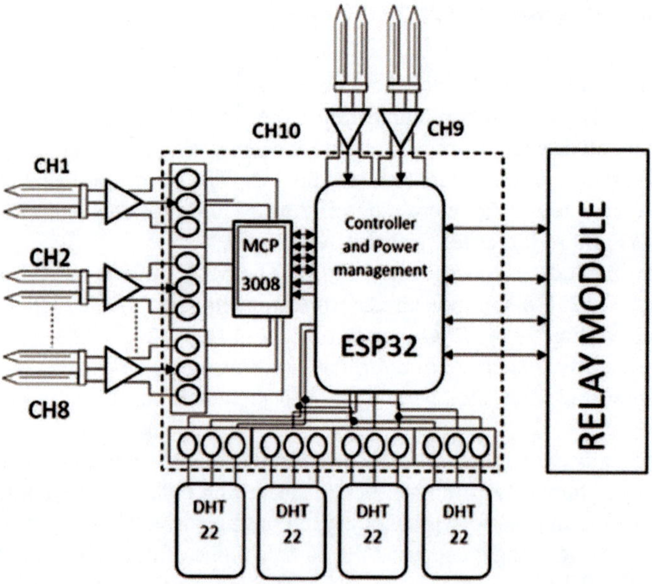


**Fig. 4** Proposed system experimental setup

Proposed system installed in the field of cucumber greenhouse is shown in Fig. 6. At onset of the process cucumber plant parameters are needed to be set for optimization of yield. A daytime temperature of 20–30 °C is optimal for the cucumber plant [26]. At temperatures above 30 °C, imbalances in plants are observed affecting the processes of photosynthesis and respiration. Due to the vast surface area of its leaves, this plant requires a lot of humidity. During the day, relative humidity should be between 60 and 70%, while at night, it should be between 70 and 90% [26].

## 3 Result

### *3.1 Test Setup*

In order to automate the proposed system in the field (the cucumber greenhouse), a set of desired parameter boundary values (minimum and maximum) (Table 1) are fed through web-application on the URL "http://smartgarden.pw".

On the web-application, user can supervise parameters (temperature, humidity and soil moisture) as well as status of the actuators (Fan and Pumps for watering and sprinkler) in the cucumber greenhouse as real-time charts. The state of various actuators (Fan and Pump) of the greenhouse can be monitored as well as manually controlled through the Internet.

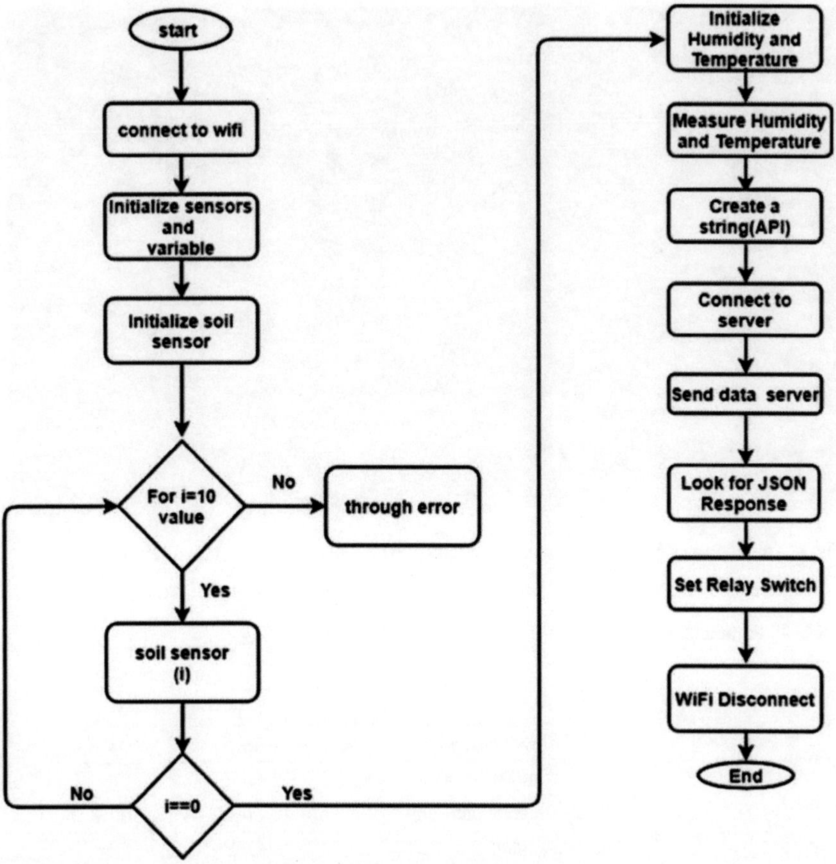


**Fig. 5** Flowchart of the proposed system

## 3.2 *Analysis of Result*

Microcontroller is logged sensor data and manipulates the status of relays to control external devices. The observed logged data is stored in Sensor.CSV file as shown in Fig. 7. The averages of 10 soil moisture sensors were recorded at an interval of 3 min for different zones to measure and control moisture, also an average of relative humidity and temperature was recorded at an interval of 3 min to control corresponding actuators.

Real time information is also logged for visual representation and analysis, which helps to take a decision. Figure 8 shows the percentage humidity Vs time plot, showing different humidity values from all 4 sensors. The micro-controller is acting on the average value (of the four sensors) to control actuator (fan) in accordance with predefined algorithm. Figure 8 also shows the temperature Vs time plot (of the four

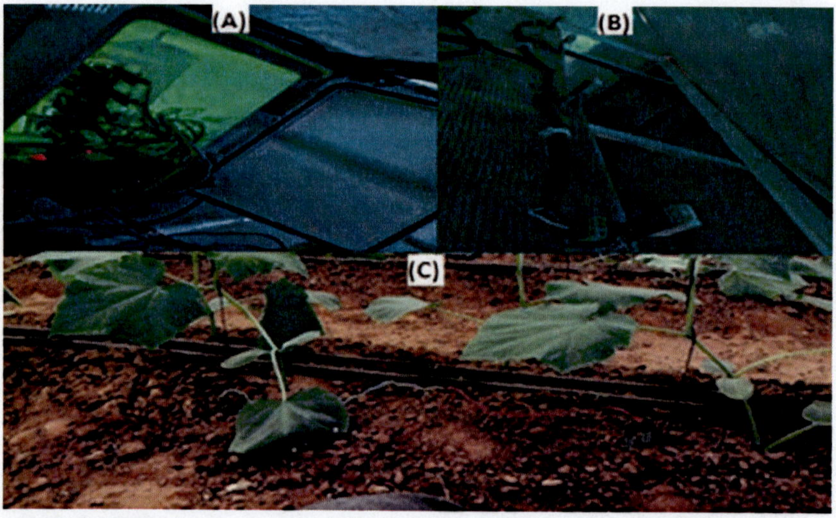


**Fig. 6** In cucumber green-house set-up **a** circuit box, **b** DHT-22, **c** soil moisture sensor

**Table 1** Parameter boundary values for automatic control

| Parameter | Predefined threshold Values obtained from sensor's | |
|---|---|---|
| | Min | Max |
| Temperature | 25 °C | 38 °C |
| Actuator (fan and pump) | OFF | ON |
| Relative humidity | 60% | 70% |
| Actuator (fan) | OFF | ON |
| Soil moisture | 70% | 80% |
| Actuator (pump) | ON | OFF |

sensors) that in turn controls actuators (fan and pump). In the case of soil moisture, the percentage moisture (of the ten sensors) Vs time plot is shown in the same Fig. 8. The average value of them is exploited to turn on/off the watering pump. The status of such actuators can also be visualized on web-application. Manual override option allows the user to have manual control of actuators, in the case needed.

## 4 Discussion

The IoT based greenhouse system permits users over the cloud network to send commands to the hub from remote location. The hub will further employ signals for the intended sensors to trigger and perform the user-requested action. Once the

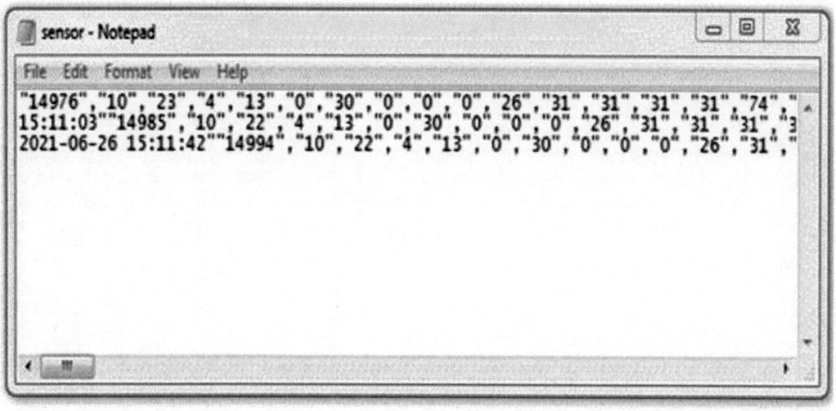


**Fig. 7** Screenshot of sensor.csv file

action is performed, web-application will update the status of the action taken to the cloud network and in this way; users can control as well as monitor the parameters manually or automatically.

Major concerns about greenhouse automation methods have been their management, installation and operational cost and efficacy. Early greenhouses had simple controls such as opening windows, turning on/off irrigation valves, etc. requiring human operator. A wired network used in large greenhouses has proven to be more expensive in terms of installation. Researchers have designed diverse wireless sensor networks to automate the greenhouse in order to facilitate the optimal climate for plant growth. The work presented depicts a scalable greenhouse that can be monitored as well as controlled from web-page. The system offers automatic as well as manual mode of control. User (admin) is provided with rights to set the parameters for different crops. Overall, the system is quite inclusive and scalable.

The system is accessed over internet, hence, unavailability of internet access, hampers the system. Also, the system is provided with 30 s delay to enable manual mode.

The system has been tested for its operation in cucumber greenhouse. The fast response exhibited by this system makes it quite efficient and results in increased yield.

## 5 Conclusion

As an emerging technology internet of thing (IoT) is explored which helps to provide the smart solution in the development of prototype greenhouse monitoring. This system is quite easy to deploy for monitoring multiple sensor parameters and controlling actuators in response. This tends to improve crop yields with easy access. This

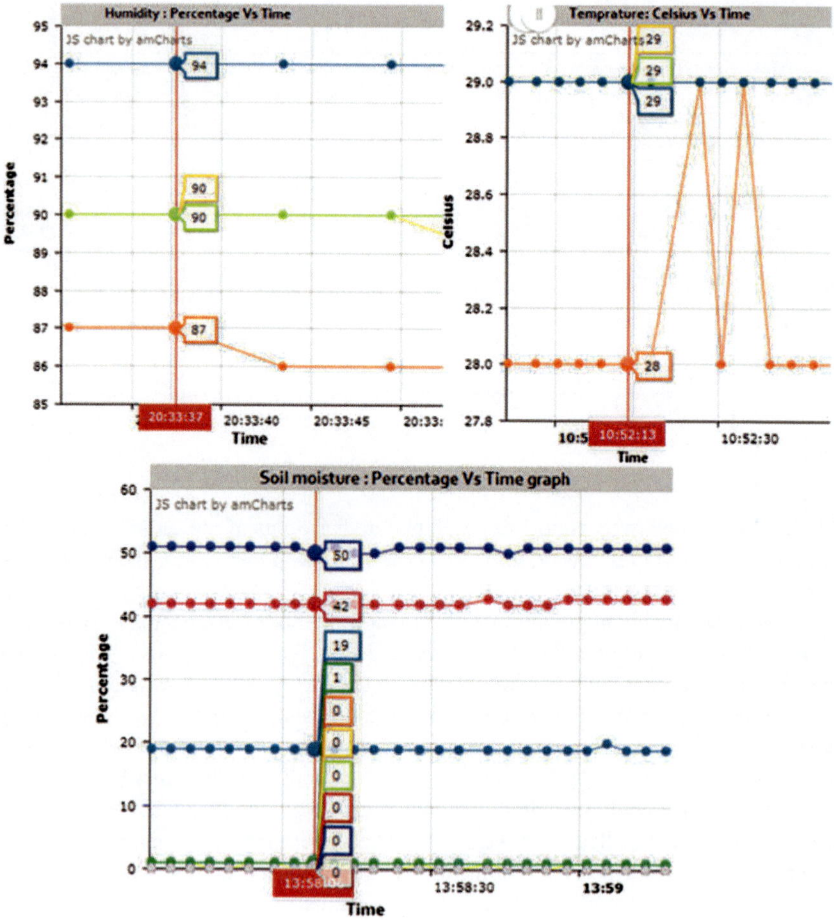


**Fig. 8** Graphically logged ambient temperature, humidity and soil moisture data in cell phone

ensures access to control the plant growth from remote places within in no time. This system works on manual as well as in auto mode with predefined values of parameter. The proposed system is extremely economic and uses water optimally, hence conserving the precious resource. This system provides consistent operation resulting in better care for plants.

Concluding, the installation of an automation system for the greenhouse will help to manage a consistent and predictable climate, i.e. ideal growing environment. One of the biggest benefit automations can provide is the ability to reduce overall production cost, minimum human power required, and improve the yield. Implementing this system in different agricultural greenhouses with different crops can be fruitful to farmers. Also, we are trying to add some additional parameters like light intensity and atmospheric Carbon dioxide to be monitored and controlled.

**Acknowledgements** Authors whole heartedly acknowledge the support from Department of Electronics and Saurashtra University, in carrying out this research.

## References

1. Ahonen T, Virrankoski R, Elmusrati M (2008) Greenhouse monitoring with wireless sensor network. In: Proceedings of the IEEE/ASME international conference on mechatronics and embedded systems and applications, Beijing, China, pp 403–408
2. Wang N, Zhang N, Wang M (2006) Wireless sensors in agriculture and food industry-recent development and future perspective. Comput Electron Agric 50(1):1–14
3. Mastalerz JW (1977) The greenhouse environment the effect of environmental factors on the growth and development of flower crops. Q Rev Biol 53(3):323
4. Bakker JC, Bot GPA, Challa H, Van de Braak NJ (1995) Greenhouse climate control (an integrated approach) II. https://doi.org/10.3920/978-90-8686-501-7
5. Paul J (1944) Kramer: Soil moisture in relation to plant growth. Botan Rev 10(9):525–559
6. Suresh M, Ashok S, Arun Kumar S, Sairam P (2019) Smart monitoring of agricultural field and controlling of water pump using internet of things. In: Proceeding of international conference on system computation, automation and networking. IEEE, Pondicherry, India, pp 1–5
7. Sreeram K, Suresh Kumar R, Vinu Bhagavath S, Muthumeenakshi K, Radha S (2017) Smart farming—a prototype for field monitoring and automation in agriculture. In: IEEE WiSPNET conference, IEEE, pp 2189–2193. 978-1-5090-4442-9/17
8. Singh TA, Chandra J (2018) IOT based green house monitoring system. J Comput Sci 14(1):639–644
9. Sri Jahnavi V, Ahamed SF (2015) Smart wireless sensor network for automated greenhouse. IETE J Res 16:1–6
10. Joaquin G, Juan Francisco V, Alejandra N, Miguel A (2014) Automated irrigation system using a wireless sensor network and GPRS module. IEEE Trans Instrument Measur 63(1):166–176
11. Shah NP, Bhatt PP (2017) Greenhouse automation and monitoring system design and implementation. Int J Adv Comput Res 8(9):468–471
12. Jaishetty SA, Patil R (2016) IoT sensor network based approach for agricultural field monitoring and control. Int J Res Eng Technol 15(6):45–48
13. Jaypal B, Afshan M, Amol B, Shweta A, Amruta C (2014) Real time monitoring and control system for greenhouse based on 802.15.4 wireless sensor network. In: 4th international conference on communication systems and network technologies. IEEE, Bhopal, India, pp 98–103
14. Nagabhushana Rao M, ChakriAjit K, Phanindra Kumar G (2018) Smart greenhouse based on IoT. Int J Eng Technol 7(2):258–261
15. Dan L, Xin C, Chongwei H, Liangliang J (2015) Intelligent agriculture greenhouse environment monitoring system based on IoT technology. In: International conference on intelligent transportation, big data and smart city. IEEE, pp 487–490
16. Mustafa A, Radosveta S (2017) An IoT-based greenhouse monitoring system with Micaz motes. Int Works IoT M2M Healthcare Proc Comput Sci 113:603–608
17. ESP32 Technical Reference Manual, Version 2.8, Espressif system, #101, Block2, 690 Bibo Road, Zhangjiang High-Tech Park, Pudong, Shanghai, China 201203 (2018)
18. BOGDAN Mihai (2016) How to use the DHT22 sensor for measuring temperature and humidity with the Arduino board. Acta UiversitatisCibiniensis Techn Ser 68(1):22–25
19. Prahlad B, Vasudha V (2019) Soil moisture, temperature and humidity measurement using Arduino. In: IEEE 9th international conference on cloud computing, data science and engineering (confluence). IEEE, Noida, India, pp 567–571

20. Brajesh D (2017) API management—an architect's guide to developing and managing APIs for your organization, 1st edn. Springer Apress, Berkeley, CA
21. Rasmus L, Kevin T, Peter M (2013) Programming PHP, 3rd edn. O'Really Media, Inc., Tokyo
22. John P (2013) Java script-A beginner guide, 4th edn. McGraw-Hill, New York
23. Thau R (1996) Design considerations for the apache server API. Comput Netw ISDN Syst 28:1113–1122
24. Williams HE, Lane D (2004) Web database applications with PHP and MySQL, 2nd edn. O'Really Media, Inc.
25. Patil P, Bhole K (2018) Real time ECG on internet using raspberry Pi. In: International conference on communication, computing and internet of things. IEEE, Chennai, India, pp 267–270
26. Introduction of environment conditions for cucumber plant. http://agriculture.infoagro.com/crops/cucumber-growing-part-i-/. Last accessed 2021/08/07

# Cancer Mammography Detection Using Four Features Extractions on Gray Level Co-occurrence Matrix with SVM Kernel Analysis

**Figo Ramadhan Hendri and Fitri Utaminingrum**

**Abstract** Cancer is one of the most dangerous diseases that often threaten human life. This study aims to detect breast cancer using the best kernel by performing a kernel analysis to obtain high accuracy breast cancer detection based on image analysis. The kind of SVM Kernel in this research uses Polynomial, Gaussian, and Radial Basis Function (RBF). The proposed method can help the medical personnel to make it easier to detect breast cancer by sending emails to doctors to immediately notice results so that patients caught with cancer can directly get special treatment. Suppose the image is detected as cancer, then the systems sending the result by e-mail to the Doctor who treats them so that patients who are detected with cancer can immediately get special treatment. This research uses a combination of Gray Level Co-occurrence Matrix (GLCM) with a distance equal to 1 and angle direction (0°, 45°, 90°, 135°). The feature extractions of the GLCM matrix are obtained from Energy, Homogeneity, Contrast, and Entropy. Furthermore, Support Vector Machine (SVM) is the classification method to classify non-cancer and cancer. Analysis, an accuracy result in different types of SVM Kernel were conducted in this experimental research. The detailed accuracy result is 93%; The sensitivity is 91%; The precision is 96%; The specificity is 95%, and The F1-score is 93%. The best accuracy of SVM Kernel is RBF. In the future, this study can be used in hospitals to make it easier to check for breast cancer.

**Keywords** Breast cancer · Mammogram · GLCM · SVM · Sending e-mail

---

F. R. Hendri
Faculty of Computer Science, Brawijaya University, Malang, Indonesia

F. Utaminingrum (✉)
Computer Vision Research Groups, Faculty of Computer Science, Brawijaya University, Malang, Indonesia
e-mail: f3_ningrum@ub.ac.id



T. Triwiyanto et al. (eds.), *Proceedings of the 2nd International Conference on Electronics, Biomedical Engineering, and Health Informatics*, Lecture Notes in Electrical Engineering 898, https://doi.org/10.1007/978-981-19-1804-9_32

# 1 Introduction

Cancer is one of the most dangerous diseases that often threaten human life. Cancer occurs when there is uncontrolled change and growth of cells in the body of a human being which results in abnormalities [1]. Breast cancer can be prevalent and often deadly among adult women. According to the World Cancer Research Found International data, in 2012, there were more than 1.7 cases of breast cancer [2]. Breast cancer can be prevented by detecting at the early stage, early detection is extremely important which reduces the time required for treatment [3]. Detection at an earlier stage can reduce mortality rate due to breast cancer to a great extent [4]. One way to identify breast cancer is to interpret mammographic images using low-dose x-ray techniques initially [5]. The resulting image is called a mammogram. Mammograms are used for screening to find changes in the breast. In addition, a mammogram is also used as a diagnostic tool if the doctor suspects a difference in the patient's breast that requires a mammogram analysis [6]. Analysis of mammograms is still done manually by doctors or radiologists. These shortcomings make this research carried out by utilizing a digital image processing system. Because the development of the medical world today cannot be separated from the development of technology. Technological developments can help the medical world to make it easier for doctors to see information from an existing image [7]. The primary purpose of image processing techniques is to recognize the image or object under consideration so that it is easier to visualize [8]. Medical imaging is a technique and process used to create images of human anatomy for clinical research, diagnosis, and treatment [9]. The use of digital images in the medical world is essential to facilitate the analysis and diagnosis of high-risk diseases. One of the technologies commonly used to identify the disease is Magnetic Resonance Imaging (MRI), Ultrasound, and Computer Tomography. Mammography is a frequently and commonly used method of detecting breast cancer. However, radiology has some variations in interpreting a mammographic image [10]. Therefore, there is a need to have an automated process for analyzing a mammographic image. The automatic method designed in this research uses feature extraction from GLCM and Support vector machine for classification.

Several studies and research are going on in this field. Such as "Statistical analysis of mammographic features and its classification using support vector machine" [9]. In this study, researchers used the same classification, SVM, where the researcher uses two different kernels from SVM, the polynomial kernel function and the Gaussian radial basis function. The classification performance was analyzed using the results of the overall accuracy, confusion matrix, and sensitivity. The overall impact of the kernel is the polynomial kernel function gets the overall best result of 92.627%, and the radial basis functions get the highest result of 92.105%. Therefore, in this study, it is proven that the use of different kernels will affect the results of the SVM classification. Another research on this field is "Comparative study on feature extraction method for breast cancer classification" [11]. This research compares three different feature extraction techniques to detect breast cancer. First, a neural network classifier is used to evaluate Gray Level Co-occurrence Matrix (GLCM) features. Second, features used in this study are histogram intensity features and intensity-based features used to detect cancer on mammograms.

Based on previous research, the problem formulation is how to get high accuracy results for detecting cancer in the mammogram image. This research uses a combination of Gray Level Co-occurrence Matrix (GLCM) with a distance equal to 1 and angle (0°, 45°, 90°, 135°). The feature extractions of the GLCM matrix are obtained from Energy, Homogeneity, Contrast, and Entropy. Furthermore, Support Vector Machine (SVM) is the classification method to classify non-cancer and cancer. This study aims to help doctors or radiologists make an easy detection and get an accurate result using SVM as classification and Gray Level Co-occurrence Matrix as feature extraction based on image analysis. Several analysis results in different SVM Kernels (Polynomial, Gaussian, and Radial Basis Function (RBF)) were conducted in the experimental research. Hence, it can help the medical personnel to make it easier to detect breast cancer by sending emails to doctors to immediately notice results so that patients caught with cancer can directly get special treatment.

The structure of this research paper contains several parts. The first is an introduction that explains the problem of research that would be to solve and analyze the previous research paper. The second part is material and method, which contains the method used and the materials needed. After that, it will proceed to the results section, which includes the experiments carried out. Next, enter the discussion stage, where it explains the results and compares the results of the article with other articles and the weaknesses of the article. The next section is the article's conclusion, which emphasizes the paper's purpose and writing down future work that can be done. The last part is the reference of this article which helps to form the basis of this article.

## 2 Materials and Method

The proposed method to identify breast cancer from Ultrasound is divided into two main parts. The first is extracting the GLCM feature for training data. The second is to implement the SVM method with various Kernel to classify data and get the best accuracy result. The training data used are non-cancer and cancer ultrasound from breast cancer patients. In this research to detect breast cancer, several steps include pre-processing, extraction feature, classification, and sending email, such as illustrated in Fig. 1.

The system will start by selecting the breast image to be tested. After that, it was pre-processing as the initial process. When the pre-processing process is complete, the image will be extracted by GLCM. In this process, the feature extraction of the image was obtained by using analysis distance and angle. Then the process continues to obtained normalized data by the average of the feature values. The SVM method uses three Kernels: Polynomial, Gaussian, and Radial Basis Functions. The image will be determined to be classified as cancer or non-cancer. If the image is detected as cancer, then the system will send an email.

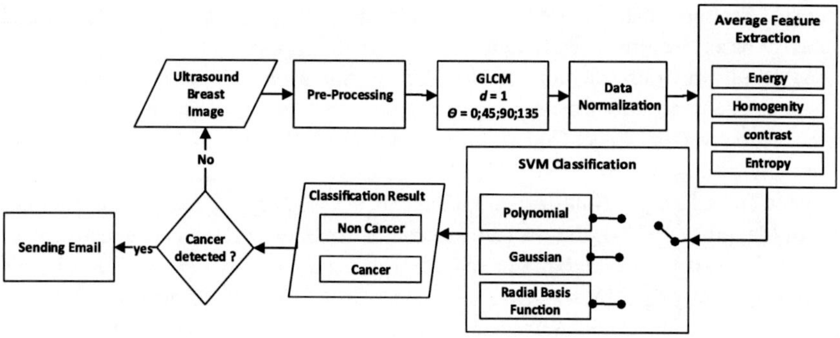


**Fig. 1** Blok diagram system

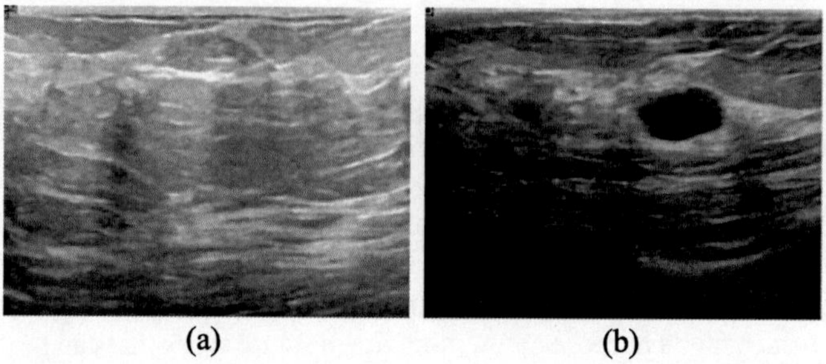


**Fig. 2** Sample data based on ultrasound breast image **a**, non-cancer and **b** cancer

## *2.1 Dataset of Ultrasound Image Breast Cancer*

Ultrasound images used in this study are provided by the website kaggel.com, containing normal and abnormal images dataset. The total data consists of 220 images, 110 as non-cancer and 110 as cancer. The example of a dataset is in Fig. 2a as non-cancer image sample data and Fig. 2b as cancer.

## *2.2 Pre-processing*

The ultrasound image was converted to a grayscale image and normalized data before the feature extraction process. This process aims to make all of the images have the same gray level and same color saturation. It is crucial to make all images in the same classification have a close-range average of extraction features.

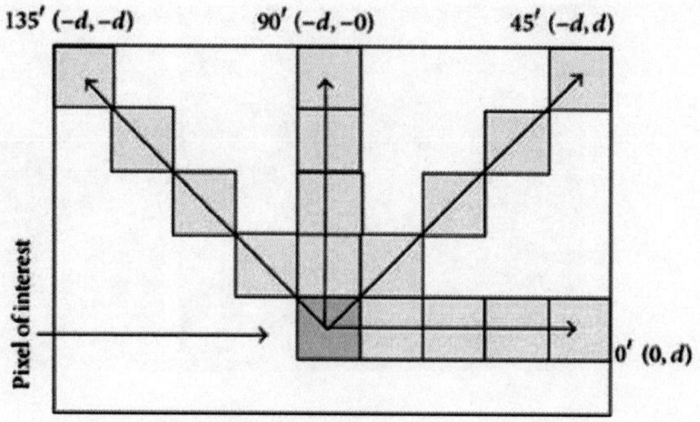


**Fig. 3** Spatial relationship of pixel

## 2.3 Gray Level Co-occurrence Matrix (GLCM)

A method that capturing visual content or an image is something called feature extraction [12]. This step plays the most vital role in the detection of breast cancer. The classification of breast cancer to the correct class depends on the result of feature extraction. The texture feature itself can distinguish between non-cancer and Cancer patterns. The feature extraction process begins when the pre-processing is done, and then some features were extracted from a non-cancer and cancer Ultrasound image.

Feature extraction in this research was performed through GLCM. Gray Level Co-occurrence Matrix is a method that is often used to analyze the texture and feature extraction of an image [13–15]. GLCM is a matrix that describes a frequency that gives rise to two pixels with intensity in a certain distance and direction in the image [16]. The coordinates of a pair of pixels have a distance d and an angular orientation Ø. GLCM angle orientation is formed from four angle directions (0°, 45°, 90°, 135°) and the distance between pixels is 1 pixel [17]. The spatial relationship of pixel and the angular orientation illustrated in Fig. 3. the process of GLCM there are several stages:

- The initial process is obtained GLCM matrix of a pair of pixels that are lined up in the direction of the 0°, 45°, 90°, and 135° angles.
- The second process calculates symmetrical matrix by adding the initial GLCM matrix with its transpose value.

## 2.4 Data Normalization

The data normalization process is one of the vital steps in this research. Normalization is a process that changes the range of image pixel intensity values [18]. This will provide image data that will be processed to have fix represent or the same dimension. The purpose of normalization is to make the image recognition process easier and improve detection accuracy [19]. Pre-processing image result are illustrated in Fig. 4. The conversion image to Gray-scale can be seen in Fig. 4a. Then the normalization

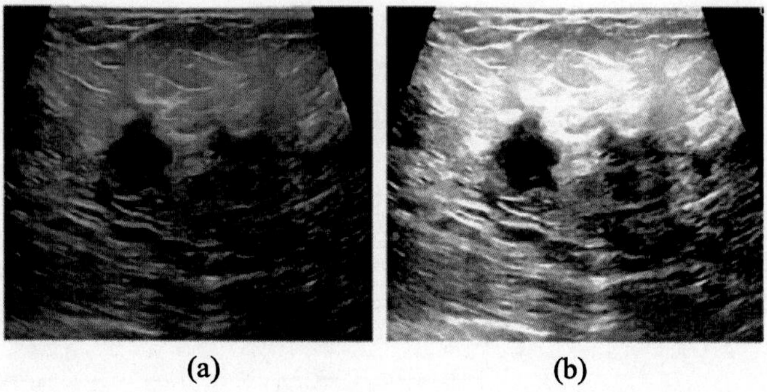

Fig. 4 Pre-processing process **a** Gray-scale image and **b** normalization image

image result is illustrated in Fig. 4b. Each element of the GLCM matrix is divided by the total data of the GLCM matrix.

## 2.5 Feature Extraction GLCM

The feature extraction in the experimental research uses contrast, entropy, homogeneity, energy. The mathematical formulation to obtain feature extraction is illustrated in Eqs. (1) upto (4).

$$\text{Energy} = \Sigma \text{i, jP(i, j)}^2 \tag{1}$$

$$\text{Homogenity} = \Sigma \text{i, j} \frac{\text{P (i, j)}}{1 + |\text{i} - \text{j}|} \tag{2}$$

$$\text{Contrast} = \Sigma \text{i, j } |\text{i} - \text{j}|^2 \text{P(i, j)} \tag{3}$$

$$\text{Entropy} = \Sigma \text{i, j} - \text{ln(P (i, j)P (i, j)} \tag{4}$$

Denotes, $(i, j)$ is pixel coordinates in the GLCM matrix and $P(i, j)$ is the normalization matrix GLCM at coordinates $(i, j)$. Each feature is calculated based on the GLCM parameter value ($d = 1$, angle direction $= 0$); ($d = 1$, angle direction $= 45°$); ($d = 1$, angle direction $= 90°$) and ($d = 1$, angle direction $= 135°$). Then the four values of each resulting feature will be averaged as the value of the basic feature.

## 2.6 Support Vector Machine (SVM)

GLCM features obtained in previous steps now will be classified using SVM. Support Vector Machine is a method derived from statistical learning theory with promising and potentially better results than other classification methods. The SVM method was done by maximizing the hyperplane limit or finding the best hyperplane separator from the two classes [20] such as illustrated in Fig. 5. Margin is the distance between the hyperplane and the closest data to each class. The most immediate data is called the support vector. Hyperplane with the maximum margin will provide better generalization in the classification process [21].

Support Vector Machine is part of a kernel-based classification that uses a pattern for variety and regression [22]. As we say in the introduction, this research used Support Vector with different kernel methods for breast detection. Using different kernels is to get and analyze the best kernel, which resulting in accuracy and precision in this method. The kernel types for analysis in this research are Gaussian radial basis function (RBF), polynomial, and Gaussian kernel. The formula of the kernel that is used in this research is illustrated in Eqs. (5) upto (7):

$$\mathrm{Polynomial} = \mathrm{K}(\mathrm{x_i},\ \mathrm{x_j}) = (\mathrm{x_i} \cdot \mathrm{x_j} + 1)^{\mathrm{d}} \quad (5)$$

$$\mathrm{Gaussian} = \mathrm{k}(\mathrm{x}, \mathrm{y}) = \exp\left(\frac{||\mathrm{x} - \mathrm{y}||^2}{2\sigma^2}\right) \quad (6)$$

$$\mathrm{RBF} = \mathrm{K}(\mathrm{x_i}, \mathrm{x_j}) = \exp(-\gamma||\mathrm{x_i}, \mathrm{x_j}||^2 \quad (7)$$

Denotes

$(x_i, x_j)$ Pair two data traning.
$k$ Number of classes.
$d$ Parameters Polynomial.

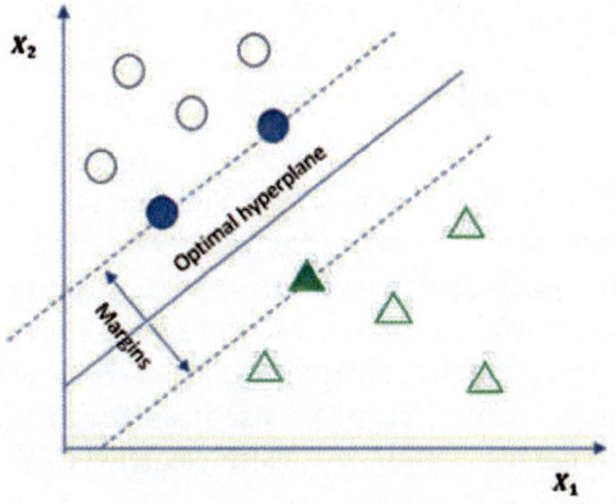


**Fig. 5** SVM classifies by finding the optimal hyperplane that has maximum margin

$\sigma$ Variance ($\sigma > 0$).
$\gamma$ Gamma RBF.

## 2.7 Sending E-mail

The sending e-mail process will be done when the classification has been carried out. The classification results will determine whether the sending e-mail process will be carried out or not because sending e-mail occurs when the classification results are declared cancer. This sending e-mail uses the simple mail transfer protocol. SMTP is the means used to sends the results from LabVIEW to the user's Gmail e-mail. SMTP has meaning as the protocol used to send e-mail between servers. When sending an e-mail, the computer will direct the e-mail to an SMTP server address to the destination e-mail server. The e-mail that will be sent contains the results of breast cancer detection and a letter of reference and information from the detected patient. This is intended so that patients can know the steps that must be taken to prevent cancer development with this sending e-mail method. Hence, that early detection and early treatment of breast cancer are more efficient in reducing breast cancer.

## 2.8 E-mail Notification Test

E-mail notification testing here serves to find out how effective and successful the e-mail system has developed. Sending e-mail in this system works when the classification results state that the cancer class includes the detection results.

The test done by testing repeatedly. For example, when the class has resulted as cancer, automatically sending e-mail is running. Meanwhile, when the testing is when the class has resulted in non-cancer and sending e-mail is not running. This test found that the sending e-mail program can generally work without the slightest problem with dependence on the classification results.

# 3 Result

The total dataset is 220 images that are considered 110 images for cancer and 110 non-cancer. It obtains from Kaggel.com dataset. We use a confusion matrix to analyze the performance of our method for classifying breast cancer. The confusion matrix is shown in Table 1. True Positive (*TP*) is the number of cancer classes detected in the cancer classes, True Negative (*TN*) is the number of non-cancer classes detected in non-cancer classes, False Positive (*FP*) is the number of cancer classes detected in non-cancer classes, False Negative (*FN*) is the number of non-cancer classes in cancer classes.

**Table 1** Table confusion matrix

| Target class | Real object | |
|---|---|---|
| | Non-cancer | Cancer |
| Non-cancer | TN | FP |
| Cancer | FN | TP |

**Table 2** Table comparison result in different Kernel

| Kernel | Confusion matrix | | | | |
|---|---|---|---|---|---|
| | Accuracy (%) | Sensitivity (%) | Precision (%) | Specificity (%) | $F1$-score (%) |
| Polynomial | 86 | 84 | 88 | 87 | 85 |
| Gaussian | 90 | 87 | 93 | 92 | 89 |
| RBF | 93 | 91 | 96 | 95 | 93 |

In our study, we analyze the performance of each Kernel in the SVM method by calculating several parameters: Accuracy, Sensitivity, Precision, Specificity, and F1-score, as illustrated in Table 2. Accuracy is the statistic formulation to measure of all the correctly identified cases [23].

## 3.1 *Kernel Analysis*

This research uses Support Vector Machine as a classification. Kernel analysis aims to get the kernel that will produce the best results. The kernel to be analyzed as before is polynomial, Gaussian, and Radial Basis Function (RBF). Datasets are prepared to apply inputs to the classifiers for training and testing. To evaluate the performance of the kernel, we use this confusion matrix defined by the Eq. (8) up to (12).

$$\text{Sensitivity} = \frac{\text{TP}}{\text{TP} + \text{FN}} \times 100\% \tag{8}$$

$$\text{Accuracy} = \frac{\text{TP} + \text{TN}}{\text{TP} + \text{TN} + \text{FP} + \text{FN}} \times 100\% \tag{9}$$

$$\text{Precision} = \frac{\text{TP}}{\text{TP} + \text{FP}} \times 100\% \tag{10}$$

$$\text{Specificity} = \frac{\text{TN}}{\text{TN} + \text{FP}} \times 100\% \tag{11}$$

$$\text{F1-Score} = \frac{2(\text{Sensitivity} \times \text{Precision})}{(\text{Sensitivity} + \text{Precision})} \tag{12}$$

Denotes

True Positive (TP) is the number of correct predictions that means non-cancer image correctly identified as non-cancer.

False Positive (FP) is the number of incorrect predictions that means non-cancer image incorrectly identified as cancer image.

True Negative (TN) is the number of incorrect predictions that means cancer image incorrectly identified as non-cancer image.

False Negative (FN) is the number of correct predictions that means cancer image correctly identified as cancer image.

F1-Score is measure of accuracy in data testing which calculated from Sensitivity and Precision.

Performance test using the confusion matrix table. The test used 30 datasets of ultrasound breast cancer patients. GLCM uses distance 1 and 4 angles orientation as 0°, 45°, 90°, 135°. The experimental research was made to calculate the performance of a test to select the best kernel for this method. The result of the test can be seen in Table 2. As shown in Table 2, the polynomial kernel has the lowest accuracy results than the others. Meanwhile, Gaussian Radial Basis Function (RBF) kernel got the best results.

**Algorithm 1** : Process Prediction Image

```
Result: determined by cancer or non-cancer
Start of prepare one prediction image do preprocessing;
    Gray-scale the image;
    Normalization the image;
    End preprocessing process;
    Calculate feature extraction using the GLCM Method;
      Calculates four values;
      Print the GLCM result;
End feature extraction process;
Into predictions weights have been learning do next;
    Used of 3 kernel SVM;
    Classified the data to the cancer non-cancer class;
    Sent the result image predictions and referral letter to email doctor;
    end prediction process;
  end process all;
```

## 4 Discussion

The results of the experiment that we did can be seen in Table 2. It can be seen that the results of this experiment have a reasonably high accuracy in each of the kernels used.

**Table 3** Classification performance of different methods

| Reference/year | Classification technique | Accuracy (%) |
|---|---|---|
| Proposed method | SVM with RBF Kernel | 93 |
| Gaike [17], 2016 | K-means | 81 |
| Saki et al. [25], 2013 | OWBPE | 89.28 |

The normalization is carried out by GLCM, so that the saturation color of each image is same [24]. The results of the study show that the RBF kernel has a higher accuracy rate. The detailed accuracy result is 93%; The sensitivity is 91%; The precision is 96%; The specificity is 95%, and The F1-score is 93%.

In this study, we also compared the performance of the accuracy results obtained from previous studies. As shown in Table 3, there is an increase in accuracy from previous research that uses other methods. The proposed method has high accuracy when compared to the previously proposed method. However, the system still cannot detect the type of cancer suffered by the patient based on the ultrasound image.

In the future, the application not only used for initial screening for classifying cancer or normal condition, but also it can be developed to obtain deep analysis, for example, the type of breast cancer based on tissue density, namely BI-RADS I, II, III, and IV with faster processing.

## 5 Conclusion

The processing images in creating a detection of breast cancer with the feature using Gray Level Co-occurrence Matrix (GLCM) with distance = 1 and teta 0°, 45°, 90°, and 135° can be a method that can get the highest accuracy. The performance of the three kernels used in this research is good enough to get high detection accuracy. But the best performance kernel in this research is kernel Gaussian radial basis function (RBF). The performance result of this kernel is high enough to call it an accurate system, and the detailed accuracy is 93%, the precision is 96%, the sensitivity is 91%, the specificity 95%, and the F1-score is 93%. Sending email programs can work very well without any problems at all. The overall result of the system is good enough but still can be improved in the future. Future work that we can add to this system is by adding the number of classifications carried out according to the level of cancer suffered by the patient and can find the position of the cancer.

**Acknowledgements** I am enormously grateful to my supervisor for her support during this research for help the exploring of ideas. Special thanks to our institution Faculty of Computer Science, Brawijaya University, Indonesia, and everyone who supports and encourages this research.

## References


1. Debelee TG, Gebreselasie A, Schwenker F, Amirian M, Yohannes D (2019) Classification of mammograms using texture and CNN based extracted features. J Biomimetics Biomater Biomed Eng 42:79–97
2. Al Rasyid MB, Yunidar FA, Munadi K (2018) Histogram statistics and GLCM features of breast thermograms for early cancer detection. In: 1st international ECTI Northern Secion. conference on electrical electronic computer telecommunications engineering ECTI-NCON, pp 120–124
3. Bhavya G, Manjunath TN, Hegadi RS, Pushpa SK (2019) A study on personalized early detection of breast cancer using modern technology. In: Sridhar V, Padma M, Rao K (eds) Emerging research in electronics, computer science and technology. Lecture notes in electrical engineering, vol 545. Springer, Singapore
4. Sara Koshy S, Jani Anbarasi L (2021) Breast cancer detection in histology images using convolutional neural network. In: International virtual conference on industry 4.0. Lecture notes in electrical engineering, vol 355. Springer, Singapore
5. Tatikonda KC, Bhuma CM, Samayamantula SK (2018) The analysis of digital mammograms using HOG and GLCM features. In: 2018 9th internatioanl conference on compututing communucation and networking technologies ICCCNT, pp 10–16
6. Sarosa SJA, Utaminingrum F, Bachtiar FA (2018) Mammogram breast cancer classification using gray-level co-occurrence matrix and support vector machine. In: 3rd international conference on sustainable information engineering technologies, pp 54–59
7. Novar Setiawan K, Suwija Putra IM. Klasifikasi Citra Mammogram Menggunakan metode K-means, GLCM, dan support vector machine (SVM). J Ilm Merpati (Menara Penelit Akad Teknol Informasi) 6(1):13
8. Mohamed Fathima M, Manimegalai D, Thaiyalnayaki S (2013) Automatic detection of tumor subtype in mammograms based on GLCM and DWT features using SVM. In: International conference information communication embedded systems, pp 809–813
9. Muthu Rama Krishnan M, Banerjee S, Chakraborty C, Chakraborty C, Ray AK. Statistical analysis of mammographic features and its classification using support vector machine. Expert Syst Appl 37(1):470–478
10. Qayyum A, Basit A (2017) Automatic breast segmentation and cancer detection via SVM in mammograms. In: International conference on emerging technologies
11. Nithya R, Santhi B. Comparative study on feature extraction method for breast cancer classification. J Theor Appl Inf Technol 33(2):220–226
12. Krishna Jothi A, Mohan P (2020) A comparison between KNN and SVM for breast cancer diagnosis using GLCM shape and LBP features. In: Proceedings of 3rd international conference smart system invention technology, pp 1058–1062
13. Utaminingrum F, Surosa SJA, Karim C, Gapsari F, Wihandika RC (2021) The combination of gray level cooccurrence matrix and back propoagation neural network for classifying stairs descent and floor. In: ICT express
14. Utaminingrum F, Johan AWSB, Somawirata IK, Risnandar AS (2021) Descending stairs and floors classification as control references in autonomous smart wheelchair. J King Saud Univ Comput Inf Sci
15. Utaminingrum F, Johan AWSB, Sari YA, Somawirata IK, Olaode AAA (2021) The improved security system in smart wheelchairs for detecting stairs descent using image analysis. In: 10th international conference on software and computer applications
16. Kathale P, Thorat S (2020) Breast cancer detection and classification. Int Conf Emerg Trends Inf Technol Eng 1:1–5
17. Htay TT, Maung SS (2018) Early stage breast cancer detection system using GLCM feature extraction and K-nearest neighbor (k-NN) on mammography image. In: 18th international symposium on communication information technology, no. Iscit, pp 345–348

18. Hiremath B, Prasannakumar SC, Praneethi K (2016) Breast cancer detection using non-invasive method for real time dataset. In: 2016 international conference advance computing communications and informatics, pp 676–681
19. Gaike V, Mhaske R, Sonawane S, Akhter N, Deshmukh PD (2016) Clustering of breast cancer tumor using third order GLCM feature. In: International conference on green computing internet of things, pp 318–322
20. Ing S (2019) Breast cancer pathological image auto-classification using weighted GLCM-SVM. In: 4th international conference mechanical control computer engineering. ICMCCE 2019, pp 475–480
21. Usha R, Perumal K (2015) SVM classification of brain images from MRI scans using morphological transformation and GLCM texture features. Int J Comput Syst Eng 5(1):18
22. Pareek M, Jha CK, Mukherjee S (2017) Classification of brain tumor using GLCM and SVM from MRI images, pp 138–145
23. Utaminingrum F, Hidayat A (2021) Bottomhat Kernel Analysisi on different shape and size using colonies extraction for counting of bacterial colonies in petri dish. Int J Comput Biol Drug Des 14(3)
24. Amin J, Sharif M, Yasmin M, Fernandes SL (2020) A distinctive approach in brain tumor detection and classification using MRI pattern recognition. Letter 139:118–127
25. Saki F, Tahmasbi A, Soltanian-Zadeh H, Shokouhi SB (2013) Fast opposite weight learning rules with application in breast cancer diagnosis. Comput Biol Med 43(1):32–41

# Phantom Simulation Model for Testing Enhancement of Image Contrast in Coronary Artery Based on Body Weight and Body Surface Area Calculations

**Gatot Murti Wibowo, Ayu Musendika Larasati, Siti Masrochah, and Dwi Rochmayanti**

**Abstract** The Houndsfield Unit (HU) on contrast media is critical in CT cardiac imaging since its arterial contrast enhancement depends on the accurate drug dosage calculation and base on a specific patient's body weight (BWp) or body surface area (BSA). The study aims to develop a model of the coronary arterial mimicking phantoms and to compare the contrast enhancement in both the BWp and BSA calculations. The 3D printing model of the coronary arterial mimicking phantoms (PLA material) was developed in the frame of experimental study design. The contrast media dosage (a mixture of 30 mL NaCl saline and 350 mg/mL Xolmetras), generated from the two different dose protocol calculations (BWp and BSA), was independently filled into the model. The simulated chest weight was varied at 37, 47, 57, 67, and 77 kg when performing CT cardiac. The averaged HU resulted from the six selected ROIs (proximal, medial, and distal area of coronary artery phantom images) was analyzed with paired t-test (95% CI). A comparison study between the BWp and BSA dose protocol calculations was deemed significant (p-value > 0.05). Both dose protocol calculations produce the same volume and weight at 57 mL and 57 kg respectively. The BSA provides the most optimal con-trast enhancement at 2148.16 HU. The coronal arterial mimicking phantom has the feasibility as a test object to estimate the suitability of contrast media drug doses on cardiac CT imaging. However, further clinical study needs to perform to test its sensitivity.

**Keywords** Body weight and body surface area protocol calculation · Coronary arterial mimicking phantoms · 3D printing model

G. M. Wibowo (✉) · S. Masrochah · D. Rochmayanti
Poltekkes Kemenkes Semarang, Semarang, Indonesia
e-mail: gatotmurtiw@gmail.com

A. M. Larasati
Doris Sylvanus Hospital, Palangka Raya, Indonesia



T. Triwiyanto et al. (eds.), *Proceedings of the 2nd International Conference on Electronics, Biomedical Engineering, and Health Informatics*, Lecture Notes in Electrical Engineering 898, https://doi.org/10.1007/978-981-19-1804-9_33

# 1 Introduction

Cardiovascular disease is a disease caused by impaired heart and blood vessel function, such as coronary heart disease, heart failure, hypertension and stroke [1]. Cardiovascular disease is the highest cause of death in the world. An estimated 13 million people died of cardiovascular disease in 2010 [2]. Risk factors for Coronary Heart Disease have been identified by various studies outside [3]. Coronary heart disease occurs as a result of a blockage in the coronary arteries [4]. Like other organs, the heart also needs nutrients and oxygen to pump blood throughout the body. If the coronary arteries are blocked or narrowed, then the blood supply to the heart will decrease, resulting in an imbalance between the need and supply of nutrients and oxygen.

In recent years, progress has been made in the development of non-invasive diagnostic alternatives to directly imaging coronary arteries. The two most promising approaches are Computed Tomography (CT) and Magnetic Resonance Imaging. Radiation dose on a CT scan is high because it get a primary dose and a secondary dose at the same time per scanning [5]. CT coronary angiography using scanners with at least 64 slices should be recommended [6]. Cardiac CT is a series of examinations using contrast media to produce cardiac imaging and aims to determine fatty deposits or calcium deposits in coronary arteries [7].

Contrast media contains iodine which has a high atomic number that can increase the attenuation (absorption) of X-rays in order to produce images of blood vessels that are brighter or more enhance than the surrounding soft tissue so that it is easy to evaluate [8]. Good attenuation is the key to evaluate various blood vessel abnormalities especially in smaller arteries. The enhancement characteristics are based on scanning techniques, patient factors, and main parameters of contrast media injection protocol such as dose (volume), concentration, viscosity, osmolality, flowrate, and saline flushing [9].

Coronary Computed Tomography Angiography (CTA) has become one of the most important diagnostic imaging modalities for the evaluation of coronary artery diseases [10]. The accuracy of the use of contrast media is an important factor in producing optimal and homogeneous enhancement along the arterial lumen. One consideration in administering a dose of contrast media is the patient's body weight. Logically, large patients need more doses than smaller patients to achieve the same enhancement. But this method does not provide an accurate estimate of contrast media. For example in obese patients who have excess fat content that is not actively metabolized in the body in circulating or weakening/diluting contrast media in the blood, this method may provide a dose of contrast media that is too high. If the dose of contrast media is made to increase along with weight gain [11], then obese patients will get an enhancement that may be higher compared to non-obese patients who receive a contrast media dose in the same body weight proportion (1 mL/kg body weight). Other parameters such as height need to be considered in determining the optimal dose of contrast media. In his research, Bae [11] found that in patients of the same weight, the value of aortic enhancement tends to decrease in patients whose body is higher. Bae concluded that the dose of contrast media should not be calculated based only on body weight but rather consider the height factor reflected in the Body Surface Area with the formula [12].

$$\sqrt{\frac{\text{height (cm)} \times \text{weight (kg)}}{3600}} \tag{1}$$

Body Surface Area (BSA) is an area of the entire surface of the human body (skin) expressed in $m^2$. Body Surface Area is a commonly used index in clinical practice to correct for patient size differences in various physiologic measurements and in calculating drugs dosage. For example BSA is used in determining the dose of anti-cancer drugs. Compared to body weight, BSA is a better indicator in describing the body's metabolic mass. That is, the use of BSA in calculating the contrast media dose makes sense. In Yanaga research, [13] concluded that aortic enhancement resulting from BSA-based contrast media dose calculation tends to be more sufficient and consistent than weight-based dose calculation (at a ratio of 1.2 mL/kg BW).

In patients with large total blood volume, the effect of dilution (weakening) of the contrast media will reduce the attenuation of coronary arteries in Cardiac CT. As the increase in blood volume is proportional to BSA, [14] assesses that if the calculation of contrast media dose is based on BSA, then this dose will be able to compensate/minimize the possibility of the dilution effect.

Administering a contrast media dose with the BSA method provides the total volume of contrast media given to the patients that different from the weight-based method. The differences in volume and concentrate will be one of the factors affecting the coronary' artery enhancement on the images, and therefore, an accurate given dose calculation of contrast media is important to obtain homogeneous image enhancement. Unfortunately, the use of the weight-based method seems to be an underdose for underweight patients and an overdose for obese patients where both contribute to less enhancement of the contrast media visualization. However, the body-weight method may replace the BSA method if it is employed to correct the failure of dose calculations, and in order to reach optimum image enhancement. By this means, our research aims to assess the difference in contrast enhancement of the arterial organ pertinent to the two methods of dose calculations (the BSA and the BWp)) and to find out which method provides optimal image enhancement the basis of a custom object test study.

## 2 Materials and Methods

This research is a quantitative research with an experimental approach. The diagram as shown in Fig. 1, describes conceptual famework of the study. The material consist of the object test model of the coronal artery and the chest mimicking phantom. The object tests was a custom of coronary artery model made of the 3D printing process of Polylactid Acid (PLA) materials. The model was filled with a mixture of 30 mL

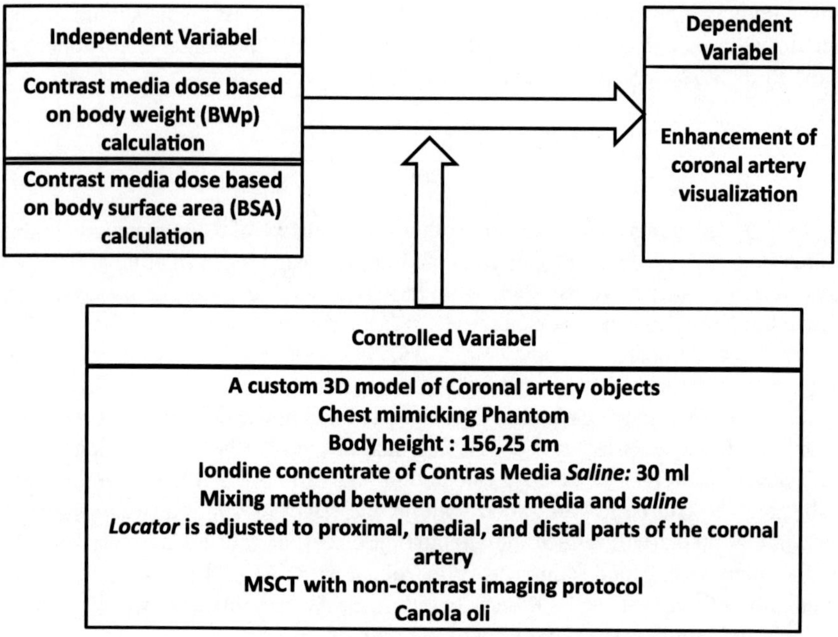


**Fig. 1** Conceptual framework

NaCl saline and 350 mgI/mL Xolmetras, and the total vol-ume of contrast media, generated from the basis of the BWp and BSA methods of dose protocol calculations.

The coronary artery phantom was attached to the heart in the chest phantom, then scanned using the CT Thorax Non Contrast protocol on the Siemens 128 Slice Somatom Perspective CT Scan tool. The chest phantom used in this study was not equipped with a head and legs so it could not be measured in weight and height. Therefore the weight and height of the phantom were obtained through calculations. Height was obtained through the formula [15] which is chest length divided by 0.288 and produced a height of 156.25 cm. This value is then used to calculate the BMI and BSA at each body weight determined. While the phantom body weight (BWp) was obtained from the formula [16] which is chest weight divided by 48.3% so that it produces a weight of 37 kg. This value was then used as the first sample and represented the underweight category based on calculation from the formula [17]. The next sample was made by added 10 kg in order to represent the normal, overweight, and obesity categories. Weight gain was defined as the addition of adipose fat in the body. In this study, a simulation of each weight gain was carried out by applying canola oil along the surface of the phantom of the chest. Canola oil was chosen because it has physical properties, composition, and density values that are similar to adipose fat [18].

The enhancement was measured using the CT Number value (HU unit) on the axial slice images of the chest by placing six ROIs in the proximal, medial and distal areas of the coronal artery. The six values were calculated on average, then the Saphiro-Wilk data normality test was performed to oversee the normal distribution. After obtaining normally distributed data, the test was continued with Paired T-Test using the SPSS programe version 24.0. An analysis was performed to examine which method that was able to provide the most optimal contrast media enhancement on the resulted images. It can be decided by interpreting the mean values from the statistical data with the level of confidence was set at 95% ($\alpha = 0.05$). We have hypothesized that there is no difference in contrast media enhancement at the location of the coronary arteries between the use of weight-based (BWp) and body area (BSA) methods of calculation. When found that the $p > 0.05$, the hypotesis is rejected.

## 3 Results

The study was begun by calculating the contrast media dose using the body weight (BWp) and Body Surface Area (BSA) methods so that the volume of contrast media for each BWp sample is obtained, as can be seen in the table 1.

The volume of contrast media produced by the two dosage calculation methods increased linearly with increasing body weight. However, in the BSA method, there was a slight decrease in the volume of contrast media at a weight of 67–77 kg when compared to the BB method. The intersection value of the two methods was on BWp 57 kg with a volume of 57 mL.

This research was conducted at the Radiology Department of Tugurejo Regional Hospital Semarang. Data retrieval was begun by calibrating the CT Scan tool so it is ready for use. Then scanned the chest phantom using the CT Thorax Non Contrast protocol. Scanning began with topogram retrieval and then continued with a scan over an area of the heart's Field of View (FOV), see in Fig. 2.

As can be seen in Fig. 3 is the position of canola oil on the top, right side, left side and bottom of the chest phantom as a simulation of weight gain. Canola oil was stored in a 30 × 40 cm plastic container and then attached using a plaster so that the oil can be spread evenly and not grouped at one point. Each side of the phantom chest

**Table 1** Comparison of the contrast media dose calculation

| BWp (kg) | BMIp category | BSAp ($m^2$) | Contrast media volume (mL) | | Volume's differences | |
|---|---|---|---|---|---|---|
| | | | Body weight method | BSA method | (mL) | (%) |
| 37 | Underweight | 1.27 | 37 | 46 | 9 | 24.30 |
| 47 | Underweight | 1.43 | 47 | 52 | 5 | 10.64 |
| 57 | Normal | 1.57 | 57 | 57 | 0 | 0 |
| 67 | Overweight | 1.70 | 67 | 62 | 5 | 7.46 |
| 77 | Obesity | 1.83 | 77 | 67 | 10 | 12.98 |

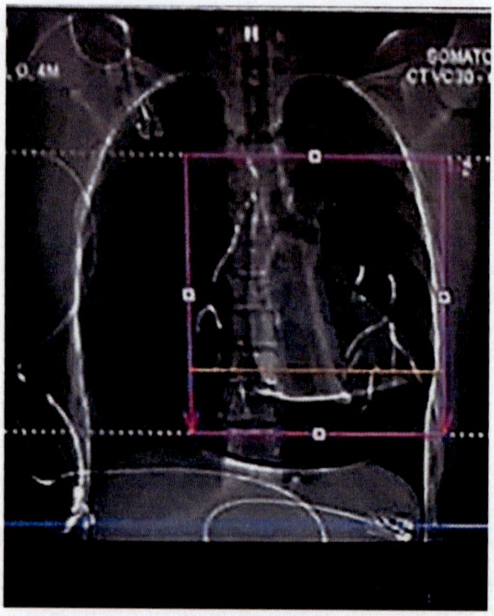

Fig. 2 Topogram

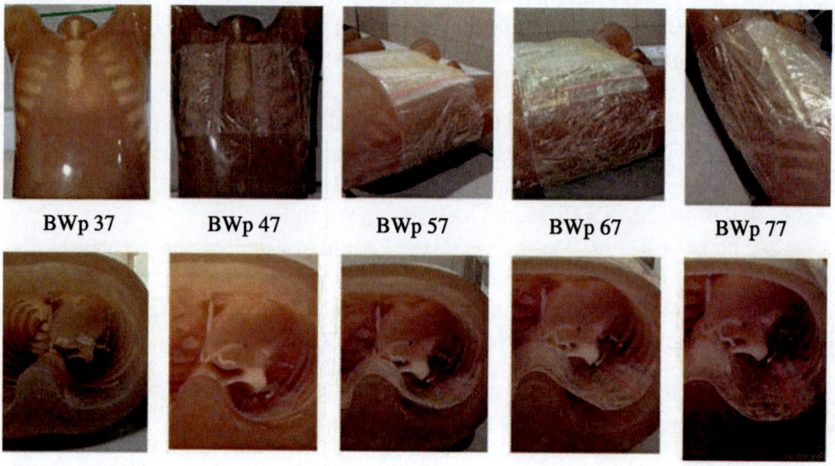


Fig. 3 Canola oil placement

was given a plastic clip. Especially for the bottom of the chest phantom, the plastic clip was placed on the inside to avoid plastic breaking of heavy crushed phantom. The picture from top to bottom starts with BWp 37, 47, 57, 67, and finally 77 kg.

In Fig. 2, BWp 37 kg didn't not use canola oil because it is the original weight of the phantom. On subsequent scans, canola oil was added in stages with the following description: BWp 47 kg used 4 plastic clips, each containing of 100 mL canola oil, placed as the first layer. BWp 57 kg, 4 more plastic clips were added, each containing of 100 mL canola oil, placed on top of the first layer. BWp 67 kg was added with 4 plastic clips, each containing of 50 mL canola oil, placed on the top of the second layer. BWp 77 kg was added again with 4 plastic clips, each containing of 50 mL canola oil, placed on the top of third layer.

## 3.1 Coronary Artery Enhancement Difference

The differences in contrast enhancement were first observed and measured using ROI locator in the proximal portion of the coronary arterial phantom (axial view) as showed on Fig. 3, where the resulted values of Average CT Number described in Table 2 and Fig. 4.

**Table 2** Average CT number value

| BWp | Average CT number (HU) | | Difference (HU) |
|---|---|---|---|
| | BW method | BSA method | |
| 37 | 891.33 | 1687.20 | 795.87 |
| 47 | 1776.63 | 1943.52 | 154.89 |
| 57 | 2096.52 | 2101.82 | 5.30 |
| 67 | 2611.45 | 2416.13 | 195.32 |
| 77 | 2935.73 | 2592.15 | 343.58 |
| Mean | 2062.33 | 2148.16 | 85.83 |

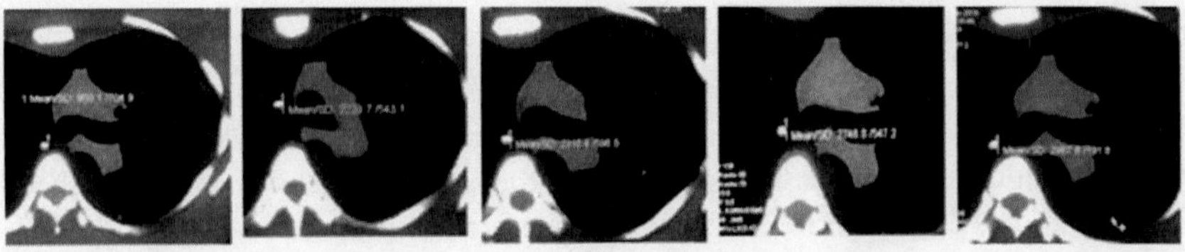

(a)

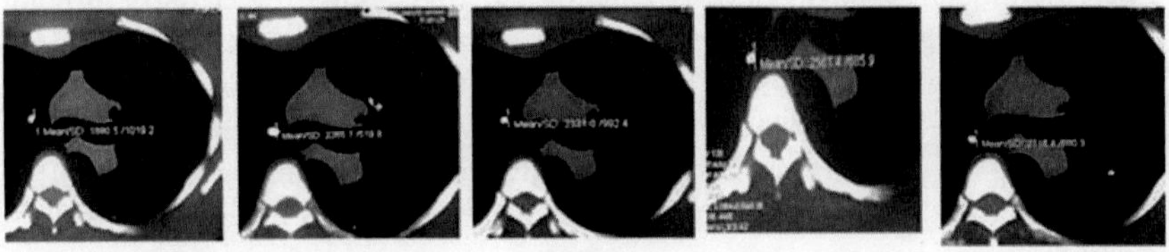

(b)

**Fig. 4** Proximal portion of the coronary artery phantom with two applications of the contrast media dose protocol methods, (**a**) Body weight method (BW), and (**b**) Body surface area (BSA) method

Table 3 Saphiro-Wilk test

| Variable | Sig. | Means |
|---|---|---|
| Body wight method | 0.854 | Normal distribution |
| BSA method | 0.903 | Normal distribution |

Table 4 Saphiro-Wilk test

| Difference | Mean | Sig. (2-tailed) |
|---|---|---|
| BW method–BSA method | −85.83 | 0.686 |

The results of average enhancement/CT Number were statistically tested to check its normality of data by using Saphiro-Wilk test.

Both methods had significance values > 0.05 (see in Table 3), which means the datas are normally distributed. Then it's continued with Paired T-Test.

Statistically, Table 4 showed that the significance value is 0.686 or >0.05 which means that there is no difference in coronary artery enhancement in the application of body weight-based and BSA-based contrast media dose calculation methods.

### 3.2 More Optimal Method

A mean value of −85.83 indicated that the mean of BSA method is higher than body weight method and this proved that the BSA method is able to produce more optimal enhancement.

## 4 Discussion

Dose calculation of the contrast media carried out by the body weight and BSA methods produced a volume that is not always the same. In the body weight method, administration of contrast media was calculated in the proportion of 1 mL/kg [7]. In this method, the volume of contrast media was only influenced by body weight so that the amount changes linearly and consistently follows the changes in body weight. Each weight gain of 10 kg would always be followed by an additional dose of 10 mL.

BSA method showed that the increase in contrast media volume is not proportional to the increase in body weight because the calculation is also influenced by height and contrast media concentration used as can be seen in the formula (mL) [13].

$$\frac{12.753 \times \sqrt{\frac{height\ (\mathrm{cm}) \times weight\ (\mathrm{kg})}{3600}}}{concentration} \tag{2}$$

At a 10 kg increase in weight (from 37 to 47 kg), the contrast media volume of the body weight method increased by 10 mL (from 37 to 47 mL) but in the BSA method, the volume increase was only as much as 6 mL (from 46 to 52 mL). In subsequent weight increases (starting at 57, 67 and 77 kg), the body weight method showed a steady increase in volume of 10 mL while in the BSA method the volume increase was only half that is 5 mL.

At 37 and 47 kg, the body weight method produced a smaller volume than the BSA method. At 57 kg, both methods produced the same volume. Then at 67 and 77 kg, the volume of contrast media based on body weight method was higher than the volume on BSA method.

The highest difference in volume of contrast media between the two calculation methods is at 77 kg, which was 10 mL. Then followed by 37 kg as much as 9 mL, then 47 and 67 kg which had the same difference of 5 mL, and finally the difference in contrast media volume at 57 kg is 0 mL.

When observed in terms of the percentage difference in the volume of contrast media, the highest difference was actually at 37 kg which is 24.30% (37: 46 mL), then followed by 77 kg at 12.98% (77: 67 mL), 47 kg at 10.64% (47: 52 mL), 67 kg at 7.46% (67: 62 mL), and finally 57 kg at 0% (both methods produced the same volume).

Through this research data, it can be seen that the thinner or fatter a person is, the volume of contrast media calculated with the BSA method will be even more different from that of the volume calculated with the BWp. In the thin people, the volume of contrast media based on the BSA method is higher than of the BWp, and vise versa. This is in accordance with the statement of Bae [11] that with the proportion of contrast media compared to 1: 1 body weight, the possibility of contrast media volume being overdosed in obese patients and under-dosed in thin patients.

The body weight method equation generated from the graph is $y = x$ which y is the volume of contrast media, and x is body weight. This equation has the same meaning as the body weight method dose of 1 mL/kg body weight.

While the BSA method produces the equation $y = 0.52x + 27.16$. This equation is faster and simpler to use. To find the volume of contrast media, technologist no longer need to calculate patient's BSA $\sqrt{}$((height (cm) × weight (kg))/3600) then proceed to calculate the volume of contrast media ((12.753 × BSA)/(350)), by adding the weight variable into the x value, it will immediately obtain the required volume. However, this equation can only be used for patients with a height of 156.25 cm, and for the use of a contrast media with the concentration of 350 mgI/mL due to the patient's BSA variation.

Canola oil has characteristics such as adipose fat [18]. Both have almost the same density, 0.92 g/mL for canola oil and 0.93–0.95 g/mL for adipose fat. In addition, both are also rich in carbon content (76.7% for canola oil and 60–70% for adipose fat). Based on this facts, the researchers used canola oil in simulating weight gain on phantom.

Researchers determined each weight gain of 10 kg, would be accompanied by the addition of canola oil of 400 mL. This applies to 47 kg (underweight) and 57 kg (normal). Whereas at 67 kg (overweight) and 77 kg (obesity), the addition of canola oil is only 200 mL.

Overweight and obesity can be interpreted as an abnormal condition caused by accumulation excess fat which might damage health. It is associated with numerous comorbidities such as cardiovascular diseases (CVD) [19]. Assuming that weight gain in the categories of overweight and obesity is indicated by an increase in abdominal fat content so that the chest area does not experience significant fat gain, the researchers set the addition of canola oil at 67 and 77 kg to only 200 mL, or half of the previous additions that reached 400 mL.

This study aims to look at the enhancement value of the coronary artery phantom in the images so that it does not necessary to employ ECG Triggering and Calcium Scoring modes when performing the Cardiac CT. Therefore, this study is sufficient to use the CT Thorax Non-Contrast protocol.

### *4.1 Coronary Artery Enhancement Difference*

Soft tissue in the phantom of the chest used is made of Polyurethane (−800 to −630 HU) and the bones are made of a mixture of epoxy resin and Calcium Carbonate [20]. This material has a HU value that is not the same as the human body. In humans, muscle tissue is valued at +50 HU and bone +1000 HU [21]. In addition, phan-tom does not have water, fat, and lung contents as contained in the human body with values: blood +20 HU, fat −100 HU, and lungs −200 HU [21] so that X-Ray attenua-tion on phantom also decreased. In addition, this phantom does not have the ability to represent vascularity and dilution of contrast media phenomenon in the human body that were affected by cardiac output and contrast media injection techniques. These factors cause the enhancement value produced by the contrast media in this study to be very high (+890 to +2900 HU). Researchers believe that this value is not sufficient to reflect the true occurrence of enhancement in humans, but still it can be used as a consideration before calculating the contrast media dose either based on body weight or Body Surface Area actually applied to Cardiac CT patients.

According to Pugliese [22] that the dose of contrast media (volume) affects the peak of enhancement. As the volume of contrast media increases, the enhancement will increase. This is proven by the tables and graphs above which show that there is an increase in coronary artery enhancement in addition to the volume of contrast media both in the body weight method and the BSA method. In the body weight method, the smallest volume of 37 mL produces the least enhancement, which is 891.33 HU. And the largest volume of 77 mL produces the highest enhancement value of 2935.73 HU. Likewise with the BSA method. The smallest volume of 46 mL resulted in enhancement of 1687.20 HU and the largest volume of 67 mL pro-duced 2592.15 HU of enhancement.

With the addition of a 10 mL volume, the resulting enhancement also increases although the magnitude of the increase is not always the same. This is influenced by the volume percentage increase with the same value for each BWp. In the body weight method, the increase in volume from 37 to 47 mL, the addition of 10 mL of contrast media means an increase in contrast media by 27% so that the increase in enhancement is also high (from 891.33 HU to 1776.63 HU or 885.30 HU difference). In the next sample, an increase in volume from 47 to 57 mL means there was an in-crease in contrast media by 21%. This shows that although the same 10 mL of contrast media were added, the second addition had a lower percentage so that the in-crease in enhancement was even smaller (1776.63 HU to 2096.52 HU or 319.89 HU difference). In addition there is attenuation factors that occur because the thickness of the object increases (weight gain is simulated by applying canola oil) which makes the CT Number value decrease. This applies to all scans on both dose calculation methods. Although the difference in the volume of contrast media is the same, the increase in the enhancement that occurs is not always the same. As was the case with the BSA method when the volume increased by 5 mL from 52 to 57 mL, from 57 to 62 mL, and from 62 to 67 mL. At 52–57 mL there was an increase in enhancement by 158.30 HU (1943.52–2101.82 HU), at 57–62 mL an in-crease of 314.31 HU (2101.82–2416.13 HU), and at 62–67 mL increased by 176.02 HU (2416.13–2592.15 HU). Whereas at 57 kg BWp, both dosage calculation methods produce the same volume of 57 mL. However, they both have a difference of 5.30 HU (2096.52 and 2101.82 HU) which is a normal thing to happen because there is a deviation in taking ROI values.

In the underweight category, the body weight method produces less enhancement than the BSA method. This is caused by the volume of contrast media calculated using the body weight method is less than the volume of contrast media calculated using the BSA method. This is in accordance with the statement that when the contrast media dose is calculated in proportion of 1: 1 compared to body weight, the volume of contrast media is under-dosed in thin patients. That's why the resulting enhancement is very low [11].

The opposite occurs in the obesity category. If the dose of contrast media is made to increase along with weight gain [11], then obese patients will get an enhancement that may be higher compared to non-obese patients who receive a dose of contrast media in the same proportion of body weight. This is evidenced by the high enhancement value produced by the body weight method at 77 kg (2935.73 HU) com-pared to the BSA method (2592.15 HU).

Through the graphical equation, the intersection of the two methods shows that the contrast media enhancement will be the same at BWp 60 kg with a value of 2210.03 HU. Even when it is manually calculated, the volume of contrast media at 60 kg is not the same (body weight method 60 mL while BSA method 58.8 mL). This shows that in the normal or ideal BMIp category, the enhancement produced by the two methods will produce values that are close to each other or even the same (keep in mind there is a deviation standard on each ROI).

## 4.2 More Optimal Method

The final results of average enhancement measurements in the SPSS test indicated that the two methods did not provide significantly different enhancements. That is, both methods are equally applicable. However, there are things that need to be underlined in the results of this study, namely that in certain categories (underweight and obesity), the enhancement produced by the two methods has a big difference. According to Scholtz and Ghoshhajra [23], optimal intravascular enhancement on Cardiac CT is between 250 and 300 HU to optimize differentiation of low-density atherosclerosis lesions in the coronary arteries (approximately 40 HU), advanced fibrous plaque (90 HU) and calcified plaque more than 130 HU. That is, CT Number values outside this range can cause radiologists to doubt interpreting fatal images which can lead to diagnostic errors. When observed one by one, the enhancement at BWp 37 kg produced by the two methods of calculating contrast media dose has a very large difference in number where the BW method produces 891.33 HU and the BSA method produces 1678.20 HU. Likewise, at 77 kg, the BW method produced 2935.73 HU while the BSA method only 2592.15 HU. Researchers believe that this value can be a consideration for technologist in the field in applying the method of calculating the exact contrast media dose for patients who are very thin (underweight) or very fat (obese) in order to provide adequate enhancement or can produce more optimal diagnostic information.

In clinical examination, optimization principle is needed, to get optimal image quality [24]. Both dosage calculation methods produce contrast media volumes which are not always the same. Because these two methods show an enhancement that is not significantly different, the researchers feel that the technologist can choose one of the two methods that has advantages in terms of effectiveness and efficiency of the contrast media (choosing a method that produces less volume of contrast media and or produces a more optimal enhancement) so it is safer for the kidney of the patient and can produce a good and accurate image of the coronary arteries.

This research has the limitation of not being able to take into account the effect of the dilution and distribution of contrast media in the body as revealed by Bae [25] that both of these factors contribute to influencing the occurrence of enhancement. In addition, the use of a saline volume of 30 mL and the addition of canola oil volume for each weight gain also needs to be validated. Likewise with a very high enhancement value (+890 to +2900 HU) which has not been able to reflect the actual enhancement of the human coronary arteries. Therefore the results in this study still need to be clinically proven.

The coronary artery phantom that is made through 3D printing is stiff/hard so that it has not been able to show physiological arteries that can flexibly dilate following the pressure or volume of blood that passes through them. Beside, the edges still cannot be perfectly closed so that there is a part of the contrast media fluid that seeps which causes the coronary artery phantom is not fully filled.

In short, the dose calculation based on body weight (BWp) method shows the equivalence of image visualization enhancement from that of the BSA method.

The proposed BWp implies an alternative approach for the contrast media dosage calculation with some advantages.

## 5 Conclusion

This study proposes to develop a model of the coronary arterial mimicking phantoms where an experiments to compare the image contrast enhancement in both of the applied methods, the BWp and BSA for calculating the contrast media doses. There was no significant difference in the coronary artery enhancement between the BWp and BSA methods of contrast media dose protocol calculation ($p > 0.05$). A more optimal method of producing coronary artery enhancement is BSA with a mean value of 2148.16 HU. Further clinical trials would be important to oversee its sensitivity for the real patients.

## References


1. Delima D, Mihardja L, Siswoyo H, Prevalensi dan Faktor Determinan Penyakit Jantung di Indonesia. Bul Penelit Kesehat 37
2. Mc Namara K, Alzubaidi H, Jackson JK (2019) Cardiovascular disease as a leading cause of death: how are pharmacists getting involved? Integr Pharm Res Pract 8:1–11
3. Saputri FB, Fauziah D, Hindariati E (2020) Prevalence proportion of patient with coronary heart disease in inpatient room of RSUD Dr. Soetomo Surabaya in 2017. Biomol Heal Sci J 3:95
4. Putri RD, Nur'aeni A, Belinda V (2018) Study of the learning needs for clients with coronary heart disease. J Nurs Care 1:60
5. Kartikasari Y, Darmini MS, Rochmayanti D (2021) Comparison of radiation dose and image noise in head computed tomography with sequence and spiral techniques. Lect Notes Electr Eng 746 LNEE, 557–566
6. Gorenoi V, Schönermark MP, Hagen A (2012) CT coronary angiography vs. invasive coronary angiography in CHD. GMS Health Technol Assess 8, Doc02
7. Desjardins B, Kazerooni EA (2004) ECG-gated cardiac CT, 993–1010
8. Van Cauteren T, Van Gompel G, Nieboer KH, Willekens I, Evans P, Macholl S, Droogmans S, de Mey J, Buls N (2018) Improved enhancement in CT angiography with reduced contrast media iodine concentrations at constant iodine dose. Sci Rep 8:1–10
9. Mihl C, Kok M, Wildberger JE, Altintas S, Labus D, Nijssen EC, Hendriks BMF, Kietselaer BLJH, Das M (2015) Coronary CT angiography using low concentrated contrast media injected with high flow rates: feasible in clinical practice. Eur J Radiol 84:2155–2160
10. Oda S, Utsunomiya D, Nakaura T, Kidoh M, Funama Y, Tsujita K, Yamashita Y (2018) Basic concepts of contrast injection protocols for coronary computed tomography angiography. Curr Cardiol Rev 15:24–29
11. Bae KT, Seeck BA, Hildebolt CF, Tao C, Zhu F, Kanematsu M, Woodard PK (2008) Contrast enhancement in cardiovascular MDCT: effect of body weight, height, body surface area, body mass index, and obesity. Am J Roentgenol 190:777–784
12. RD M, Simplified calculation of body-surface area. N Engl J Med 22
13. Yanaga Y, Awai K, Nakaura T, Utsunomiya D, Oda S, Hirai T, Yamashita Y (2010) Contrast material injection protocol with the dose adjusted to the body surface area for MDCT aortography. Am J Roentgenol 194:903–908

14. Pazhenkottil AP, Husmann L, Buechel RR, Herzog BA, Nkoulou R, Burger IA, Vetterli A, Valenta I, Ghadri JR, Von Schulthess P, Kaufmann PA (2010) Validation of a new contrast material protocol adapted to body surface area for optimized low-dose CT coronary angiography with prospective ECG-triggering. Int J Cardiovasc Imaging 26:591–597
15. Karimi G, Jahani O (2012) Genetic algorithm application in swing phase optimization of AK prosthesis with passive dynamics and biomechanics considerations. Genet Algorithms Appl
16. Shah Y, Patel N, Patel N, Patel S, Surani P (2021) Design and fabrication of wheelchair CUM stretcher. Int J Eng Adv Technol 10:210–214
17. Nuttall FQ, Body mass index obesity, BMI, and Health: A Critical Review
18. Fitzgerald PF, Colborn RE, Edic PM, Lambert JW, Bonitatibus PJ, Yeh BM (2017) Liquid tissue surrogates for X-ray and CT phantom studies
19. Poirier P, Giles TD, Bray GA, Hong Y, Stern JS, Pi-Sunyer FX, Eckel RH (2006) Obesity and cardiovascular disease: pathophysiology, evaluation, and effect of weight loss: an update of the 1997 American heart association scientific statement on obesity and heart disease from the obesity committee of the council on nutrition. Phys Circulation 113:898–918
20. Murata K, Nitta N, Multipurpose chest phantom N1 "LUNGMAN."
21. Bontrager KL (2018) Textbook of positioning and related anatomy. CV. Mosby Company, St. Louis (2018)
22. Pugliese FD (2008) Which contrast agent for. https://repub.eur.nl/pub/13655/Francesca_Appendix.pdf
23. Scholtz JE, Ghoshhajra B (2017) Advances in cardiac CT contrast injection and acquisition protocols. Cardiovasc Diagn Ther 7:439–451
24. Masrochah S, Wibowo AS, Ardiyanto J, Fatimah SAN (2021) The optimal scan delay of contrast media injection for diagnosing abdominal tumors (image quality and radiation dose aspects of abdominal CT scan), presented at the BT—proceedings of the 1st international conference on electronics, biomedical engineering, and health Inf.
25. Bae KT (2010) Intravenous contrast medium administration and scan timing at CT: considerations and approaches. Radiology 256:32–61

# Optimization of Battery Management System with SOC Estimation by Comparing Two Methods

**Lora Khaula Amifia, Moch. Iskandar Riansyah, Benazir Imam Arif Muttaqin, Adellia Puspita Ratri, Firman Adi Rifansyah, and Bagas Wahyu Prakoso**

**Abstract** Electric vehicles are currently being developed where the battery is the main driver. SOC (State of Charge) is one of the determinants of the success of electric vehicles. It is the current battery capacity expressed in per cent and provides information about the battery's state. One method to measure SOC is to use Coulomb Counting; the integration of current against time. Kalman Filter is also a very suitable method for estimating SOC to obtain an effective and efficient BMS. SOC estimation requires accurate battery modelling to create a reliable BMS enabling the battery to be able to operate optimally. The important thing in electric vehicles is to optimize BMS performance with an accurate SOC estimation algorithm. This research is oriented to the estimation of the state of charge on the BMS to optimize the BMS performance with an accurate SOC estimation algorithm. In this research, 2 battery models were proposed, i.e., the simple and Thevenin battery models. SOC estimation based on those battery models was done with coulomb counting, open-circuit voltage, and Kalman Filter. The results showed that the estimated final SOC value with Model 1 was 20.04%, while the estimated final SOC value with Model 2 was 19.42%. The direct impact or consequence of the findings in this study is that the coulomb counting method is easier to use in calculating battery capacity.

**Keywords** State of charge · Battery modelling · Coulomb counting · Kalman filter

## 1 Introduction

State of Charge (SOC) is the ratio of the available battery capacity to the nominal capacity of the battery in an electric vehicle. It is one of the components in the Battery Management System (BMS), which cannot directly be measured [1]. The determination of SOC value can be done using methods and algorithms to estimate

L. K. Amifia (✉) · Moch. I. Riansyah · B. I. A. Muttaqin · A. P. Ratri · F. A. Rifansyah · B. W. Prakoso
Faculty of Electrical Engineering and Intelligent Industry, Institut Teknologi Telkom Surabaya, Jalan Ketintang Selatan No.156, Surabaya, Indonesia
e-mail: loraamifia@ittelkom-sby.ac.id



T. Triwiyanto et al. (eds.), *Proceedings of the 2nd International Conference on Electronics, Biomedical Engineering, and Health Informatics*, Lecture Notes in Electrical Engineering 898, https://doi.org/10.1007/978-981-19-1804-9_34

the exceeding parameters such as voltage and current. The estimation of battery SOC is an important focus in Electric Vehicles, i.e. by measuring the availability in the current cycle and using the battery before recharging [2, 3].

Battery modelling is one of the most important aspects to maximize the estimation process. It is needed to help the SOC estimation process to make the results accurate and the battery optimal when being operated [4]. Based on previous research, the nonlinear battery model (Thevenin) is the battery model that was successful in estimating SOC with high accuracy using the Kalman Filter supported by experimental data [5]. The battery model was then parameterized using the recursive least square (RLS) algorithm to obtain the characteristics of its recursive parameters. Knowing the parameters can facilitate to estimate the SOC while guaranteeing a longer BMS life [6].

In another study, the OCV method was used to estimate SOC by modifying the OCV-SOC relationship that was applied with Kalman Filter to improve algorithm performance in overcoming any battery modelling problems [7]. In this method, it was explained that this method was very accurate, but it needed a rest to estimate SOC and the Kalman Filter method as an optimal adaptive algorithm based on recursive estimation based on model parameters [8, 9]. In other studies, overcharging and discharging lithium batteries could cause a permanent damage and to maintain battery safety and performance, battery reliability and accuracy, it was necessary to estimate the SOC of the battery management system [10–12].

In addition to the estimation methods above, the value of a battery model help to get an accurate SOC [13]. Based on the references that have been obtained, this study used a battery model that has been selected from the results of research that has been previously developed in which it succeeded in estimating SOC with high accuracy based on a nonlinear battery model (Thevenin) using the Kalman Filter supported by experimental data [14]. This battery model was then parameterized using the recursive least square (RLS) algorithm [15]. The use of this method was because with RLS, the characteristics of its recursive ability could be obtained [16, 17]. Knowing the parameters can facilitate to estimate the SOC while guaranteeing a longer BMS life. Thus, from the battery model, the SOC estimation algorithm was then developed using several battery models purposely for obtaining the precise and accurate SOC estimates [18].

Based on this explanation, this study focused on optimizing BMS with SOC estimation by comparing the Rint battery model with the Thevenin battery model so that it can produce a precise and accurate SOC estimate.

# 2 Methodology

## 2.1 Estimation Method

Accurate SOC estimation can maintain an effective battery operation to the desired battery operating limit and minimize battery failure caused by overcharge and overdischarge. An overcharge will cause the battery to burn easily [3, 19]; meanwhile, overdischarge conditions can reduce the capacity of battery cells due to chemical reactions that cannot be changed (irreversible). Battery parameters, such as ambient temperature, charge rate and discharge rate, and self-discharge rate are required to achieve a high level of accuracy when estimating SOC [20, 21].

The most precise and accurate SOC estimation methods include OCV (Open Circuit Voltage), Coulomb Counting, and Kalman Filter [22]. Coulomb Counting and Kalman Filter methods can be implemented for linear systems with nonlinear battery models [7]. Another adaptive method for estimating battery SOC is based on Coulomb Counting and OCV. This estimation method can be stated to be accurate when the battery is operating [23].

This process aims to get an accurate battery SOC so that battery usage lasts longer and does not get damaged quickly. In addition, the use of an effective method for estimating battery SOC can encourage the development of the electric vehicle industry using intelligent vehicle exhaust emission-free technology (Fig. 1).

In this study, the estimation of SOC was carried out by several methods: Coulomb Counting, Open Circuit Voltage, and Kalman Filter. Then, a comparative study and analysis were carried out for an accurate SOC estimation for optimal performance of the battery. In addition, the system design was made to facilitate researchers in experiments. The main components in the experiment included Charge–Discharge-Open Circuit, Dummy Load as a loading circuit, Control Circuit connected to current and voltage sensors to measure current and battery voltage data. Furthermore, the data recorded on the two sensors were connected directly to the PC so that researchers were able to find out firsthand how the current and voltage data obtained could then be directly handled or taken action. The research procedure carried out in this study is presented as follows.

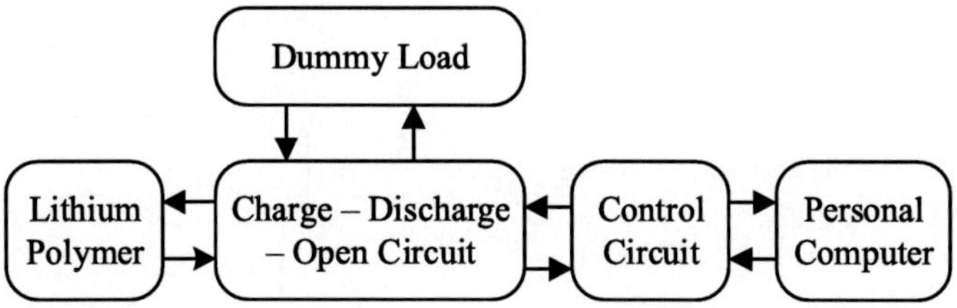


**Fig. 1** Block diagram

**Data Collection**. An important main thing to do in this research was the data collection of Lithium Polymer batteries to make it simple in the treatment of the program design.

**Designing an Estimation Algorithm**. After obtaining valid battery data, the next step was to design an approximate SOC estimate for the battery using several methods as described above.

**Simulation and Experiment**. The results of the research simulation were used for the validation of experimental data and analysis of the success of the methods used and repeated testing.

**Testing and Analysis**. The design of the SOC estimates on the BMS has been completed and testing has been carried out to prove the hypotheses that have been made previously with the appropriate parameters for the problem to be solved.

**Decision Logic**. The final part of the research was to draw a conclusion or decision making from the test results and the results that have been achieved.

## 2.2 *Battery Modelling*

Experiments were carried out for battery testing. The Lithium Polymer battery became the object of research which was tested to determine its characteristics by charging, discharging, and open circuit. The switching circuit used was a tool to connect the battery, dummy load, charger and controller (Arduino UNO 32) for switching and storing data to a computer via serial communication. ACS712 current sensor (−5 to 5 A) was with a sensitivity of 185 mV/A. When the current reading was 0 A in the circuit, the sensor voltage output was 2.5 V. When the sensor read a positive current from the circuit, the sensor output was more than 2.5 V indicating current flows from IP+ to IP−. Conversely, when current flowed from IP− to IP+, a negative current would be read (voltage on sensor $< 2.5$ V). The simple battery model (Rint) and Thevenin battery model described the battery process in detail, making it accurate for modelling battery characteristics. Here, the Rint model consisted of resistance, capacitor, and capacitor voltage and resistance voltage. As for the Thevenin battery model (Fig. 2).

**Fig. 2** Rint battery model

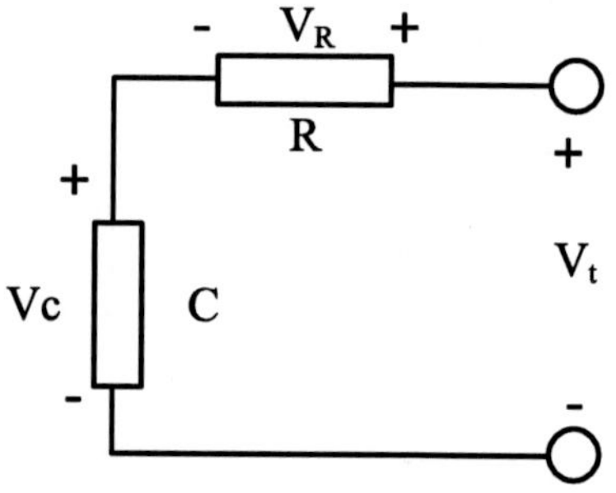

Fig. 3 Thevenin battery model

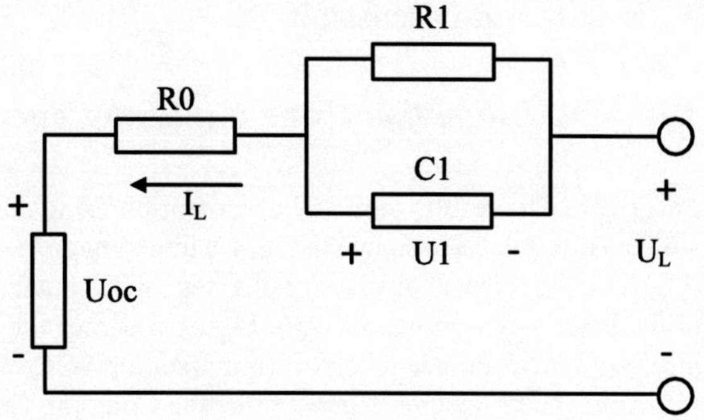


The capacitors in the RC battery model are presented as follows.

$$I = -C\frac{dV_C}{dt} \tag{1}$$

$$\frac{dSOC}{dt} = -\frac{I}{C_n} \tag{2}$$

$$C = C_n\frac{dSOC}{dOCV} \tag{3}$$

The initial SOC obtained from the OCV-SOC relationship, by providing the initial terminal voltage as the initial OCV from the SOC information and Eq. (2) was critical; the battery SOC was calculated using the Coulomb Counting method (Fig. 3).

$U_{OC}$ was modeled as C so that the parameters in this model became 4; C, $R_0$, $R_1$, and $C_1$. Based on this model a number of equations could be derived.

$$U_C = \frac{1}{C}\int I_L dt \tag{4}$$

*with* $\boldsymbol{U_C = U_{OC}}$,

$$\dot{U_{OC}} = \frac{1}{C}I_L \tag{5}$$

Based on (5) a state space model can be formed.

$$\begin{bmatrix} \dot{U}_1 \\ \dot{U}_{OC} \end{bmatrix} = \begin{bmatrix} -\frac{1}{R_1C_1} & 0 \\ 0 & 0 \end{bmatrix}\begin{bmatrix} U_1 \\ U_{OC} \end{bmatrix} + \begin{bmatrix} \frac{1}{C_1} \\ \frac{1}{C} \end{bmatrix} I_L \tag{6}$$

# 3 Result and Discussion

## 3.1 SOC Estimation Using Coulomb Counting Method

***Pulse Test.*** The results of the SOC estimation using the Coulomb Counting method with pulse test data are shown in Fig. 4. The estimation results were used as a reference (SOC true) for error analysis. The test was carried out from a full battery (SOC 100%) to the battery ran out (SOC 0%). Figure 5 shows the simulation performed if the initialization was made incorrect (initialization SOC = 80%, which should be SOC = 100%). These results indicated that the Coulomb Counting method was not able to correct errors in the initialization of the SOC value so that the estimate continued to go wrong.

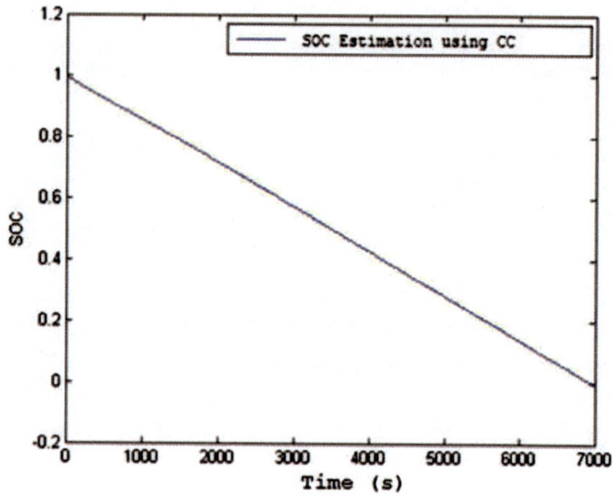


**Fig. 4** SOC estimation using coulomb counting

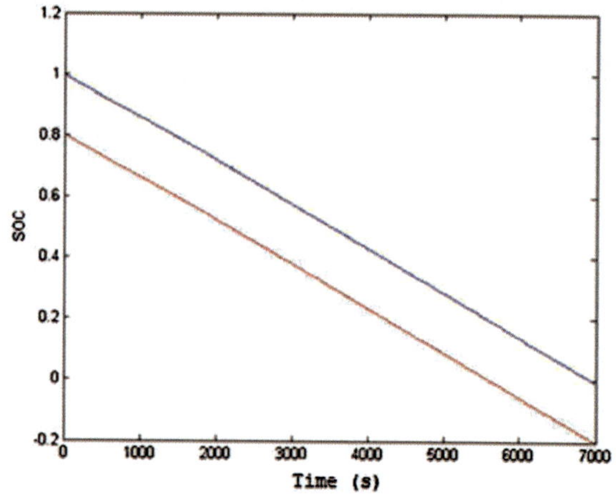


**Fig. 5** SOC initialization error using coulomb counting

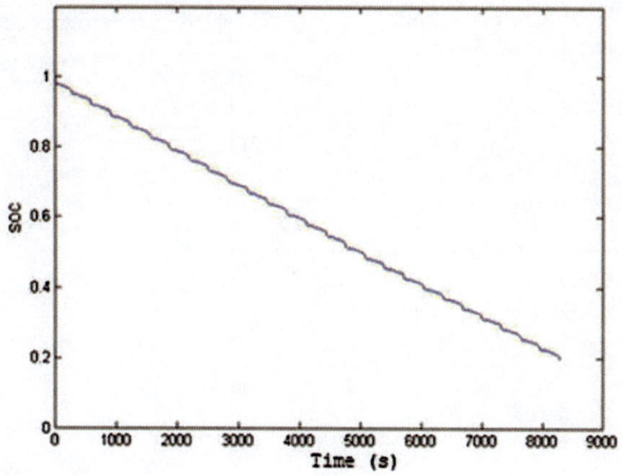


**Fig. 6** SOC estimation using coulomb counting

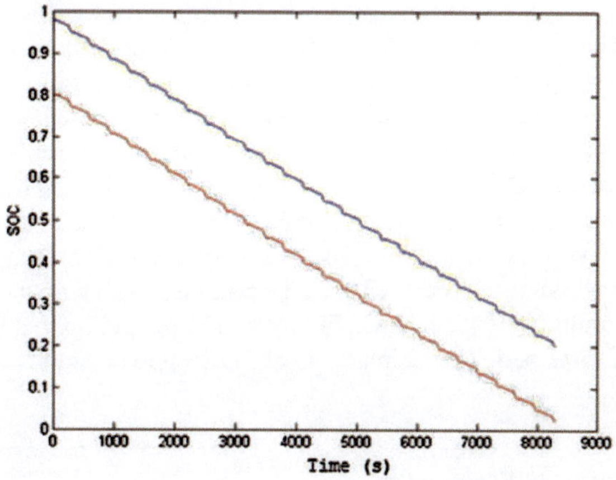


**Fig. 7** SOC initialization error using coulomb counting

***Variable Load Test***. Figure 6 shows the results of the SOC estimation using the Coulomb Counting method. These results were used as a reference (SOC true) for error analysis. The test was carried out from full battery (SOC 100%) to SOC 20%. Figure 7 depicts a simulation that was done if the initialization was made wrong (initialization SOC = 80%, which should be SOC = 100%). These results indicated that the Coulomb Counting method was unable to correct errors in the initialization of the SOC value so that the estimate continued to be wrong.

## 3.2 SOC Estimation Using Kalman Filter

***Pulse Test***. Figure 8 presents the results of SOC estimation using the Kalman Filter method from the Thevenin battery model using pulse test data with the CC method.

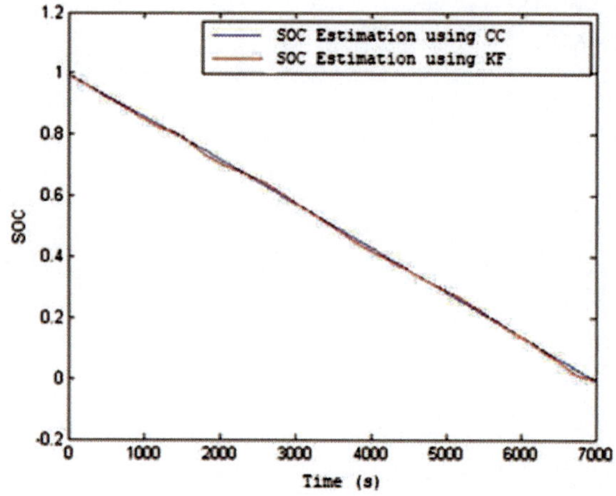


**Fig. 8** SOC estimation using Kalman Filter

The estimation results of the Kalman Filter method were close to the CC method estimation. The estimated final SOC value with this method was 0.00%.

Figure 9 shows the simulation performed if the initialization was made incorrect (initialization SOC = 80%, which should be SOC = 100%) and Fig. 10 with initialization SOC 0%. These two results indicated that the Kalman Filter method was able to correct the SOC initialization error.

***Variable Load Test.*** The results of the SOC estimation using the Kalman Filter method were compared with the pulse test data with the CC method. The estimation results using the Kalman Filter method were close to the estimation results using the CC method. The estimated final SOC value using this method was 19.42%.

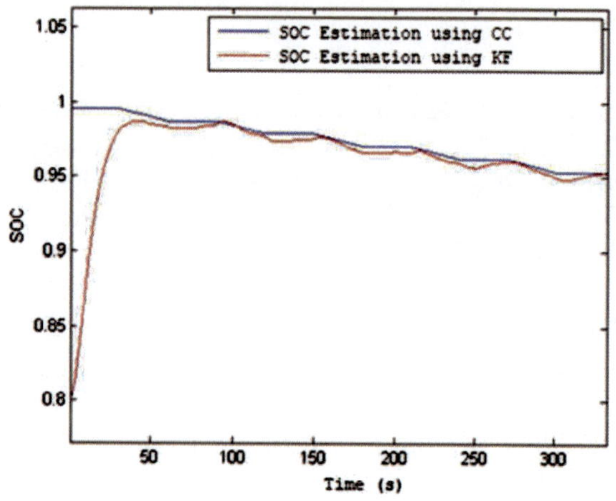


**Fig. 9** SOC initialization error using Kalman Filter

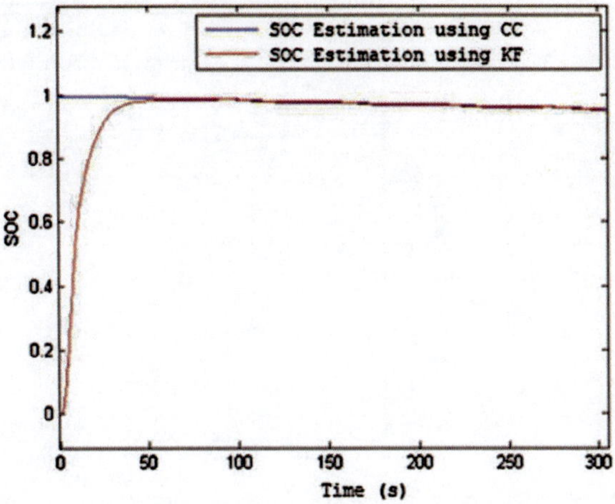


**Fig. 10** SOC initialization error using Kalman Filter

Figure 9 shows the simulations performed if the initialization was made wrong (SOC initialization = 80%) and Fig. 10 with 0% SOC initialization. These two results indicated that the Kalman method could correct the SOC initialization error.

Battery testing was carried out with varying loads with the results of SOC estimation using the OCV method compared to the CC method as shown in Fig. 11. The final SOC value was 20.04% adrift from the CC method, which was 19.77%. While Fig. 12 shows the SOC Initialization Error using Kalman Filter Method with a final value of 19.42%.

Table 1 shows the value of the average error, MSE, Max–Min error, and RMSE of the two models at the time of testing. Model 1 had a larger average value than did Model 2 but the error range was smaller. While Model 2 had an MSE value greater than Model 1 and the mean error was smaller than Model 1.

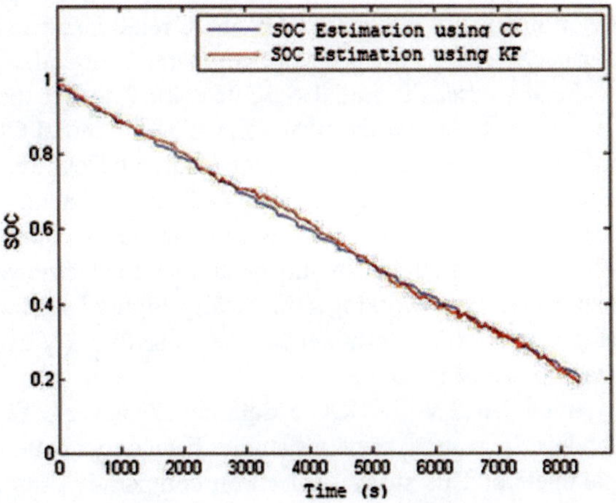


**Fig. 11** SOC estimation using Kalman Filter

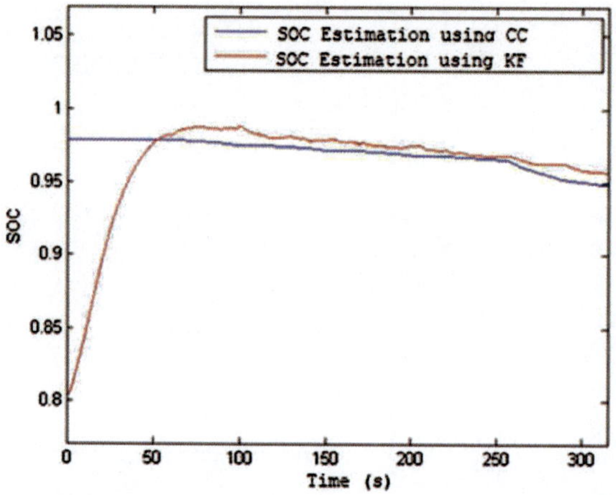


**Fig. 12** SOC initialization error using Kalman Filter

**Table 1** Mean error, MSE, range, and RMSE both models during discharge testing

| Model | Mean error | MSE | Range | RMSE |
|---|---|---|---|---|
| Model 1 | 11.345513e-03 | 9.45229e-04 | 2.987658 | 2.97634752e-02 |
| Model 2 | 8.0987575e-03 | 7.11123e-05 | 3.451317 | 7.09876303e-03 |

## 3.3 Discussion

In the next study, it is deemed necessary to estimate SOC using battery modelling methods and models other than those carried out in this study. In addition, the implementation of the algorithm generated on the actual BMS also needs to be done to see the results of good and accurate battery reliability [24, 25]. SOC estimation and determination of nonlinear OCV–SOC relationship in Lithium Polymer battery with a capacity of 2.2 Ah need to be compared using other non-linear methods.

In this case, the initial SOC is critical to get the OCV-SOC relationship. By providing the initial terminal voltage as the initial OCV of the battery SOC, SOC information is calculated using the Coulomb Counting method [26]. In electric vehicles, the estimation method using OCV is important, but it is difficult to apply when the electric vehicle is running because the OCV condition requires time for rest time [27]. So, this method can only be applied to electric vehicles at a stop, not when the battery system is working dynamically. Figure 13 shows that the OCV-SOC relationship has an OCV—terminal voltage value of 4.3 V using a lookup table or obtained from the OCV function.

In the BMS study, SOC estimation has never been done by comparing 2 battery models. In general, previous studies have only applied 1 battery model with various parameters. This study focused on comparative studies for 2 battery models: the Rint battery model and the Thevenin battery model with a 2.2 Ah Lithium Polymer

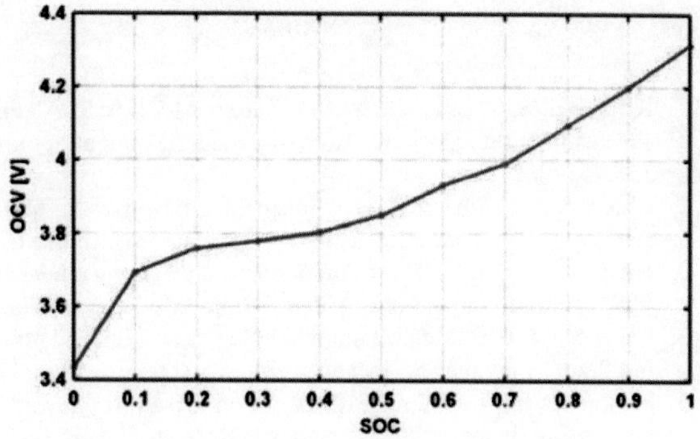


**Fig. 13** OCV–SOC

battery that has been tested and validated previously. The results of this study were by the initial hypothesis, namely that both battery models could help to analyze the exact value of SOC accuracy to produce BMS in electric vehicles that functioned optimally.

The weaknesses of the Coulomb Counting method are related to its sensitiveness to the precision of the current sensor at the input, and the initial value of SOC is unknown. While the weakness of the Kalman Filter method is that it demands accuracy in system modelling.

The author realized that this research has future work and needs to be improved in several ways; estimated SOC using battery modelling and methods other than those carried out in this study and implementation of the resulting algorithm on the actual BMS.

## 4 Conclusion

The SOC estimation of the battery could produce a good performance and avoid overcharge or undercharge so that the battery life could last longer. The purpose of this study is to produce a BMS with an accurate SOC estimation and work optimally by comparing 2 models, namely the Rint battery model and the Thevenin battery model. SOC estimation of 2.2 Ah Lithium Polymer battery using the Rint and Thevenin battery models produced an equally good quality of accuracy. The estimated final SOC value with Model 1 was 20.04%. While the estimated final SOC value with Model 2 was 19.42%. For future research, it is deemed necessary to estimate SOC using an online system and implement the resulting algorithm on a BMS system close to the real thing.

## References


1. Klee Barillas J, Li J, Günther C, Danzer MA (2015) A comparative study and validation of state estimation algorithms for Li-ion batteries in battery management systems. Appl Energy 155:455–462
2. Unterrieder C, Zhang C, Lunglmayr M, Priewasser R, Marsili S, Huemer M (2015) Battery state-of-charge estimation using approximate least squares. J Power Sources 278:274–286
3. Hu X, Sun F, Zou Y (2013) Comparison between two model-based algorithms for Li-ion battery SOC estimation in electric vehicles. Simul Model Pract Theory 34(5):1–11
4. Lai X et al (2020) Mechanism, modeling, detection, and prevention of the internal short circuit in lithium-ion batteries: recent advances and perspectives. Energy Storage Mater
5. Hu C, Youn BD, Chung J (2012) A multiscale framework with extended Kalman filter for lithium-ion battery SOC and capacity estimation. Appl Energy 92:694–704
6. Chen J, Xu C, Wu C, Xu W (2018) Adaptive fuzzy logic control of fuel-cell-battery hybrid systems for electric vehicles. IEEE Trans Ind Inform 14(1):292–300
7. Hemmati R, Mehrjerdi H (2020) Stochastic linear programming for optimal planning of battery storage systems under unbalanced-uncertain conditions. J Mod Power Syst Clean Energy 8(5):971–980
8. Hong J, Yin J, Liu Y, Peng J, Jiang H (2019) Energy management and control strategy of photovoltaic/battery hybrid distributed power generation systems with an integrated three-port power converter. IEEE Access 7:82838–82847
9. Carkhuff BG, Demirev PA, Srinivasan R (2018) Impedance-based battery management system for safety monitoring of lithium-ion batteries. IEEE Trans Ind Electron 65(8):6497–6504
10. Xing Y, He W, Pecht M, Tsui KL (2014) State of charge estimation of lithium-ion batteries using the open-circuit voltage at various ambient temperatures. Appl Energy 113:106–115
11. He Y, Liu XT, Bin Zhang C, Chen ZH (2013) A new model for State-of-Charge (SOC) estimation for high-power Li-ion batteries. Appl Energy 101:808–814
12. Belhani A, M'Sirdi NK, Naamane A (2013) Adaptive sliding mode observer for estimation of state of charge. Energy Proc 42:377–386
13. Gangatharan S, Rengasamy M, Elavarasan RM, Das N, Hossain E, Sundaram VM (2020) A novel battery supported energy management system for the effective handling of feeble power in hybrid microgrid environment. IEEE Access 8:217391–217415
14. Liu X et al (2020) Online identification of power battery parameters for electric vehicles using a decoupling multiple forgetting factors recursive least squares method. CSEE J Power Energy Syst 6(3):735–742
15. Tariq M, Maswood AI, Gajanayake CJ, Gupta AK (2018) Modeling and integration of a lithium-ion battery energy storage system with the more electric aircraft 270 v DC power distribution architecture. IEEE Access 6:41785–41802
16. Kim M, Kim K, Han S (2020) Reliable online parameter identification of Li-Ion batteries in battery management systems using the condition number of the error covariance matrix. IEEE Access 8:189106–189114
17. Xiong R, Cao J, Yu Q, He H, Sun F (2017) Critical review on the battery state of charge estimation methods for electric vehicles. IEEE Access 6:1832–1843
18. Kong X, Zheng Y, Ouyang M, Lu L, Li J (2018) Fault diagnosis and quantitative analysis of micro-short circuits for lithium-ion batteries in battery packs. J Power Sources 395(May):358–368
19. Hung MH, Lin CH, Lee LC, Wang CM (2014) State-of-charge and state-of-health estimation for lithium-ion batteries based on dynamic impedance technique. J Power Sources 268:861–873
20. Duong VH, Bastawrous HA, Lim KC, See KW, Zhang P, Dou SX (2015) Online state of charge and model parameters estimation of the LiFePO4 battery in electric vehicles using multiple adaptive forgetting factors recursive least-squares. J Power Sources 296:215–224
21. Corno M, Pozzato G (2020) Active adaptive battery aging management for electric vehicles. IEEE Trans Veh Technol 69(1):258–269

22. Kim KD, Lee HM, Hong SW, Cho GH (2019) A noninverting buck-boost converter with state-based current control for li-ion battery management in mobile applications. IEEE Trans Ind Electron 66(12):9623–9627
23. Mastali M, Vazquez-Arenas J, Fraser R, Fowler M, Afshar S, Stevens M (2013) Battery state of the charge estimation using Kalman filtering. J Power Sources 239:294–307
24. Zhong F, Li H, Zhong S, Zhong Q, Yin C (2015) An SOC estimation approach based on adaptive sliding mode observer and fractional order equivalent circuit model for lithium-ion batteries. Commun Nonlinear Sci Numer Simul 24(1–3):127–144
25. Chun CY et al (2015) Current sensor-less state-of-charge estimation algorithm for lithium-ion batteries utilizing filtered terminal voltage. J Power Sources 273:255–263
26. Hua Y, Yurkovichb S (2012) Battery cell state-of-charge estimation using linear parameter varying system techniques. J Power Sources 198:338–350
27. Feng X, Pan Y, He X, Wang L, Ouyang M (2018) Detecting the internal short circuit in large-format lithium-ion battery using model-based fault-diagnosis algorithm. J Energy Storage 18(February):26–39

# EMG Based Classification of Hand Gesture Using PCA and SVM

**Limcoln Dela, Daniel Sutopo, Sumantri Kurniawan, Tegoeh Tjahjowidodo, and Wahyu Caesarendra**

**Abstract** Biomechanics is a field of science that studies the movement of living things, especially humans. Bio-mechanical science produces new technology, namely electromyography (EMG). Electromyography (EMG) is a technique for recording signals originating from human muscles during contraction or relaxation, so it is widely used as a control medium. One of the applications of the EMG is in controlling the robotic arm. To do this task the recognizing the signal of the EMG for hand gestures is needed. This study aims to identify five finger movement patterns using a Myo Armband sensor based on electromyography (EMG) signals. This equipment is located on the forearm of the user's right hand to get a signal from the EMG. The 70 percent EMG signal is used as training to get the weight of the results for each movement. Then, the weight of the training results is tested using 30% of the EMG signal data and grouped using the Support Vector Machine (SVM) method. At the classification stage, a success percentage of 60% was obtained for sensor 3, 73% for sensor 4, and 53% for sensor 8. Furthermore, after receiving a percentage of the success of this study, the authors hope this research can become a reference for the development of making hand robots for medical purposes.

**Keywords** EMG · Hand gesture classification · PCA · SVM

L. Dela · D. Sutopo · S. Kurniawan
Department of Electrical Engineering, Politeknik Negeri Batam, Batam, Indonesia

T. Tjahjowidodo
Department of Mechanical Engineering, De Nayer Campus, Leuven, KU, Belgium

W. Caesarendra (✉)
Faculty of Integrated Technologies, University Brunei Darussalam, Bandar Seri Begawan, Brunei Darussalam
e-mail: wahyu.caesarendra@ubd.edu.bn



T. Triwiyanto et al. (eds.), *Proceedings of the 2nd International Conference on Electronics, Biomedical Engineering, and Health Informatics*, Lecture Notes in Electrical Engineering 898, https://doi.org/10.1007/978-981-19-1804-9_35

# 1 Introduction

Robotics technology is growing. Many people innovate to help their activities, including making robot manipulators pick up things in hard-to-reach places or move stuff with very high precision. The indirect benefit resulting from this system is to reduce the risks of the operator because they do it remotely [1]. Robots are not only used in industry but can help humans in the medical field. In the medical field, many applications and tools are used to support medical science, such as in diagnosing [2], treating [3], and preventing disease or injury to parts of the human body [4, 5]. In the medical field, there is a field of science that studies the movement of living things, especially in humans, namely biomechanics. Biomechanics applies the concept of technology, treatment, and diagnosis related to the movement of human activities to produce new technology, namely electromyography (EMG). Electromyography (EMG) is a signal that comes from human muscles during contraction or relaxation which is called electrophysiological in the field of medicine because it is a basic method for understanding the normal and pathological conditions of human muscle cells, so it is widely used and developed as a control medium for electric devices, for example in the field of prosthetics [6].

These signals are used as a control medium in human individuals who have limited muscle movement in everyday life. For example, people with physical disabilities, especially those who do not have wrists, are congenital or have an accident so that the hand is amputated [6]. This makes it difficult to carry out daily activities [7]. For this reason, a prosthetic or artificial hand aid is needed to replace the lost role of the wrist by utilizing the EMG signal generated by muscle contraction based on the forearm muscle in hand. The EMG sensor raw signal requires other methods to be processed. Thus, the practice of the technique to recognition of the pattern, which enables to read the activity of the muscle is a necessary matter [8].

The features of EMG's signals are be grouped into three main domains. The time domain, the frequency domain, and time–frequency domain are the significant features domain. These feature domains have been used by researchers to identify the pose of the hand of the subjects. For examples of the features in the time domain is Root Mean Square (RMS), Mean Absolute Value (MAV), and wavelength of the signal [9]. In the other hand, Mean Frequency, Median Frequency [10], Fast Fourier Transforms (FFT) [7], and Octave Band [11], are the example of the frequency domain. In comparison, Wavelets and Wavelets Packet Transforms [12, 13] are the samples of the features in the time–frequency domain.

To recognize the poses of the hand, several algorithms have been studied. For instance, Linear Discriminant Analysis (LDA) [14], K-Nearest Neighbor (K-NN) [15, 16], Fuzzy [17], Neural Network (NN) [18], and Artificial Neuro-Fuzzy Inference System (ANFIS) [6]. The electrodes to read the EMG signal are divided into two depending on where the electrodes are placed. The first place of the electrodes is in the skin of the human. This mode is called the invasive mode [18]. The electrodes could be located in the human skin, known as the non-invasive method. The successful percentage rates of those algorithms and techniques vary between 70 and 90%. We establish this study to accomplish the higher percentage.

This system is comprised of non-invasive sensors. The SVM algorithm, also combines with PCA methods, will be used to identify five hand gestures based on the signal of EMG. Sixteen features in the time domain are used for the feature extraction process. PCA is used as a feature reduction in these 16 features.

# 2 Methodology

## 2.1 Features Extraction

The raw EMG signal is generated from several electrodes located on a muscle that contains a vast amount of data but only has little information. If the EMG raw data is used as input in the identification process, the identification accuracy will be low, and the calculation time will increase. So that in pattern recognition, EMG raw data requires the transformation of representative features. In this research, only the time-domain feature is used. Time-domain (TD) features are the most popular which utilized in the classification of the signal process. The advantage over other features is that TD is fast to calculate because TD does not require a mathematical transformation [15, 19]. EMG time-domain features used are as follows:

Integrated EMG (IEMG) corresponds to the sequence of the EMG signal firing points. This feature is defined as the sum of the absolute value of the signal's amplitude [20].

$$\mathrm{IEMG} = \sum_{i=1}^{N} |x_i| \tag{1}$$

Mean absolute value (MAV) is used as an onset index, particularly in the signal surface EMG for prosthetic control.

$$\mathrm{MAV} = \frac{1}{N}\sum_{i=1}^{N} |x_i| \tag{2}$$

Root mean square (RMS) is modeled as the amplitude of the Gaussian random modulation process, which corresponds to constant force and non-fatiguing contraction [20]. The RMS is very similar to the calculation of Standard Deviation [21].

$$\mathrm{RMS} = \sqrt{\frac{1}{N}\sum_{i=1}^{N} x_i^2} \tag{3}$$

Difference Absolute Standard Deviation Value (DASDV) is the standard deviation value of the wavelength [20].

$$\mathrm{DASDV} = \sqrt{\frac{1}{\mathrm{N}-1}\sum_{\mathrm{i}=1}^{\mathrm{N}\text{-}1}(\mathrm{x}_{\mathrm{i}+1} + \mathrm{x}_{\mathrm{i}})^2} \tag{4}$$

The simple square integral (SSI) can be defined as the sum of the squared value of the signal amplitude or can be defined as an energy index [20].

$$\mathrm{SSI} = \sum_{\mathrm{i}=1}^{\mathrm{N}} \mathrm{x}_{\mathrm{i}}^2 \tag{5}$$

Variance of EMG (VAR) is the average of the cubes of the deviation variable. The mean value of the EMG signal is near zero [20].

$$\mathrm{VAR} = \frac{1}{\mathrm{N}-1}\sum_{\mathrm{i}=1}^{\mathrm{N}} \mathrm{x}_{\mathrm{i}}^2 \tag{6}$$

Modified mean absolute value type 1 (MAV1) can be defined as the extension or extension of the MAV feature. The weighted window function wi is put into the Equation to increase the robustness of the MAV feature [20].

$$\mathrm{MAV1} = \frac{1}{\mathrm{N}}\sum_{\mathrm{i}=1}^{\mathrm{N}} \mathrm{w}_{\mathrm{i}}|\mathrm{x}_{\mathrm{i}}|$$

$$w_i = \begin{cases} 1, & if\, 0.25N \le i \le 0.75N \\ 0.5, & else\, if \end{cases} \tag{7}$$

Modified mean absolute value type 2 (MAV2) is an extension of the MAV feature. However, the weighted window function $w_i$ is included in the Equation as a continuous function. This feature enables to raise the smoothness of the weighted window function [20].

$$\mathrm{MAV2} = \frac{1}{\mathrm{N}}\sum_{\mathrm{i}=1}^{\mathrm{N}} \mathrm{w}_{\mathrm{i}}|\mathrm{x}_{\mathrm{i}}|$$

$$\mathrm{w}_{\mathrm{i}} = \begin{cases} 1, & \text{if } 0.25\mathrm{N} \le \mathrm{i} \le 0.75\mathrm{N} \\ 4\mathrm{i}/\mathrm{N}, & \text{else if } \mathrm{i} \le 0.25\mathrm{N} \\ \frac{4(\mathrm{i}-\mathrm{N})}{\mathrm{N}}, & \text{otherwise} \end{cases} \tag{8}$$

Waveform length (WL) is defined as the cumulative length of the signal waveform over a time segment [20].

$$WL = \sum_{i=1}^{N-1} |x_{i+1} - x_i| \tag{9}$$

Activity parameters represent signal power, the variation of the time function so that it can indicate the surface of the power spectrum in the frequency domain [22, 23].

$$Hjorth\_1 = \sigma_x^2 = \frac{1}{N}\sum_{i=1}^{N}(x_i - 1)^2 \tag{10}$$

Mobility parameters represent the mean frequency or proportion of standard deviations in the power spectrum [22, 23].

$$Hjorth\_2 = \frac{\sigma_{x'}}{\sigma_x} \tag{11}$$

The complexity parameter represents the change in frequency. This parameter compares the signal similarity to a pure sine wave, where the value is centered on the number 1 if the many signals are similar [22, 23].

$$Hjorth\_3 = \frac{\sigma_{x''}/\sigma_{x'}}{\sigma_{x''}/\sigma_x} \tag{12}$$

An autoregressive coefficient is a general approach to univariate time series modeling in Equation [15, 22].

$$y_t = a_1 y_{t-1} + a_2 y_{t-2} + \cdots + a_n y_{t-n} + \varepsilon_t = \sum_{i=1}^{N} a_1 y_{t-1} + \varepsilon_t \tag{13}$$

## 2.2 *Feature Reduction Using PCA*

PCA, in general, is a technique that uses the basics of sophisticated mathematical principles to convert a number of variables that may be correlated into a small number of significant uncorrelated variables, which are called main components [24, 25]. The PCA technique lies in multivariate data analysis. However, this method has a lot of applications; one of them is to recognize the patterns.

The procedure for performing PCA is as follows:

1. Calculating the Covariance Matrix

   Vector input $x_t(t = 1, \ldots, 1$ and $x_t = 0)$ with dimensions m $x_t = [x_t(1), x_t(2), \ldots, x_t(m)]^T$ usually $m < 1$, each vector $x_t$ is transformed linearly into a new vector $s$ which is expressed as in (14)

$$S_t = U^T \cdot x_t \tag{14}$$

   where $U$ is the $m \times m$ orthogonal matrix with the column to $i$, $u_i$ is the eigenvector value of the sample covariance matrix C. The C matrix can be calculated using (15)

$$C = \frac{1}{1}\sum_{t=1}^{1} x_t \cdot x_t^T \tag{15}$$

2. Calculating the Eigenvalue and Eigenvector of the Covariance Matrix

$$\lambda_t U_t = C \cdot u_i, i = 1, \ldots, m \tag{16}$$

   where i is one of the eigenvalues of $C$, $u_i$ is the eigenvector.

3. Calculating the value of orthogonal transformation

   Based on the estimated value $u_i$ and the component $s_t$, which is then calculated as an orthogonal transformation of $x_t$

$$S_t(i) = u_t^T x_t, \quad i = 1, \ldots, m \tag{17}$$

   The new component is called a principal component. By using only the first few eigenvector values that have been sorted according to their eigenvalues, the number of principal components of $s_t$ can be reduced.

### 2.3 *Feature Classification Using SVM*

SVM is a classification method that requires model training to test samples [26]. SVM provides training as a supervised learning technique. In this case, the first trained model learns according to the class that needs to be classified and reduced by PCA [12]. This classification is simple because it builds a hyperplane. This hyperplane is to differentiate the classes. The classification could be linear or non-linear. For the linear, the samples of the training class can be separated linearly. But for some cases, the sample cannot be classified linearly. For such cases, non-linear classification is exploited [26].

Kernel functions are used to construct linear through non-linear transformations or mappings to find the best class for the output field [26]. This algorithm applies that input vector non-linearly mapped to a high-dimensional feature space. Input data is xi $(i = 1, 2, \ldots, M)$M the number of samples. If we have two classes, namely the positive class and the negative class, they are defined by $y1 = 1$ for the positive one and $y1 = -1$ for another class. The hyperplane plane function of $f(x) = 0$ separating the given data as in (18) for linear data.

$$f(x) = w^T x + b = \sum_{i=1}^{M} w_i x_i + b = 0 \tag{18}$$

Dimensional $-M$ vector $w$ and scalar $b$ are used to determine the position of the separating hyperplane. Identifying both classes can be done by the decision function or the sign f(x). The formula (19) is the formula for the constraint for separating the hyperplane.

$$y_i f(x_i) = y_i\left(w^T x_i + b\right) \geq 1 \text{ for } i = 1, 2, \ldots, M \tag{19}$$

The optimal hyperplane separation can be defined as the maximum distance between the plane and the closest data. Figure 1 shows the sample of the optimal hyper-plane.

In Fig. 1, there are two classes, namely a positive class and a negative class. One of the objectives of the SVM algorithm is to create a linear boundary to separate both classes and orient it so that dashed dashes are maximized. In addition, SVM aims to direct the optimal hyper-plane in every class. The boundary is in the middle of the margin between two points. The support vector is the closest data point used

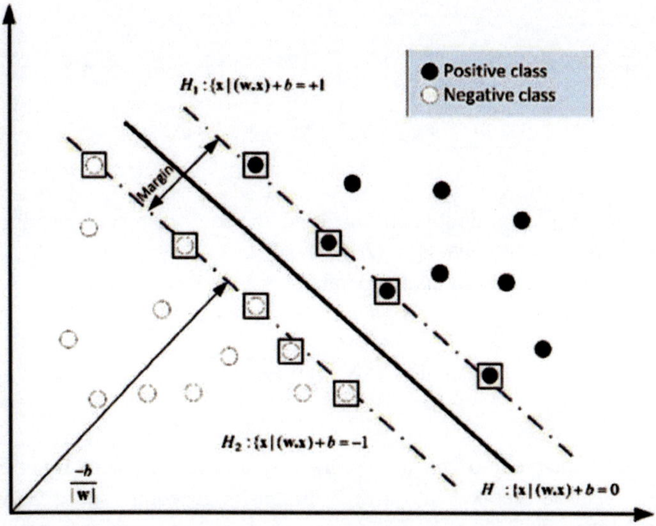


**Fig. 1** Classification of two classes that can be separated linearly using SVM

to determine the margin. The support vector is represented by the black circle in a square and the white circle in a square. The normal vector to the hyperplane is w and the perpendicular distance from the hyperplane to the origin is $\frac{-b}{|w|}$.

Noise with the slack variable $\xi_i$ and error penalty $C$, the optimal hyperplane that separates the data can be calculated using Eqs. (20) and (21)

$$\text{Minimize} \quad \frac{1}{2}||w||^2 + C\sum_{i=1}^{M}\xi_i \tag{20}$$

$$\text{Subject to} \quad \begin{cases} y_i\left(w^T x_i + b\right) \geq 1 - \xi_i, & i = 1, \ldots, M \\ \xi_i \geq 0, & i = 1, \ldots, M \end{cases} \tag{21}$$

$$\text{Min} \quad L(w, b, \alpha) = \frac{1}{2}||w||^2 - \sum_{i=1}^{M}\alpha_i y_i (w \cdot x_i + b) + \sum_{i=1}^{M}\alpha_i \tag{22}$$

Its task is to minimize Eqs. (20) and (21) concerning w and b. The saddle point at the optimal point can be found using Eqs. (23) and (24)

$$\text{Maximize} \quad L(\alpha) = \sum_{i=1}^{M}\alpha_i - \frac{1}{2}\sum_{i=1}^{M}\alpha_i\alpha_j y_i x_i x_j \tag{23}$$

$$\alpha_i = 0, i = 1, \ldots, M$$

$$\text{Subject to} \sum_{i=1}^{M}\alpha_i y_i \tag{24}$$

To solve the problem of double optimization, the coefficient $\alpha i$ is obtained, which is needed to express $w$ to solve Eqs. (20) and (21).

Equation (25) is the non-linear decision

$$f(x) = \text{sign}\left(\sum_{i,j=1}^{M}\alpha_i y_i \left(x_i\ x_j\right) + b\right) \tag{25}$$

SVM is also enabled to use in non-linear classification with function kernel applications. Data is mapped into a high-dimensional feature space using a non-linear vector function of $\Phi(x) = (\phi_1(x), \ldots, \phi_i(x))$. The decision function can be calculated using Eq. (26)

$$f(x) = \mathrm{sign} \sum_{i,j=1}^{M} \alpha_i \cdot y_i \left(\Phi^T(x_i) \cdot \Phi(x_j)\right) + b \tag{26}$$

The problem that can be arisen with high dimensions will cause overfitting and computational. This problem will occur due to a large vector. These issues can be resolved with the kernel function $K(x_i, x_j) = \left(\Phi^T(x_i).\Phi_j(x_j)\right)$. Decision function such as Eq. (27)

$$f(x) = \mathrm{sign}\left( \sum_{i,j=1}^{M} \alpha_i y_i K\left(x_i\ x_j\right) + b \right) \tag{27}$$

## 2.4 Experimental Setup

The EMG data were generated from all the gestures, as shown in Fig. 4. The subjects are people with non-neurological or muscular disorders. The subject conducting the test is seated in an armchair with the arm supported on the armchair, and carefully leveled. This is to prevent the variation generated by arm position. The EMG signal is obtained using a Myo motion control ring with a 200 Hz sampling rate. The sensor is installed close to the superficial flexor digitorium. Figure 2 shows the Myo device that is attached to the lower arm of the subject. This device consists of eight EMG sensors. This article examines the outputs of the signal from EMG3, EMG4, and

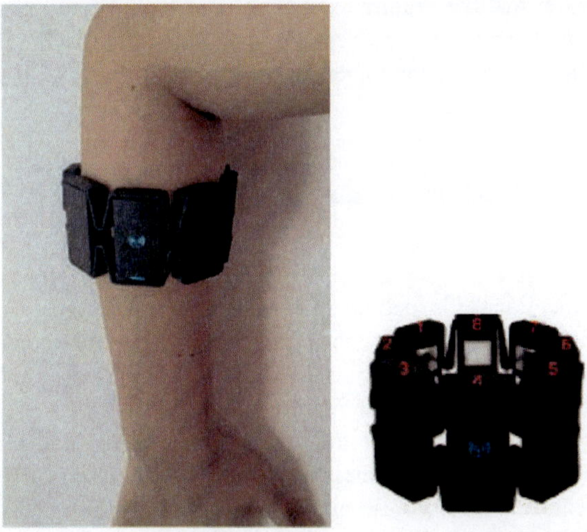

**Fig. 2** **a** Myo Armband position on the arm; **b** assignment of the Myo sensor position

(a) (b)

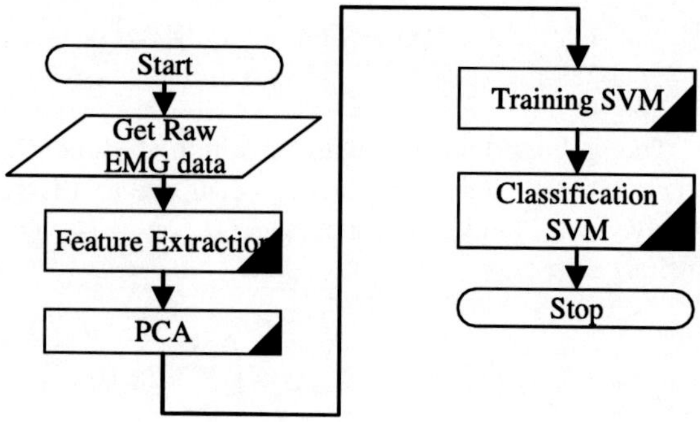


**Fig. 3** Flowchart of the system

EMG8 sensors. Subjects doing the test were instructed to obtain the contraction data (flexor) of the finger movement pattern and hold that position for five seconds, followed by relaxation (extensor) for approximately five seconds. These processes were repeated ten times. From this experiment was obtain ten flexor and ten extensor data were for each movement.

# 3 Result and Discussion

## 3.1 Design System

The process of the flowchart of the system is illustrated in Fig. 3. The first process is reading the raw EMG signal. Next, the raw signal is processed in feature extraction. After that the feature extraction process, the data is reduced using PCA. Then the data from PCA is trained and finally classified by the SVM method. Figure 4 shows the gestures of the fingers and a sample of the raw signal for each finger.

## 3.2 Features Reduction Using PCA

PCA is a technique that is often referred to as dimensionality reduction or feature reduction. This method enables to generation number of new features that minimizes from the previous number. This technique aims to obtain new features that provide more dense classification information than the original features.

In the research, the final result of PCA is in the form of matrix data that has the same order. The order number of PCA is the row-column of the data to be reduced by PCA. This can be seen in Table 1, the example of the PCA process in the extraction feature data from the first data retrieval on the EMG 3 sensor from all movement patterns.

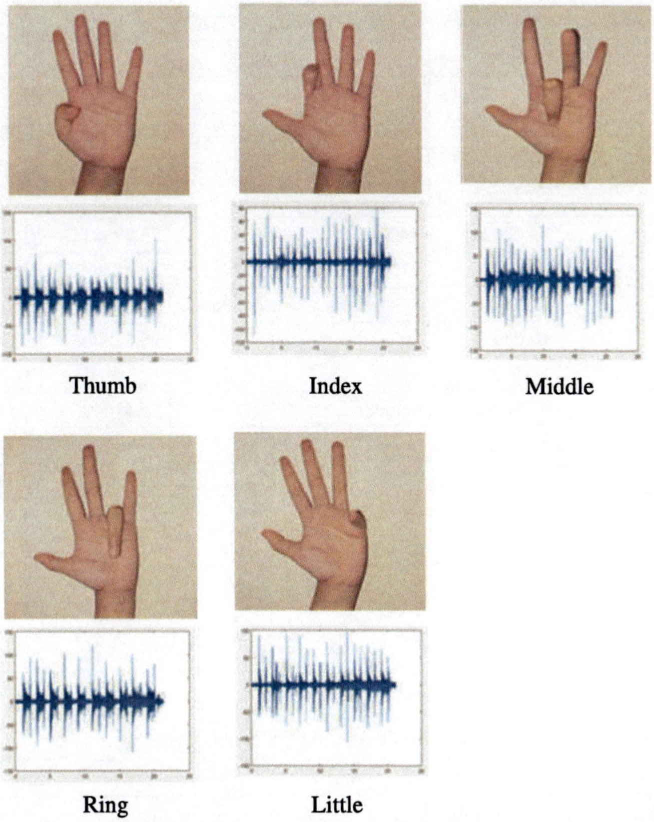


**Fig. 4** Finger movements when EMG signal data is obtained

Table 2 exhibits the number of orders from the data matrix before processing on the PCA reduction feature is 5 × 17. After the PCA reduction feature processes the data, the number of orders from the data matrix after PCA becomes 5 × 5 in Table 2. The data from the 13 extraction features turn into data for new variables called Principal Component (PC). The new variables are the combination of the original linear variables. The new variable p shows the maximum variance that has not been calculated on the previous variable $p - 1$. For example, the PC1 or the first new variable corresponds to the maximum variance of the data. PC2 or the second new variable shows the maximum variance that has not been calculated on the first variable.

**Table 1** Features extraction of the first capture from signal EMG 3

| | Thumb | Index | Middle | Ring | Little |
|---|---|---|---|---|---|
| RMS | 15.55912 | 9.280703 | 24.17389 | 21.49282 | 10.03496 |
| VAR | 242.3293 | 86.21241 | 584.8235 | 462.3799 | 100.7984 |
| MAV2 | 5.063523 | 1.579404 | 8.636478 | 6.496462 | 1.963773 |
| MAV2 | 10.68606 | 5.3277 | 15.65038 | 14.5351 | 5.531128 |
| DASDV | 24.82424 | 14.58035 | 38.68314 | 35.72881 | 15.22451 |
| SSI | 241,360 | 91,730 | 765,534 | 486,886 | 103,520 |
| MAV1 | 7.523069 | 3.306103 | 10.84198 | 10.18311 | 3.429475 |
| IE | 10,654 | 5674 | 20,502 | 15,320 | 5686 |
| AR | 1 | 1 | 1 | 1 | 1 |
| AR | 0.389562 | 0.269283 | 0.297154 | 0.541049 | 0.318027 |
| AR | 0.232912 | 0.099587 | 0.079483 | 0.318665 | 0.325677 |
| AR | 0.243009 | 0.106825 | 0.022233 | 0.290908 | 0.329941 |
| AR | 0.224073 | 0.055334 | 0.136696 | 0.256522 | 0.260899 |
| Hjorth1 | 241.7985 | 85.9396 | 584.7086 | 462.1344 | 100.5384 |
| Hjorth2 | 1.597229 | 1.57353 | 1.600361 | 1.662798 | 1.519109 |
| Hjorth3 | 1.117717 | 1.135298 | 1.122543 | 1.08759 | 1.134777 |
| Waveform length | 3 | 2 | 10 | 2 | 2 |

**Table 2** Result PCA of data capture from signal EMG 3 first experiment

| PC# | Thumb | Index | Middle | Ring | Little |
|---|---|---|---|---|---|
| PC1 | 0.25422 | 0.599045 | 0.037573 | 0.749074 | −0.1183 |
| PC2 | 0.096561 | 0.50934 | −0.37983 | −0.31043 | 0.700435 |
| PC3 | 0.806815 | −0.39924 | −0.43013 | 0.06289 | −0.02628 |
| PC4 | 0.513048 | 0.139464 | 0.781022 | −0.30658 | 0.115517 |
| PC5 | 0.108996 | 0.450413 | −0.24354 | −0.49455 | −0.6938 |

## 3.3 Feature Classification

The SVM algorithm is one of the most powerful classification techniques based on statistical theory. In research, testing on the SVM classification feature was carried out by five subjects, with ratio7:3 for training and testing.

Figure 5 is the training process carried out on the EMG 3 signal. In the training process, the weight or area of each movement pattern is obtained. The blue color is for the thumb pattern area, the red color is the index pattern area, then green is the middle pattern area, while the black color is for the ring pattern area, and the turquoise color is the little finger area.

Figure 6 is the training process carried out on the EMG 4 signal. In the training process, the weight or area of each movement pattern is obtained. The blue color

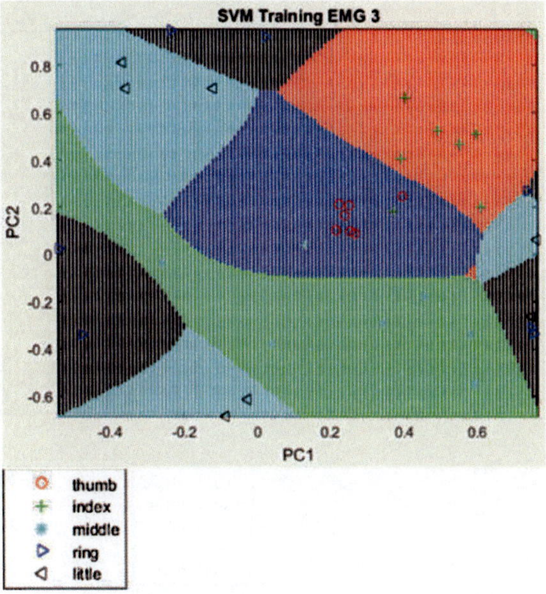


**Fig. 5** Training process SVM EMG 3

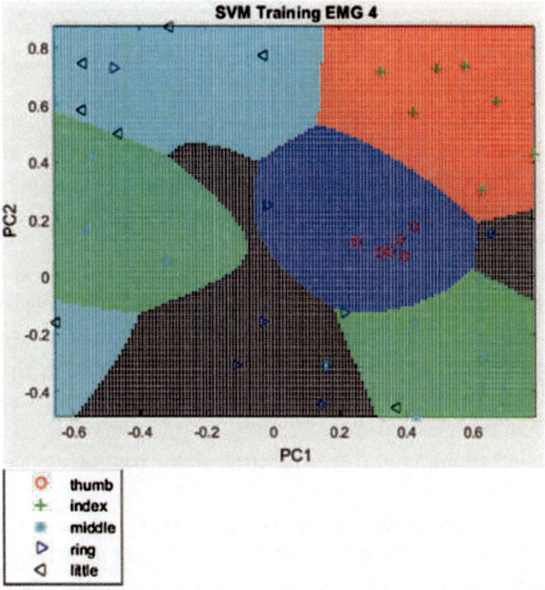


**Fig. 6** Training process SVM EMG 4

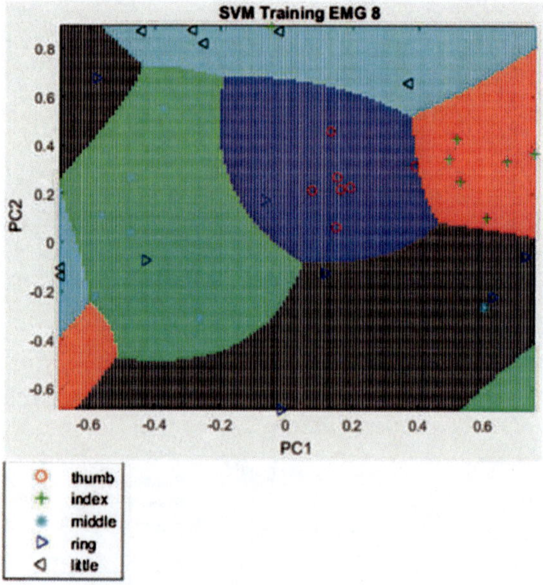


**Fig. 7** Training process SVM EMG 8

is for the thumb pattern area, the red color is the index pattern area, then green is the middle pattern area, while the black color is for the ring pattern area, and the turquoise color is the little finger area.

Figure 7 is the training process carried out on the EMG 8 signal. In the training process, the weight or area of each movement pattern is obtained. The blue color is for the thumb pattern area, the red color is the index pattern area, then green is the middle pattern area, while the black color is for the ring pattern area, and the turquoise color is the little finger area.

Figure 8 is the testing process carried out on the EMG 3 signal. In the testing process, the testing data will be classified in their respective classes according to the classes in the training stage. In the testing process carried out on the EMG 3 signal, the percentage of success can be seen in Table 3, for the blue box is a successful experiment. At the same time, the red one is a failed experiment and the yellow one is an error experiment. From the results obtained, there were 9 successful trials, 5 failed attempts, and an error trial, so the percentage of success for the EMG 3 signal is 60%.

Figure 9 is the testing process carried out on the EMG 4 signal. In the testing process, the testing data will be classified in their respective classes according to the classes at the training stage. In the testing process carried out on the EMG 4 signal, the percentage of success can be seen in Table 4, for the blue box is a successful experiment. At the same time, the red one is a failed experiment, and the yellow one is an error experiment. From the results obtained, the number of successful trials was 11, the failed three trials, and the error one trial, so the percentage of success for the EMG signal 4 was 73%.

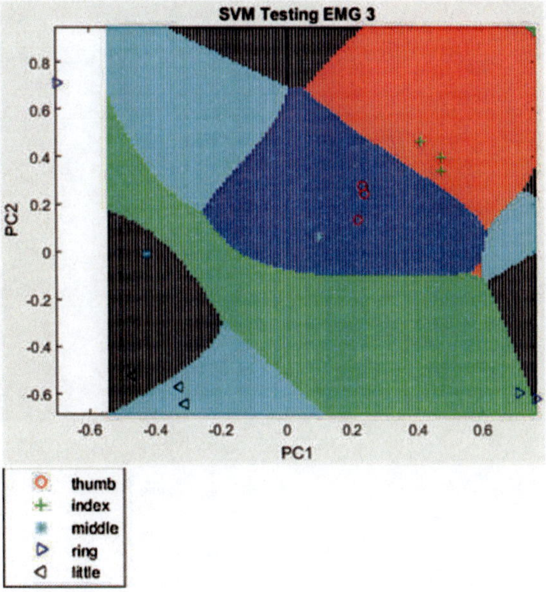


**Fig. 8** Testing process SVM EMG 3

**Table 3** Comparison between results and actual data at EMG 3

| Movement pattern (actual data) | Experiment and result | | |
|---|---|---|---|
| | 1 | 2 | 3 |
| Thumb | Thumb | Thumb | Thumb |
| Index | Index | Index | Index |
| Middle | Thumb | Ring | Little |
| Ring | Ring | Middle | – |
| Little | Little | Little | Ring |

Figure 10 is the testing process carried out on the EMG 8 signal. In the testing process, the testing data will be classified in their respective classes according to the classes at the training stage. In the testing process carried out on the EMG 8 signal, the percentage of success can be seen in Table 5, for the blue box is a successful experiment and the red one is a failed experiment. From the results obtained, the number of successful attempts was 8, and the number of failed attempts was 7, so the percentage of success for the EMG 8 signal was 53%.

According to Tables 3, 4 and 5, the successful participation of each sensor is obtained, which is shown in Table 6. From Table 6, the results of the sensor that has the highest level of accuracy are received, is sensor EMG 6 with a success rate of 70%. However, these results still do not reach a higher percentage compared with other methods.

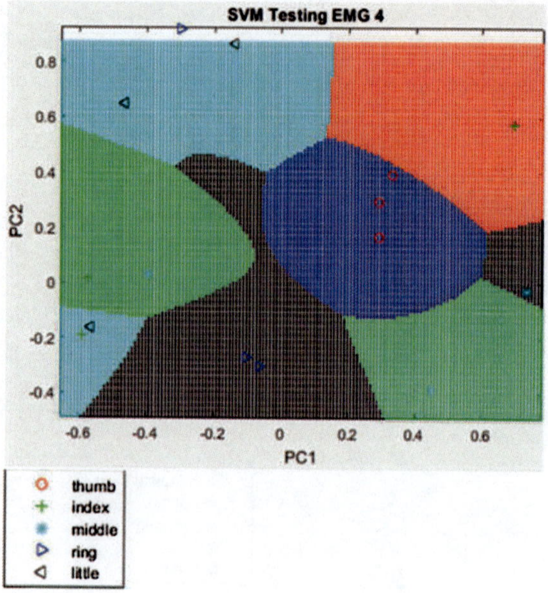


**Fig. 9** Testing process SVM EMG 4

**Table 4** Comparison between results and actual data at EMG 4

| Movement pattern (actual data) | Experiment and result | | |
|---|---|---|---|
| | 1 | 2 | 3 |
| Thumb | Thumb | Thumb | Thumb |
| Index | Index | Middle | Little |
| Middle | Middle | Ring | Middle |
| Ring | Ring | Ring | – |
| Little | Little | Little | Little |

## 4 Conclusion

This proposed system is able to classify finger movement patterns with an accuracy rate of 60% for EMG 3, 73% for EMG 4, and 53% for EMG 8. In this study, the middle and little finger patterns were the most difficult to classify. This can be seen during the data retrieval process. When we close our middle finger to retrieve data, the other finger will almost close, as well as the little finger pattern. The results of this study will be used for possible hardware implementation in the future.

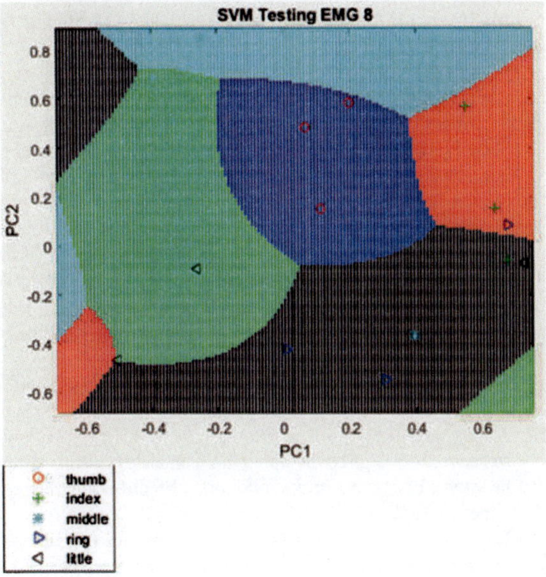


**Fig. 10** Testing process SVM EMG 8

**Table 5** Comparison between results and actual data at EMG 8

| Movement pattern (actual data) | Experiment and result | | |
|---|---|---|---|
| | 1 | 2 | 3 |
| Thumb | Thumb | Thumb | Thumb |
| Index | Index | Index | Manis |
| Middle | Ring | Middle | Little |
| Ring | Ring | Ring | Index |
| Little | Middle | Middle | Ring |

**Table 6** Success rate of prediction result on EMG sensor

| Sensor# | Accuracy (%) |
|---|---|
| EMG3 | 60 |
| EMG4 | 73 |
| EMG8 | 53 |

## References

1. Caiza G, Garcia C, Naranjo JE, Garcia M (2020) Flexible robotic teleoperation architecture for intelligent oil fields. Heliyon 6
2. Mariappan M, Ramu V, Khoo B, Ganesan T, Nadarajan M (2014) Medical tele-diagnosis robot (MTR)—internet based communication & navigation system. Appl Mech Mater 490–491:1177–1189

3. Yu S, Perez H, Barkas J, Mohamed M, Eldaly M, Huang T, Yang X, Su H, Cortes M, Edwards DJ (2019) A soft high force hand exoskeleton for rehabilitation and assistance of spinal cord injury and stroke individuals. ArXiv, abs/1902.07112
4. Simo A, Nishida Y, Nagashima K (2006) A humanoid robot to prevent children accidents
5. Triwiyanto T, Sari L, Sumber S, Andjar P, Abd K, Bedjo U, Triana R, Dyah T (2021) A review: sensory system data processing, actuator type on a hand exoskeleton design. J Biomimetics Biomater Biomed Eng (50):39–49
6. Anwar T, Jumaily AA (2016) Estimation of angle based on EMG using. ANFIS In: conference 2016, IEEE symposium series on computational intelligence (SSCI), Sydney, Australia, p 1
7. Hasan HN (2016) A wearable rehabilitation system to assist partially hand paralyzed patients in repetitive exercises. In: Frist international scientific conference Al-Ayen University, Iraq
8. Õunpuu S, DeLuca PA, Bell KJ, Davis RB (1997) Using surface electrodes for the evaluation of the rectus femoris, vastus medialis and vastus lateralis muscles in children with cerebral palsy. Gait Posture 5:211–216
9. Esa NM, Zain AM, Bahari M (2018) Electromyography (EMG) based classification of finger movements using SVM. Int J Innov Comput 8(3)
10. Angelova S, Ribagin S, Raikova R, Veneva I (2018) Power frequency spectrum analysis of surface EMG signals of upper limb muscles during elbow flexion—a comparison between healthy subjects and stroke survivors. J Electromyogr Kinesiol Official J Int Soc Electrophysiol Kinesiol 38:7–16
11. Hayder AY et al (2019) Assessment of muscles fatigue based on surface (EMG) signals using machine learning and statistical approaches: a review. IOP Conf Ser Mater Sci Eng
12. Pancholi S, Joshi A (2020) Improved classification scheme using fused wavelet packet transform based features for intelligent myoelectric prostheses. IEEE Trans Industr Electron 67:8517–8525
13. Guo X, Yang P, Li Y, Yan WL (2006) The SEMG analysis for the lower limb prosthesis using wavelet transformation. In: Conference proceedings: annual international conference of the IEEE engineering in medicine and biology society. IEEE engineering in medicine and biology society. Annual conference, pp 341–344
14. Zhang D, Xiong A, Zhao X, Han J (2012) PCA and LDA for EMG-based control of bionic mechanical hand. In: 2012 IEEE international conference on information and automation, pp 960–965
15. Phinyomark A, Phukpattaranont P, Limsakal C (2011) A review of control methods for electric power wheelchair based on electromyography signals with special emphasis on pattern recognition. IETE Tech Rev 28(4):316–326
16. Simatupang I, Pamungkas D, Risandriya S (2021) Naïve Bayes classifier for hand gestures recognition. In: Proceedings of the 3rd international conference on applied engineering—ICAE, pp 110–114
17. Kaya E, Kumbasar T (2018) Hand gesture recognition systems with the wearable Myo Armband. In: 2018 6th international conference on control engineering & information technology (CEIT), pp 1–6
18. Gogić A,N Miljkovic N, Đurđević Đ (2016) Electromyography-based gesture recognition: fuzzy classification evaluation
19. Kurniawan S, Pamungkas D (2018) MYO Armband sensors and neural network algorithm for controlling hand robot. In: International conference on applied engineering (ICAE), pp 1–6
20. Phinyomark A, Phukpattaranont P, Limsakal C (2012) Feature reduction and selection for EMG signal classification. Expert Syst App 39(3):7420–7431
21. Toledo-Perez DC, Rodriguez-Resendiz J, Gomez-Loenzo RA, Jauregui-Correa JC (2019) Support vector machine-based EMG signal classification techniques a review
22. Arijanto M, Caesarendra W, Mustaqim KA, Irfan M, Pakpahan JA, Setiawan JD (2015) Finger movement pattern recognition method using artificial neural network based on electromyography (EMG) sensor. In: Proceedings of international conference on automation, cognitive science, optics, micro electro-mechanical system, and information technology, 29–30 Oct

23. Khushaba RN, Kodagoda S, Takruri M, Dissanayake G (2012) Toward improved control of prosthetic finger using surface electromyogram (EMG) signals. Expert Syst Appl 39:10731–10738
24. Theodoridis S, Koutrombus K (2009) Pattern recognition, 4th ed. Academic Press, US
25. Meena P, Bansal M, Classification of EMG signal using SVM–kNN. Int J Adv Res Electron Commun Eng (IJARECE) 6
26. Caesarendra W, Irfan M (2018) Classification method of hand gesture based on support vector machine. Comput Eng Appl 7(3):179–190

# A Review for Designing a Low-Cost Online Lower Limb Monitoring System of a Post-stroke Rehabilitation

**Andi Nur Halisyah, Reza Humaidi, Moch. Rafly, Cut Silvia, and Dimas Adiputra**

**Abstract** The physical therapy generally requires direct assistance from therapists continuously, however, the time is very limited. Moreover, the social distancing policy in the COVID-19 pandemic period made the patient could not come to rehabilitation center for physical therapy. Remote physical therapy is suggested to reduce dependency of therapist for conducting the physical therapy. However, there is few information about the necessary parameters in lower limb monitoring of post-stroke patient. Therefore, in this paper, a review for designing a low-cost online home-care physical therapy monitoring system is proposed. Article finding had been done using online search engine Google Scholars to conclude the design of the online monitoring system. Several keywords had been used, such as "online stroke rehabilitation monitoring," "stroke rehabilitation parameters," "stroke monitoring Internet of Things," and "lower limb stroke monitoring." The results show that the necessary monitor parameters are lower limb kinematics and dynamics, which can be complimented by bio-signal data, such as EMG. The lower limb monitoring system can use IMU, muscle sensor, and footswitches to measure the necessary parameters. IMU measures the lower limb kinematics because it provides wide range of measurement. Muscle sensor, which compatible to microcontroller, measures the EMG. Lastly, the footswitches detect the gait phases, which classify the measured data for more in-depth analysis. The mentioned sensors are cheap and available in the online market of Indonesia, which is suitable to realize a low-cost lower limb monitoring system. The research finding also suggests quick and accurate feedback mechanism for improving the training quality, which the feedback is combination of therapist opinion and artificial intelligence prediction.

**Keywords** Internet of things · Post-stroke patients · Online monitoring · Post-stroke rehabilitation · Low-cost

A. N. Halisyah · R. Humaidi · Moch. Rafly · C. Silvia · D. Adiputra (✉)
Institut Teknologi Telkom Surabaya, Jalan Ketintang Selatan No. 156, Surabaya, Indonesia
e-mail: adimas@ittelkom-sby.ac.id

 
T. Triwiyanto et al. (eds.), *Proceedings of the 2nd International Conference on Electronics, Biomedical Engineering, and Health Informatics*, Lecture Notes in Electrical Engineering 898, https://doi.org/10.1007/978-981-19-1804-9_36

# 1 Introduction

Stroke is still one of the main causes of disability worldwide [1]. In Indonesia, the number of stroke patients has increased every year. Because of this the stroke has been nominated as the number one cause of death for more than decades. The stroke also leads to disabilities [2]. For instance, patients who survive the acute phase of stroke completely lose their ability to walk or having a gait impairment [3]. Others have moderate to severe walking disabilities. This condition results in a foot drop. Foot Drop is a symptom of neuromuscular disorders, which can be temporary or permanent, and experience decreased walking speed, shortened stride length, increased metabolism when walking, and a high risk of falling and the muscle anterior tibialis weak, so the patient cannot perform movements dorsiflexion to lift the forefoot off the runway.

One way to overcome the condition of foot drop is rehabilitation with ankle foot orthosis therapy. After a stroke, the command signal pathways from the brain become disrupted. New command-sending ways are needed for signals from the brain to reach parts of the body such as the ankles. The more often the patient trains with the correct gait, the faster the body can find the new pathway. Thus, the key to successful rehabilitation is the duration and intensity of physical therapy exercise [4]. Physical therapy generally requires continuous, direct assistance from therapists. However, continuity (duration and intensity) exercise therapy has limited time therapists coupled to the pandemic Covid-19 required for social distancing.

Talking about the rehabilitation of patients with post-stroke, we certainly envisage the exercise is handled directly by the therapist to restore speech and motion. But for patients living in remote areas, hundreds of kilometres from the specialists they need, such therapy is hard to come by. Also, with the widespread outbreak of COVID-19, the government is implementing social distancing, where social distancing is an act of self-isolation to prevent and control the spread of COVID-19. The goal is to reduce the possibility of contact between infected and uninfected people to minimize the transmission of COVID-19 and even prevent death. So many things have to be done from home, be it school, college, work or other activities. Not also spared for post-stroke patients who have to do physical therapy directly with the therapist. Physical therapy generally requires continuous, direct assistance from therapists. However, the continuation of therapeutic exercise has limited time. Some patients also stated that they needed to do independent activities at home and practice time [5]. Coupled with the current COVID-19 pandemic, which requires social distancing, independent training is the main option before face-to-face training. Thus, to reduce dependence on physical therapist activities, an alternative form of remote rehabilitation is needed.

Aside from supporting the patient, the therapist also monitors the patient's progress, usually in terms of limb functional. Based on the progress, the therapist can decide whether the patient needs further training or new orthosis prescription [6]. Figure 1 shows the positioning of progress monitoring in the post-stroke rehabilitation. Previous literature reviews regarding post-stroke rehabilitation monitoring have been done by several researchers. The physiological monitoring is important

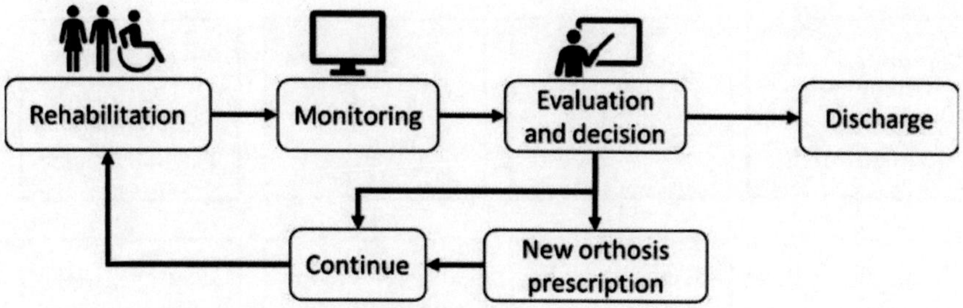


**Fig. 1** General process of a post-stroke rehabilitation

in post-stroke rehabilitation [7]. However, previous researches had show that the monitoring is not solely limited to that, but also covers other aspects, such as stroke registries status [8, 9] and stroke risk factor monitoring [10]. Technology used in this field comprise of wearable technologies [11–13] and mobile application [14], which is integrated in Internet of Things (IoT) environment to enable remote rehabilitation [15]. The data types, devices types, key features, challenges of IoT platform for stroke rehabilitation monitoring has been reported in previous researchers [15–17]. Despite that, there were less literature review that had been focusing on online lower limb monitoring system for post-stroke patient, especially the necessary monitoring parameter. Therefore, this paper aims to reviews the previous studies on lower limb monitoring system both online and offline types to conclude the necessary parameters of an online lower limb monitoring system.

## 2 Materials and Methods

The research aims to do literature review for designing a low-cost online lower limb monitoring system of a post-stroke rehabilitation. Here, the literature review must provide the information of the necessary monitoring parameters in a physiological therapy. Then, the prototype can be designed based on the results of the literature review.

The literature review is carried out by collecting various references in the journal articles, scientific papers, and other sources that can be used to analyze making tools using online search engine, Google Scholars. The search used several keywords, such as "online stroke rehabilitation monitoring," "stroke rehabilitation parameters," "stroke monitoring Internet of Things," and "lower limb stroke monitoring." Each keywords resulted in more than 100.000 results, but only the results in the first three pages are considered. Therefore, there were 30 sources for each keyword. The initial search strategy is to review by title and abstract. The inclusion criteria for the considered articles reviewed were: (1) discussing post-stroke rehabilitation monitoring, (2) rehabilitation type discussed is physiological therapy on lower limb, (3) there is a qualitative or quantitative measurement of the rehabilitation. Meanwhile,

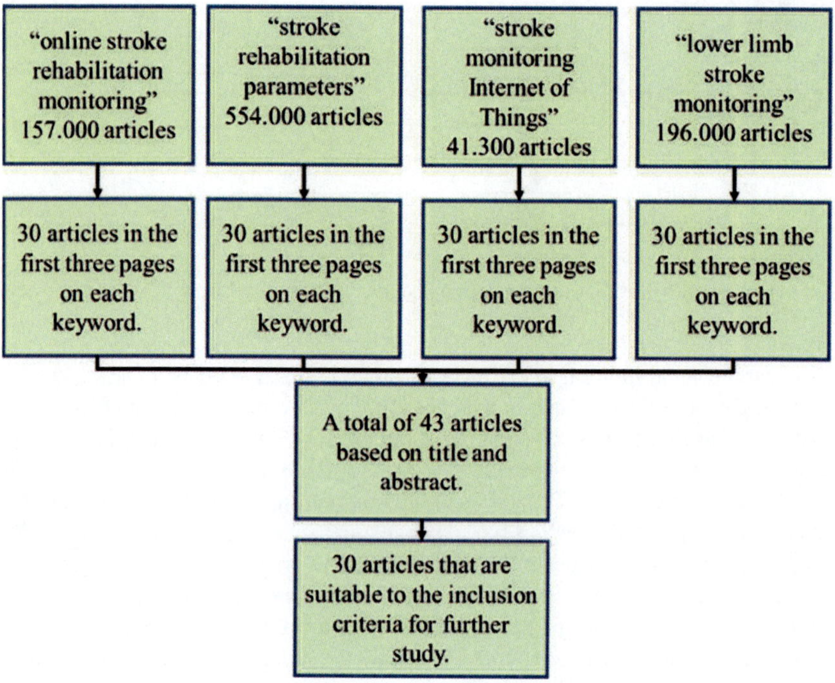


**Fig. 2** Selecting review articles flowchart

documents that do not contain inclusion criteria are not taken into account in this study. At the end, only 30 articles from a total of 120 articles are considered for further study. Figure 2 shows the flow of selecting the review articles.

From the 30 articles, the research extracts informations of monitoring methods, qualitative parameters, and quantitative parameters of the rehabilitation monitoring. After knowing the necessary parameters to assess the patient's condition, the search for tools and sensors to measure each of these parameters is carried out. Reliability, dimensions, and price are the main benchmarks in determining what sensor to use to develop the prototype as a portable, reliable, and affordable design for most people. In addition to sensors, a microcontroller is needed to receive, process, and display reading data from each sensor used. The chosen microcontroller is prioritized to have built-in wifi connectivity, sufficient connection ports for each sensor, good computing power. It has a size that is not too large so that the value of prototype portability does not decrease. Availability and prices of sensors and microcontrollers in the Indonesian market are checked through e-commerce. Then the sensor's reading data will be displayed on the IoT platform to be accessed remotely by doctors/therapists. Ease of use and access are the main considerations in choosing the IoT platform to be used. Finally, the proposed designed a low-cost online lower limb monitoring system of a post-stroke rehabilitation is presented.

## 3 Results

The research categorizes the result into two categories, which are monitoring methods and parameters of stroke rehabilitation, as shown in Table 1. *Common monitoring methods are manual measurement, instrumentation measurement, and online instrumentation measurement. The manual measurement means that rehabilitation data monitoring is conducted directly by the therapist using non-electronic device* [18, 19], *visual observation* [20, 21] *and interview with check list* [22, 23], *such as measuring the duration of walking and walking distance* [24]. *The data collection obtained by using sensors, such as wearable device* [12, 25] *or non-wearable device* [26] *belongs to instrumentation measurement group. The non-wearable device is motion capture system* [27, 28], *while the wearable devices mostly have Inertial Measurement Unit (IMU)* [5], *force sensor* [29] *and bio-signal sensor* [30]. *Lastly, the online instrumentation measurement is using instrumentation device in an Internet of Things platform, which then enable remote rehabilitation monitoring* [31].

**Table 1** List of stroke rehabilitation monitoring methods and parameters

| References | Methods | Quantitative parameter | Qualitative parameter |
|---|---|---|---|
| [18–24, 44] | Manual measurement | Lower limb kinematics and dynamics | Walking ability, support needed and pain |
| [40, 42, 43] | Wearable instrumentation measurement | Bio-signal (ECG/EEG/EMG) | – |
| [30, 39, 41] | | Lower limb kinematics and dynamics, bio-signal (ECG/EEG/EMG) | – |
| [12, 25, 35, 38, 46] | Wearable instrumentation measurement | Lower limb kinematics and dynamics | – |
| [27, 28, 45] | Non-wearable instrumentation measurement | Limb kinematics | – |
| [33, 37, 47] | Instrumentation measurement and manual measurement | Lower limb kinematics and dynamics | Walking ability, support needed and comfortability |
| [29, 31] | Online wearable instrumentation measurement | Lower limb kinematics and dynamics | – |
| [5] | | lower limb kinematics and bio-signal (ECG) | – |
| [36] | | Lower limb kinematics | Activity quality |

*The main concern in rehabilitation monitoring is to see patient's improvement rate over the time, which can be observed through quantitative and qualitative parameters. The limb kinematics and dynamics are often reported as the quantitative monitoring parameters, whether in short term* [32] *and long term* [19]. *The joint range of motion (ROM)* [33], *the stride and step length* ("Real-time Gait Monitoring System for Consumer Stroke Prediction Service," no date; Chang et al. 2021), *walking speed and distance* [34], *foot steps number* [35], *phase duration* [36], *foot torque* [37] *and foot pressure* [38] *are the example of limb kinematics and dynamics parameter. The bio-signals, such as EEG* [39], *EMG* [40], *ECG* [41], *and blood flow* [42] *are monitored whether to see the improvement or predict the upcoming stroke occurrence* [43]. *Previous study also reports walking ability and support needed as the qualitative parameter that are being measured using scoring system, such as Functional Independence Measured (FIM)* [33] *and Barthel Index* [44]. *Other reported qualitative parameter reported is comfortability of the patient with the robot intervention that they are using* [33].

*Each method have their own advantages and disadvantages. The manual measurement by* [18–24, 44] offers a complete monitoring of the limb functional including the pain, but takes time in the process as it cannot be done simultaneously with the training. Wearable instrumentation measurement enable simultaneous training and measurement of the limb functional, but it requires combination of lower limb kinematics-dynamics and bio-signal to obtain comprehensive data as shown by [30, 39, 41]. Therefore, lots of sensors should be attached on the patient. Non-wearable instrumentation method by [27, 28, 45] shows that monitoring without attaching any sensors to the patient, which is more comfortable. However, the method is restricted to be done in a one room with motion capture system. The monitoring is also limited to limb kinematics only. Lastly, the online monitoring system has integrated the wearable instrumentation system with the internet. However, previous studies only report ECG as the measured bio-signal [5], which is only correlated to patient's stamina during training instead of monitoring the limb functionality.

## 4 Discussion

In rehabilitation monitoring shown Table 1, some methods are conducted onsite and the others are online. Onsite monitoring is done face-to-face between the patient and the therapist. This method allows the therapist to perform various measurements and exercises to determine and improve the patient's condition. Onsite monitoring can be done by manual measurement or instrumentation measurement. Based on the findings, only few studies that report combination of instrumentation and manual measurement [33, 37, 47]. The advantage is both quantitative and qualitative data can be monitored. However, the onsite monitoring is less accessible and time restricted both the patient and the therapist. The online monitoring enable stroke rehabilitation to be done remotely, so patients do not need to come in person to carry out rehabilitation. But, the measurement methods and exercises are limited because the therapist/doctor cannot guide the patient directly. Interactive platform, such as serious games can be used to guide the patient's training without the needs of therapist [5, 48].

The most popular quantitative parameter is the lower limb kinematics and dynamics because. This parameter directly inform the stroke improvement with variety of sensor and instrument for the measurement. Combination of accelerometer and gyroscope, in the form of IMU, is the most used sensor as it provides wide range of measurement type, such as the join angle [30] and spatiotemporal parameter [34]. The IMU is also usually small and wearable, which can be used to monitor patient's data during the daily activity or outside the training context. The non-wearable instrumentation, such as the motion capture is comfort way to measure the limb kinematics without attaching any sensor to the patient. But, it requires a set up, which is not as flexible as the IMU. The other sensor is force sensor, which is used to measure the foot pressure and torque [39]. The higher the torque indicates improvement on the patient. Force measurement is mostly done in rest position, which means it can be used in a context of training only. Meanwhile, the bio-signal also explain the patient's improvement, but mostly it has been used as countermeasure to detect stroke occurrence in advance [42, 43].

The qualitative parameters put emphasize on the patient's walking ability and support needed. Indication of patient's improvement is more walking ability and less support needed. The other qualitative parameter is the user's comfort to the wearable devices instead of stroke improvement, as reported by [33]. The data collection from the wearable instrumentation can be converted into qualitative data like in manual measurement, such as the walking ability. But, only the therapist can translates the quantitative data into the qualitative data accurately at the moment. As reported by [38], the collected lower limb kinematics data is translated into the activity quality by the therapist. The information regarding the pain also cannot be collected using instrumentation method, unless by utilizing the brain signal [49] or reported by the patient through an application [14, 27].

The Monitoring of stroke rehabilitation is important as it can affect the outcome positively [50]. A good monitoring should have a feedback based on the monitored parameter. By doing so, the patient can know what do they wrong during the training activity and what do they should do to improve their training [31]. In conventional rehabilitation, the feedback number is few due to restriction in time allocation of onsite monitoring. The feedback is actually can be artificially created by using the data collected by instrumentation monitoring method. But again, only the therapist can suggest an accurate feedback. The artificial intelligence can be occupied to give feedback regarding the trainings explicitly or implicitly like in game feedback [5]. Also, it needs to be improved from time to time. Combining the feedback from therapist and artificial intelligence is the way to go in providing real-time feedback, which will improve the outcome of the rehabilitation as a whole [36].

The Internet of Things can be the solution as shown by [45, 51, 52]. The sensors attached through a wearable device collects the real time data. Then, the data can be processed in the cloud to generate feedback to the patient. Meanwhile, the therapist can also access the patient's data and revise the feedback as needed. By doing so, the patient can get feedback accurately in a relatively short time. However, currently reported study in Table 1. Only focusing on sending the training data to the therapist, such as classifying the task type [31] and stroke prediction [29] rather than the training feedback. The bio-signal has been used by [5] to monitor the patient condition, but has not been used to monitor petient's progress in the rehabilitation as suggested by [40].

Based on the findings, the research concludes that the necessary monitor parameters are lower limb kinematics and dynamics, which can be complimented by bio-signal data, such as EMG. The findings also suggest that an online stroke monitoring should full fill some categories. Firstly, it has to be wearable, so it is possible to monitor the daily activity also outside the training activity. Secondly, the wearable device should uses sensors that has wide range measurement such as the IMU that can measures a lot of limb kinematics and dynamics parameters. By doing so, the number of attached sensors can be optimized. Thirdly, the wearable device should utilized bio-signal sensors, such as the muscle sensors to get better representation of the patient's improvement instead of limb kinematics and dynamics data only. For instance, previous studies had shown that dorsiflexion capability is reflected in Tibialis Anterior (TA) muscle activity [53]. It means, if the TA muscle's activity start to appear, then it is a good indication about the patient's rehabilitation progress. Lastly, the wearable device should be equipped with monitoring application that combines feedbacks from therapist and artificial intelligence. Here, gait classification using footswitches can enrich the data for the therapist and artificial intelligence to generate the feedback accurately. By doing so, the patient is expected to get a fast feedback for improving their training performance.

There were a number of limitations in this review. Firstly, the sources are limited to one search engine only, which is the Google Scholars. If other search engine is included, such as Scopus and Web of Science, then more impactful sources can be obtained for enriching the literature review. Secondly, the point of interest of this review is the monitoring methods and parameters types, which mention in the previous researches. Other concern, such as accuracy, sensitivity, and specificity of the method will be explored in the future study. Lastly, although some methods applied in the upper-limb might also suitable for lower limb, the study only considers articles that explain stroke monitoring on lower limb part.

## 5 Conclusion

In this research, a literature review for designing a low—cost online lower limb monitoring system of a post-stroke rehabilitation has been done. The research finding suggest that the necessary monitor parameters are lower limb kinematics and dynamics, which can be complimented by bio-signal data, such as EMG. The lower limb monitoring system can use IMU, muscle sensor, and footswitches to measure the necessary parameters. IMU measures the lower limb kinematics because it provides wide range of measurement. Muscle sensor, which compatible to microcontroller, measures the EMG. Lastly, the footswitches detect the gait phases, which classify the measured data for more in-depth analysis. The mentioned sensors are cheap and available in the online market of Indonesia, which is suitable to realize a low-cost lower limb monitoring system. The research finding also suggests quick and accurate feedback mechanism for improving the training quality, which the feedback is combination of therapist opinion and artificial intelligence prediction.

## References

1. Alam M, Choudhury IA, Bin Mamat A (2014) Mechanism and design analysis of articulated ankle foot orthoses for drop-foot. Sci World J 2014:1–14.https://doi.org/10.1155/2014/867869
2. Widjaja KK et al (2020) Knowledge of stroke and medication adherence among patients with recurrent stroke or transient ischemic attack in Indonesia: a multi-center, cross-sectional study. Int J Clin Pharm 43(3):666–672. https://doi.org/10.1007/s11096-020-01178-y
3. Adiputra D et al (2019) Control reference parameter for stance assistance using a passive controlled Ankle Foot Orthosis-A preliminary study. Appl Scie (Switzerland) 9(20). https://doi.org/10.3390/app9204416
4. Adib MAHM et al (2021) Development of physiotherapy-treadmill (PhyMill) as rehabilitation technology tools for kid with cerebral palsy. Lect Notes Electrical Eng 730:829–838. https://doi.org/10.1007/978-981-33-4597-3_74
5. Agyeman MO, Al-Mahmood A, Hoxha I (2019) A home rehabilitation system motivating stroke patients with upper and/or lower limb disability. https://doi.org/10.1145/3386164.3386168
6. Kane K, Manns P, Lanovaz J, Musselman K (2019) Clinician perspectives and experiences in the prescription of ankle-foot orthoses for children with cerebral palsy. Physiother Theory Pract 35(2):148–156. https://doi.org/10.1080/09593985.2018.1441346
7. Jones SP, Leathley MJ, McAdam JJ, Watkins CL (2007) Physiological monitoring in acute stroke: a literature review. J Adv Nurs 60(6):577–594. https://doi.org/10.1111/j.1365-2648.2007.04510.x
8. Cadilhac DA et al (2016) National stroke registries for monitoring and improving the quality of hospital care: a systematic review. Int J Stroke 11(1):28–40. https://doi.org/10.1177/1747493015607523
9. Meretoja A et al (2010) Stroke monitoring on a national level: Perfect stroke, a comprehensive, registry-linkage stroke database in Finland. Stroke 41(10):2239–2246. https://doi.org/10.1161/STROKEAHA.110.595173
10. Chew DS, Rennert-May E, Spackman E, Mark DB, Exner DV (2020) Cost-effectiveness of extended electrocardiogram monitoring for atrial fibrillation after stroke a systematic review. Stroke 51(7):2244–2248. https://doi.org/10.1161/STROKEAHA.120.029340
11. Kim GJ, Parnandi A, Eva S, Schambra H (2021) The use of wearable sensors to assess and treat the upper extremity after stroke: a scoping review. Disabil Rehabil, 1–20. https://doi.org/10.1080/09638288.2021.1957027
12. Gebruers N, Vanroy C, Truijen S, Engelborghs S, de Deyn PP (2010) Monitoring of physical activity after stroke: a systematic review of accelerometry-based measures. Arch Phys Med Rehabil 91(2):288–297. https://doi.org/10.1016/j.apmr.2009.10.025
13. Peters DM et al (2021) Utilization of wearable technology to assess gait and mobility post-stroke: a systematic review. J Neuroeng Rehabil 18(1):1–18. https://doi.org/10.1186/s12984-021-00863-x

14. Lobo EH et al (2021) mHealth applications to support caregiver needs and engagement during stroke recovery: a content review. Res Nurs Health 44(1):213–225. https://doi.org/10.1002/nur.22096
15. Tun SYY, Madanian S, Mirza F (2021) Internet of things (IoT) applications for elderly care: a reflective review. Aging Clin Exp Res 33(4):855–867. https://doi.org/10.1007/s40520-020-01545-9
16. Ulloa M, Prado-Cabrera D, Cedillo P (2021) Systematic literature review of internet of things solutions oriented to people with physical and intellectual disabilities, no. Ict4awe, pp 228–235. https://doi.org/10.5220/0010480902280235
17. Elmalaki S et al (2021) Towards internet-of-things for wearable
18. van Bloemendaal M, Bus SA, Nollet F, Geurts ACH, Beelen A (2021) Feasibility and preliminary efficacy of gait training assisted by multichannel functional electrical stimulation in early stroke rehabilitation: a pilot randomized controlled trial. Neurorehabil Neural Repair 35(2):131–144. https://doi.org/10.1177/1545968320981942
19. Kwakkel G (2002) Long term effects of intensity of upper and lower limb training after stroke: a randomised trial [Online]. Available: www.jnnp.com
20. Fulk GD, Echternach JL, Nof L, O'Sullivan S (2008) Clinometric properties of the six-minute walk test in individuals undergoing rehabilitation poststroke. Physiother Theory Pract 24(3):195–204. https://doi.org/10.1080/09593980701588284
21. Shariat A et al (2021) Effect of cycling and functional electrical stimulation with linear and interval patterns of timing on gait parameters in patients after stroke: a randomized clinical trial. Disabil Rehabil 43(13):1890–1896. https://doi.org/10.1080/09638288.2019.1685600
22. Ward AB et al (2014) Evaluation of the post stroke checklist: a pilot study in the United Kingdom and Singapore. Int J Stroke 9(A100):76–84. https://doi.org/10.1111/ijs.12291
23. Kalichman L, Alperovitch-Najenson D, Treger I (2016) The impact of patient's weight on post-stroke rehabilitation. Disabil Rehabil 38(17):1684–1690. https://doi.org/10.3109/09638288.2015.1107640
24. Watanabe H, Tsurushima H, Yanagi H (2021) Effect of hybrid assistive limb treatment on maximal walking speed and six-minute walking distance during stroke rehabilitation: a pilot study. J Phys Ther Sci 33(2):168–174. https://doi.org/10.1589/jpts.33.168
25. Mudge S, Stott NS, Walt SE (2007) Criterion validity of the stepwatch activity monitor as a measure of walking activity in patients after stroke. Arch Phys Med Rehabil 88(12):1710–1715. https://doi.org/10.1016/j.apmr.2007.07.039
26. Mortazavi F, Nadian-Ghomsheh A (2019) Continues online exercise monitoring and assessment system with visual guidance feedback for stroke rehabilitation. Multimed Tools Appl 78(22):32055–32085. https://doi.org/10.1007/s11042-019-08020-2
27. Webster D, Celik O (2014) Systematic review of Kinect applications in elderly care and stroke rehabilitation [Online]. Available: http://www.jneuroengrehab.com/content/11/1/108
28. Abreu J et al (2017) Assessment of microsoft kinect in the monitoring and rehabilitation of stroke patients. Adv Intell Syst Comput 570:167–174. https://doi.org/10.1007/978-3-319-56538-5_18
29. Park H, Hong S, Hussain I, Kim D, Seo Y, Park SJ (2020) Gait monitoring system for stroke prediction of aging adults. Adv Intell Syst Comput 973:93–97. https://doi.org/10.1007/978-3-030-20476-1_11
30. He Y et al (2014) An integrated neuro-robotic interface for stroke rehabilitation using the NASA X1 powered lower limb exoskeleton. https://doi.org/10.0/Linux-x86_64
31. Bisio I, Garibotto C, Lavagetto F, Sciarrone A (2019) When eHealth Meets IoT: a smart wireless system for post-stroke home rehabilitation. IEEE Wirel Commun 26(6):24–29. https://doi.org/10.1109/MWC.001.1900125
32. Hornby TG, Moore JL, Lovell L, Roth EJ (2016) Influence of skill and exercise training parameters on locomotor recovery during stroke rehabilitation. Curr Opin Neurol 29(6): 677–683. Lippincott Williams and Wilkins. https://doi.org/10.1097/WCO.0000000000000397

33. Cherry COB et al (2017) Expanding stroke telerehabilitation services to rural veterans: a qualitative study on patient experiences using the robotic stroke therapy delivery and monitoring system program. Disabil Rehabil Assist Technol 12(1):21–27. https://doi.org/10.3109/17483107.2015.1061613
34. Wonsetler EC, Bowden MG, A systematic review of mechanisms of gait speed change post-stroke. part 1: spatiotemporal parameters and asymmetry ratios. Topics Stroke Rehab 24(6):435–446. https://doi.org/10.1080/10749357.2017.1285746
35. Stepien JM, Cavenett S, Taylor L, Crotty M (2007) Activity levels among lower-limb amputees: self-report versus step activity monitor. Arch Phys Med Rehabil 88(7):896–900. https://doi.org/10.1016/j.apmr.2007.03.016
36. Dobkin BH (2017) A Rehabilitation-internet-of-things in the home to augment motor skills and exercise training. Neurorehabil Neural Repair 31(3):217–227. https://doi.org/10.1177/1545968316680490
37. de Vlugt E, de Groot JH, Schenkeveld KE, Hans Arendzen J, van der Helm FC, Meskers CG (2010) The relation between neuromechanical parameters and Ashworth score in stroke patients [Online]. Available: http://www.jneuroengrehab.com/content/7/1/35
38. Rusu L et al (2021) Brain sciences plantar pressure and contact area measurement of foot abnormalities in stroke rehabilitation
39. Newton JM et al (2008) Reliable assessment of lower limb motor representations with fMRI: use of a novel MR compatible device for real-time monitoring of ankle, knee and hip torques. Neuroimage 43(1):136–146. https://doi.org/10.1016/j.neuroimage.2008.07.001
40. Hong YNG, Ballekere AN, Fregly BJ, Roh J (2021) Are muscle synergies useful for stroke rehabilitation? Curr Opin Biomed Eng 19:100315.https://doi.org/10.1016/j.cobme.2021.100315
41. Blas HSS, Mendes AS, Encinas FG, Silva LA, González GV (2021) A multi-agent system for data fusion techniques applied to the internet of things enabling physical rehabilitation monitoring. Appl Sci (Switzerland) 11(1):1–19. https://doi.org/10.3390/app11010331
42. Treger I, Streifler JY, Ring H (2005) The relationship between mean flow velocity and functional and neurologic parameters of ischemic stroke patients undergoing rehabilitation. Arch Phys Med Rehabil 86(3):427–430. https://doi.org/10.1016/j.apmr.2004.09.004
43. Choi YA et al (2021) Machine-learning-based elderly stroke monitoring system using electroencephalography vital signals. Appl Sci (Switzerland) 11(4):1–18. https://doi.org/10.3390/app11041761
44. Sulter G, Elting JW, Langedijk M, Maurits NM, de Keyser J (2003) Admitting acute ischemic stroke patients to a stroke care monitoring unit versus a conventional stroke unit: a randomized pilot study. Stroke 34(1):101–104. https://doi.org/10.1161/01.STR.0000048148.09143.6C
45. Mortazavi F, Nadian-ghomsheh A (2019) Continues online exercise monitoring and assessment system with visual guidance feedback for stroke rehabilitation, 32055–32085
46. Real-time Gait Monitoring System for Consumer Stroke Prediction Service.
47. Chang MC, Lee BJ, Joo NY, Park D (2021) The parameters of gait analysis related to ambulatory and balance functions in hemiplegic stroke patients: a gait analysis study. BMC Neurol 21(1). https://doi.org/10.1186/s12883-021-02072-4
48. Hocine N, Gouaïch A, Cerri SA, Mottet D, Froger J, Laffont I (2015) Adaptation in serious games for upper-limb rehabilitation: an approach to improve training outcomes. User Model User Adapt Interaction, 65–98. https://doi.org/10.1007/s11257-015-9154-6
49. Nezam T, Boostani R, Abootalebi V, Rastegar K (2021) A novel classification strategy to distinguish five levels of pain using the EEG signal features. IEEE Trans Affect Comput 12(1):131–140. https://doi.org/10.1109/TAFFC.2018.2851236
50. Cavallini A, Micieli G, Marcheselli S, Quaglini S (2003) Role of monitoring in management of acute ischemic stroke patients. Stroke 34(11):2599–2603. https://doi.org/10.1161/01.STR.0000094423.34841.BB
51. Li X, Ren S, Gu F (2021) Medical internet of things to realize elderly stroke prevention and nursing management. J Healthcare Eng 2021. https://doi.org/10.1155/2021/9989602

52. Shaaf ZF et al (2021) Home-based online multisensory arm rehabilitation monitoring system. J Phys Conf Ser 1793(1). https://doi.org/10.1088/1742-6596/1793/1/012017
53. Adiputra D, Rahman MAA, Ubaidillah, Mazlan SA (2020) Improving passive ankle foot orthosis system using estimated ankle velocity reference. IEEE Access 8:194780–194794. https://doi.org/10.1109/access.2020.3033852

# Real-Time Field Segmentation and Depth Map Using Stereo, Color and Ball Pattern

**Ardiansyah Al Farouq, Ahmad Habibi, Putu Duta Hasta Putra, and Billy Montolalu**

**Abstract** We present a real-time field segmentation in recognizing the object ball, field lines, and goalpost that have the same color. The same color on these objects make it difficult to be segmented. Then the system we build is using stereo cameras to vision sensors and a neural network for the object classification process. With the stereo camera and neural network, the object ball, field lines, and goalposts can be recognized easily. This is because the results of the value of the stereo camera and the neural network are unique. This is evident from the 10 times trials in recognizing all the white objects, gaining an error of 10%. The entire system runs an average time-consuming process for 0.08523 s.

**Keywords** Segmentation · Neural network · Stereo camera · Recognizing · Real-time

## 1 Introduction

Technological developments in highly developed Humanoid Robot. To improve and test the Humanoid Robot technology that we have built, it requires the existence of events or competition related. One of the existing competitions of robotics, especially Humanoid Robot, is RoboCup Humanoid League [1]. In the last two years, there are significant additions and updates rules developed by the technical committee at RoboCup Humanoid League. Additions and updates are initiated from the dimensions of the robot, a technical challenge, objects soccer game, and others. It has the intention to encourage the researchers of this field to develop quickly [2]. Segmentation becomes one of the problems that must be solved to equip the robot to be able to recognize these objects with fast processing time [3]. Problems on the segmentation of the ball, the field lines and goalposts arise. This is because all three objects have the same color, while in previous year rule all three objects have a different color. Although the rules concerning these things have been run in the last two

A. Al Farouq (✉) · A. Habibi · P. D. H. Putra · B. Montolalu
Fakultas Teknik Elektro, Institut Teknologi Telkom Surabaya, Surabaya, Indonesia
e-mail: alfarouq01@gmail.com; alfarouq@ittelkom-sby.ac.id

 
T. Triwiyanto et al. (eds.), *Proceedings of the 2nd International Conference on Electronics, Biomedical Engineering, and Health Informatics*, Lecture Notes in Electrical Engineering 898, https://doi.org/10.1007/978-981-19-1804-9_37

years, there are still many obstacles in the implementation of segmentation on these objects. Therefore, the purpose of this paper is to optimize results of segmentation and processing time is still fast enough. So that the robot can perform all sorts of obstacles and challenges in the RoboCup Humanoid League. The approach taken to optimize results of segmentation on these objects are using Stereo Vision and Neural Network.

Stereo Vision and Neural Network processed to improve the knowledge of those objects and processing time is still fast enough. Segmentation problems that often arise is a disorder that occurs in the image. Especially on objects that have the same color in a single image. This causes the system of robots to trouble locating objects. The result is the slow execution or incorrect execution and because the robot can not resolve the obstacles and tasks to RoboCup Humanoid League game. Of these problems, this paper discusses the process of segmentation algorithms built on T-FLOW robot. T-FLOW is a Humanoid Robot that we designed to solve all kinds of challenges in the RoboCup Humanoid League [4]. Vision sensors on the T-FLOW using Stereo Camera. While the process of classifying objects is using Neural Network.

Each object has a different segmentation process. In the field lines are segmented using depth data to ensure the lines are above ground and plane figure. An object is said to be a ball, if the object is colored white base and is on the field, solid figure, and has a unique color motif. To determine the color motif attached to the ball is to use the classification process Neural Network. When the output of the Neural Network classification process is not a ball, then the object is a goalpost or any other object that should not be on the field. An object is said to be a goalpost if the object is on field and is a solid figure, the classification process with Neural Network when the output is not a ball, and height of the goalposts is greater than width.

## 2 Introduction

Technological developments in highly developed Humanoid Robot. Many ways to segment already been done by another researcher. We demonstrate the use of the method on other research such as color segmentation, neural networks, and stereo matching.

### *2.1 Color Segmentation*

Color segmentation is an important part in the stages of computer vision or image processing related tasks. Color segmentation is very important and influential in the world of robotics such as the RoboCup, which includes environmental features important for color-coding, is still unfinished as a challenge related to irregular illumination condition [5]. Choosing the type of color space is the first step in the color segmentation, which is expected to determine the level of resistance of a color variation. Color space is a method in which there are specify, create, and visualize the color features of the image. Shape color space used RoboCup, such as RGB to classify image pixels into a ball, the goal, and the field line.

### 2.2 *Neural Network*

CogV system provides robust basic frame work very Disparate objects can be targeted. Extend this work to color environment and 3D space, this is very important to include the ability to pay attention to special sections scene so as to reduce the complexity of the search [6, 7]. The human eye allows for conceptualizing complex scenes into a simple scene that contains a collection of objects far more abstract and various other examples. Details of the scene that is often forgotten unless they become a necessity. Examples of human analogy to illustrate the ability to tie your shoes or wear buttons, also do not need to consider how many holes in clothing and how the number of fasteners required to wear clothes.

## 3 System Design for Segmentation in Robot

This system design is built to solve problems of segmentation on the objects that have similar colors. The algorithm is built must also have time process that is fast enough. Faster processing time is needed in building software on Humanoid Robot. This happens because the system is built to be approached in a human way of thinking and have knowledge of objects in the environment with a short processing time. Therefore we use stereo camera to determine the distance of each object and Neural Network to recognize knowledge of objects. System design to solve the problems of this segmentation is described in Fig. 1.

Neural Network is a process used for object classification process. The specific function of the neural network is to recognize the ball from motives which had owned in ball dataset. Ball dataset is a collection of images of balls from all sides. Each image has been mapped and extracted into sections as in Fig. 2.

Then sum of the color at each pixel of the parts of map will be extracted into a scale between 0 and 1. Exemplified color is white. While the color other than white is done in the same way as before. Then added as features of other color of ball. After that the dataset used for training process. By using a Neural Network in the training process will produce output weights. Training process is the process to obtain optimal weights or the best weight. The value of weights are used to test the color data from color extraction process. So white it can be recognized as a ball or not. When the results of the test are not ball then the white color data are lines or goalposts.

In Fig. 3 is a model of artificial Neural Networks are used for the classification process. Color extraction is the result from extraction of the colors in ball features.

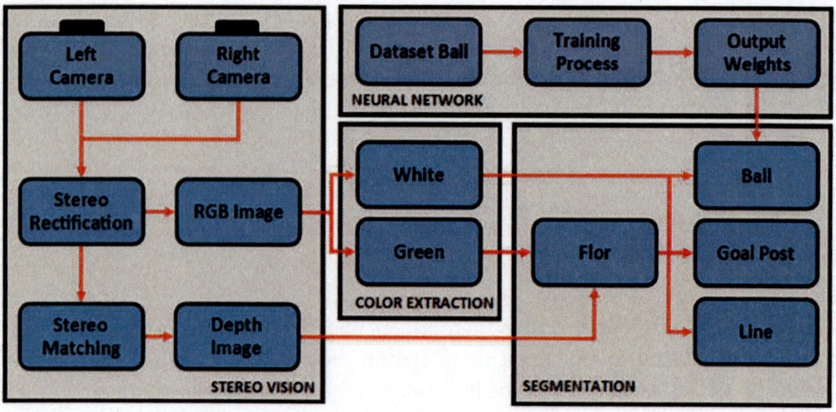


**Fig. 1** System design for segmentation objects in robot

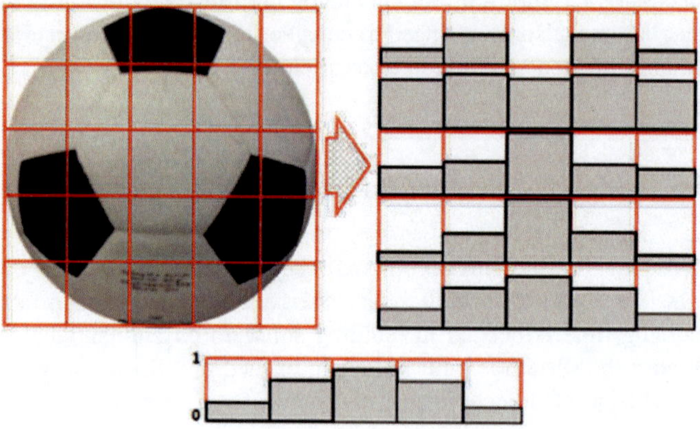


**Fig. 2** Image of ball extraction

**Fig. 3** Model of artificial neural networks

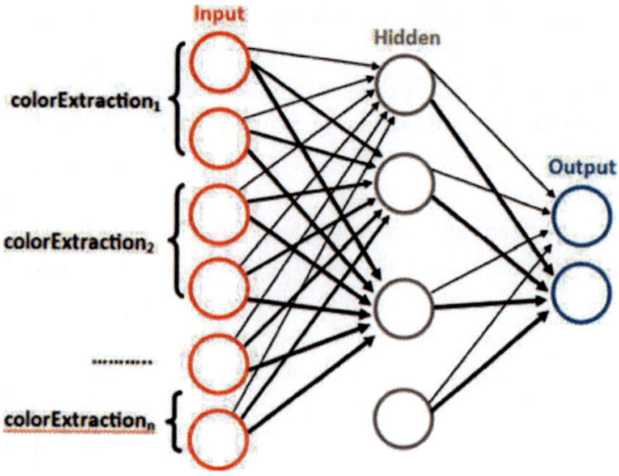

## 4 Experimental Result

In this section, experiments are designed to demonstrate the performance of a segmentation system that we developed. Performance shown is the system can complete the whole process of segmentation by the time consumption is still quite fast. Segmentation is performed on each object and the object that has the combination of all basic colors of white and green. White objects it is a ball, field lines and goalposts. While green object is field. Segmentation is done not only using the basic colors, but using depth data. Depth data be able reinforce the results of the segmentation of these objects. There are three experiments, it is field segmentation, ball segmentation, and all white objects segmentation.

In this experiment is to do segmentation of images experiments to determine the field area. The images size used is $640 \times 480$ and specification on computer is using Intel NUC. Field area images is taken from a wide variety of possible positions. The results of field area on each image segmentation is considered successful if it can map the most field area are possible by combination color extraction process and floor detection. Figure 4 is one of the results of experiment segmentation field. There is appear field area that has a region of interest line. The next experiment is to demonstrate the processing time used. Experiment conducted by processing multiple images is the percentage of total pixels when the pixels is the field then compared with the total pixels of the overall image sizes. The result of that experiment is in Table 1.

In next experiment is to do segmentation of images experiments to determine the ball. First experiment is to find the correct weight using Neural Network. The first thing is to prepare a dataset of images ball position are possible. The number of datasets are 200 images. In input layer for Artificial Neural Network is 25 neurons.

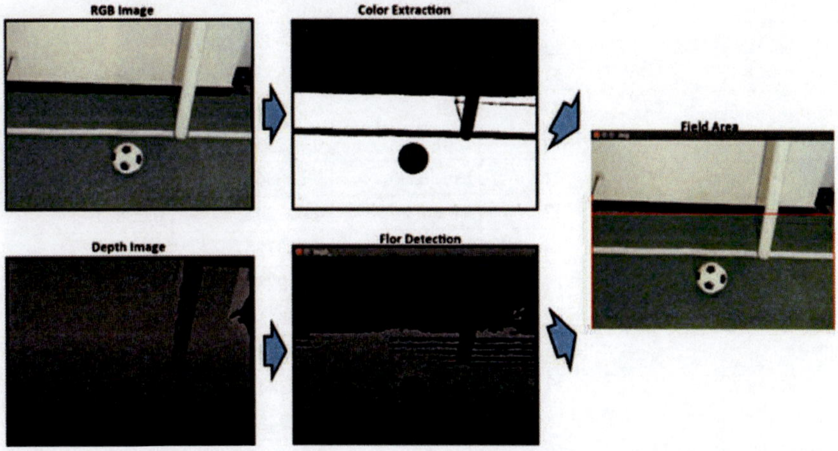


**Fig. 4** Simulation of field segmentation

**Table 1** Experiment of processing time used

| Field pixels (%) | Runtime (s) |
|---|---|
| 10 | 0.029895 |
| 20 | 0.029897 |
| 30 | 0.029902 |
| 40 | 0.02981 |
| 50 | 0.029789 |
| 60 | 0.029768 |
| 70 | 0.029741 |
| 80 | 0.029745 |
| 90 | 0.02976 |
| 100 | 0.030483 |

In hidden layer is 9 neurons. In output layer is 1 neurons. The next step is weight training process to get the correct weight. Then prepare test data consisting of 10 images of different ball pose and 10 images not ball. It aims to test the correctness weight gained. The experimental of data set results listed in Table 2. If the value from output layer is close to 1, then that value is a ball.

**Table 2** The experimental of data set results

| No | Object | Output NN | Runtime(s) |
|---|---|---|---|
| 1 | Ball | 0.999828 | 0.00187 |
| 2 | Ball | 0.928019 | 0.00837 |
| 3 | Ball | 0.873882 | 0.00234 |
| 4 | Ball | 0.798273 | 0.00236 |
| 5 | Ball | 0.990938 | 0.00237 |
| 6 | Ball | 0.89823 | 0.00423 |
| 7 | Ball | 0.97837 | 0.00324 |
| 8 | Ball | 0.638235 | 0.00324 |
| 9 | Ball | 0.982933 | 0.00873 |
| 10 | Ball | 0.782938 | 0.00234 |
| 11 | Line field | 0.118342 | 0.00238 |
| 12 | Line field | 0.097341 | 0.00837 |
| 13 | Line field | 0.013725 | 0.00238 |
| 14 | Line field | 0.019283 | 0.00213 |
| 15 | Line field | 0.028452 | 0.00234 |
| 16 | Goalpost | 0.394352 | 0.00423 |
| 17 | Goalpost | 0.293842 | 0.00387 |
| 18 | Goalpost | 0.112484 | 0.00753 |
| 19 | Goalpost | 0.692846 | 0.00234 |
| 20 | Goalpost | 0.103482 | 0.00633 |

## 5 Discussion

Table 1 shows the experimental process speed of the algorithm developed when detecting field area conditions ranging from 10 to 100% of the frame. From the table, there is no significant difference in processing time. This happens because the algorithm created does not recognize every pixel in the image and uses the concept of cellular automata. Cellular automaton algorithms allow the system to quickly find objects in an image. This happens because the system does not search for objects in every pixel of the image, but based on the properties of each identified object.

Table 2 shows an experiment to measure the processing speed of the developed system. This table shows the differences between balls, goal posts and field lines. In this experiment, when output NN approaches number one, the object becomes a ball, when output NN approaches 0.1, the object becomes a field line, and when output NN 0.6 approaches, the object becomes a goal post.

This algorithm, which was developed, is intended only for soccer games in RoboCup. The properties of the stadium objects are known. The object in question is definitely a round ball, the goal post is definitely a rectangle, and the field line object is a flat area. If you use this algorithm on an object whose properties are not specified, you will not be able to run this algorithm.

The purpose of this algorithm is to mimic the way humans quickly recognize existing objects after they already know the properties of the object. When it comes to recognizing objects, humans are not like computers that calculate all aspects of an object, they are just some of the main criteria for an object. Using this algorithm as an example of an experiment, you can already know the differences between objects in the arena, just by knowing the basic properties and colors of the objects. The integration of the object reading algorithm into the game strategy algorithm and the robot movement algorithm represents further development.

## 6 Conclusion

The system built has gotten to know the ball, the field lines, and the goal despite having the same color. With the Stereo Vision and Neural Network can sharpen segmentation results of the three objects. This is caused information that is excluded from the process of Stereo Vision and Neural Network has a unique value. The final output of Stereo Vision be able recognize an object that is plane figure and solid figure. Therefore, in recognizing the field lines can be done easily, because the field lines are plane figure and equal with floor. Remaining other objects that are not plane figure is ball and goal posts. By using the Neural Network, two objects be able do the training process to obtain the corresponding weights. The weights can be used to calculate the object being tested is a ball or the goalpost. Of the 10 times the experiment the error rate obtained when the three objects in one image is 10%.

While processing time required to perform the entire system only takes an average of 0.08523 s.

## References

1. Burkhard HD, Duhaut D, Fujita M, Lima P, Murphy R, Rojas R (2002) The road to RoboCup 2050. IEEE Robot Autom Mag 9(2):31–38
2. Waskitho SA, Alfarouq A, Sukaridhoto S, Pramadihanto D (2016) FloW vision: depth image enhancement by combining stereo RGB-depth sensor. In: 2016 international conference on knowledge creation and intelligent computing (KCIC). IEEE, pp 182–187
3. Al-Farouq A et al (2017) Merging of depth image between stereo camera and structure sensor on robot "FloW" vision. Int J Adv Sci Eng Inf Technol 7(2). https://doi.org/10.18517/ijaseit.7.2.2176
4. Al-Farouq A et al (2014) Simultaneous localization and mapping (SLAM) pada humanoid robot soccer games. In: Politeknik Elektronika Negeri Surabaya, international electronics symposium (IES). ISBN: 978-602-0917-14-6
5. Zhang X, Wang, H, Chen Q (2014) Evaluation of color space for segmentation in robot soccer. In: 2014 IEEE international conference on system science and engineering (ICSSE). IEEE, pp 185–189
6. Zhang X, Tay ALP (2007) Fast learning artificial neural network (FLANN) based color image segmentation in RGBSV cluster space. In: International joint conference on neural networks, IJCNN 2007. IEEE, pp 563–568
7. Mirante E, Georgiev M, Gotchev A (2011) A fast image segmentation algorithm using color and depth map. In: 3DTV conference: the true vision-capture, transmission and display of 3D video (3DTV-CON). IEEE, pp 1–4

# Investigation of the Unsupervised Machine Learning Techniques for Human Activity Discovery

**Md. Amran Hossen, Ong Wee Hong, and Wahyu Caesarendra**

**Abstract** Human activity recognition has been considered as the main capability of an intelligent system in understanding of human activities. Human activity recognition focuses on classifying activities with predefined models learned from labelled data based on supervised or semi-supervised approaches. These approaches have assumed the availability of abundant labelled activity observations. In real-world scenarios, labelled activity observations are difficult to obtain given the undefined number of human activities and their wide variation between different subjects. The desirable approach is an un-supervised one in which an intelligent system can discover new activities from unlabeled observations. This work aimed to evaluate the performance of several clustering algorithms to effectively distinguish different daily activities for human activity discovery. Clustering algorithms used include k-means, spectral, hierarchical and BIRCH clustering. Activity observations were represented as a sequence of postures with 3D skeletal joint locations derived from the Kinect depth map, and then different clustering algorithms were applied to the data. The approach is evaluated on a lab recorded dataset and a publicly available dataset. Overall mean precision, recall and F1-score for both datasets were above 58%, 68%, 61% respectively. K-means and agglomerative clustering with ward linkage achieved highest precision, recall and f1-score on both datasets which demonstrated the potential of using clustering algorithms to distinguish and group different activities for activity discovery without using labeled data.

**Keywords** Human activity discovery · Clustering human activities · Machine learning · Unsupervised learning

Md. A. Hossen · O. W. Hong
Faculty of Science, Universiti Brunei Darussalam, Bandar Seri Begawan, Brunei Darussalam

W. Caesarendra (✉)
Faculty of Integrated Technologies, Universiti Brunei Darussalam, Bandar Seri Begawan, Brunei Darussalam
e-mail: wahyu.caesarendra@ubd.edu.bn

 
T. Triwiyanto et al. (eds.), *Proceedings of the 2nd International Conference on Electronics, Biomedical Engineering, and Health Informatics*, Lecture Notes in Electrical Engineering 898, https://doi.org/10.1007/978-981-19-1804-9_38

# 1 Introduction

Human activity analysis has been an important area of computer vision research for the past few decades.

It has a wide range of applications in various domains, including human–robot interaction, video surveillance, gesture recognition, home behavior analysis and healthcare monitoring. Most of the research works in human activity analysis have focused on human activity recognition (HAR). The HAR systems mainly use supervised or semi-supervised approaches to recognize a limited set of activities they have been trained on. It's a challenging task to train models for each and every activity as human activity can be numerous and be carried out with wide variation. Another challenge is labelling all learning data, which is required for supervised learning. With supervised learning approaches, it is assumed that there are abundant la-belled observations of activities. However, in real life due to the wide variety of human activities, it is impossible to acquire labelled sample of all possible daily activities. A much less studied aspect in human activity analysis is the human activity discovery. Eunju et al. [1] has pointed out that human activity analysis comprises of different aspects including human activity discovery and human activity recognition. Human activity discovery is the ability of an intelligent system to find new activities from a pool of unlabeled and unknown activities. From the pool of unknown activities, human activity discovery groups the same or similar activities using unsupervised learning, and each group of a new activity can then be used for human activity recognition with the help of active learning (ask human). In other words, human activity discovery requires the ability to autonomously differentiate or distinguish between different activities without knowing their labels.

Survey papers on HAR have shown that the majority of the approaches on HAR are focused on supervised, semi-supervised and hybrid learning approaches [2–5]. Many research works have applied unsupervised learning in HAR. Clustering algorithms have been used to determine crucial postures for constructing activity feature vectors to recognize human activities with high precision [6, 7]. Unsupervised learning algorithms have been used in various contexts for mapping temporal motion dynamics from a fixed or varying length of skeleton sequences [8, 9]. These approaches have used unsupervised learning algorithms to extract features to improve the accuracy of their HAR systems, which were eventually trained using labelled data.

A few researchers have proposed the use of unsupervised algorithms for human activity discovery. They have predominantly used data from accelerometer [10–13] and smart home systems [14, 15]. Their approaches either require attaching sensors on different parts of the human limbs or attaching sensors to the household objects such as chairs, cupboards and doors. The requirement to attach sensors on human body is cumbersome, uncomfortable, and not desirable in human's everyday life. The use of objects to indirectly label the activities, for example going out of home when the door sensor has detected the movement of the doors, has limited the use of such approach to identifying highly distinguishable activities and demanding large number of environment sensors to be installed.

Consequently, very few works have studied unsupervised human activity discovery based on visual data, particular the skeleton data from a single depth sensor. To the authors' knowledge, the most related research on human activity discovery based on skeleton data is done by Ong et al. [16]. Incremental k-means clustering was used by Ong et al., for the discovery of human activity using human range of movement features which were extracted from skeleton data of the postures in consecutive frames of each activity sample. Though they were able to distinguish several unknown activities using their technique, they have only used k-means clustering in their method. K-means clustering has assumed that the data distribution is spherical. The nature of the distribution of human activities data is unknown. Investigation with other clustering algorithms to solve the problem is desirable. In this paper, we investigated the effectiveness of four widely used clustering algorithms in human activity discovery.

In this work, different unsupervised machine learning techniques were evaluated to group different activities within a pool of unlabeled and unknown activities. For the investigation, methods preferred were based on visual data that do not require people to wear sensors or devices to capture motion data, as in daily living environment it is unlikely for a person to wear sensors. Specifically, we obtained human skeleton data from a depth vision sensor as the features for the unsupervised learning algorithms. It's worth pointing out that recording skeleton data from depth sensor, i.e. without the color images, has the advantage of preserving a good degree of privacy for the person being recorded by the sensor. The main contributions of this study are that it investigates the application of different clustering algorithms in human activity discovery based on visual data without labels, and highlights areas for further research.

The paper is structured as follows. Section 2 explains how human activity discovery was portrayed as a clustering problem. Section 3 describes the experiments carried out for the investigation. The findings of this study are summarized in Sect. 4. Brief discussion is presented in Sect. 5 and finally, this work is concluded in Sect. 6.

## 2 Application of Clustering for Human Activity Discovery

In this section we describe the formulation of human activity discovery as a clustering problem. Assume the data points in Fig. 1a represent different samples or instances of human activities. There are three different activities, for examples standing, walking and waving right hand, represented with different symbols in the figure. Each activity instance comprises of a set of features extracted from depth images, which will be described in detail in the following paragraph. A clustering algorithm is applied on all the activity instances without knowing their label. The objective of the clustering is to distinguish and separate the three different activities into three coherent groups as shown in Fig. 1b.

These groups of activities discovered by the clustering algorithm can then be used for human activity recognition by using active learning and state of the art HAR

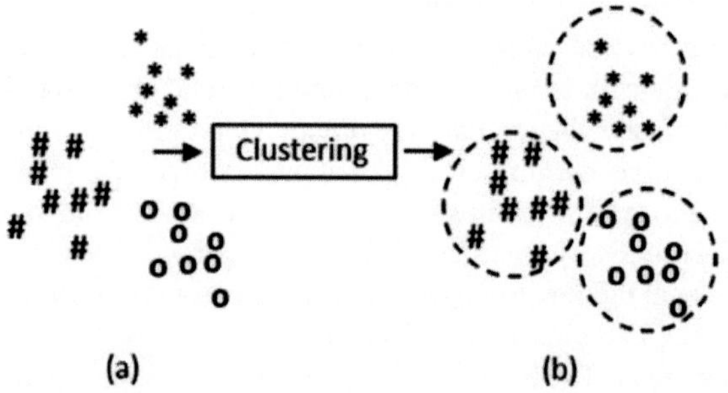


**Fig. 1** Application of clustering for human activity discovery **a** unlabeled activity sequences, **b** similar activities grouped into respective clusters

techniques. Depending on the clustering algorithm, the number of clusters may be specified by human, or determined by the clustering algorithm. In this study, we have defined an activity instance as a fixed duration of an activity. This assumption has been widely used in HAR research. Based on HAR literatures, an activity can be recognized from an observation of within a few seconds duration. For activity that may last longer, such as walking, an observation of 1–3 s is sufficient to recognize the activity. If the sensor data is 30 fps, that will translate to an instance of 30 to 90 frames. Each frame is a single posture of the activity represented as a skeleton comprising of various body joints. The number of joints is depending on the algorithm that has been used to extra skeleton data from the depth images. Each joint is represented by its 3D position in XYZ coordinates. An activity instance is, therefore, represented by a feature vector comprising of $f$ frames $\times$ $j$ joints $\times$ 3 coordinates features. A geometric transformation Fig. 2 was used to translate the skeleton in each frame, with hip center joint being translated to the center of the coordinate frame (0, 0, 0) to make the activity instances view invariant. Figure 2b, d are the translation of Fig. 2a, c respectively which shows two different frames of walking that were recorded at different locations in the sensor's field of view.

## 2.1 *Clustering*

In this sub section, we briefly describe the four clustering algorithms we have investigated in this work. In general clustering is the process of grouping comparable objects from a given set of objects based on certain measure of resemblance, so that intra-class similarity is enhanced, and inter-class similarity is reduced.

**K-means**. Clustering looks for a finite number ($K$) of clusters in a dataset by categorizing $n$ data points in $d$ dimensions into $K$ clusters while maintaining the cost function low in Eq. 1

$$J = \sum_{k=1}^{K} \sum_{i=1}^{n} X_i^{(j)} - C_k^2 \tag{1}$$

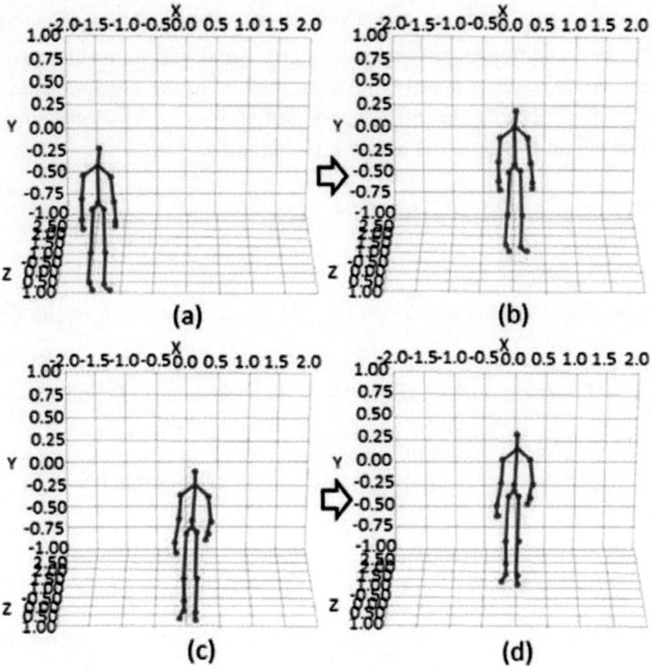


**Fig. 2** **a, c** are frames of same activity performed at different positions in the sensor's field of view. **b, d** are the translation of **a, c**

$J$ is the objective function, number of clusters is denoted with $K$, $n$ is the number of objects in the dataset, $X_i^{(j)} - C_k^2$ is a chosen distance metric between a data point $X_i^{(j)}$ in cluster $k$ and the centroid $c_k$ of cluster $k$.

**Spectral.** Clustering is a technique for identifying groups of nodes in a graph by looking at the edges that connect them. Given data points $X = X_1, X_2, \ldots, X_n$, for each pair of data points $i, j \in X$, a similarity (weight) $S_{ij} = S_{ji} \geq 0$ is assigned. In Spectral clustering, a graph $G = (V, E, W)$ is composed with $V$ containing the vertices (data points), $E$ containing the edges and $W$ containing the edge weights. $W$ is also known as the adjacent matrix. Spectral clustering applies k-means clustering on the eigenvalues of the graph Laplacian of the neighboring matrix $W$ to obtain the clusters.

**Hierarchical.** Clustering constructs nested clusters by combining (agglomerative) or splitting (divisive) data points in a tree or dendrogram. Divisive clustering begins with all data points in single cluster known as the root, which is then split into a set of child clusters until each cluster is a single data point. Agglomerative clustering begins with each data point as a cluster and proceed to combine the most similar pair of clusters until all the data points are unified into a single cluster. For this study, investigations were performed using agglomerative clustering with ward, complete and average linkages methods.

**Balanced Iterative Reducing and Clustering Using Hierarchies (BIRCH).** Clustering creates a compact summary of the original dataset as clustering feature (CF) entries, which is subsequently clustered instead of the given dataset. For a set of $N$ $d$-dimensional objects, the clustering feature $CF$ is a 3-D vector encapsulating characteristics about the data points and it is defined as

$$CF = \left(N, \overrightarrow{LS}, SS\right) \tag{2}$$

where $N$ is number of objects, $\overrightarrow{LS} = \sum_{i=1}^{N} \vec{X}_i$ is the linear sum of the data points $\vec{X}_i$ and $SS = \sum_{i=1}^{N} \left(\vec{X}_i\right)^2$ is the squared sum of the data points $\vec{X}_i$. BIRCH operates agglomerative clustering on the CF starting with each data point being a cluster. For two separate clusters, $C_1$ and $C_2$ with clustering feature $CF_1 = \left(N_1, \overrightarrow{LS_1}, SS_1\right)$ and $CF_2 = \left(N_2, \overrightarrow{LS_2}, SS_2\right)$, the clustering feature for the cluster that has been created by combining $C_1$ and $C_2$ will be

$$CF_1 + CF_2 = \left(N_1 + N_2, \overrightarrow{LS_1} + \overrightarrow{LS_2}, SS_1 + SS_2\right) \tag{3}$$

## 3 Experiments

There are a few publicly accessible human activities datasets with skeletal data which include MSR daily activity Dataset [17], UTKINECT dataset [7] and CAD60 dataset [18]. In the MSR daily activity dataset and the UTKINECT dataset, subjects completed each activity only once for most of the activities. To perform clustering, we require sufficient data points for each activity. Table 1 shows the summary of

**Table 1** Summary of publicly available datasets and our dataset

| Datasets | Total samples | Samples/class | Classes | Subjects | Modalities |
|---|---|---|---|---|---|
| MSRDailyActivity3D | 320 | 20 | 16 | 10 | RGB + D + 3DJoints |
| CAD60 | 1200 | 120[a] | 12 | 4 | RGB + D + 3DJoints |
| UTKINECT | 150 | 15 | 10 | 10 | RGB + D + 3DJoints |
| Our dataset | 2295 | 135 | 17 | 3 | RGB + D + 3DJoints |

[a] For 10 of the activities in CAD60

the characteristics of the three publicly available datasets and a dataset that we have collected. Among the three publicly available dataset, we have chosen to evaluate clustering performance on the CAD60 dataset.

The CAD60 dataset comprises of 12 daily activities performed by four subjects with skeleton data of 15 joints. We have eliminated two activities that have only a few observations. We used 10 activities from the CAD60 dataset that we could sample sufficient instances, i.e. 120 instances for each activity. Activities from the CAD60 dataset that we have used are standing, brushing teeth, talking on phone, drinking water, cooking (chopping), cooking (stirring), talking on couch, relaxing on couch, writing on whiteboard and working on computer. Figure 3 shows sample RGB images of the ten activities from CAD60 dataset. We have only used the skeleton data provided in the dataset. Data in CAD60 were obtained from OpenNI library that provides skeleton data with 15 joints. For CAD60, we have sampled 30 instances consisting of 30 frames each for each subject giving 120 instances for each activity. The feature vector for each activity instance comprised of 30 frames $\times$ 15 joints $\times$ 3 coordinates, i.e. 1350 features.

To evaluate human activity discovery on more activities, we have collected a dataset ourselves. We have intentionally added activities that have locomotion activity, i.e. the walking and are motion intensive such as jumping, kicking and

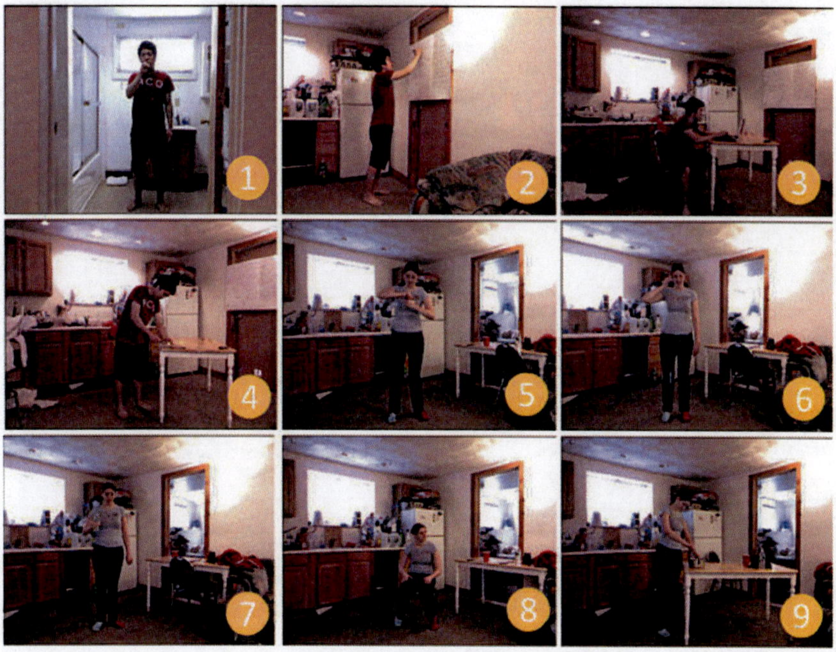


**Fig. 3** Instances of activities from the CAD60 dataset [18]. (1) brushing teeth, (2) writing on the board, (3) working in computer, (4) cooking (chopping), (5) opening pill container, (6) making phone calls, (7) having a drink, (8) sitting, (9) cooking (stirring)

waving hands. We note activities in CAD60 have limited motion. We have collected the datasets using the Microsoft Kinect SDK that provides skeleton data with 20 joints, in contrast to the 15 joints in CAD60. For our dataset, three subjects in an indoor environment performed seventeen activities: standing, raising the right hand, raising the left hand, kicking the right leg, kicking the left leg, waving the right hand, waving the left hand, doing jumping jacks, walking, sitting down, being seated, standing up, making a phone call, drinking, picking up, sitting, and reading a book, and sweeping the floor. We recorded a sequence of each activity using a single stationary Kinect at 30 frames per second for at least 2 min. We have recorded both RGB and depth images, however we have only used the skeleton data derived from the depth images in this work. Sample RGB images from the dataset are shown in Fig. 4. For each action, 45 observations consisting of 70 frames each were sampled from the recording of each individual giving 135 instances for each activity. The feature vector for each activity instance comprised of 70 frames $\times$ 20 joints $\times$ 3 coordinates, i.e. 4200 features. This differs from the feature vectors of CAD60 for the purpose of investigation.

In Fig. 5, we have summarized the process involved in the experiment. The input to the clustering algorithm is all the transformed instances in a dataset. In this study,

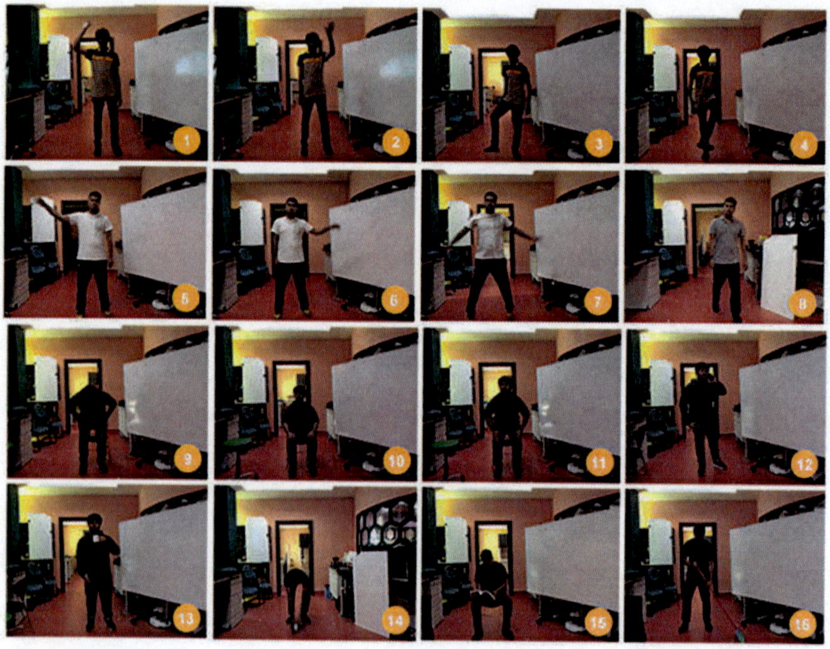


**Fig. 4** Sample images from 16 activities in our dataset. (1) raising right hand, (2) raising left hand, (3) kicking right leg, (4) kicking left leg, (5) waving right hand, (6) waving left hand, (7) jumping jacks, (8) walking, (9) sitting down, (10) seated, (11) standing up, (12) phone call, (13) having a drink, (14) picking up from the floor, (15) seated and reading book, (16) sweeping the floor

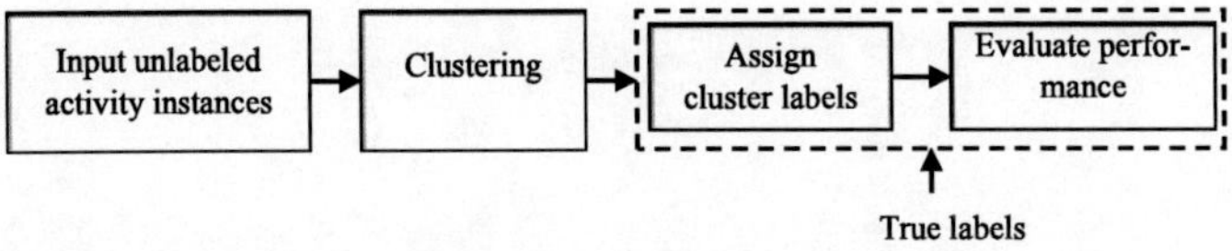


**Fig. 5** Experimental flow. True labels were only used for evaluation purposes

we have specified the number of clusters. Each of the clusters generated by the clustering technique was anticipated to be a group of the instances for an activity. True labels of the activity instances were used to evaluate the performance of the clustering algorithm. For evaluation purpose, each cluster was labelled as one of the activities in the dataset based on the label of its majority instances. For instance, if true labels for a dataset comprising of six instances from two activities were [0, 0, 0, 1, 1, 1] and the instances were clustered into two clusters as [***1***, ***1***, ***0***, ***0***, ***0***, ***1***]. There were one activity 0 and two activity 1 in cluster ***0***; two activity 0 and one activity 1 in cluster ***1***. Based on majority, cluster ***0*** would be labelled activity 1, and cluster ***1*** would be labelled activity 0 giving the predicted labels as [0, 0, 1, 1, 1, 0]. Then we compared the predicted labels with ground truth, i.e. true labels, to evaluation the performance of the clustering. Evaluations were performed applying the K-means, Spectral, Agglomerative clustering with several linkage techniques (ward, average and complete linkage) and BIRCH clustering on both datasets. Random centroid initialization was used in K-means and spectral clustering. The K-means and spectral clustering algorithms were repeated ten times and average results are reported. For agglomerative and BIRCH clustering, the clustering results do not change in each run. Precision, recall and F1-score were computed for each result.

## 4 Results

Figure 6 summarizes the result of each clustering algorithm performed on our dataset. Each bar represents the average precision, recall and F1-score of the clustering results for all the 17 activities. The rightmost bar shows the overall mean precision, recall and F1-score of all clustering algorithms, which were 58%, 68%, and 61% respectively. The agglomerative clustering with ward linkage and BIRCH clustering have achieved the same precision, recall and F1-score were 62%, 70% and 63% respectively, which was the highest performance among the clustering algorithms used.

Figure 7 shows the precision, recall and F1-score for the results on CAD60 dataset. Overall mean precision, recall and F1-score for all clustering algorithms were 61%, 69% and 63% respectively as shown by the rightmost column. Similar to the results on our dataset, agglomerative clustering (using ward and average linkage) and BIRCH clustering have achieved the highest precision, recall and F1-score at 62%, 70% and 64% respectively.

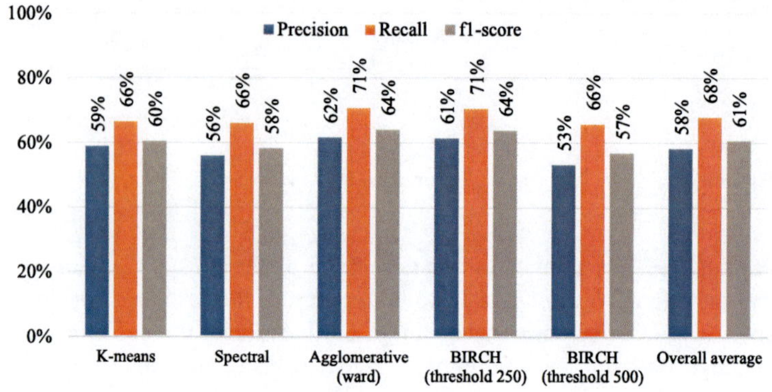


**Fig. 6** Precision, recall and F1-score of different clustering algorithms on our dataset

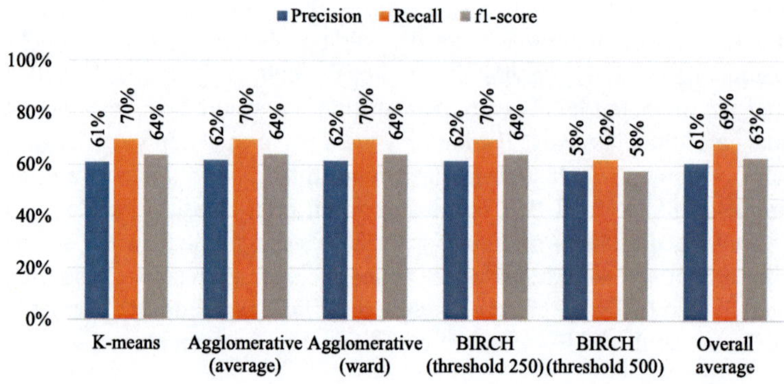


**Fig. 7** Precision, recall and F1-score of different clustering algorithms on CAD60 dataset

Comparing the results on both datasets, we observe that precision, recall and F1-score of k-means, agglomerative clustering with ward linkage and BIRCH clustering results were consistent and relatively high. However, clustering results for spectral clustering differed significantly on the two datasets. Determining two of the required parameters for BIRCH clustering (branching factor and threshold) was challenging. We have determined these parameters empirically for both datasets. Figure 8 summarizes the overall clustering performance on the two datasets. It can be observed that overall precision, recall and F1-score on our dataset was lower than that on CAD60 dataset. This is due to that our dataset contains more activities with more variation and a few highly similar activities. Figure 9 shows the precision, recall and F1-score achieved by k-means, spectral, agglomerative with ward linkage and BIRCH (threshold of 250) clustering for every activity in our dataset.

For brevity, we have omitted the results of the other agglomerative and BIRCH clustering that were lower. It can be observed that activities which were grouped well by all of the clustering algorithms were: raise left hand, kick right leg, kick left leg,

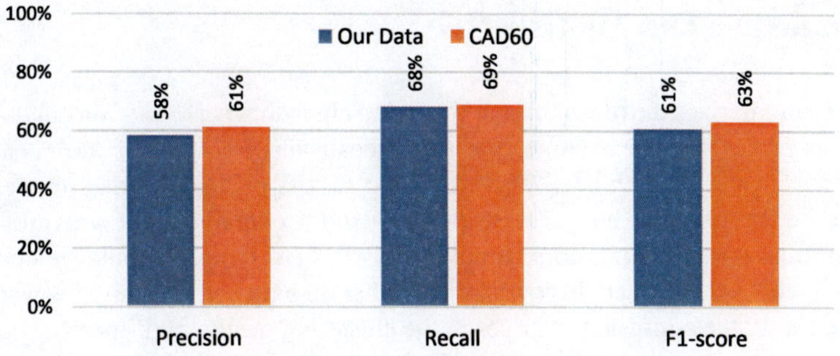


**Fig. 8** Average precision, recall and F1-score achieved on both datasets

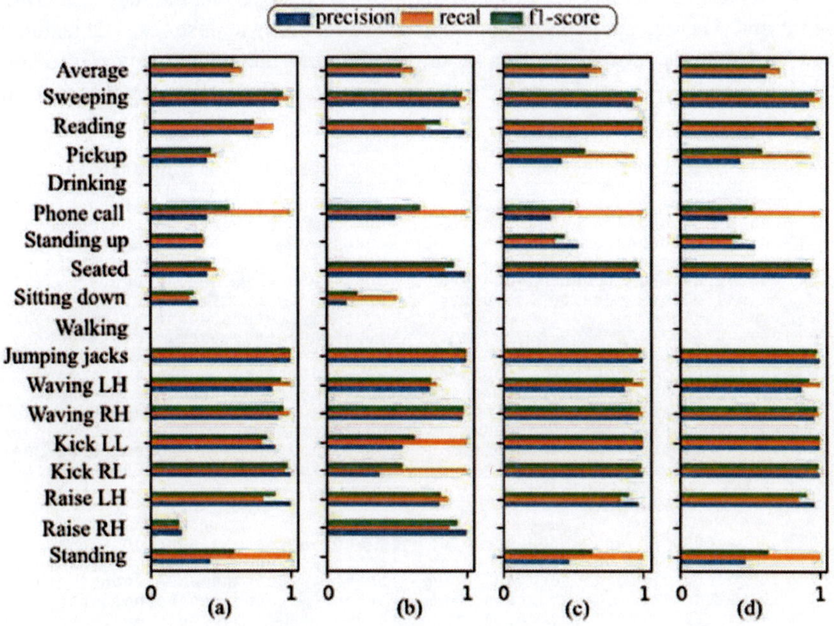


**Fig. 9** Precision, recall and f1-score for every activity in our dataset. **a** k-means, **b** Spectral, **c** Agglomerative with ward linkage, **d** BIRCH with threshold of 250

waiving right hand, waiving left hand, jumping jacks, seated, sitting and reading and sweeping floor. A few activities were poorly clustered including walking, drinking and sitting down. There were activities which were clustered well by some clustering algorithms while other clustering algorithms had poorly grouped them. For example, standing was clustered well by k-means, agglomerative and BIRCH clustering while with spectral clustering it was confused with other activities.

## 5 Discussion and Analysis

Figure 6 summarizes the result of each clustering algorithm performed on our dataset. Each bar represents the average precision, recall and F1-score of the clustering results for all the 17 activities. The clustering results on CAD60 dataset were on average better than that on our dataset. Our dataset contains more activities with more similar activities and more complex activities (walking, jumping) in comparison to the CAD60 dataset. To investigate further on why certain activities were not clustered well, the confusion matrices of the clustering results for k-means, spectral, agglomerative with ward linkage and BIRCH (threshold 250) clustering performed on our dataset are shown in Fig. 10a–d respectively. The activities are enumerated as in Fig. 4 and standing is enumerated as 0. It can be observed that walking (label 8) and standing (label 0) were grouped in the same cluster by all the four clustering algorithms. The two activities appear similar when looking at postures. The features used in this study lack the motion or time series information. Raising right hand (label 1), drinking (label 13) and talking on the phone (label 12) were grouped in

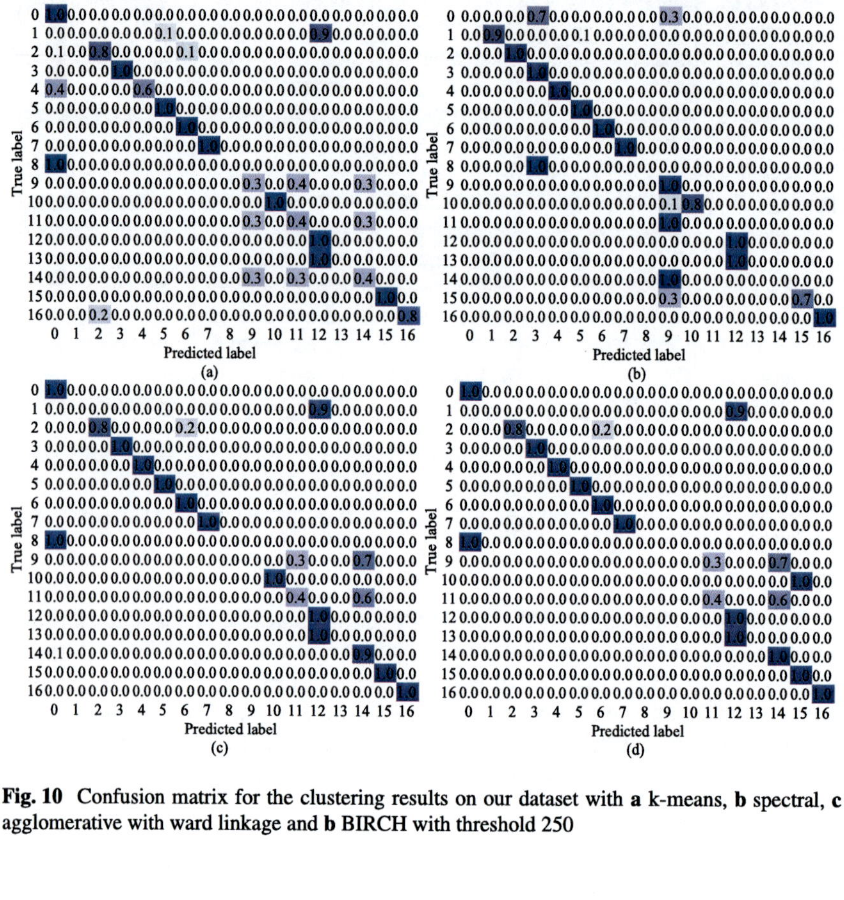

**Fig. 10** Confusion matrix for the clustering results on our dataset with **a** k-means, **b** spectral, **c** agglomerative with ward linkage and **b** BIRCH with threshold 250

the same cluster by k-means, agglomerative and BIRCH as shown in Fig. 10a, c, d respectively, however spectral clustering could effective cluster raising right hand (label 1) as shown in Fig. 10c. Drinking and talking on the phone appear similar when looking at the postures. Raising right hand shares similarity in terms of right hand being raised. Coincidently, all subjects are right-handed hence drinking and talking on the phone were performed with right hand.

Figure 11 shows the confusion matrices for the results on CAD60 dataset. The activities labels are as shown in Fig. 3. It can be seen that drinking (label 3), brushing teeth (label 4) and talking on the phone (label 1) were confused by all clustering algorithms. These three activities are highly similar with their hands raised to the head. Cooking (chopping, label 7) was confused with cooking (stirring, label 8) by all clustering algorithms. The two activities are similar when viewed as postures.

The confusion matrices for the clustering results on both datasets show that k-means, agglomerative clustering (ward linkage) and BIRCH clustering (thresh hold

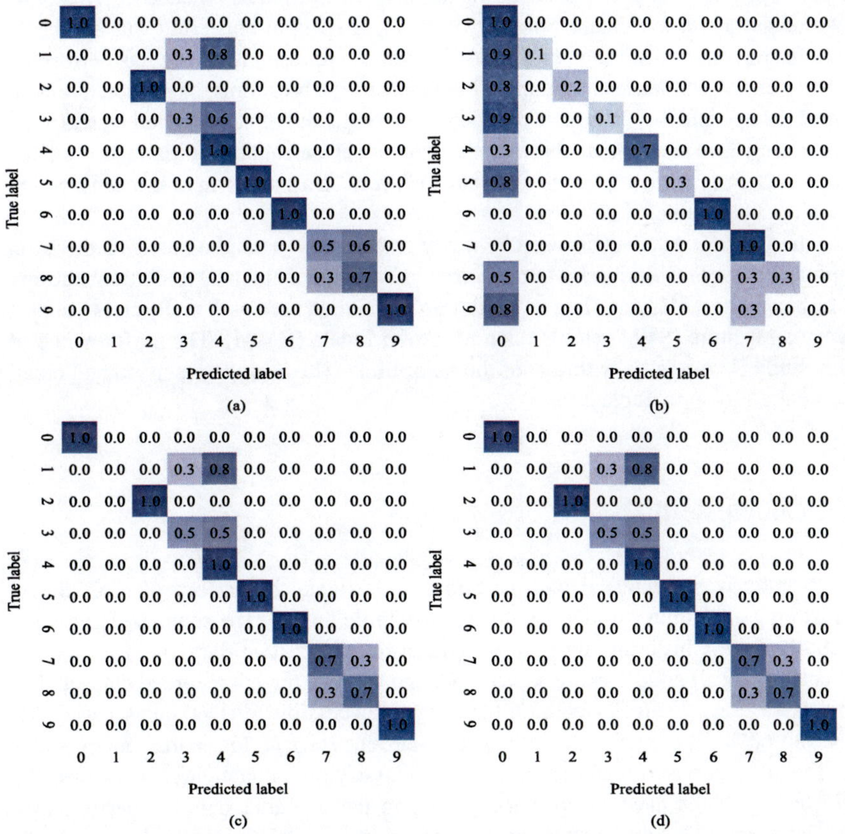


**Fig. 11** Confusion matrix for the clustering results on **a** k-means, **b** spectral, **c** agglomerative with ward linkage and **b** BIRCH with threshold of 250

**Table 2** Overall precision and recall score of this study compared with other methods

| Authors | Method | Precision (%) | Recall (%) |
|---|---|---|---|
| Sung et al. [17] | Supervised with MEMM | 68 | 56 |
| Gaglio et al. [19] | Supervised with HMM and SVM | 77 | 77 |
| Shan and Akella [20] | Supervised with SVM and BoW | 94 | 95 |
| Cippitelli et al. [6] | Supervised with SVM and BoW | 94 | 94 |
| Proposed | Unsupervised/k-means/agglomerative | 61 | 69 |

250) performed consistently on both datasets. However, BIRCH clustering performance varied significantly with different threshold values. It was challenging to determine the optimum threshold value. We experimented with different threshold values to find the threshold value that produced the best result. This is not feasible in real life application when the algorithm does not know the true labels to evaluate the clustering outcome. Spectral clustering performance varied significantly between the two datasets. On our dataset, the performance of spectral clustering was similar to that of the other clustering algorithms. However, spectral clustering has performed poorly on CAD60 dataset. Among all the clustering algorithms, agglomerative with ward linkage and k-means have produced consistent and relatively good results. One issue with k-means is that the result is dependent on random initialization of the centroids. In real life application, we can only rely on a single run of k-means, which may not be reliable.

The CAD60 dataset was used by many researchers to validate their methods on human activity recognition. Methods used by researchers include maximum entropy Markov model (MEMM), bag of words (BoW) method used with multi-class Support Vector Machine (SVM) and Hidden Markov Models (HMM). The performance of this study is compared with few of the algorithms. The average precision and recall score are shown in Table 2.

## 6 Conclusion

This study was conducted with an aim to investigate the performance of several clustering algorithms to identify the most suitable one to explore unlabeled human activity data. Clustering algorithms were evaluated on two datasets. The average precision, recall and F1-score was 58, 68, and 61% on the lab recorded dataset. The precision, Recall and F1-score on the publicly accessible CAD60 dataset were 61, 69 and 63%. The overall performance at current stage is lower than many states of the art supervised methods available to classify human activities. However, the clustering results have shown performance in par or better than the performance of classifiers trained with supervised learning on the CAD60 dataset (see Table 2). The results from this work have demonstrated the potential of clustering algorithms for human activity discovery without requiring labels. From the results, spectral clustering performed poorly, BIRCH clustering requires setting of parameters that would be difficult without the knowledge of the dataset, and k-means is subject to uncertainty of random centroids initialization. Agglomerative clustering with ward linkage appears to be the preferred clustering algorithm given the features based on joint positions in fixed number of frames.

As this is an exploratory work, a number of assumptions and conditions have been used to simplify the experiments. This study highlights that more problems need to be addressed besides improving the clustering performance which will be carried out as extension of this study. Firstly, the assumption of knowing the number of clusters or activities will be an issue in real life application. It is necessary to explore clustering algorithms that do not require knowing the number of clusters. Secondly, it is necessary to deal with the different durations of different activities. This is an unsolved problem even in HAR using supervised learning. In many cases, HAR has made assumption on activity duration based on the dataset. Thirdly, more useful features need to be extracted that capture the motion and time series information of the activities. Current set of features was effective to distinguish activities that are different in the postures involved, however failed to distinguish activities that have similar postures that are distinguished by their motion (e.g. stirring food and chopping food).

## References


1. Kim E, Helal S, Cook D (2010) Human activity recognition and pattern discovery. IEEE Pervasive Comput 9:48–53
2. Aggarwal JK, Xia L (2014) Human activity recognition from 3D data: a review. Pattern Recognit Lett 48:70–80
3. Baisware A, Sayankar B, Hood S (2019) Review on recent advances in human action recognition in video data. In: 2019 9th international conference on emerging trends in engineering and technology—signal and information processing (ICETET-SIP-19). IEEE, pp 1–5. https://doi.org/10.1109/ICETET-SIP-1946815.2019.9092193
4. Chen L, Wei H, Ferryman J (2013) A survey of human motion analysis using depth imagery. Pattern Recognit Lett 34:1995–2006
5. Trong NP, Minh AT, Nguyen H, Kazunori K, Le Hoai B (2017) A survey about view-invariant human action recognition. In: 2017 56th annual conference of the society of instrument and control engineers of Japan (SICE), pp 699–704. https://doi.org/10.23919/SICE.2017.8105762
6. Cippitelli E, Gasparrini S, Gambi E, Spinsante S (2016) A human activity recognition system using skeleton data from RGBD sensors. Comput Intell Neurosci 2016
7. Xia L, Chen C, Aggarwal JK (2012) View invariant human action recognition using histograms of 3D joints. In: 2012 IEEE computer society conference on computer vision and pattern recognition workshops. IEEE, pp 20–27. https://doi.org/10.1109/CVPRW.2012.6239233
8. Mohammadzade H, Tabejamaat M (2020) Sparsness embedding in bending of space and time; a case study on unsupervised 3D action recognition. J Vis Commun Image Represent 66:102691
9. Zheng N et al (2018) Unsupervised representation learning with long-term dynamics for skeleton based action recognition. In: 32nd AAAI conference on artificial intelligence AAAI 2018, pp 2644–2651
10. Abdallah ZS, Gaber MM, Srinivasan B, Krishnaswamy S (2016) AnyNovel: detection of novel concepts in evolving data streams: an application for activity recognition. Evol Syst 7:73–93

11. Fang L, Ye J, Dobson S (2019) Discovery and recognition of emerging human activities using a hierarchical mixture of directional statistical models. IEEE Trans Knowl Data Eng 14:1–1
12. Gjoreski H, Roggen D (2017) Unsupervised online activity discovery using temporal behaviour assumption. In: International symposium on wearable computers. ISWC Part F1305, pp 42–49
13. Kwon Y, Kang K, Bae C (2014) Unsupervised learning for human activity recognition using smartphone sensors. Expert Syst Appl 41:6067–6074
14. Huynh T, Fritz M, Schiele B (2008) Discovery of activity patterns using topic models. In: Proceedings of the 10th international conference on Ubiquitous computing—UbiComp '08 10. ACM Press. https://doi.org/10.1145/1409635.1409638
15. Ye J, Fang L, Dobson S (2016) Discovery and recognition of unknown activities. In: UbiComp 2016 Adjunct—Proceedings of the 2016 ACM international joint conference on pervasive and ubiquitous computing, pp 783–792. https://doi.org/10.1145/2968219.2968288
16. Ong WH, Koseki T, Palafox L (2013) Unsupervised human activity detection with skeleton data from RGB-D sensor. In: Proceedings of 5th international conference on computational intelligence, communication systems and networks, pp 30–35. https://doi.org/10.1109/CICSYN.2013.53
17. Sung J, Ponce C, Selman B, Saxena A (2012) Unstructured human activity detection from RGBD images. In: Proceedings of international conference on robotics and automation, pp 842–849. https://doi.org/10.1109/ICRA.2012.6224591
18. Wang J, Liu Z, Wu Y, Yuan J (2012) Mining actionlet ensemble for action recognition with depth cameras. In: Proceedings of the IEEE computer society conference on computer vision and pattern recognition, pp 1290–1297. https://doi.org/10.1109/CVPR.2012.6247813
19. Gaglio S, Re G, Morana M (2015) Human activity recognition process using 3-D posture data. IEEE Trans Hum Mach Syst 45:586–597
20. Shan J, Akella S (2014) 3D human action segmentation and recognition using pose kinetic energy. In: 2014 IEEE international workshop on advanced robotics and its social impacts. https://doi.org/10.1109/arso.2014.7020983

# The Development of an Alarm System Using Ultrasonic Sensors for Reducing Accidents for Side-By-Side Driving Alerts

**Krunal Suthar, Harikrishna Parikh, Haresh Pandya, and Mahesh Jivani**

**Abstract** On the road, safety of vehicles and passengers, along with other moving vehicles on the road, is the responsibility of the driver. Crashing into a vehicle from the side is a most common problem for the driver due to lack of maintaining a safe distance by other vehicle drivers. To avoid crashing from side one need view side mirrors frequently, causing distraction. Distracted driving is another leading cause of a car accident. Aim of designing the side-by-side assistant system is alerts the driver with a beep sound for an oncoming vehicle near to the forward driver and vice versa for the trailing vehicle if the vehicle leads to a forward vehicle with unsafe distance. The system utilizes a set of six ultrasonic sensor arrays. The Arduino board in the system generates trigger signal and processes the echo signals received from each of 3 sensors mounted on each side of the vehicle to estimate distance between adjacent vehicles. If the distance is less than the critical limit set (adjustable), audible alarm will be generated. This alarm will be life saving for the driver and all passengers along with other vehicles on the road. During the laboratory tests, the alarms are generated in a time period less than 1 s for optimum distance. 100 such tests were carried out, and it showed no failure in the lab test conditions. Further field tests are to be carried out post permission from the Road Transportation Authority. Reduced distraction from frequent viewing of the side mirrors, help to reduce accidents by increasing driver efficiency.

**Keywords** Ultrasonic sensors · Arduino · Smart vehicle · Side-by-side assistance · Road safety

## 1 Introduction

Day by day, the large number of vehicles are dumped on the road, increasing vehicle density like never before. The overall annual average production and sale of vehicles for the year 2010 to 2019 is 71 million globally [1]. Comparing to the increasing

K. Suthar (✉) · H. Parikh · H. Pandya · M. Jivani
Department of Electronics, Saurashtra University, Rajkot, Gujarat, India
e-mail: krunalsuthar85@gmail.com



T. Triwiyanto et al. (eds.), *Proceedings of the 2nd International Conference on Electronics, Biomedical Engineering, and Health Informatics*, Lecture Notes in Electrical Engineering 898, https://doi.org/10.1007/978-981-19-1804-9_39

number of vehicles, the available driving lanes, have increased only a little owing to diverse reasons. In the 20th Century era time is a precious resource, and hence, everyone wishes to reach the destination as early as possible, leading to overtakes and traffic jams [2]. The high density of vehicles on the road causes collisions between vehicles. A side-by-side collision of the vehicle isn't uncommon in case of insecure overtaking. This mandates a system alerting a driver, in case, the trailing vehicle overtakes unsafely or vice versa. The vehicles outside rear view mirrors (ORVM) are maximally used by drivers on a highway for overtaking and for giving side to another vehicle [3]. But frequent watching in ORVM while driving, leads to distraction and in turn, to an accident [4].

Researchers have been working on the issue to help reduce the risk, employing various techniques. Adamu Murtala Zungeru has tested and utilized Microwave-based detectors for the front and rear side of vehicle safety [5], while, Shinde [6] has reported use of infrared detectors for the same purpose. The optical waves are prone to scattering and absorbance by shape, material, and the dimension of a reflecting surface. Shival Dubey & Abdul Wahid Ansari used Ultrasonic sensors for the front and back side safety of vehicles [7] but not for the side-by-side. Ultrasonic sensors are also used in reverser parking alerts systems [8, 9] which provide alerts for tail only. An ultrasonic sensor measures the distance of a target object by emitting ultrasonic sound waves and measuring the time for echo [10] but for batter accuracy Temperature & humidity values are not calculated in any research for vehicle.

In contrast of side-by-side safety systems for vehicles, reverse parking systems are quite common. Even, there is no alert system available for safe distance measurement from both the side of the vehicle during driving on multiple lanes of the road and parking. Ultrasonic waves travel faster than the speed of audible sound and their speed largely depend on humidity, air pressure, and temperature [11, 12]. From morning to night times and even during different seasons of the year and different geographical locations, humidity and temperature varies [13]. In spite of temperature and humidity variation, the need to measure accurate distance, mandates correction against such changes. No reference could be found for accurate distance calculation, with compensation against temperature and humidity variation, for such vehicle safety systems.

In this research paper Arduino UNO [14] is used as the core, with ultrasonic sensor and humidity sensor for accurate distance measurement. The same Arduino UNO is used to continuously monitor the distance from each of the sensor and generate alerts upon alert conditions set [15]. Arduino IDE is used for writing and compiling codes to control the inputs and outputs on the board. Purpose of this system development is reduced the driver distraction, property loss/damage and save the time significantly because reduction in traffic jam due to reduction in accidents.

## 2 Materials and Method

### 2.1 Hardware Design

Electronics systems are an important integral part of all vehicles. Majority of the mechanical parts are operated or controlled by electronic control systems driven by feedback from different automobile sensors. Figure 1, shows the block diagram of the Side-by-side protection and alerts system. The circuit is realized using an Arduino Uno development board, an array of 06 ultrasonic sensors HR-SC04 [16], one DHT 11 digital humidity & temperature sensor [17], a buzzer, LEDs and some switches. For adjusting a safe distance for alert, four push button switches are provided: up arrow key (+), down arrow key (−), left arrow key (No) and right arrow key (Yes). Furthermore, for visualization of the vehicle-to-vehicle safe distance in international unit meter, one 16 X 2 alphanumeric LCD is employed [18].

DHT 11 sensor is connected to measure humidity and temperature [17] around the vehicle. The output data pin 3 of DHT 11 sensor is connected as input mode for Arduino UNO Analog pin (A0) [19]. This ultra-low-cost digital temperature and humidity sensor uses a capacitive humidity sensor and a thermistor to measure the surrounding air humidity and temperature [17]. Time to echo is measured to know the distance travelled by the ultrasound waves. Figure 1 illustrates well the distance measurement process using the ultrasonic sensor.

An array of 6, HRSC04 sensors, transmitting ultrasonic (40 kHz) pulses in omni direction of the vehicle are employed here. All sensors (HRSC04) are triggered to generate a common and simultaneous 10-microsecond pulse by pin D9. The pulse, reflected from any rigid surface (echo), will be detected by the sensors generating an echo pulse on pin 3 of the respective sensor. HRSC04 sensor Echo pin output pulse width will be in range of 150 microseconds to 25 ms, due to its range of detection. Echo pin of each HRSC04 sensor is connected to Arduino Uno pins as tabulated in Table 1. The time to echo is measured, which is further processed to calculate the exact distance of travel after carrying out temperature and humidity compensation

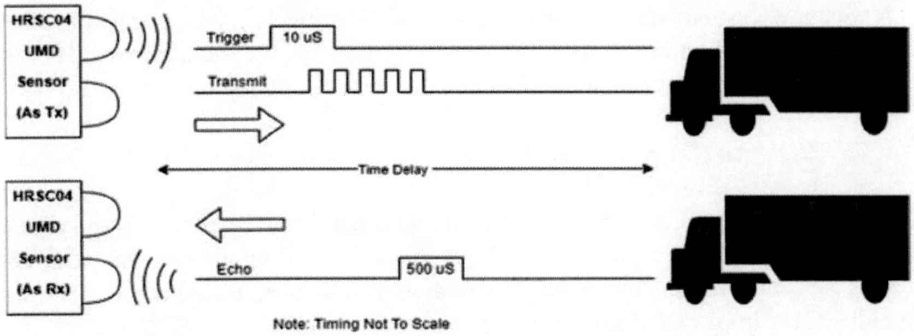


**Fig. 1** Distance measurement process using Arduino UNO to HR-SC04 sensor

**Table 1** I/O pin configuration and connections

| Arduino pin number | Function | Peripheral pin connection |
|---|---|---|
| Analog (A0) | Input | DHT-11 Pin-2 (Data) |
| Analog (A1) | Input | HR-SC04 Sensor 1 pin 3 (echo), Front Right (FR) |
| Analog (A2) | Input | HR-SC04 Sensor 2 pin 3 (echo), Center Right (CR) |
| Analog (A3) | Input | HR-SC04 Sensor 3 pin 3 (echo), Back Right (BR) |
| Analog (A4) | Input | HR-SC04 Sensor 4 pin 3 (echo), Front Left (FL) |
| Analog (A5) | Input | HR-SC04 Sensor 5 pin 3 (echo), Center Left (CL) |
| Digital (D0) | Input | HR-SC04 Sensor 6 pin 3 (echo), Back Left (BL) |
| Digital (D1) | Input | Initially use as arrow key Left |
| | Output | Alerts for HR-SC04 Sensor 1, Front Right (FR) |
| Digital (D2) | Input | Initially use as arrow key Right |
| | Output | Alerts for HR-SC04 Sensor 2, Center Right (CR) |
| Digital (D3) | Input | Initially use as arrow key Down |
| | Output | Alerts for HR-SC04 Sensor 3-BR, Back Right (BR) |
| Digital (D4) | Input | Initially use as arrow key Up |
| | Output | Alerts for HR-SC04 Sensor 4-FL, Front Left (FL) |
| Digital (D4) | Input | Alerts for HR-SC04 Sensor 5, Center Left (CL) |
| Digital (D6) | Output | Alerts for HR-SC04 Sensor 6, Back Left (BL) |
| Digital (D7) | Output | LCD RS pin to digital pin |
| Digital (D8) | Output | LCD Enable pin to digital pin |
| Digital (D9) | Output | Pin 2 -trigger, pin for all HR-SC04 Sensor 01 to 06 |
| Digital (D10) | Output | LCD D4 pin |
| Digital (D11) | Output | LCD D5 pin |
| Digital (D12) | Output | LCD D6 pin |
| Digital (D13) | Output | LCD D7 pin |

[20]. Ultrasonic signal travels at the speed of the sound (343 m/S) at 20 °C. The pulse width of the echo pin is utilized to calculate the distance [10].

If we know the velocity of sound (C) and travelling time (T), we can calculate the distance (D). Considering the transmittance and reflection, the wave travels distance double the actual distance, hence, the actual distance can be represented by Eq. 1.

$$Distance\ (D) = \left[Travel\ time\ (T) \times Velocity\ of\ sound\ (C)\right]/2. \tag{1}$$

The velocity of sound varies considerably with humidity, air pressure, and especially at temperature. To incorporate the temperature and humidity compensation DHT11 sensor is used. The speed of sound at, atmospheric temperature (T) with humidity (H) can be calculated using Eq. 2.

$$Velocity\ of\ Sound\ (C) = [331.4 + (0.606 \times T) + (0.0124 \times H)] \tag{2}$$

Here, the velocity of ultrasonic wave (C) is a function of humidity and temperature, and will provide an accurate distance. For a safe distance of 4-m, the system needs 23.323 ms to detect the signal. A single one-way travel time (T/2) by ultrasonic wave is calculated, which is further processed using Eqs. (1) and (2) to calculate temperature and humidity compensated distance. In this calculation we assume air pressure is constant.

Figure 2 depicts the block diagram of the complete system designed with label and placement of ultrasonic sensors. User is provided with enabling/disabling switches to avoid annoying alerts (the blinking light during the night-time or continuous sound of beep in a heavy traffic jam). This hardware uses limited I/Os and interface, making the system cost effective and simple. The pin numbers of sensors connected to various pins of Arduino Uno and their configuration as well as functions are tabulated in Table 1, while Fig. 3 depicts the actual circuit diagram of the system.

The Side-by-Side protection circuit drains power from the vehicle's battery. A voltage regulator ensures constant voltage is being provided to the circuit and in turn safe and prolonged operation [21]. Most power supply module also ensures isolation of any reverse leakage and short-circuited power toward the main battery [22]. All ultrasonic sensors are sourced from +Vcc of the Arduino UNO. As shown in diagram the main power supply switch is also used as the restart switch of the system.

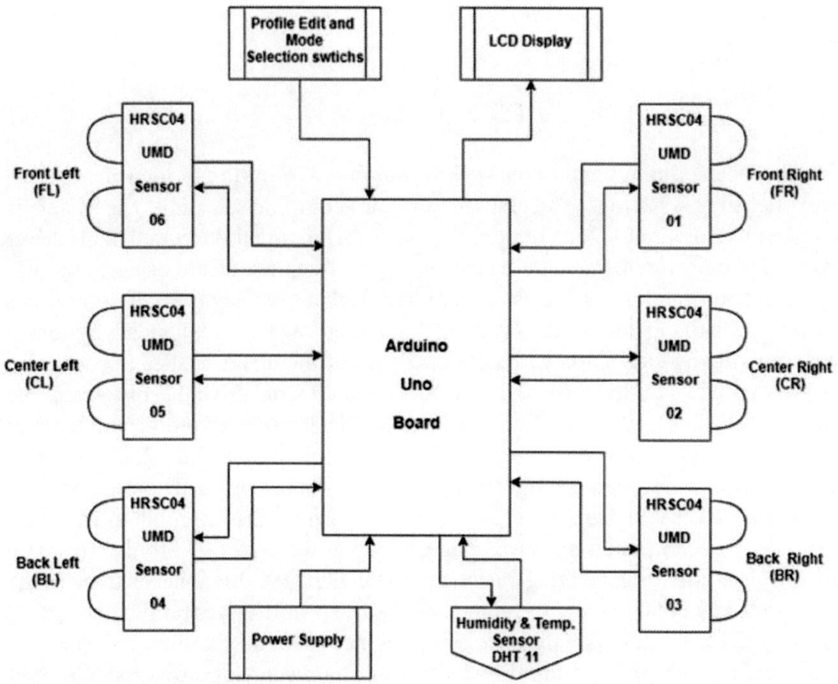


**Fig. 2** Block diagram of side-by-side system

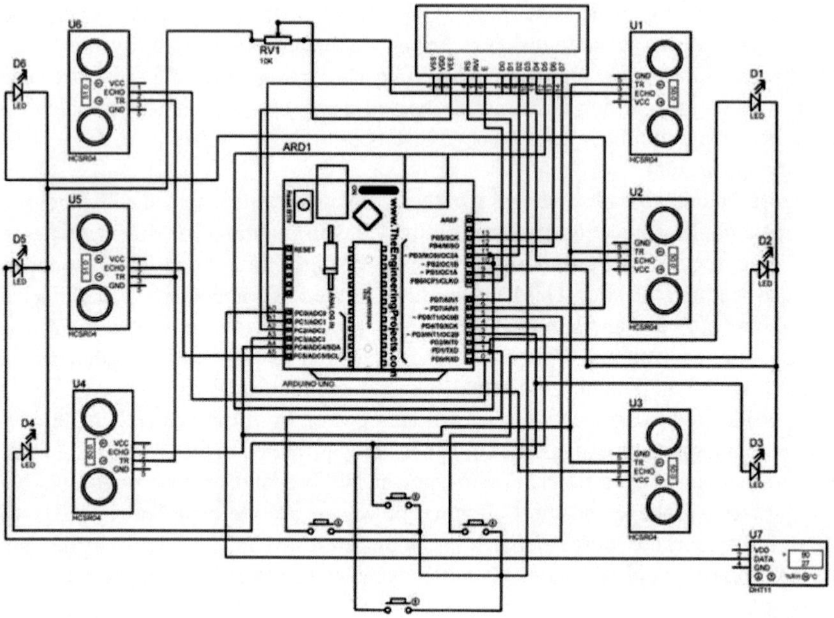


**Fig. 3** Circuit diagram

## 2.2 *Software*

Flowchart depicting program flow is shown in Fig. 4. Working of the software can be explained in 4 sections. The first section is driver profile selection. The system is designed to store up to 3 custom profiles for 3 drivers in addition to default driver profile. Once powered, the system enables default (maximum safe distance setting) profile as shown in Fig. 5a and asks to press the right arrow key (yes), if user wishes to continue with default profile. Pressing the right arrow key (yes), means system is ready for side-by-side alerts with default profile. If the driver wishes to customize the preset profiles of driver 01 or driver 02 or driver 03, the driver needs to press the left arrow key (No), to cancel loading default profile and select a profile number. For illustration purpose shown in Fig. 5b driver 01 profile initiate and asked for use of the driver profile 01, press the right arrow key (yes) for use driver 01 profile or if the driver pressed the left arrow key (No) will lead to load the driver profile 02 as shown in Fig. 5c, and the same way driver can reach up to the driver 03 profile. To set up any driver profile for generating customized safe alerts the driver needs to press the right arrow key (yes) to enter the edit mode. Once specific driver profile is selected, it is required to set new safe distance values in meters for all six ultrasonic sensors.

As shown in Fig. 5f, if the driver 01 profile is displaying now, and the right arrow key (yes) is pressed, it activates setup of driver 01 profile. It will allow editing threshold value for sensor 1, named front right (FR). One can edit the value using up

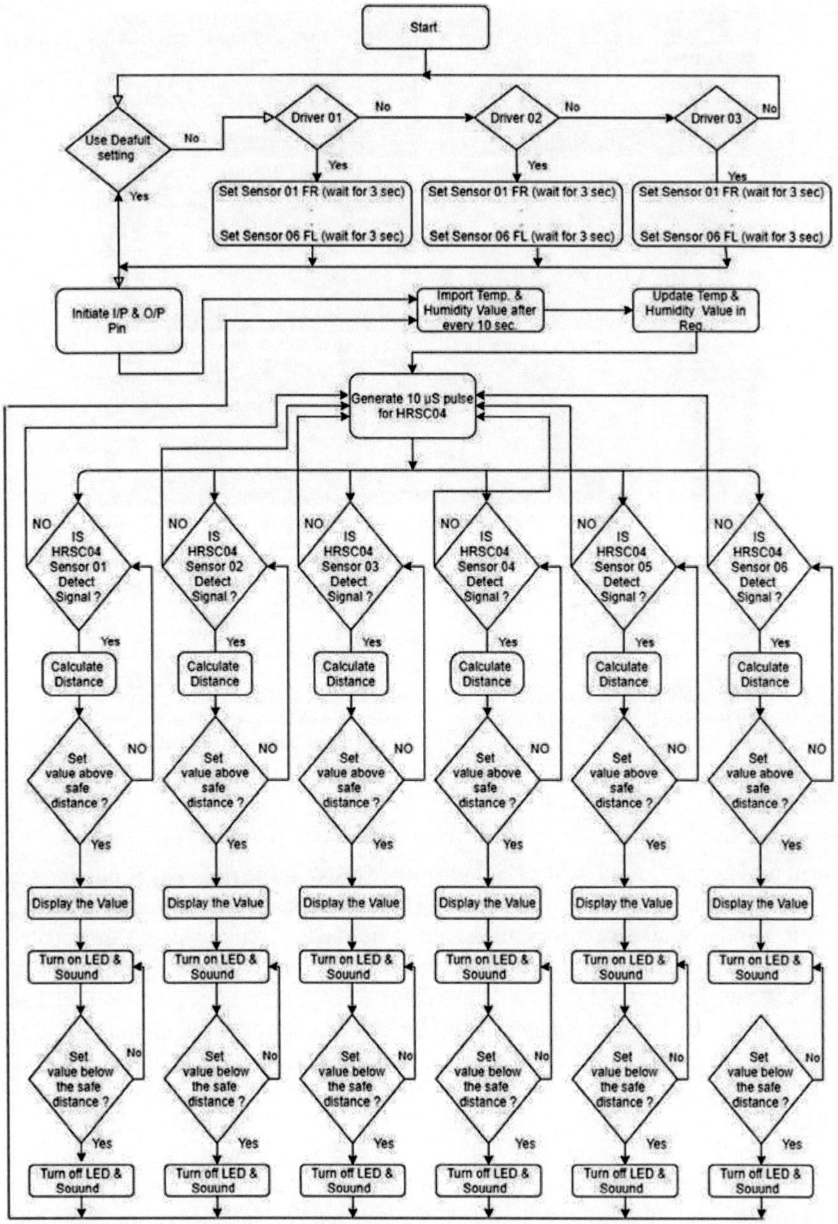


**Fig. 4** Flowchart representing embedded software written using Arduino IDE

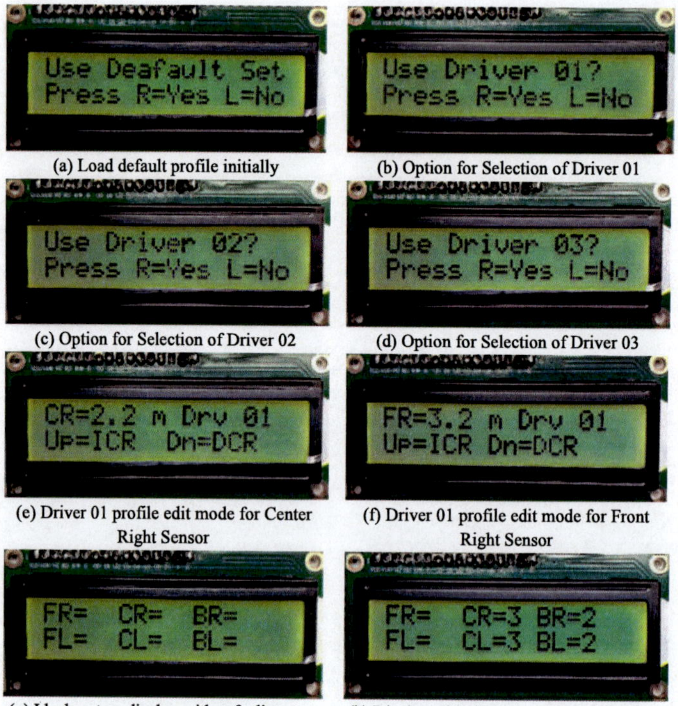


(a) Load default profile initially
(b) Option for Selection of Driver 01
(c) Option for Selection of Driver 02
(d) Option for Selection of Driver 03
(e) Driver 01 profile edit mode for Center Right Sensor
(f) Driver 01 profile edit mode for Front Right Sensor
(g) Ideal system display with safe distances
(h) Display with distance value, while alerts for unsafe distance are generated

**Fig. 5** Program execution on display

and down keys, followed by the right arrow key (Yes). If the right key is not pressed for 03 s after up or down arrow key, the last value displayed is saved against that sensor. Similarly, all six sensors' threshold values (safe distance values) are updated and then the system is ready to work on the road with a new driver's profile.

Once the driver profile is set, the second section of the program is executed configuring (A0) Arduino pin as input for temp & humidity sensor, digital pin D9 as trigger output for all ultrasonic sensors, analog pins (A1 to A5) & digital pin (D0) as echo inputs for six ultrasonic sensors, digital pins (D1-D6) for alert from each ultrasonic sensor, and pins (D7, D8, D10, D11, D12 & D13) to drive LCD.

For the third task, each individual ultrasonic sensor waits for detection of the reflected signal, measuring time of reflection. Humidity and temperature data are sampled and updated every 10 s, for corresponding compensation. Now, the calculation of distance is carried out using Eqs. 1 and 2.

The fourth section is for the alert generation. The calculated distances from each sensor are compared to the current safe distance value preset by the driver in the first section of software. If the calculated distance is below the preset safe distance, the calculated value is displayed on the alphanumeric LCD as well as the buzzer and corresponding LED are turned on to generate visible and audible alerts. These alerts continue until the side-by-side system finds the car in the safe distance zone.

Section two and three are looped to run indefinitely. In order to avoid annoying sound of buzzer during a traffic jam and distracting flashing of LED during the night, there is provision of disabling alerts, although it is not advisable to disable these alerts.

## 3 Result

The side-by-side system is tested for its operation in laboratory conditions. This side-by-side system is tested for a range of distances (1–4 m), for all six sensors individually. We carried out measurement of accuracy in the distance and time to detect the distance followed by the generation of alert. Also, we have tested the system for various sound reflecting surfaces. All the observations were initially carried out at 25 °C temperature with humidity <30%, and later in a closed cool environment with differing humidity.

The measured accuracy of all 6 sensors is penned in Table 2. We carried out measurement of distance for at least 3 times for a sensor at a distance to find the average value of error in measurement and accuracy in turn. Table 2 indicates measured distances (average), error and accuracy of measurement. The sensors offered least accuracy (98.5%) for distance 4 m, while the highest accuracy was recorded for a distance of 1.5 m (100%). The result also reveals that, the accuracy achieved in calculation is attributed to the compensation against change in temperature and humidity using DHT 11 sensor. The observations reveal the maximum amount of error not more than 15 mm/m. Also, delay in the generation of alert was measured for each distance in the range specified.

Table 3 indicates time of travel for ultrasonic waves for different distances as well as time to generate alert for the same distance. Here, it is found that travel time is in

**Table 2** Distance accuracy measurement

| Sr. no. | Manually applied Distance from sensor to object ($D_M$) (m) | System calculated distance from object to sensor ($D_s$) (m) | Mean difference of $\lvert D_M \sim D_s \rvert$ (m) | Accuracy of readings in percentage (%) |
|---|---|---|---|---|
| 1 | 4.00 | 3.94 ± 0.0216 | 0.06 | 98.5 |
| 2 | 3.50 | 3.46 ± 0.0251 | 0.04 | 98.8 |
| 3 | 3.00 | 2.99 ± 0.0081 | 0.01 | 99.6 |
| 4 | 2.50 | 2.47 ± 0.0163 | 0.03 | 98.8 |
| 5 | 2.00 | 1.99 ± 0.0057 | 0.01 | 99.5 |
| 6 | 1.50 | 1.5 ± 0.0416 | 0.00 | 100 |
| 7 | 1.00 | 0.99 ± 0.0057 | 0.01 | 99.0 |

**Table 3** Distance time observation and calculation

| Sr. no. | Manually applied distance from sensor to object ($D_M$) (m) | System calculated one-way travelling time ($T_s$) (ms) | Actual observed time take for alert generation ($T_{AL}$) (ms) |
|---|---|---|---|
| 1 | 4.00 | 13.56 | 27.78 |
| 2 | 3.50 | 12.01 | 23.18 |
| 3 | 3.00 | 10.31 | 21.32 |
| 4 | 2.50 | 08.57 | 18.11 |
| 5 | 2.00 | 06.88 | 14.71 |
| 6 | 1.50 | 05.14 | 12.34 |
| 7 | 1.00 | 03.42 | 7.47 |

**Table 4** Testing of the ultrasonic wave on different material used for automobile

| Sr. no. | Type of material tested | The system response for ultrasonic waves |
|---|---|---|
| 1 | Metal | Yes |
| 2 | Glass | Yes |
| 3 | Fiber/plastics | Yes |
| 4 | Chromium surface | Yes |
| 5 | Paper graphics | Yes |
| 6 | Rubber | Moderately |

proportion with the distance. Delay in the generation of alert is also increasing with distance.

Travel time and Delay in the generation of alert measurement were carried out using a digital oscilloscope. The travel time was found to be quite in line with the calculated value from Eqs. 1 and 2, considering ambient temperature and humidity.

This side-by-side system is also tested for different surface materials used in automobiles and surrounds the road environment to detect the reflection of sound waves. The result is satisfactory for reflection of ultrasonic waves as per listed in Table 4. The result reveals that the system works quite well with metal, glass, fiber, plastic, paper graphics, and chrome surfaces. On the other hand, rubber works as moderate reflector and sensors exhibit difficulty in calculating distance from echo signals.

## 4 Discussion

Accuracy and reliability are very important parameters because the system is expected to save lives. Any undetected warning or non-generated alert can lead to accident. Result tabulated above makes it sure that the system has performed well in test conditions and is reliable enough.

Distance measurement between the vehicles showed accuracy $\geq$98.5%, which is maximum $\pm$6 cm for the largest distance 4 m. For smaller distances $\leq$2 m the accuracy remains $\geq$99%, counting not more than 2 cm. This ensures reliable measurement and guarantees faithful alerts. Travelling time of waves match that of the theoretically calculated time and maximum delay in the generation of alert for a distance of 4 m was recorded to be 27.78 ms. For smaller distance the risk increases exponentially. For a distance of 1 m, the alert is generated in only 7.47 ms, giving a chance of safe survival. The time to alert in order of milliseconds (<30 ms) is considered very good. Hamdy Youssef Hussein Aly and Saud Salem Almusallam have reported a system with extended range of distance measurement up to 5 m [23]. Our system has been tested for distance up to 4 m with adequate accuracy, which is considerably sufficient for vehicle safety. The distance accuracy measurement carried out by Neeraja Soni et. al. exhibited 3.397% average error in distance measurement [24]. Our system design for ultrasonic distance measurement is inspired from previous work sited by P. Ramesh et. al. [25] and a web-based article [26]. Table 1 reveals an average error <1%, while our raw observations for the same table ensures maximum error of 2.34%. Another technique for distance measurement presented with title using IR Sensor for Distance Measurement in Mobile Robot [27] and Distance Measurement Systems Using Lasers and Their Applications [28], both researches required specific reflectance angle to detector for the reflected energy to measure accurate distance, this limitation is overcome by ultrasonic sensor. This means a significant improvement in accuracy of distance measurement. For side-by-side alerts system all materials tested for reflection response, except rubber, have shown good refection, resulting in quite good response of the sensors in terms of accuracy as well as alert time.

This System is tested in a laboratory environment. The results obtained from Laboratory test setup of side-by-side system alert are very accurate and promising with the level of satisfaction and serves purpose for which it is designed. The system is designed at very low cost. Such cost-effective system can be of great help to large scale transportations. On road testing is yet to be performed, and further permission of road transport authorities is to be obtained before deploying the system in cars on the road. As power is consumed from vehicle batteries, some electrical modifications are also required. As well detection of malfunctioning of any ultrasonic sensor and alert about the failure of said sensor to driver need to be integrated.

## 5 Conclusion

The system is proven in the laboratory and achieved the goal of safe distance alerts, this alert system generated faithful alerts in time and in turn to help reduce the number of accidents on roads. This system is applicable to vehicles with 4 or more wheels with construction material form fiber, metal, glass even chromium plating and paper graphics. We are in the process of improving the system with the interface of CAN network. In future, we are planning to connect & integrate the camera to create virtual graphics for the vehicle and show on the driver's floating display as an actual scenario of the safe distance. This Side-by-Side alert system will prove to be game changer for safety of vehicle, driver, passengers and loaded goods. This system will surely reduce on road accident, provide safe alerts in traffic jam, and financial burden on vehicle insurance company as well.

## References

1. Statista Homepage, https://www.statista.com/statistics/200002/international-car-sales-since-1990. Last accessed 30 Aug 2021
2. Bull AF (2013) Traffic congestion the problem and how to deal with it. United Nation Publication, Chile
3. Ministry of Road Transportation. https://transport.delhi.gov.in/content/rules-road. Last accessed 30 Aug 2021
4. Belcher RSF (2018) King of the road. Macmillan Publisher, New York
5. Zungeru AMF (2012) Development of an anti-collision model for vehicles. Int J Embedded Syst Appl (IJESA) 2(4):21–34
6. Shinde TF (2013) Car anti-collision and intercommunication system using communication protocol. Int J Sci Res (IJSR) 2(6):187–191
7. Shival DF, Abdul Wahid AS (2013) Design and development of vehicle anti-collision system using electromagnet and ultrasonic sensors. Int J Theoret Appl Res Mech Eng (IJTARME) 2(1):80–83
8. Carullo AF, Parvish MS (2001) An ultrasonic sensor for distance measurement in automotive applications. IEEE Sens J 1(2):143–149
9. Christofer NF, Cid Mathew SAS (2017) Analysis of obstacle detection using ultrasonic sensor. Int Res J Eng Technol (IRJET) 4(1):1015–1019
10. Manpreet KF, Jai PS (2015) Distance measurement of object by ultrasonic sensor HC-SR04. Int J Sci Res Dev 3(5):503–505
11. Takahiro MF, Naoto WS (2013) Simultaneous measurement of air temperature and humidity based on sound velocity and attenuation using ultrasonic probe. Jpn J Appl Phys 52(7)
12. Vadim AZF, Dimitrov LS (2018) Application of ultrasonic sensor for measuring distances in robotics. In: International conference information technologies in business and industry 2018, Journal of Physics Conference Series 1015, pp 1–9. IOP Publishing
13. Matthews TF (2018) Humid heat and climate change. Prog Phys Geogr Earth Environ 42(3):391–405
14. Arduino uno hardware detail, https://docs.arduino.cc/hardware/uno. Last accessed 23 Aug 2021
15. Anju Latha N, Rama Murthy B, Bharat Kumar K (2016) Distance sensing with ultrasonic sensor and Arduino. Int J Adv Res Ideas Innov Technol 2(5):1–5
16. L. Shenzhen PENPOS Technology Co. (2014) HR-Sc04 Datasheet. Last accessed 11 Aug 2021
17. Shenzhen PENPOS Technology Co., DHT11 Humidity & Temprature Sensor Data sheet. Last accessed 11 Aug 2021
18. XIAMEN AMOTEC DISPLAY CO., Specification of LCD Module, ADM1602K-NSW-FBS/3.3V Data sheet. Last accessed 11 Aug 2021
19. Kamweru Paul KF, Owino Ochieng RS, Mutinda Mutava GT (2020) Monitoring temperature and humidity using Arduino Nano and Module-DHT11 sensor with real time DS3231 data logger and LCD display. Int J Eng Res Technol (IJERT) 9(12):466–422
20. Deeksha SF, Awanish KS, Shivani DT (2018) Measurement of temperature and humidity by using Arduino. Int Res J Eng Technol (IRJET) 5(12):876–878

21. Vikram KF, Viswaprakash BS (2017) Embedded smart car security system on face detection. Int J Comput Commun Technol 5(3):176–180
22. Sunitha MF, Vinay Kumar VS, Raghu GT (2014) Embedded car security system. Int J Eng Dev Res 2(1):1126–1131
23. Hamdy Youssef Hussein AF, Saud Salem AS (2019) Maximizing range using ultrasonic sensor and Arduino. J Eng Res Appl 9(3):17–27
24. Neeraja SF, Sarita CS, Garima ST (2017) Distance measurement using ultrasonic sensor and Arduino. Int J Eng Sci Comput 7(3):5991–5992
25. Ramesh PF, Sudheera SS, Vinay Reddy DT (2021) Distance measurement using ultrasonic sensor and Arduino. J Adv Res Technol Manage Sci 3(2):1–5
26. Allied Electronics, Arduino Uno Datasheet A00066. Last accessed 11 Aug 2021
27. Benet GF, Blanes FS, Simó JET (2020) Using Infrared sensors for distance measurement in mobile robots. Robot Auton Syst 40(4):255–266
28. Fonseca JA, Baptista A, Martins MJ, Torres JP (2017) Distance measurement systems using lasers and their applications. Appl Phys Res 9(4):33–43

# Diagnosis of Epilepsy Disease with MRI Images Analysis and EEG Signal Processing

**Golnoush Shahraki and Elyas Irankhah**

**Abstract** Today, brain signals (EEG), CT Scans, and MRI images are the methods for diagnosing Epilepsy disease, and methods such as surgery, medication, and electrode implants are used to treat the disease, but there is not diagnosis exactly. At this time, we have tried to find a way for early diagnosing by combining the features of image processing and EEG signal processing with each other. At first, linear and nonlinear features have been extracted from the brain signals and MRI images, and then the degree of similarity and compatibility of features with each other has been examined and finally are evaluated by the neural networks. Based on the obtained results, the percentage of neural network (Elman) accuracy of brain signals between normal and mild persons is 73.8%, between normal and severe persons is 78.2% and between mild and severe persons is 72.9%. Also, the percentage of neural network (MLP) accuracy in image processing between normal and mild persons is 81.3%, between normal and severe persons is 84.3% and between mild and severe persons is 79.3%. Finally, the results of the combination in the percentage of accuracy between normal and mild persons is 84%, between normal and severe persons is 89% and between mild and severe persons is 85.7%. Hopefully, based on these results, this method will be developed by different methods in EEG signal processing and MRI image processing in the disease.

**Keywords** Epilepsy disease · MRI images · EEG signals · Neural networks

G. Shahraki
Department of Biomedical Engineering, Islamic Azad University of Mashhad, Mashhad, Iran

E. Irankhah (✉)
Department of Mechanical Engineering, University of Massachusetts Lowell, Lowell, MA, USA
e-mail: Elyas_Irankhah@student.uml.edu

 
T. Triwiyanto et al. (eds.), *Proceedings of the 2nd International Conference on Electronics, Biomedical Engineering, and Health Informatics*, Lecture Notes in Electrical Engineering 898, https://doi.org/10.1007/978-981-19-1804-9_40

# 1 Introduction

Epilepsy is a neurological disease, known as a disorder of the central nervous system and is associated with loss of consciousness and seizures. This disease is caused by unusual electrical discharge in this group of people, which leads to uncontrollable movements, seizures, and loss of consciousness[1].

According to researches, this disease is one of the disorders caused by the central nervous system [2], also genetic, familial, and metabolic disorders play a major role in this disease [3]. Epilepsy can be diagnosed through neurological tests, blood tests, brain signals [4], CT scans, MRI images, PET scans (SPECT MEG) [5], and magnetoencephalography [6].

There are several ways to reduce the prevention of this disease, but it cannot be said that treatment is definitive, including medication [7], surgery [8], Vagus nerve stimulation, ketogenic diet [9], deep brain stimulation [10]. Nowadays, because the brain signals measurement methods are generally cost-effective and it is easier to diagnose this disease on the frequency of brain signals, it has been used more in the treatment of such diseases. In this case, in the processing of brain signals, the importance of neural networks in processing is considered a lot, most of which are implemented by MATLAB or Python softwares. Based on all previous researches in this field, in which they have been presented their methods, it looks like one of the intuitive disadvantages among them is accuracy percentage. Where in this study, tried to improve it by more sufficient results and achieve high accuracy percentage, however, because of running this method in this paper, we had to do more process and get more details, whereas, they could be so useful for achieving the main purpose [11]. Obviously, the procedure based on combination of medical image processing with the brain signals is able to utilize in another diseases like Alzheimer, Parkinson as well as Apnea [12].

Finally, using medical images, especially MRI, along with brain signals can speed up processing in neural networks and give us important results [13]. Moreover, as probably you know, when we are using the combination of biomedical image/signal processing, we are able to extract more details such as statistical features in the signals frequency, or even images color features, where they enter in neural networks as per inputs, the results percentage will be outcome from the neural networks. Hence, these methods are so important for us for utilizing by developing and also implementing them in the upcoming researches.

# 2 Materials and Method

## *2.1 Dataset*

In this paper with the optimal EEG signal and MRI image processing and also the combination of features together, we will feature an appropriate solution for

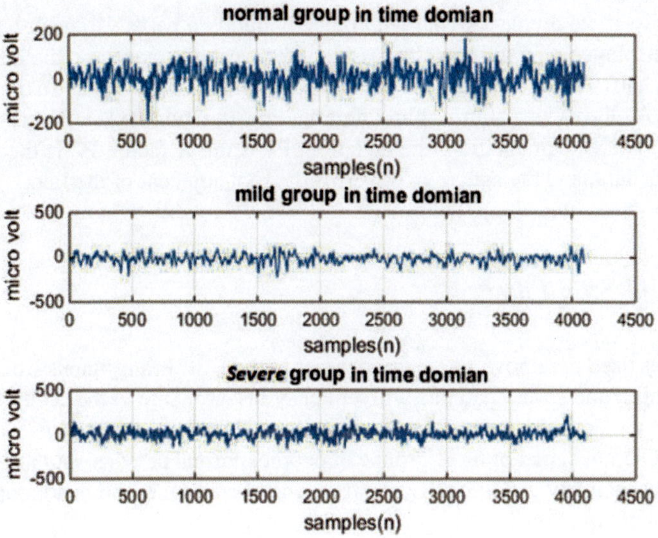


**Fig. 1** The performance of the EEG brain signal in the time domain (from above, respectively, normal persons, mild, and severe patients)

early diagnosing epilepsy disease. In order of data that is utilized in this study, the EEG signal/MRI images data set are from the public online data set which is called physionet[1] where we have extracted the data from 20 people in three group of normal people, mild patients and, severe patients. The all data have been processed by MATLAB software.

## 2.2 *Display the EEG Brain Signals in the Time Domain 5*

The EEG brain signals are important vital signals in humans that can be processed to obtain a lot of information about brain function. Figure 1 shows the EEG brain signals of normal persons, mild, and severe patients with epilepsy disease over time.

As mentioned earlier, by processing these vital signals and transmitting them into the frequency domain, brain function can be studied and analyzed.

## 2.3 *Segmentation*

Generally, the first step for signal processing is using the Segmentation filter, due to the volume of the data set. This will greatly help a researcher in signal processing.

[1] https://physionet.org/.

Accordingly, if we divide a signal with range X into two parts X1 and X2, and both parts are displayed on a different basis, this information is placed on the line X = Y in the first half. This means that the X1 and X2 signals are the same. To do this, just use TCF (Toolbox Curve Fitting) and find the line equation f(x) = P1 (x) + P2 (x) where f(x) is the segmentation line equation, P1 is the X factor, P2 is the width of origin, X is data, and the square of the error the root adjacent of the line.

## 2.4 *Band-Stop Filter*

This filter is used to remove single frequencies in the EEG brain signals from normal persons, mild, and severe patients with epilepsy disease. Due to the accuracy of the single-frequency component, is an accurate filter. Therefore, we have used this filter on the EEG brain signal of three groups of people, normal persons, and mild, severe patients, respectively. Additionally, the frequency response of the band-stop filter is in the form of equation.

$$H(jw) = \begin{cases} k & f_c = 50 \\ 0 & f\langle 50,\ f\rangle 50 \end{cases} \tag{1}$$

## 2.5 *Band-Stop Filter*

The composition of a low-pass filter with a high-pass filter will create a band-pass filter. The band-pass filter is used to separate the frequency bands, which are performed in five frequency bands of the EEG brain waves (according to Table 1).

Also, in this section, to eliminate low-frequency noise (transpiration) and eliminate municipal power noise, a filter with a cut-off frequency of 0.001–45 Hz has been utilized, which increases the quality and performance accuracy of the processing for the next steps. The frequency response of this filter is as follows in Eq. (2).

**Table 1** Maximum EEG brain signals power in frequency bands

| Frequency bands | Maximum power | | | | |
|---|---|---|---|---|---|
| | Delta | Theta | Alpha | Beta | Gamma |
| Normal people | 3/25 | 1/84 | 4/12 | 0/11 | 0/0014 |
| Mild patients | 1/48 | 4/13 | 1/00 | 1/22 | 0/0018 |
| Severe patients | 2/81 | 1/00 | 1/28 | 0/50 | 0/005 |

$$H(jw): \begin{cases} K, & f_H < f < F/L \\ 0, & f > F/L\,and\,f < F/L \end{cases} \quad (2)$$

In accordance with the three groups, the frequency bands in the EEG brain signals have been shown in order of a, b and c groups.

a. Normal group **2**: The brain of this group are so healthful and intact without any problem in their EEG brain signals (Fig. 2).

b. Mild group **3**: In this group there are some problems and unhealthful signs in their EEG brain signals (Fig. 3).

c. Severe group **4**: In the group, their EEG brain signals have shown so many harmful signs and problems (Fig. 4).

In Table 1 we have maximum power results from the bands, which is shown in three groups.

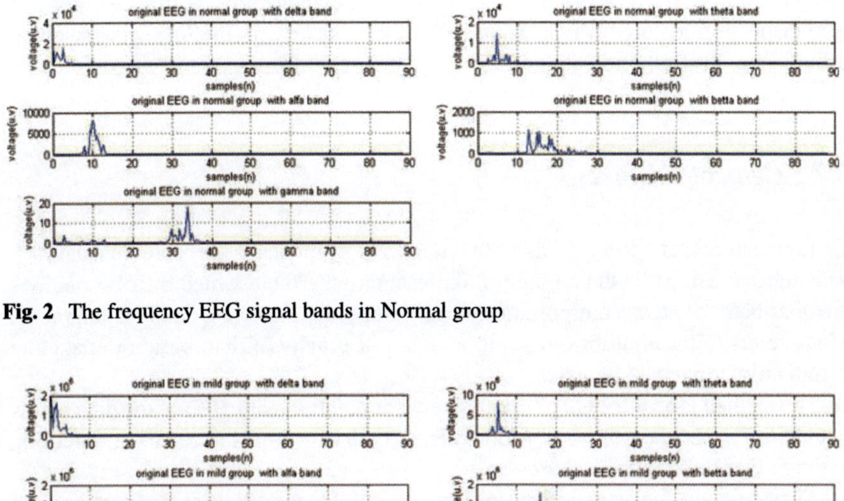


**Fig. 2** The frequency EEG signal bands in Normal group

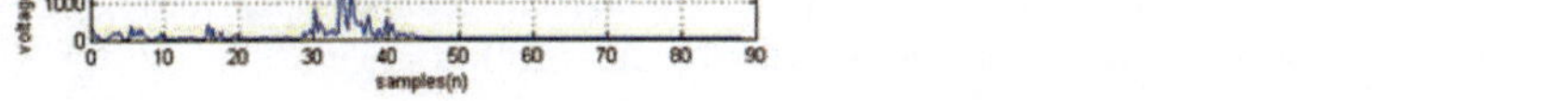


**Fig. 3** The frequency EEG signal bands in Mild group

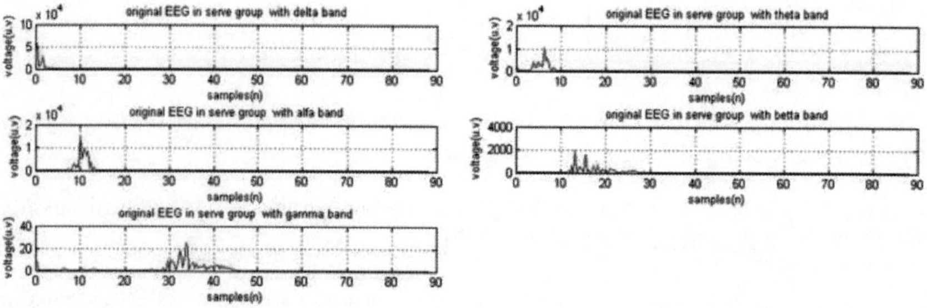


**Fig. 4** The frequency EEG signal bands in Severe group

## 2.6 *Statistical Features*

Statistics is a scientific method used to collect, analyze, interpret, and generally to study and evaluate observations. Statistical features are divided into two general categories. In terms of these features, it has been extracted the central features and also dispersion features which they are described clearly. In the following, we will provide more information about these two statistical features.

## 2.7 *Central Features*

Central features refer to any numerical criterion that represents the center of a data set. This means that this is the amount of representation around which the observations are distributed. The most important central features are the mean, median, and mode. Mean refers to the equilibrium point or center of gravity of distribution in data that is regularly aligned on an axis.

The median is an attribute of the statistical population with 50% of the data below it and 50% of the data above it. Mode refers to the value that has the most repetition among other distribution values.

As mentioned above, one of the important central features is mean. Mean is one of the first indicators that is calculated for random variables and statistical models so that it can be used to approximate the expected value of a random variable. The calculation of the mean can be defined based on the mathematical expectation operator and for the number of $N$ samples for the random variable $X$ as follows (3):

$$E[X] = \int_{-\infty}^{\infty} xf(x)dx \ and \ \mu_x = \frac{1}{N}\sum_{i=1}^{N} x_i \tag{3}$$

where $N$ indicates number of case samples in which for random variable $X$ indicator.

## 2.8 Dispersion Features

Dispersion features are indices that show the average distance and proximity of distribution data to their average. This helps to describe a series of data more accurately and also helps to compare two or more sets of data. Among the most important scattering features, we can mention the maximum, minimum, standard deviation, and variance. Maximum refers to the maximum amount of data and vice versa refers to the minimum amount of data.

The standard deviation shows how far the average data is from the average value. This index is used to correct the defects of previous indicators. The variance in this mean deviation index from the mean is used instead of the absolute value of the square of two deviations. Another case of extracting statistical features of variance is that a random variable based on the mathematical hope operator is defined as the central second anchor where $M_2$ has been known as variance and $\mu_x$ as a mean indicator (4).

$$M_2 = E\left[(x - \mu_x)^2\right] = \int_{-\infty}^{\infty} (x - \mu_x) f(x) \tag{4}$$

In addition, for the number of $N$ samples of variance, a random variable is defined as follows (5):

$$\frac{1}{N-1}\sum_{i}^{N}(x_i - \overline{x})^2 \; and \; \frac{1}{N}\sum_{i}^{N}(x_i - \overline{x})^2 \tag{5}$$

## 2.9 Conformity

Conformity determines the degree of similarity in the frequency domain, in which the horizontal axis determines the frequency component and the vertical axis determines the percentage of similarity. This value will be obtained to simultaneously measure the phase difference between two recorded signals regardless of their amplitude. This value will be obtained from Eq. (6).

$$Coh(f) = \left| \frac{\sum_{i=1}^{N} F_1(f).F_2^*(f)}{\sum_{i=1}^{N} |F_1(f)|^2 . \sum_{i=1}^{N} |F_1(f)|^2} \right|^2 \tag{6}$$

## 2.10 Covariance (7)

In probability theory, the magnitude of the coordinated changes of two variables is random. (If the two variables are the same, the covariance will be equal to the variance). For random variables X and Y whose mathematical expectation is E (x) = μ and E (y) = v, covariance is defined as follows:

$$E(X.Y) = E(X).E(Y), Cov(X, Y) = 0 \tag{7}$$

It should be noted that the opposite is not true, meaning that the covariance of two random variables may be zero, but the two random variables are not independent.

## 2.11 Correlation (Temporal Similarity)

Operational correlation is mathematical which is very similar to convolution. On the interrelationship between two energy signals, the intensity of similarity between these two signals is measured.

If a signal is correlated with itself, it is called self-correlated. Assume that x (n) and y(n) each have a certain energy, the correlation between which is calculated as Eq. (8).

$$\begin{cases} \sum\limits_{n=0}^{n-m-1} (X_n + mY_N) & m \geq 0 \\ R_{x,y}(-m) & m \leq 0 \end{cases} \tag{8}$$

In this regard, m = ..., −2, −1, 0, 1, 2, ... and an index that shows time changes and possible delays. On the other hand, according to the subtitle x, y, which one is written first, shows the direction of changes of one variable in terms of another. These characteristics are the maximum value of the moment when the maximum value occurs.

The center of gravity, the equivalent width, and the mean square of the length represent the correlation fraction in R(m).

## 2.12 Return Map

The purpose of drawing a Return map is to find the points of the collision on the vital signals relative to the previous samples, current samples, and next samples. The Return map is called the phase diagram, which according to the drawing in three-dimensional space if it is on a straight line in the drawing of the diagram, means that the previous sample and the next sample are similar.

The farther the phase diagram is from the straight-line curve and the closer it is to the circle, the more the current signal is dissimilar to the before and after signals. When these samples are placed on a straight line, it means that the signal becomes linear, which indicates disease, and the farther they are from the straight line, the more similar the frequency, so the lower the similarity (Fig. 5).

## 3 Image Processing

As mentioned earlier, another indicator that can help diagnose epilepsy disease is the use of MRI images. First, we show MRI images of a normal person and a patient with epilepsy disease. These images are shown in Fig. 6.

### *3.1 Noise Remove in MRI Images 7*

This optimizer and filter eliminates all kinds of noise in an image to an acceptable level and gives us a clearer image. The way to eliminate noise in this command is to check the multi-pixel system next to each other and get the average color.

The most color in the image is the main color of the image, and noise is always the least amount of color in an image, so the color of the pixels that are far from the average color in a part of the image is the same as the color of the noise. The software changes them to the average color (Fig. 7).

### *3.2 Binary Images 8*

Images that have only two colors black and white and only the numbers zero and one are in their matrix are called binary images. The simplest processing is done on these images because it has reduced volume and increased speed processing, and this is only due to the single-bit pixels of these types of images (Fig. 8).

### *3.3 Square Matrix Mean Filter 9*

Commonly, we cannot filter an entire image at the same time. Thus, an image should be divided into small networks and each network should be filtered individually. This filtering is done on the whole image, so for a filter, we just need to design a square matrix grid of the desired size and then use this filter with functions.

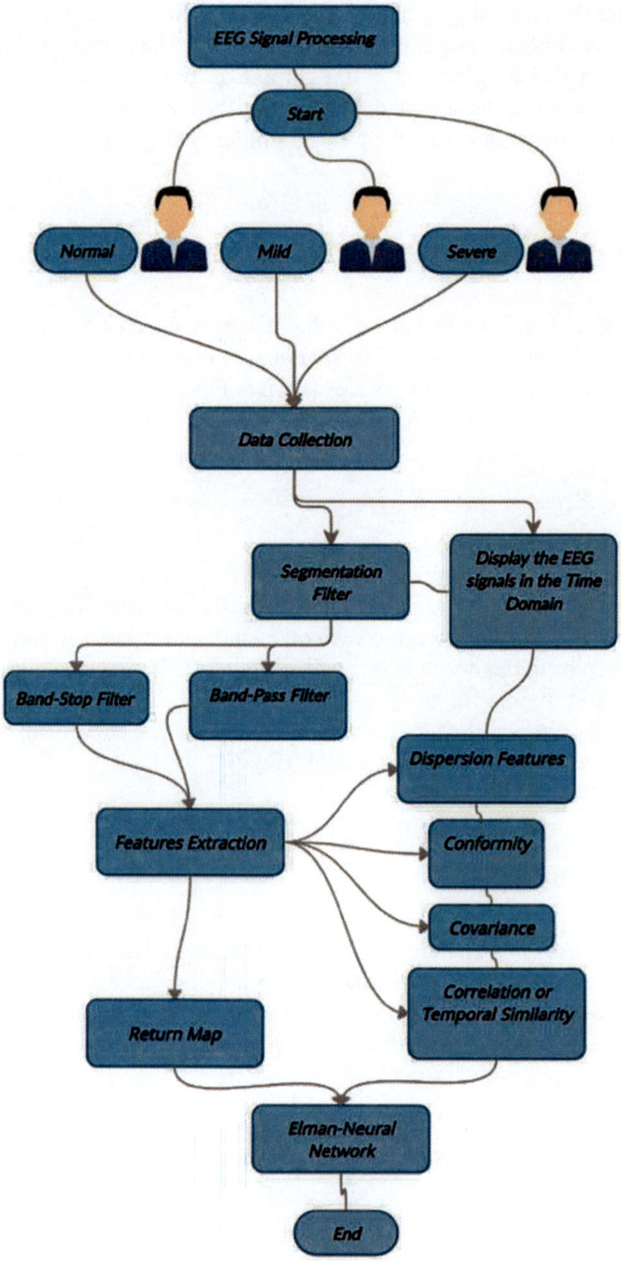


**Fig. 5** The block diagram of signal processing section

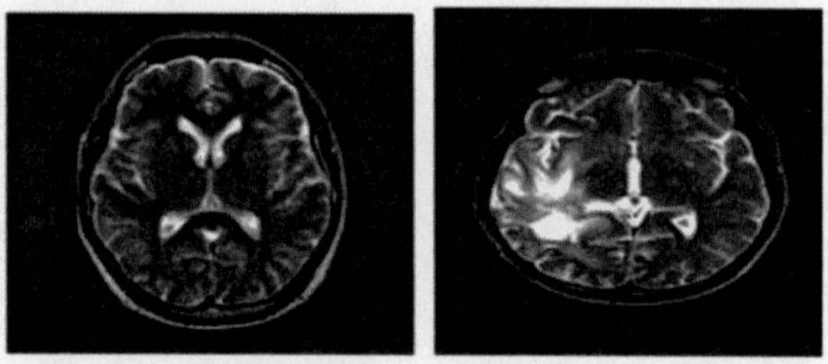

**Fig. 6** Left image (normal person), right image (epileptic patient)

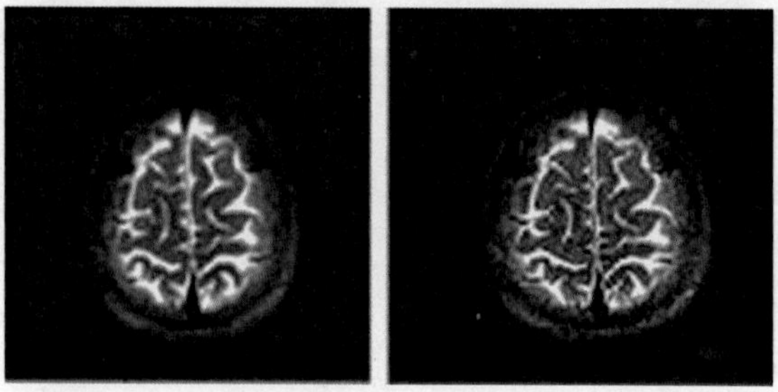

**Fig. 7** Left image (after noise remove), right image (with noise)

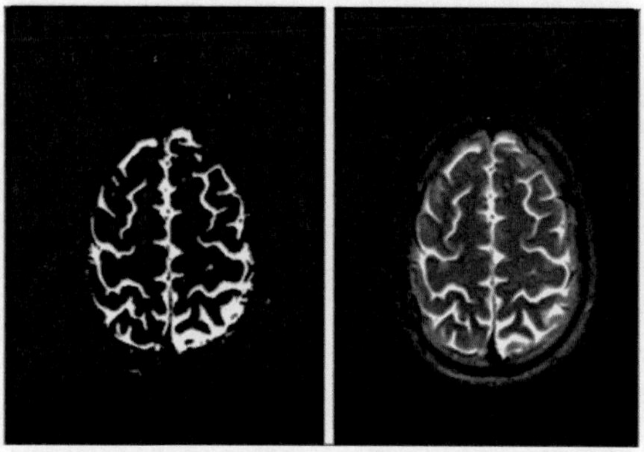

**Fig. 8** Left image (after binary image), right image (before binary image)

This filter causes the image to blur. The larger the size of our square matrix in the average algorithm, the larger the filter matrix grid and the more blur the image (Fig. 9).

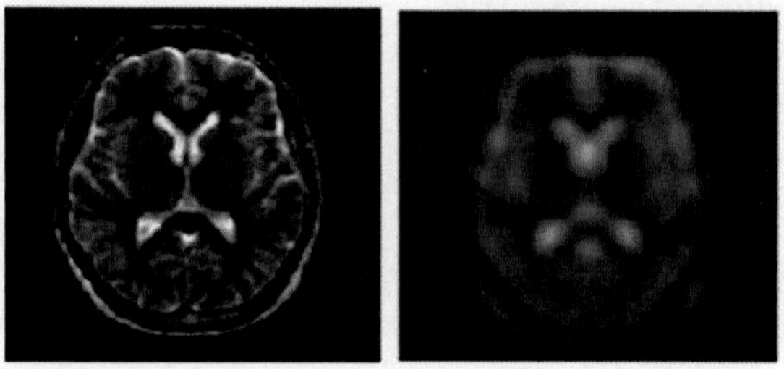

**Fig. 9** Left image (before SMM filter), right image (after SMM filter)

## 3.4 Filters to Increase Light Intensity and Edge (9)

This filter works the reverse algorithm of the average and increases the light in the image and its edges. The sharpness and brightness of the image can be determined by a value of a. This value can be changed between zero and one.

The value of a is the alpha in the following algorithm. The value of $\alpha$ is 0.2 by default.

$$Filter = \frac{1}{\alpha + 1}\begin{bmatrix} -\alpha & \alpha - 1 & -\alpha \\ \alpha - 1 & \alpha + 5 & \alpha - 1 \\ -\alpha & \alpha - 1 & -\alpha \end{bmatrix}. \tag{9}$$

## 3.5 Compression

The goal of real compression is to minimize the number of bits needed to display it, which will help a lot in image processing. This is while storing information of acceptable quality. In this study, we saved the image in matrix mode after compression.

## 3.6 Neural Networks

Neural networks are one of the most widely used and valid methods in engineering applications today. In the following, we have utilized neural networks to evaluate the performance and investigate these methods and the neural networks are Elman Neural Network and MLP Neural Network.

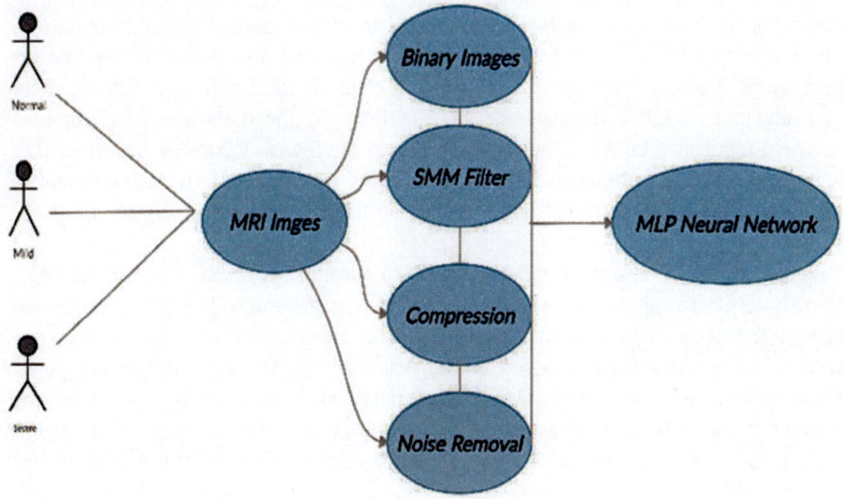


**Fig. 10** The block diagram of image processing

## *3.7 Elman Neural Networks*

Elman neural network generally have two layers, with one feedback from the output of the first layer (hidden) to the input of the first layer. This feedback to the network helps to detect and generate time-varying patterns. The reason for using the Elman neural network is the recursive feature because at each stage the weights are modified and there are also several features in the hidden layer of the neural network. The more use the neurons in the hidden layer, the more it adapts to the case function and causes to increase accuracy.

## *3.8 MLP Neural Network 10*

In this neural network, the number of latent neurons are about 28. The neural network is three-layer and recurrent and the error regulation range is 5% (Fig. 10).

# 4 Results

Since there is no definitive treatment for this disease, this study has tried to help the early diagnosis of the disease by combining two methods of EEG brain signal processing and MRI image processing by examining the statistical features central and scattering. The statistical feature of mode has shown these changes more noticeably. Examination of frequency characteristics in five brain bands shows that on average, the highest value in all three normal states is mild and severe in the delta band, and the lowest value in these three states is in the theta band. In scattered statistical features (standard deviation, variance) the lowest values in all three cases are normal persons, mild, and severe patients in the gamma band. In the image statistical features, MAT image property have been used to evaluate the percentage of information accuracy [14].

According to the results, the percentage of neural network accuracy on the EEG brain signals between the two classes of normal persons and mild patients is 73.8%, between the two classes of normal persons and severe patients is 78.2% and between the two classes of mild and severe patients is 72.9%. Besides, the percentage of neural network accuracy on the MRI image processing between the two classes of normal persons and mild patients is 81.3%, and between the two classes of normal persons and severe patients is 84.3% and between the two classes of mild and severe patients is 79.3%.

Eventually, the percentage of neural network accuracy on the EEG brain signals and their combination with image processing between two classes of normal persons and mild patients is 84%, between two classes of normal persons and severe patients is 89%, and between two classes of mild and severe patients is 85.7% (Fig. 11).

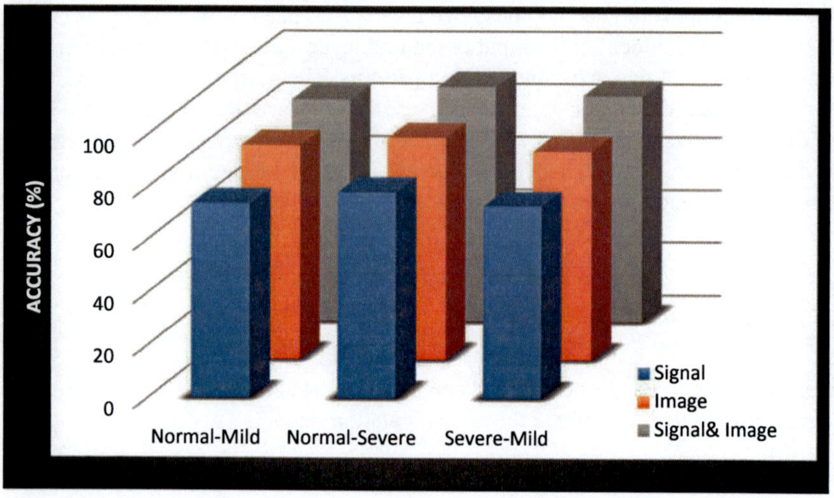


**Fig. 11** The output of NN accuracy percentage between the groups

## 5 Discussion

Based on the studies in this field, a lot of research has been done on brain signals. Among them, we can mention the study [15] in which using EEG signals and conversion of discrete-wavelet-transform (DWT) into several sub-bands in EEG signals by Shannon entropy and k-nearest neighbor (KNN) to classify data to diagnose Autism and Epilepsy diseases [16, 17].

In other research, researchers have tried to automatically diagnose epilepsy using convolutional neural networks and find a way to help doctors speed up the diagnosis. One of the most important point in this research is the use of combining convolutional neural network with brain signals [18, 19].

One of the diagnostic goals in epilepsy is to extract features that can be obtained from the patient's brain signals. Such as research [20] which uses low density-electrical source imaging (LD-ESI) and high density-electrical source imaging (HD-ESI) methods from 82 patients, gives useful results. Researchers are always trying to diagnose the disease through brain signals using a convenient and low-cost method. And they are always looking for a model in this field to present it [21].

In addition to research on brain signals, some researchers have tried to use medical images to provide a diagnostic model for the disease. One of the medical images used in this regard is MRI images. Feature extraction from such images gives us valuable results and they could help us to early diagnosis [22, 23]. Today, epilepsy is one of the diseases that researchers believe that extracting the features of brain signals along with medical images is a way forward in this field [24].

Applying these methods along with clinical trials is a big step in diagnosing this disease. The use of methods such as surgery and medicine is currently practical, but therapeutic and diagnostic methods in research are moving towards early diagnosis by combining image processing with the brain signals [25, 26].

As you see, in evaluating the other studies, this study was able to improve the results such as results of neural networks in the three groups on different frequency bands based on this method (Fig. 12).

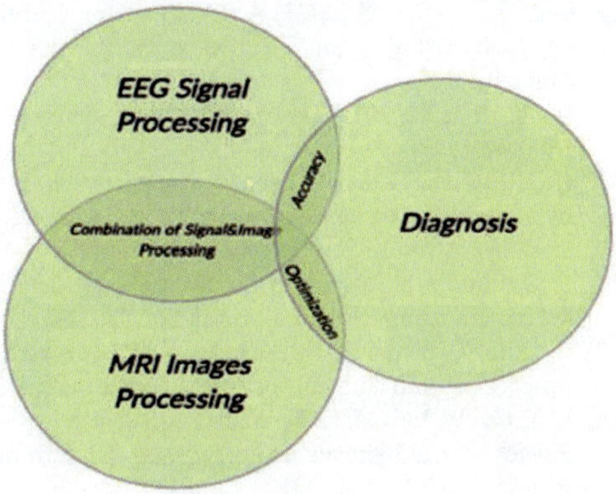


**Fig. 12** Combination of image and signal processing

## *5.1 Conclusion*

In this study, due to the combination of the EEG brain signals characteristics and MRI images features, the percentage of accuracy has improved and increased, but compared to the separate case, the percentage of accuracy has not changed significantly. Obviously, for having a high accuracy percentage, it would be to process more on the dataset to gain more details as well as results. To improve the accuracy of neural network function, the filters implemented in the images can be replaced or an optimization algorithm can be used to extract optimal features in the EEG brain signals and MRI images, such as GA, PCA, or analysis as well as ANOVA.

## References


1. Peker M, Sen B, Delen D (2016) A novel method for automated diagnosis of epilepsy using complex-valued classifiers. IEEE J Biomed Heal Inf
2. Annegers JF, Rocca WA (1996) Causes of epilepsy: Contributions of the rochester epidemiology project. In: Mayo clinic proceedings
3. Shorvon SD (2011) The causes of epilepsy: changing concepts of etiology of epilepsy over the past 150 years. Epilepsia
4. Chen G, Xie W, Bui TD, Krzyżak A (2017) Automatic epileptic seizure detection in EEG using nonsubsampled wavelet–fourier features. J Med Biol Eng
5. Ramli N, Rahmat K, Lim KS, Tan CT (2015) Neuroimaging in refractory epilepsy. Current practice and evolving trends. Eur J Radiol
6. Anderson CT, Carlson CE, Li Z, Raghavan M (2014) Magnetoencephalography in the preoperative evaluation for epilepsy surgery. Curr Neurol Neurosci Rep
7. Moshé SL, Perucca E, Ryvlin P, Tomson T (2015) Epilepsy: new advances. PubMed J
8. Blümcke I et al (2016) International recommendation for a comprehensive neuropathologic workup of epilepsy surgery brain tissue: a consensus task force report from the ILAE Commission on Diagnostic Methods. Epilepsia
9. Guerrini R et al (2015) Diagnostic methods and treatment options for focal cortical dysplasia. Epilepsia
10. McIntyre CC, Chaturvedi A, Shamir RR, Lempka SF (2015) Engineering the next generation of clinical deep brain stimulation technology. Brain Stimulation
11. Brari Z, Belghith S (2021) A novel machine learning model for the detection of epilepsy and epileptic seizures using electroencephalographic signals based on chaos and fractal theories. Math Probl Eng
12. Irankhah E (2020) Evaluation of early detection methods for alzheimer's disease. Bioprocess Eng
13. Ge HW, Qian F, Liang YC, Du W, Wang L (2008) Identification and control of nonlinear systems by a dissimilation particle swarm optimization-based Elman neural network. Nonlinear Anal Real World Appl
14. S. Saminu et al., A recent investigation on detection and classification of epileptic seizure techniques using eeg signal. Brain Sci, (2021).
15. Ibrahim S, Djemal R, Alsuwailem A (2018) Electroencephalography (EEG) signal processing for epilepsy and autism spectrum disorder diagnosis. Biocybern Biomed Eng
16. Li Y, Cui W, Luo M, Li K, Wang L (2018) Epileptic seizure detection based on time-frequency images of EEG signals using gaussian mixture model and gray level co-occurrence matrix features. Int J Neural Syst

17. Choubey H, Pandey A (2019) A new feature extraction and classification mechanisms For EEG signal processing. Multidimens Syst Signal Process
18. Wei Z, Zou J, Zhang J, Xu J (2019) Automatic epileptic EEG detection using convolutional neural network with improvements in time-domain. Biomed Signal Process Control
19. Acharya UR, Oh SL, Hagiwara Y, Tan JH, Adeli H (2018) Deep convolutional neural network for the automated detection and diagnosis of seizure using EEG signals. Comput Biol Med
20. Foged MT et al (2020) Diagnostic added value of electrical source imaging in presurgical evaluation of patients with epilepsy: a prospective study. Clin Neurophysiol
21. Sharmila A (2018) Epilepsy detection from EEG signals: a review. J Med Eng Technol
22. Rüber T, David B, Elger CE (2018) MRI in epilepsy: clinical standard and evolution. Curr Opin Neurol
23. Wiest R, Beisteiner R (2019) Recent developments in imaging of epilepsy. Curr Opin Neurol
24. Xiong Z et al (2021) A study on seizure detection of eeg signals represented in 2d. Sensors
25. Lopes MA, Perani S, Yaakub SN, Richardson MP, Goodfellow M, Terry JR (2019) Revealing epilepsy type using a computational analysis of interictal EEG. Sci Rep
26. Yao X, Li X, Ye Q, Huang Y, Cheng Q, Zhang GQ (2021) A robust deep learning approach for automatic classification of seizures against non-seizures. Biomed Signal Process Control

# AutoSpine-Net: Spine Detection Using Convolutional Neural Networks for Cobb Angle Classification in Adolescent Idiopathic Scoliosis

**Wahyu Caesarendra, Wahyu Rahmaniar, John Mathew, and Ady Thien**

**Abstract** The Cobb angle measurement in adolescent idiopathic scoliosis is prone to inter- and intra-observer variations. This paper proposes a deep learning architecture for detection of spine vertebrae from X-ray images to automatically evaluate the Cobb angle, and to assess for the presence of scoliosis and severity of the curvature. The public AASCE MICCAI 2019 anterior–posterior X-ray image dataset was used for training and testing of the proposed convolutional neural network architecture. Seventeen vertebrae were detected from the input image to obtain 68 landmark features of the spine. The obtained landmarks were processed to measure the Cobb angle and to assess whether scoliosis was present. The severity of the curvature was further classified into mild, moderate and severe, if scoliosis was present. The results showed that the proposed algorithm has a classification accuracy of approximately 0.9 (90%). This architecture may be used as a tool to augment Cobb angle measurement in X-ray images of patients with adolescent idiopathic scoliosis in a real-world clinical setting.

**Keywords** Convolutional neural network · Deep learning · Scoliosis · Cobb angle · Vertebrae

W. Caesarendra (✉)
Faculty of Integrated Technologies, Universiti Brunei Darussalam, Jalan Tungku Link, Bandar Seri Begawan 1410, Brunei Darussalam
e-mail: wahyu.caesarendra@ubd.edu.bn

W. Rahmaniar
Department of Electrical Engineering, National Central University, Zhongli, Taoyuan, Taiwan

J. Mathew · A. Thien
Department of Neurosurgery, Brunei Neuroscience, Stroke and Rehabilitation Centre, Pantai Jerudong Specialist Centre, Jerudong, Brunei Darussalam

 
T. Triwiyanto et al. (eds.), *Proceedings of the 2nd International Conference on Electronics, Biomedical Engineering, and Health Informatics*, Lecture Notes in Electrical Engineering 898, https://doi.org/10.1007/978-981-19-1804-9_41

# 1 Introduction

Adolescent idiopathic scoliosis (AIS) is an abnormal curvature, in which the spine curves abnormally from side to side and rotates. The Cobb measuring method is the gold standard used in quantifying the curve. The Cobb angle (CA) is measured from the most tilted vertebra (end vertebra) above and below the apex (most laterally placed vertebra) of the curve on radiographs taken either in the anterior–posterior or the posterior-anterior view on the coronal plane [1]. Generally, the manual procedure requires lines to be drawn onto a hardcopy of radiographic films and the angle between the two lines are measured using a protractor (Fig. 1).

In addition to being time consuming, CA measurement of spine is unreliable [2] and is associated with inter-observer and intra-observer variations [3]. Reported accuracies of measuring CA vary from 2° to 11° [4–6] with measurements differing up to 5° even with the same end vertebrae selected [4, 7]. The emergence of computerized digitization of radiographs has allowed for semi-automatic assessment of CA where the picture archiving and communications system (PACS) allows for an in-built function enabling the user to digitally draw the lines for the end vertebrae and the system automatically measures the CA. This has shown to have good reliability and

**Fig. 1** Measurement of Cobb angle (CA)

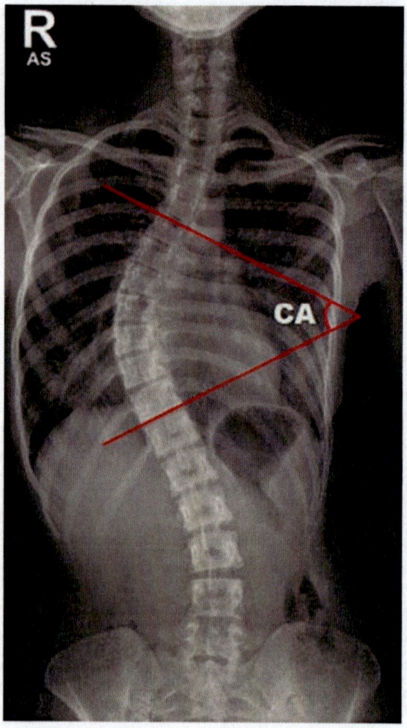

less variations compared to the manual method [6, 8]. However, this is method is still dependent on the manual inputs from the user.

The availability of an accurate reproducible CA measurement method is important as the assessment of the CA is used to diagnose AIS and to guide decisions regarding curve progression as well as therapeutic options including surgical interventions. In addition, the method has be user-friendly and takes less time compared to the manual and semi-automatic methods.

The development of computer vision technologies [9], machine learning methods [10, 11], and deep learning methods [12–14] led to attempts for the transition from traditional and semi-automatic CA assessment to automated CA measurement. In this instance, the X-ray images were processed by means of computerized learning method to enable CA measurement and prediction. The various machine learning methods used in scoliosis clinical practice, including screening, diagnosis and classification, have previously been reported [11]. Vertebrae detection is an important stage to identify the landmarks of interest on the spine image for CA measurement. Studies on the vertebrae and spine detection based on machine learning methods [10, 11] and deep learning methods [12–14] have been previously reported. Bernstein et al. showed that a neural network (NN) can be applied to automatically train the vertebrae centroids detection [10]. However, automatic detection of the vertebrae in X-ray images can be difficult. Computer vision task is challenging in X-rays compared to computed tomography (CT) and magnetic resonance imaging (MRI) images due to multiple overlapping shadows of the ribs and pelvis, as well as, a differences in contrast between thoracic and lumbar vertebrae regions [15, 16]. Convolutional neural network (CNN) architecture can help overcome this problem [10]. Researchers in the field of deep learning (DL) have previously develop fully automated methods for Cobb angle measurement (Table 1). The methods had successfully detected and segmented the vertebrae and the spine. However, most of the studies

**Table 1** Brief summary of selected papers in CA measurement using deep learning methods

| References | Image processing methods and the procedures | Method |
|---|---|---|
| [12] | 1. Vertebrae isolation and detection<br>2. Drawing spinal curve line<br>3. Vertebra rectangle segmentation | CNN |
| [13] | 1. Usage of Moire screening system to obtain the curve<br>2. Fitting the curve to the 17 position using cubic B-spline<br>3. Calculate the two contact points of three lines perpendicular to the curve<br>4. Define the middle vertebrae<br>5. Calculate the angle | CNN |
| [14] | 1. Use picture archiving and communication systems<br>2. Consider the orientation of the overall spinal curve<br>3. Identify the max angle between the superior perpendicular of the cranial<br>vertebrae and the inferior perpendicular of the caudal vertebrae at the longitudinal central lines of the vertebral bodies | R-CNN |

were not collaborated with the clinicians and the results obtained were not compared with measurements made in the real-world setting.

In this paper, we propose a CNN for spine vertebra detection, CA evaluation and curve severity classification in AIS. The main objective is to automate and augment (1) the detection and the assessment of the CA, and (2) the confirmation of presence of scoliosis, based on standard spine X-ray images. The severity of the scoliosis is also classified into mild (10°–25°), moderate (>25° to 40°), and severe (> 40°).

## 2 Proposed Method

### 2.1 Datasets

The collection and labelling of spinal images were performed by the public AASCE MICCAI 2019 anterior–posterior X-ray images dataset [17]. The input images vary in sizes from 359 × 973 to 1427 × 3755. Each image contains 17 vertebrae from the thoracic (upper spine) and lumbar (lower spine). The image input resolution is set to 1024 × 512 for the algorithm development. A total of 962 images are used as follows, 481 images for training, 323 images for validation, and 158 images for testing are used. Each vertebrae is located by 4 corner landmarks. The ground-truth of the 68 landmarks or points in each image is provided by the dataset.

### 2.2 System Overview

The 50-layer ResNet [18] is used to classify 68 landmarks to obtain the corner offset of spine. This CNN consists of several convolutional layers that learn the local features of the images and generate the classifications. The proposed network (Fig. 2) includes

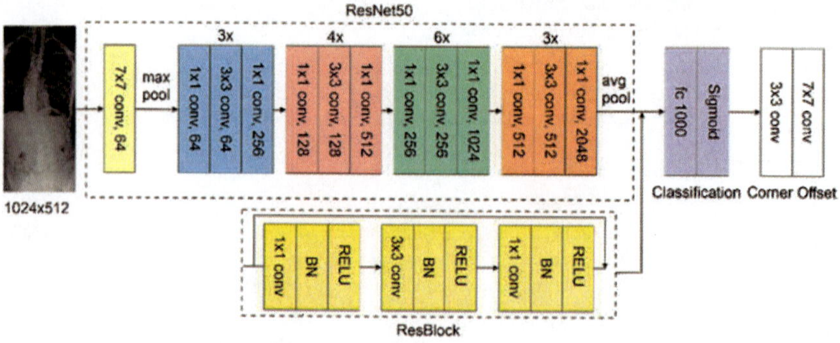


**Fig. 2** Vertebrae detection network

pooling layers (average pool and max pool), classification, and corner offset. Combination of semantically similar features into a single feature reduces the dimensions of the extracted features and fully connected layers, and gives a final probability value for the class. Network depth has been previously shown to be beneficial to classification accuracy [19]. However, its performance can become saturated with resultant rapid decrease in performance as the network gained greater depth. This issue can be fixed by the ResNet framework [20] where a shortcut connection is added for every three convolution layers across the deep network. These shortcut connections performed identity mapping without additional parameters which can increase computational complexity. This simplification of network optimization during the training process enables ResNet to achieve a higher accuracy from deeper networks when performing image classification tasks.

The ResNet50 architecture is mainly composed of residual blocks (Fig. 2). Residual connection in ResNet architecture maintains connection to gain knowledge during training and speed up model training time by increasing network capacity. Batch normalization with ReLU activation is added for each convolutional layer. Bi-cubic interpolation is used as upscaling method. The skip connection technique is performed to exploit high-level semantic information and low-level fine details to improve model performance.

During the training process, a fine-tuning technique is applied to transfer the connection weights from the pre-trained model to our model and retrain the model to the current task. This model accepts an image as input and performs a fully connected layer as a final assessment. Finally, the model outputs the bounding box of each target object as well as the corresponding category label.

The X-ray images used contain 17 vertebrae, where each vertebrae has 4 corner landmarks: top-left, top-right, bottom-left and bottom-right. Therefore, each image has a total of 68 landmarks. The order of the landmarks is used to accurately localize the vertebrae, so that the slope of each can be known. The landmarks were separated into different groups to obtain an output feature map with a channel number of 68. Then, a heat map of the center point [21] is constructed to obtain a corner offset maps using a convolutional layers for landmark localization.

Landmarks of each corner of the vertebrae were obtained using the corner offset. The corner offset was obtained from the center of the heat map to the vertebrae margin using L1 loss to optimize the corner offset at the midpoint.

### 2.3 Cobb Angle Measurement for Classification

A review study on the classification of AIS is presented in [22]. The Author reviewed the clinical classification of AIS from a few previous studies. It mentioned that the classification provides a better and more reliable tool to assist surgeons in determining the appropriate method of treatment for certain curve pattern. In addition, with the developing methods in 3D reconstruction may be used as a basis classification for new therapeutic concepts [22].

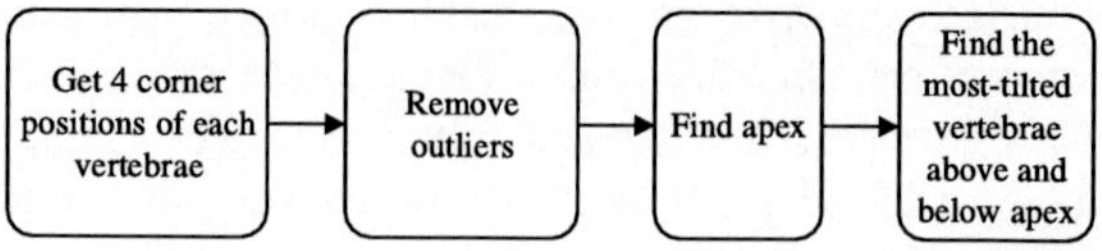


**Fig. 3** CA measurement for classification

In this study, the application of CNN for AIS classification is presented. The steps to calculate the CA from the position of each corner found is presented in Fig. 3. After detecting an object on the X-ray image, detected bounding boxes are displayed on the spine. Boxes with a score of more than 0.5 were extracted. From the location of the detected boxes, the center point of each vertebrae is found to remove some outliers based on the anatomy of spine, where the adjacent vertebrae should not be far apart from each other. If the x-axis center of the detected bounding box is more than half the width of the box from the x-axis center of its two closest neighbors (top and bottom), the box is rejected as an outlier. Otherwise, the position of the box is reconsidered based on the position of the nearest boxes.

Following this, the depth of the curve at the found position of the corner box is calculated. For each of the two vertebrae, the distance between the bottom-left point of the upper box and the top-left of the lower box, and the bottom-right point of the upper box and the top-right of the lower box is calculated. The apex of the spinal is found as the deepest part of the curve.

For each box above the apex, the slope of each vertebrae is measured based on the position between top-left and top-right to detect the most-tilted vertebrae above the apex. For each box below the apex, the slope of each vertebrae is measured based on the position between bottom-left and bottom-right to detect most-tilted vertebra below the apex. The Cobb angle is then calculated as the angle of the intersection between two lines from the most-tilted vertebrae above the apex and most-tilted vertebrae below the apex.

## 3 Results

The datasets was trained on the RTX2060 GPU with Intel Core-i7 processor. Figure 4 shows the performance of the training dataset and the validation dataset when training the network. The models are initialized from the pre-trained weights on ImageNet. The network was trained with a learning rate of 0.0001 with Adam optimizer during training. The batch and epoch sizes are set as 2 and 100, respectively.

Figure 5 shows the result of the detection of vertebrae in the spine on the X-ray images. The condition of the patient's spine is classified as normal if the measured CA is less than 10°. For mild, moderate, and severe AIS, the CA measurements are 10° to 25°, >25° to 40°, and >40°, respectively.

The performance metrics comparison of the four classes is summarized in Table 2. *Precision rate* (*PR*), *Recall*, and *F*1-*measure* [23] can be computed as follows:

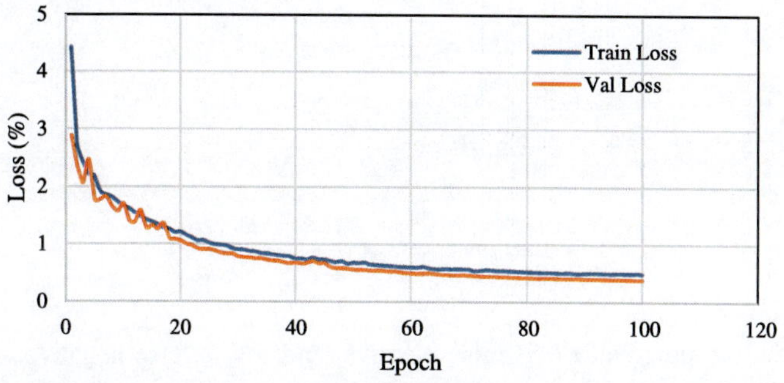


**Fig. 4** Performance of the dataset in network training

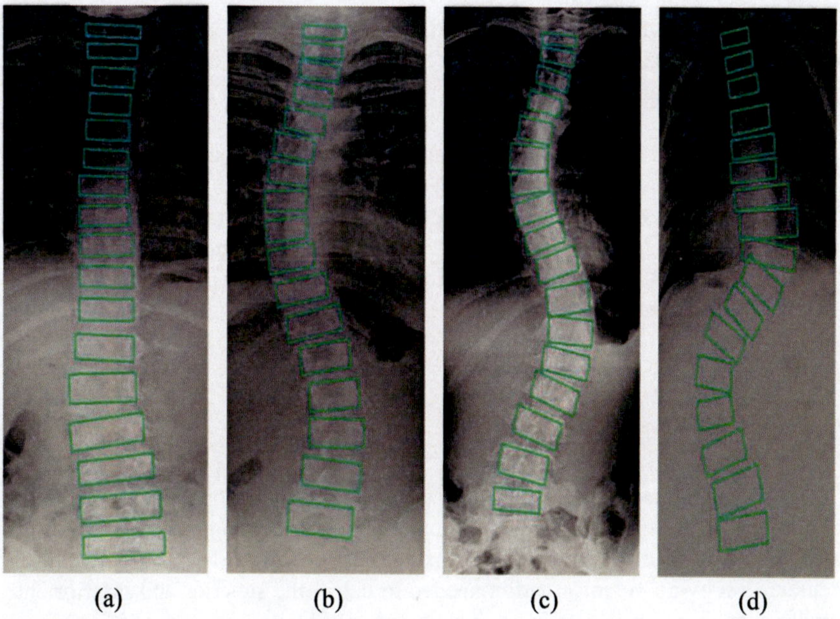


**Fig. 5** Detection results: **a** normal, **b** mild, **c** moderate, and **d** severe

**Table 2** Performance metrics comparison

| Class | Accuracy results | | |
|---|---|---|---|
| | PR | Recall | F1-measure |
| Normal | 0.92 | 0.89 | 0.9 |
| Mild | 0.95 | 0.93 | 0.94 |
| Moderate | 0.94 | 0.89 | 0.91 |
| Severe | 0.9 | 0.8 | 0.84 |
| Average | 0.92 | 0.87 | 0.9 |

$$PR = \frac{TP}{TP + FP} \tag{1}$$

$$Recall = \frac{TP}{TP + FN} \tag{2}$$

$$F1 - measure = 2 \times \frac{PR \times Recall}{PR + Recall} \tag{3}$$

where *TP* is true positive, *FP* is false positive, and *FN* is false negative. *TP* is the detected area of the vertebrae and corresponds to the associated class. *FP* is the detected area not associated with the vertebrae. *FN* is the area associated with the vertebrae that is not detected.

Severe AIS has the lowest *PR*, *Recall*, and $F1$-*measure* compared to the other classes. The increase in the curvature made it difficult for the vertebrae to be detected in the area of the arch. In some cases, the vertebrae is completed undetected or misrepresented.

Mild AIS has the highest *PR*, *Recall*, and *F1-measure* compared to other classes. The network can detect the vertebrae well as the spine is not too curved. In addition, the X-ray images have good lighting and contrast conditions for this class of spine in our dataset. Normal spine has lower accuracy than mild AIS as some image conditions for this class are not optimum. This resulted in a high number of *FP* and *FN* in the detection.

## 4 Discussion

The proposed architecture using CNN accurately detected the location of each of the 17 vertebrae in the spine X-ray. In addition to this, the bounding box was evaluated to be sufficient in its accordance with the vertebra positions. Its performance was accurate to provide the information needed to detect the superior and inferior end vertebrae, enabling the CA to be evaluated correctly.

The detection results also showed that the proposed architecture can be used to identify the vertebrae in X-ray images of different contrast and lighting conditions. Our test on several images with poor contrast and lighting conditions yielded good results. Importantly, CA measurements and curve classification were able to be accurately accomplished even when the detection process failed to identify one or two vertebrae. This is was a key part of the algorithm as X-ray images may come in different contrast and lighting qualities in the clinical setting, depending the severity of the curve as well as the patient's body habitus.

Previous studies using CNN [12–14] focus on vertebrae detection and measurement of CA under certain conditions but did not classify the severity of scoliosis. The method we proposed was able to measure CA from normal to severely scoliotic spine (up to 81°). This was an important step as severely abnormal curvatures were often difficult to detect.

There are some limitations to our study. In this proposed CNN, more errors in detection had occurred in images where the X-ray were of different sizes and when it involved larger areas from the neck to the hip which were not important landmarks for vertebrae detection. Further improvements with automatic image cropping to satisfy the conditions for optimal vertebrae detection is ongoing. Lastly, the results from this CNN were not validated against the clinicians' CA measurements (which remains the gold standard). This important final step will be crucial in confirming that this CNN will be capable in augmenting the specialist clinician's ability to accurately measure CA and may be used as a tool for non-specialist clinicians and nurses to assess CA in AIS patients.

## 5 Conclusions

A convolutional neural network for vertebrae spine detection, Cobb angle measurement and curvature severity classification in X-ray images of adolescent idiopathic scoliosis is proposed in this paper. The detection of vertebrae and classification had an accuracy of 0.9 (90%). Upon clinical validation, this architecture may be used as tool to augment Cobb angle measurement in X-ray images of patients with adolescent idiopathic scoliosis in a real-world clinical setting. A developed CNN method is also possible to be implemented for the real-time assessment or monitoring of scoliosis patients in the future [24].

**Funding** This project was supported by The AO Spine National Research Grant 2020 [AOSEA(R)2020–05].

## References

1. Cobb J (1948) Outline for the study of scoliosis. Instr Course Lect 5:261–275
2. Wu H, Bailey C, Rasoulinejad P, Li S (2018) Automated comprehensive adolescent idiopathic scoliosis assessment using MVC-Net. Med Image Anal 48:1–11
3. De Carvalho A, Vialle R, Thomsen L, Amzallag J, Cluzel G, le Pointe HD, Mary P (2007) Reliability analysis for manual measurement of coronal plane deformity in adolescent scoliosis. Are 30 × 90 cm plain films better than digitized small films? Eur Spine J 16(10):1615–1620
4. Carman DL, Browne RH, Birch JG (1990) Measurement of scoliosis and kyphosis radiographs: intraobserver and interobserver variation. J Bone Joint Surg 72(3):328–333
5. Cheung J, Wever DJ, Veldhuizen AG (2002) The reliability of quantitative analysis on digital images of the scoliotic spine. Eur Spine J 11:535–542
6. Shea KG, Stevens PM, Nelson M (1998) A comparison of manual versus computer-assisted radiographic measurement intraobserver measurement variability for Cobb angles. Spine 23:551–555

7. Morrissy RT, Goldsmith GS, Hall EC, Kehl D, Cowies GH (1990) Measurement of the Cobb angle on radiographs of patients who have scoliosis. Evaluation of intrinsic error. The J Bone Joint Surg Am 72(3):320–327
8. Chockalingam N, Dangerfield PH, Giakas G, Cochrane T, Dorgan JC (2002) Computer-assisted Cobb measurement of scoliosis. Eur Spine J 11:353–357
9. Aroeira RM, de Las Casas EB, Pertence AE, Greco M, Tavares JM (2016) Non-invasive methods of computer vision in the posture evaluation of adolescent idiopathic scoliosis. J Bodyw Mov Ther 20(4):832–843
10. Bernstein P, Metzler J, Weinzierl M, Seifert C, Kisel W, Wacker M (2021) Radiographic scoliosis angle estimation: spline-based measurement reveals superior reliability compared to traditional COBB method. Eur Spine J 30:676–685
11. Chen K, Zhai X, Sun K, Wang H, Yang C, Li M (2021) A narrative review of machine learning as promising revolution in clinical practice of scoliosis. Ann Transl Med 9(1):1–16
12. Horng MH, Kuok PC, Fu M (2019) Cobb angle measurement of spine from X-ray images using convolutional neural network. Comput Math Methods Med 19(2019):6357171
13. Choi R, Watanabe K, Jingufi H (2017) CNN-based spine and Cobb angle estimator using Moire images. IIEEJ Trans Image Electron Vis Comput 5(2):35–144
14. Pan Y, Chen Q, Chen T (2019) Evaluation of a computer-aided method for measuring the Cobb angle on chest X-rays. Eur Spine J 28(12):3035–3043
15. Huang SH, Chu YH, Lai SH, Novak CL (2009) Learning-based vertebra detection and iterative normalized-cut segmentation for spinal MRI. IEEE Trans Med Imaging 28(10):1595–1605
16. Glocker B, Zikic D, Konukoglu E, Haynor DR, Criminisi A (2013) Vertebrae Localization in Pathological Spine CT via Dense Classification from Sparse Annotations. In: Mori K, Sakuma I, Sato Y, Barillot C, Navab N (eds) Medical image computing and computer-assisted intervention—MICCAI 2013. MICCAI 2013. Lecture Notes in Computer Science 8150. Springer, Berlin, Heidelberg, pp 262–270
17. AASCE—Grand Challenge Hompage. https://aasce19.grand-challenge.org/. Last accessed 30 Aug 2021
18. He K, Zhang X, Ren S, Sun J (2016) Deep residual learning for image recognition. In: 2016 IEEE conference proceedings on computer vision and pattern recognition (CVPR). IEEE, Las Vegas, NV, USA, pp 770–778
19. Szegedy C, Liu W, Jia Y, Sermanent P, Reed S, Anguelov D, Erhan D, Vanhouche V (2015) Going deeper with convolutions. In: 2015 IEEE conference proceedings on computer vision and pattern recognition (CVPR). IEEE, Boston, MA, USA, pp 1–9
20. He K, Sun J (2015) Convolutional neural networks at constrained time cost. In: 2015 IEEE conference proceedings on computer vision and pattern recognition (CVPR). IEEE, Los Alamitos, CA, USA, pp 5353–5360
21. Yi J, Wu P, Huang Q, Qu H, Metaxas DN (2020) Vertebra-focused landmark detection for scoliosis assessment. In: 2020 IEEE 17th international symposium on biomedical imaging (ISBI). IEEE, Iowa City, IA, USA, pp 736–740
22. Ovadia D (2013) Classification of adolescent idiopathic scoliosis (AIS). J Children's Orthop 7:25–28
23. Rahmaniar W, Wang W-J (2019) Real-time automated segmentation and classification of calcaneal fractures in CT images. Appl Sci 9(1):3011–3028
24. Jung JY, Bok SK, Kim BO, Won Y, Kim JJ (2015) Real-time sitting posture monitoring system for functional scoliosis patients. Lecture Notes Electr Eng 339:391–396

# Upper Limb Exoskeleton Using Voice Control Based on Embedded Machine Learning on Raspberry Pi

**Triwiyanto Triwiyanto, Syevana Dita Musvika, Sari Luthfiyah, Endro Yulianto, Anita Miftahul Maghfiroh, Lusiana Lusiana, and I. Dewa Made Wirayuda**

**Abstract** Generally, upper limb exoskeletons are controlled using the EMG signal; however, the EMG signal is influenced by the position of the electrodes, as well as muscle fatigue. Therefore, another alternative to control the upper limb exoskeleton is required. The purpose of this study is to develop an upper limb exoskeleton based on voice control using embedded machine learning on Raspberry Pi. Moreover, this study compared two feature extraction methods namely mel-frequency cepstral coefficient (MFCC) and zero-crossing (ZCR). Two classifiers, namely K-nearest Neighbor (K-NN) and Decision Tree (DT) were evaluated to obtain the best model in recognition of voice command. The exoskeleton development consists of 3D upper limb exoskeleton, microphone, Raspberry Pi 4B+, PCA9685 servo driver, and servo motor. Microphone was used to record the given voice commands. This study found that the combination between MFCC feature and K-NN classifier resulted the highest accuracy ($96 \pm 4.0\%$). Additionally, when the model was embedded on the Raspberry Pi to execute the voice command, the accuracy of the classifier is $92.0 \pm 7.37\%$ and $84.0 \pm 4.97\%$ for up and down command, respectively. The development of an upper limb exoskeleton based on voice control can be used for rehabilitation purposes whether it is applied in a hospital or privately at home.

**Keywords** Exoskeleton · Strokes · Machine learning · Feature extraction · Mel-frequency cepstral coefficient · Zero-crossing rate

## 1 Introduction

Upper-limb consists of shoulder complexity, elbow complexity, wrist complexity [1]. Movement disorders of the hands and arms in general can be caused by stroke, fractures and damage to ligaments [2]. According to the results of the 2018 Basic

T. Triwiyanto (✉) · S. D. Musvika · S. Luthfiyah · E. Yulianto · A. M. Maghfiroh · L. Lusiana · I. D. M. Wirayuda
Poltekkes Kemenkes Surabaya, Jl. Pucang Jajar Tengah No. 56, Surabaya 60282, Indonesia
e-mail: triwi@poltekkesdepkes-sby.ac.id



T. Triwiyanto et al. (eds.), *Proceedings of the 2nd International Conference on Electronics, Biomedical Engineering, and Health Informatics*, Lecture Notes in Electrical Engineering 898, https://doi.org/10.1007/978-981-19-1804-9_42

Health Research (RISKESDAS) conducted by the Health Research and Development Agency of the Ministry of Health of the Republic of Indonesia. Facts prove that the prevalence of stroke patients is increasing from year to year [3]. According to the World Health Organization (WHO), stroke is the third leading cause of paralysis [4], where the possibility of paralysis in the upper extremities is very high. Stroke sufferers require continuous medical care and therapy. Repetitive functional movement is one of the safe and effective methods to regain limb mobility [5]. In addition, exoskeletons have the potential to be used in providing therapy for a long period of time regardless of skill and fatigue compared to manual therapy. Furthermore, the exoskeleton is a tool that can increase human performance [6]. These assistive devices can be in the form of lower extremities (legs), upper extremities (hands), back or the whole body that can be controlled via actuators, such as electric motors, pneumatics, hydraulics, or a combination of technologies [7]. In the medical field, the exoskeleton can help with the rehabilitation process from stroke or spinal cord injury. The hardware design of existing exoskeletons often causes user discomfort and is not designed as a permanently wearable device [1]. Therefore, the design has to be improved so that it is comfortable to wear the exoskeleton for a longer period of time without discomfort. Generally, the EMG signal is widely used as an input signal to the exoskeleton controller [8].

There have been many studies that have developed various exoskeletons that can assist the rehabilitation process for upper extremity paralysis recovery, such as the NEUROBOTICS elbow exoskeleton (NEUROExos) which uses a passive-compliance control system and torque control [9]. This system is equipped with a load cell sensor to measure the pressure on the bowden cable which is used to move the artificial exoskeleton. Yong-Kwun Lee used a remote controller or RS485 communication from the main computer to control the movement of the exoskeleton robotic hand/arm and fingers [2]. The cable actuated dexterous glove used a PCI-6229 data acquisition board to drive the motor, but it was used on healthy subjects and controls the middle finger, index finger and thumb [10]. Seo and Lee designed an upper limb exoskeleton using a pressure sensor to detect the pressure interaction of the user's arm movement [11]. From the interaction of pressure, the movement to drive the motor will be estimated. This exoskeleton has a total weight of 4 kg and has problems with torque transmission which reduces the control performance of this tool. In the research conducted by Wan et al. [12] and Priyadarshini et al. [13], they used electromyography (EMG) as a control actuator in their designed upper limb exoskeleton.

In addition to using the EMG signal, several studies have developed a rehabilitation device using sound as a control signal. Sahar et al. made a voice-controlled prosthetic hand using the VR3 voice recognition module. This device records seven voice commands, namely "drink", "easy", "hello", "grab", "leave", "up" and "down" which were given to control the movement of the prosthetic hand design. The VR3 voice recognition module was also used by Nasrin Aktar, Israt Jahan and Bijoya Lala as a wheelchair controller in their research [14]. This wheelchair was equipped with a GPS marker so that its position can be tracked. The commands used are "forward", "reverse", "right", "left", "stop", "high" and "low". In this study, they used the NodeMCU as a microcontroller, GSM module, VR3 voice recognition module, infrared sensor, and L298N motor driver. However, this research was limited to the implementation of the hardware system. Megalingam et al. also used voice as an exoskeleton control [15]. This device can be controlled in 3 ways, through a voice recognition module, an Android application connected by Bluetooth and through a computer with text input. All commands are "open" and "close".

In several previous studies, there were several control systems used to control the exoskeleton, including remote controls, torque and pressure control systems, EMG signals, and voice control using the VR3 voice recognition module. Previous studies widely used EMG signals as a control signal. However, the EMG signal is influenced by several parameters, namely subject, electrode position, and muscle fatigue [16]. In addition, the use of EMG as an exoskeleton control has limited capabilities due to fatigue muscles [17]. Therefore, as an alternative, human voice can be used as control signal for the exoskeleton device. Therefore, the purpose of this study is to develop an upper limb exoskeleton device based on voice control using k-nearest neighbor-hood (KNN) and decision tree (DT).

# 2 Materials and Method

## 2.1 *Experimental Setup*

This study used 10 healthy people as respondents. The voice command (up and down) for each respondent was recorded 20 times. After the recording process, an online process was carried out to determine the accuracy level of the machine learning model that has been embedded in the Raspberry Pi. In the implementation, this study used a microphone to record the voice commands. Furthermore, the feature extraction and machine learning implementation were carried out in the Raspberry Pi machine. The servo driver used is PCA9685. In this study, after the training and testing of the classifier was completed, the model was embedded in the Raspberry Pi. In the real time assessment, the upper limb exoskeleton system based on voice control was tested using 10 respondents. In the testing process, each respondent was given 10 times to say "up" and "down" command. Additionally, the performance of the upper limb exoskeleton system was calculated for each command.

## 2.2 *Proposed Method*

The main part in the developing of an upper limb exoskeleton based on voice control using embedded machine learning is shown in Fig. 1. Voice commands were detected using a USB microphone. So that the pattern of the voice signal can be recognized, the voice signal was extracted using feature extraction, both MFCC and ZC. Furthermore, the feature extraction results were identified using machine learning which was embedded in the minicomputer Raspberry Pi. The results of the speech pattern recognition carried out at the machine learning stage were then processed using motion classification to determine whether the upper limb exoskeleton must perform an up or down movement.

Then, the model was tested using direct voice commands that have been extracted and the model predicts the class or label of the given voice signal. This label or class was then used as an exoskeleton control by moving the actuator or servo, depending on the class results predicted by the model according to Fig. 1. Figure 2 below is a flowchart of the application of the feature extraction method with the best prediction

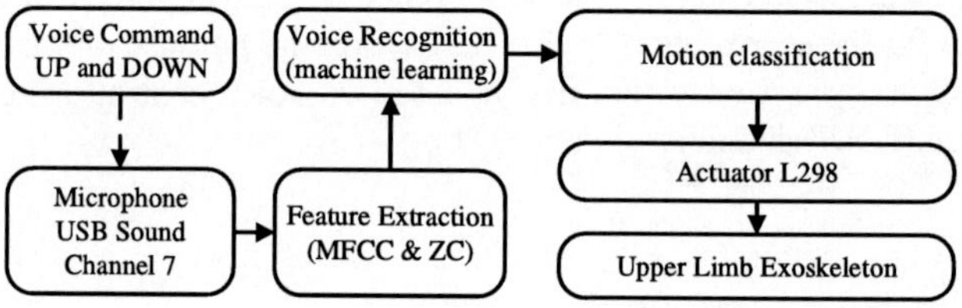


**Fig. 1** Upper limb exoskeleton based on voice control using embedded machine learning on Raspberry Pi

**Fig. 2** Machine learning model testing flowchart

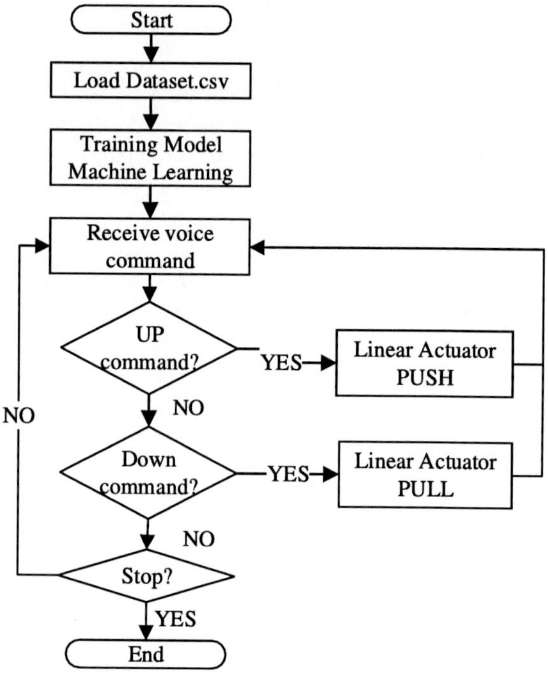

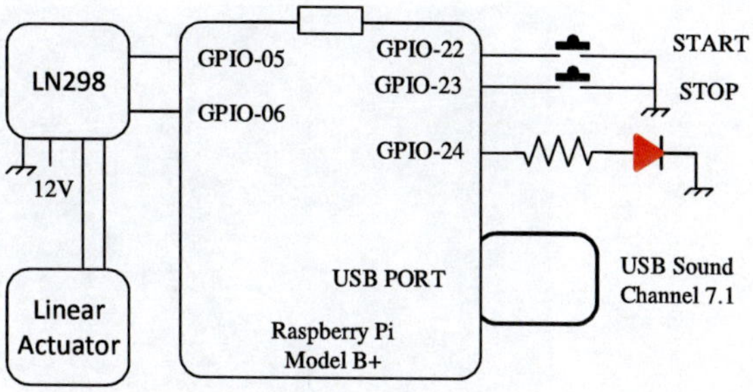


**Fig. 3** Raspberry Pi circuit

accuracy results in real time on the exoskeleton. Based on the Fig. 3, the process began with loading the dataset, then it went through one training process. When given a new voice command, the model that has gone through the training process then extracted new voice data and then the model classified the new command. When the model classification generated an "up" command, it will control the actuator to push the arm mechanics. Meanwhile, when it generated a "down" command, it will control the servo to pull the arm mechanic.

## 2.3 *System Design*

Figure 3 shows that the upper limb exoskeleton system was composed of Raspberry Pi, LN298N driver to control the linear actuator. A start, stop button, and a LED indicator were connected to the GPIO-22, GPIO-23, and GPIO-24, respectively. A voice sensor made of a condenser mic was connected to a USB sound recorder. Additionally, the plug and play USB sound recorder was connected to the Raspberry Pi B+ USB ports. Furthermore, the LN298 driver was connected to the GPIO-05 and GPIO-06. This high current input–output driver was used to drive the linear actuator which can provide push and pull motion for the exoskeleton device. When the start button was pressed, the exoskeleton system was ready to receive a command to move the exoskeleton (flexion or extension). Figure 4 shows the implementation of an exoskeleton device control system using embedded machine learning on a Raspberry Pi B+ device. The figure shows that the Raspberry Pi module was connected to a shield printed circuit board (PCB) for input output connection.

The shield was then connected to several modules, including the LN298 driver and the USB sound recorder. In this design, the exoskeleton framework was made using 3D printing technology. Furthermore, the prime mover of the exoskeleton framework used linear actuators. The exoskeleton device (Fig. 5) was constructed using the main component linear actuator (ZS 200310) with a stroke length of 150 mm, 12 V power supply and a maximum torque of 1500 N. The linear actuator was connected to the upper arm which was made of 3D printing and the support was fastened with a strap around the biceps and triceps. The actuator portion was connected to a 3D printed material (arm) which is attached to the forearm via a strap. When the actuator pushed

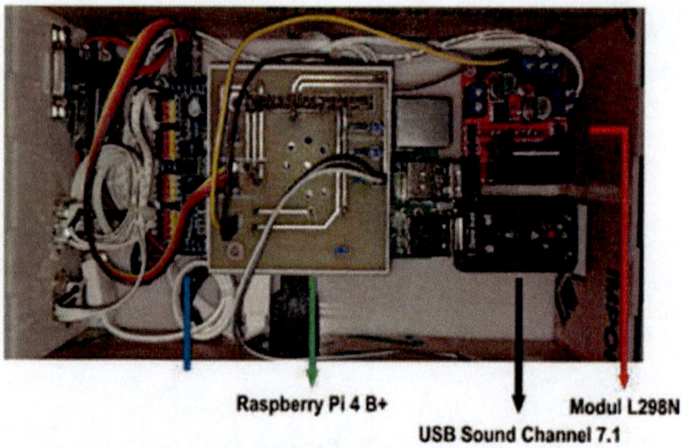


**Fig. 4** Implementation of an exoskeleton device control system design using embedded machine learning

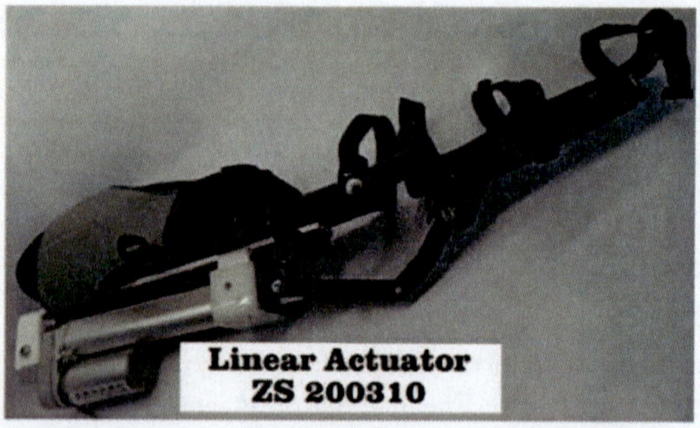


(a)

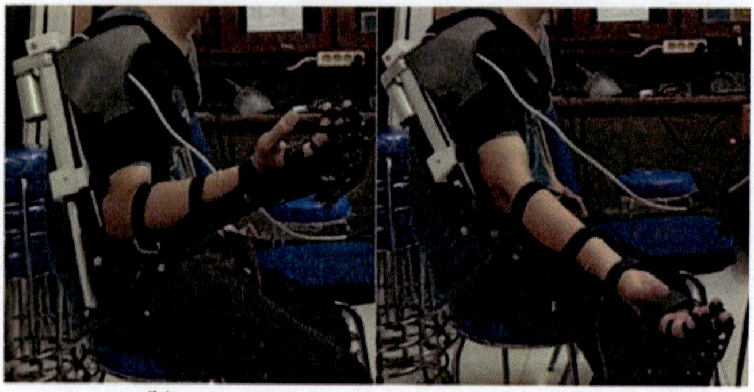

(b) (c)

**Fig. 5** **a** Elbow exoskeleton design using linear actuator, **b** linear actuator push the arm (flexion position), and **c** linear actuator pull the arm (extension position) the arm lever, the elbow then performs a 0–100 flexion movement. On the other hand, when the actuator performed a pull motion, the arm was in a state of extension.

# 3 Result

## 3.1 Voice Pattern

Sound signals were recorded using a microphone connected to USB Sound channel 7.1 on the Raspberry Pi B + system. There are two sounds used to control the movement of the exoskeleton, namely "up" (in bahasa: "*naik*") and down (in bahasa: "*turun*"). In this study, the voice command was spelled in Indonesian language. The sound signal recording results are saved in wav format. The wav format can be opened by using the Python program through the audio library. So that the sound signal pattern can be seen visually on the computer screen. The sound signal stored in wav format was taken and plotted using a Python program as shown in Fig. 6.

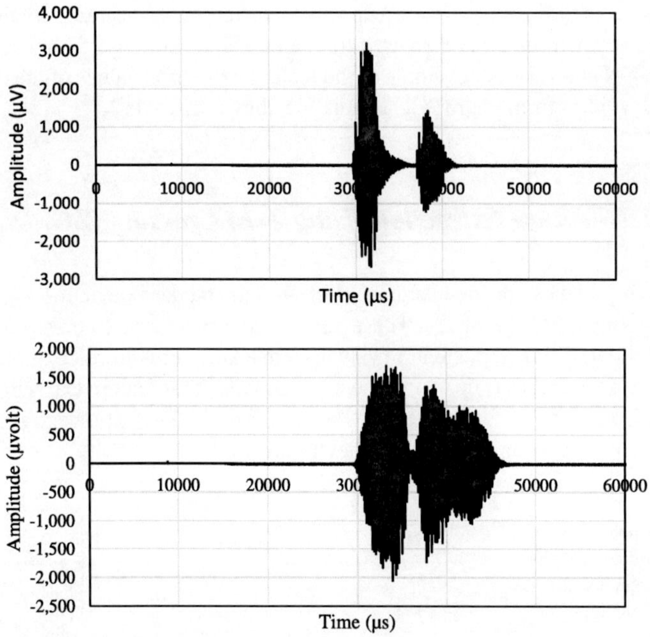


**Fig. 6** Voice pattern recording for UP (in bahasa = "*naik*") and DOWN (in bahasa = "*turun*")

Table 1 Samples of MFCC feature-extraction values

| Mean [1] | Mean [2] | Mean [3] | Std [1] | St d[4] | Std [6] | Label |
|---|---|---|---|---|---|---|
| − 8.7 | 4.8 | − 4.6 | 67.0 | 8.6 | 13.8 | Up |
| − 6.3 | 5.0 | − 6.1 | 67.3 | 8.9 | 15.4 | Up |
| 13.8 | 11.9 | 6.4 | 71.7 | 20.8 | 6.9 | Down |
| 10.1 | 8.7 | 9.5 | 67.2 | 18.6 | 5.5 | Down |

## 3.2 Voice Feature Extraction Using MFCC

The following values are the examples of feature extraction results which were collected from single respondent for "up" and "down" commands voice. The feature extraction process was performed using a Python program. The 13 MFCC coefficients was extracted in this study. Additionally, the mean and standard deviation (SD) values were calculated based on 13 coefficients. After an evaluation, the three MFCC coefficients from thirteen coefficients were taken. Specifically, the mean values from coefficients 1, 2, 3 were selected. Furthermore, the standard deviation values from coefficients 1, 4, 6 were chosen. This selection was made based on the values that showed the most differences between up and down voices. All features obtained were then stored in csv format and then used for the machine learning training and testing process (KNN and DT). An example of the feature extraction values of the mean and standard deviation from the MFCC feature are shown in Table 1.

## 3.3 Voice Feature Extraction Using Zero Crossing (ZC)

The following values are the example of mean and standard deviation value based on zero crossing (ZC) (Table 2). These values were then used to train and test the classifier model. This sample feature values were taken from the voice of one patient while the respondent said "up" and "down" command. This feature extraction values were calculated using Python program. The results of the ZC feature extraction were then calculated the mean and standard deviation (SD).

Table 2 Samples of zero crossing feature extraction from voice signal while the respondent said "up" and "down"

| Mean | STD | Label |
|---|---|---|
| 0.013838 | 0.030187 | Up |
| 0.017251 | 0.034905 | Up |
| 0.016923 | 0.023555 | Down |
| 0.018826 | 0.026921 | Down |

### 3.4 Classes Classification Using K-NN and DT

The performance of the KNN and DT classifiers can be known through a two-dimensional scatter visualization based on two classes. Before the training process, the parameter k was determined at the beginning. The value of **k** was determined based on the experiment that produces the highest accuracy value. Furthermore, after carrying out the experimental process, the parameter value k = 5 can be generated. Figure 7a, b show the two classification areas shown in black and yellow. The scattering plot shown in Fig. 7 is based on mean and standard deviation values of the MFCC.

### 3.5 Comparison of the Machine Learning Performance

Machine learning (KNN and DT) were trained and tested using datasets derived from offline recordings of ten respondents. The process of training and testing was carried out alternately using the same dataset. Accuracy was measured and compared for two different feature extractions, namely MFCC and ZC. Furthermore, based on the training and testing process, four accuracy results were produced based on different combinations of machine learning and feature extraction as shown in Table 3.

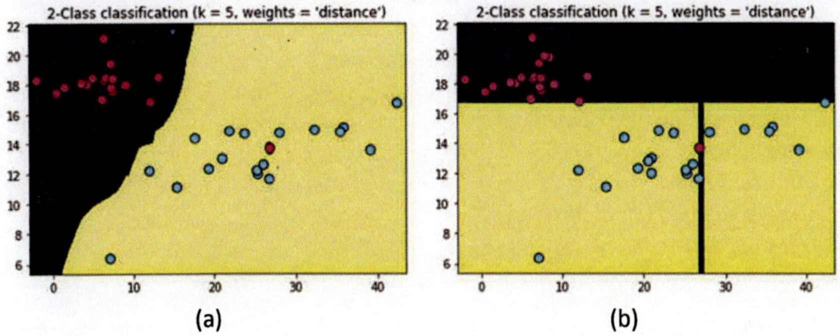


**Fig. 7** An offline two-dimensional scattering plot visualization for machine learning using parameter constants k = 5 **a** K-NN and **b** Decision tree

**Table 3** Comparison of the accuracy (mean ± standard deviation) of K-NN and DT for the two feature extractions MFCC and ZC based on datasets from 10 respondents conducted offline

| MFCC KNN (%) | MFCC DT (%) | ZC KNN (%) | ZC DT (%) |
|---|---|---|---|
| 96 ± 4.0 | 74.5 ± 1.50 | 69.5 ± 1.99 | 64.5 ± 1.27 |

**Table 4** Summary of the results of machine learning model testing (MFCC-KNN) conducted directly to ten respondents (mean standard ± deviation) for voice Up and Down

| Accuracy (%) | |
|---|---|
| Up voice | Down voice |
| 92.0 ± 7.37 | 84.0 ± 4.97 |

Table 3 shows that machine learning with a combination of feature extraction MFCC-KNN, MFCC-DT, ZC-KNN, and ZC-DT resulted in an accuracy of 96 ± 4.0%, 74.5 ± 1.50%, 69.5 ± , respectively. 1.99% and 64.5 ± 1.27%.

Based on the investigation of the accuracy of the model conducted offline by combining machine learning and feature extraction, it can be seen that the combination of KNN machine learning and MFCC feature extraction resulted in better accuracy during the training and testing process (Table 3). Furthermore, the model (MFCC-KNN) is used for the direct use of the voice control-based exoskeleton device. The model testing process was carried out online using ten respondents. Each respondent gave instructions to the exoskeleton by saying Up and Down. Every voice that succeeds in moving the exoskeleton device was recorded as True and every voice that fails was recorded as False. All recordings were calculated with the average value and standard deviation for voice Up and voice Down. Table 4 shows a summary of online accuracy measurements for voice Up and Down.

To determine the response of the exoskeleton movement to sound, it is necessary to test the range of angles that can be reached and the time it takes to perform these movements. The angle measurement was carried out using a mini digital protractor placed on the mechanical arm to measure the angle of the arm inclination at the time of the rising position 10 times and an average of 85.8° ± 2.56° was obtained. Time measurement was carried out using a stopwatch by measuring the time of arm movement from one position for 10 times and obtained a total time of 30.74 ± 1.56 s. So that the angular velocity of the mechanical arm starting from the full extension position to the maximum flexion is 27.91°/s.

## 4 Discussion

In this study, a comparison of two extraction methods, namely MFCC and ZCR and two machine learning methods (KNN and DT) has been done. MFCC feature extraction is an adaptation of the human auditory system. In performing MFCC feature extraction, researchers have used the librosa library available in python. The researchers have used the default mode from the library and took 13 coefficients from the MFCC. This is because the first 13 coefficients of the MFCC contain the most important information needed for speech recognition [18]. After getting the value of the 13 MFCC coefficients, then the selection of three coefficients from the 13 coefficients was carried out, which were then used as training data for machine learning [19, 20]. In a study conducted by Soheil Shafiee, it was said that the value of the mean MFCC for the coefficient values (1, 2, 3, 4, 5, 6, 7, and 8) produced the best results [21]. So, the researchers conducted a trial to find out how many good coefficients were used to produce the highest accuracy in machine learning. The researcher did this by comparing the use of the mean and SD values of the 13 coefficients by using the mean and SD values of several coefficients. In addition to using MFCC extraction, researchers have also used ZC feature extraction.

Based on Table 3, it can be seen that by using 3 mean and 3 SD from the MFCC extraction and the K-NN algorithm, the highest accuracy value is $96 \pm 4.0$. Furthermore, based on Table 3, accuracy using feature extraction MFCC has better accuracy results than using feature extraction ZC for either KNN or DT machine learning. This is because MFCC extraction is an extraction by converting sound signals into the form of a mel scale where the mel scale is a unit for human hearing, in contrast to ZC extraction which calculates the number of signal changes that cross the zero threshold. So, this makes MFCC extraction obtained higher accuracy than ZC. After the best model was obtained (MFCC-KNN), the next step was to implement the model to be applied to exoskeleton devices using voice control. The results of direct testing with respondents obtained performance values of $92.0 \pm 7.37\%$ and $84.0 \pm 4.97\%$, respectively for up and down movements (Table 4). These results showed a decrease when compared to the results obtained during the offline training and testing process using recorded voice datasets. This result is due to the difference in voice intonation when the respondent says up and down as a command for the exoskeleton device.

In this study, both offline and online testing to respondents was only carried out in a quiet laboratory environment with the sound of air conditioning (50 dB noise). However, this study has not been tested in other environments where there is greater environmental noise, for example there is a conversation around the respondent. Testing in different environments is very important to determine the ability of machine learning to distinguish voices in the midst of large noise. Furthermore, this research can be used for post-stroke patients who need an independent therapy process that can be done at home. Before its use, it is necessary to conduct a training process using a special voice from the user so that the accuracy of the exoskeleton device is expected to be even better.

## 5 Conclusion

The purpose of this study is to make an arm exoskeleton device with movement control using voice pattern recognition using machine learning K-nearest neighborhood (KNN) and Decision tree (DT). It is known that MFCC extraction produces better accuracy than ZC when training was carried out against the model. In this study, the number of coefficients used in MFCC is 6. The coefficients include mean (1), mean (2), and mean (3), SD (1), SD (4) and SD (6). The results of offline testing using datasets from 10 respondents obtained the highest accuracy in the KNN-MFCC machine learning model, which is 96 ± 4.0%. The results of the online test to the user obtained that the performance value of the voice control-based exoskeleton device was 92.0 ± 7.37% and 84.0 ± 4.97%, respectively for the Up and Down commands. Developments that can be done by researching more deeply about MFCC extraction and the coefficients used to train machine learning. Development can also be done using deep learning in the speech recognition process by utilizing libraries such as Keras which are commonly used in biomedical signal pattern recognition applications.

## References


1. Gopura RARC, Bandara DSV, Kiguchi K, Mann GKI (2016) Developments in hardware systems of active upper-limb exoskeleton robots: a review. Rob Auton Syst 75:203–220
2. Lee Y (2014) Design of exoskeleton robotic hand/arm system for upper limbs rehabilitation considering mobility and portability, [Urai], pp 540–544
3. Balitbangkes. Hasil Utama Riskesdas (2018) Jakarta, Indonesia
4. Johnson W, Onuma O, Owolabi M, Sachdev S (2016) WHO stroke a global response is needed. Bull World Health Organ, pp 633–708
5. Gopura RARC, Kiguchi K, Bandara DSV (2011) A brief review on upper extremity robotic exoskeleton systems. In: 6th International conference on industrial and information systems, ICIIS, vol 8502, pp 346–351
6. Young AJ, Ferris DP (2016) State-of-the-art and future directions for lower limb robotic exoskeletons. IEEE Trans Neural Syst Rehabil Eng 25(2):171–182
7. McGowan B (2018) Industrial exoskeletons what you're not hearing. Occup Health Saf, pp 1–5
8. Solihin AK, Yulianto E, Ariswati HG (2021) Design of an electromyograph equipped with digital neck angle elevation gauge. J Electron Electromed Eng Med Informatics. 3(3):141–148
9. Vitiello N, Lenzi T, Member S, Roccella S, Marco S, De RM et al (2013) NEUROExos : a powered elbow exoskeleton for physical rehabilitation. IEEE Trans Robot 29(1):220–235
10. Kim DH, Park H (2018) Cable Actuated Dexterous (CADEX) glove for effective rehabilitation of the hand for patients with neurological diseases. In: 2018 IEEE/RSJ international conference on intelligent robots and systems (IROS). Madrid, Spain, pp 2305–2310
11. Seo H, Lee S (2017) Design and experiments of an upper-limb exoskeleton robot. In: 14th International conference on ubiquitous robots and ambient intelligence (URAI). Jeju, South Korea, pp 807–808
12. Wan GC, Zhou FZ, Gao C, Tong MS (2017) Design of joint structure for upper limb exoskeleton robot system. In: Progress in electromagnetics research symposium-fall (PIERS—FALL), pp 19–22
13. Priyadarshini RG, Suryarajan R, Prasad J (2018) Development of electromyogram based rehabilitation device for upper limb amputation using neural network. In: 2018 3rd international conference on communication and electronics systems. IEEE, Coimbatore, India, p. 826–830
14. Aktar N, Jaharr I, Lala B (2019) Voice recognition based intelligent wheelchair and GPS tracking system. In: 2nd International conference on electrical, computer and communication engineering ECCE 2019, pp 7–9
15. Megalingam RK, Vijay E, Naveen PNVK, Reddy CPK, Chandrika D (2019) Voice-based hand orthotic device. In: Proceedings of 2019 IEEE international conference on communication signal process ICCSP 2019, pp 496–500
16. Triwiyanto T, Wahyunggoro O, Nugroho HA, Herianto H (2018) Muscle fatigue compensation of the electromyography signal for elbow joint angle estimation using adaptive feature. Comput Electr Eng [Internet] 71(July):284–293

17. Sahar SG, Nisar R, Arshad S, Fatima M, Hafeez SA, Syah SMJ et al (2018) Voice controlled 6-DoF prosthetic arm for the patients with shoulder disarticulation. In: 2018 IEEE-EMBS conference on biomedical engineering and sciences (IECBES). Sarawak, Malaysia: IEEE, pp 233–238
18. Patel KH (2018) Accent recognition using machine learning methods. California State Polytechnic University, Pomona
19. Shirani A (2016) Speech emotion recognition based on SVM as both feature selector and classifier, vol 4, pp 39–45
20. Ranjan R, Thakur A (2019) Analysis of feature extraction techniques for speech recognition system. Int J Innov Technol Explor Eng. 8(7):197–200
21. Shafiee S, Almasganj F, Jafari A (2008) Speech/non-speech segments detection based on chaotic and prosodic features, vol 1, pp 111–114